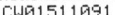

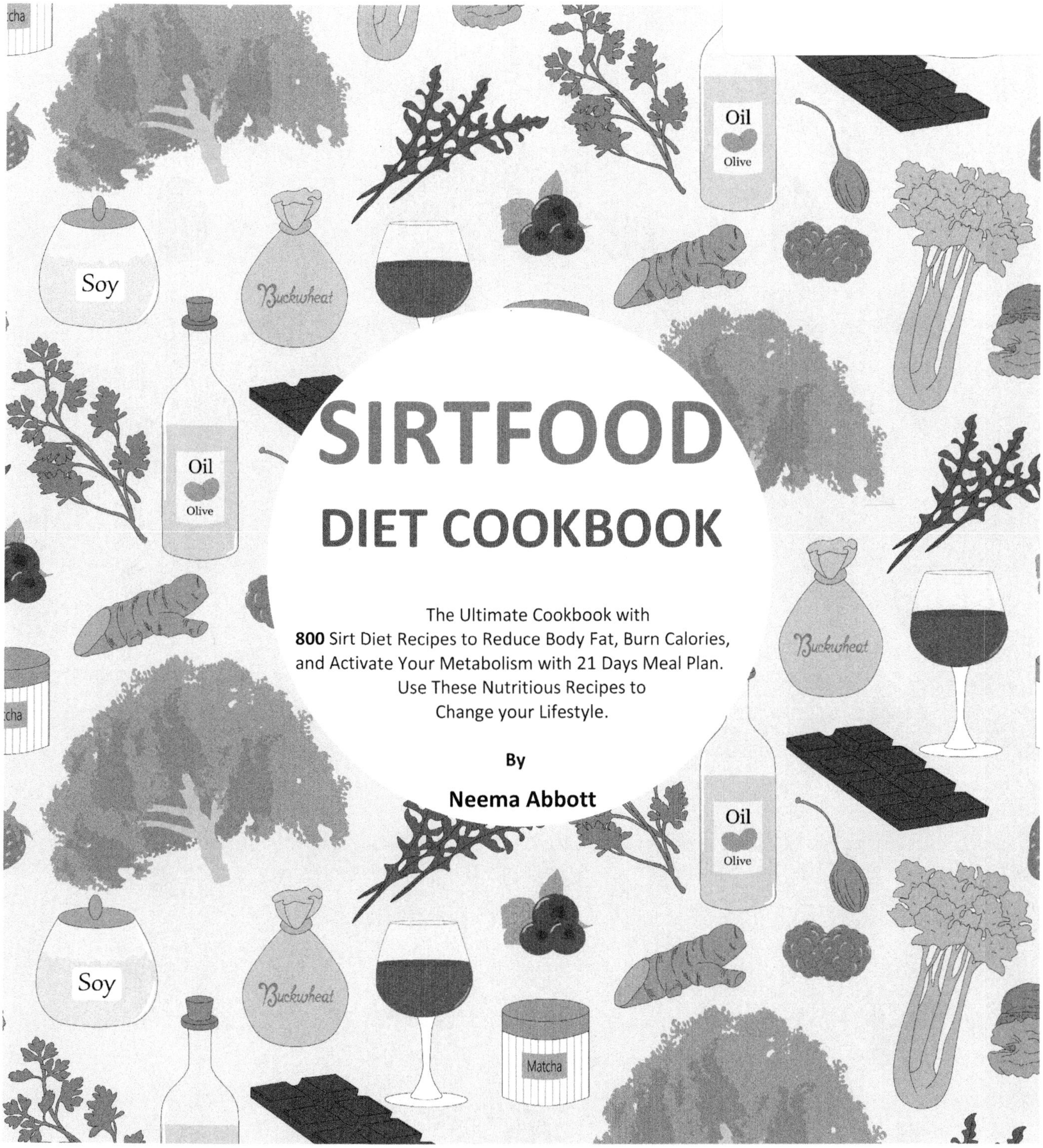

SIRTFOOD
DIET COOKBOOK

The Ultimate Cookbook with
800 Sirt Diet Recipes to Reduce Body Fat, Burn Calories,
and Activate Your Metabolism with 21 Days Meal Plan.
Use These Nutritious Recipes to
Change your Lifestyle.

By

Neema Abbott

Sirtfood Diet Cookbook

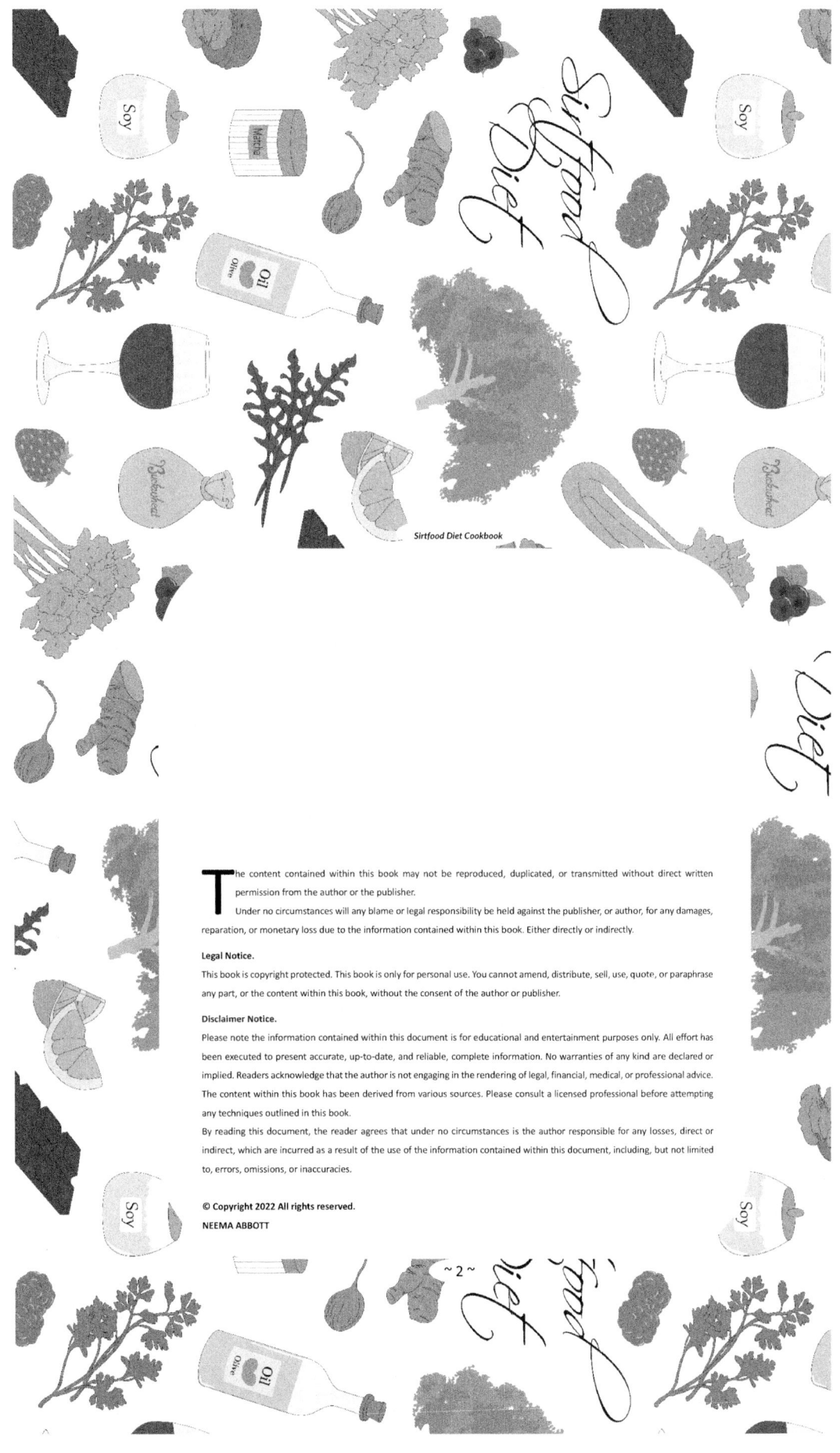

Sirtfood Diet Cookbook

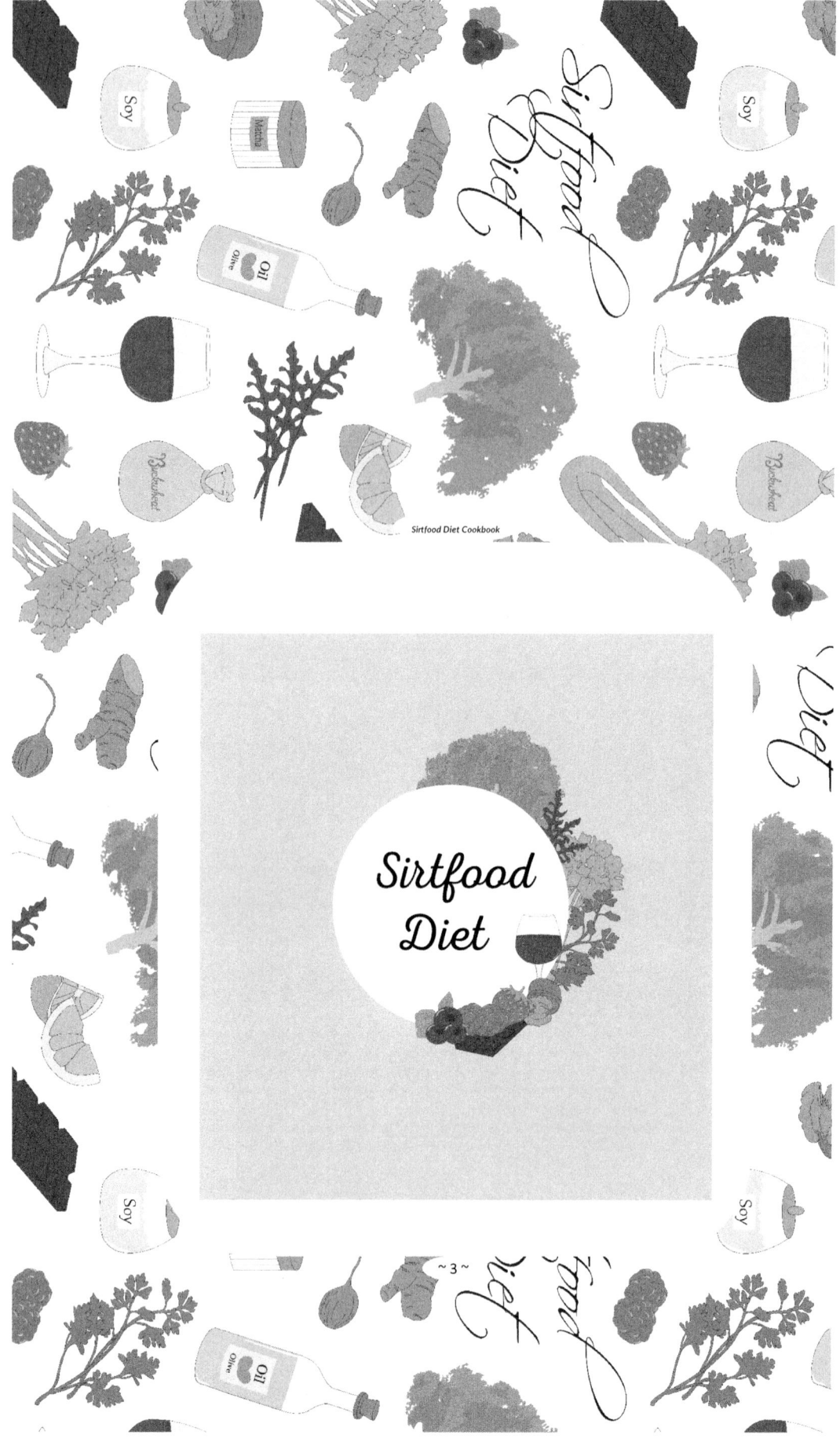

Sirtfood Diet Cookbook

Sirtfood Diet

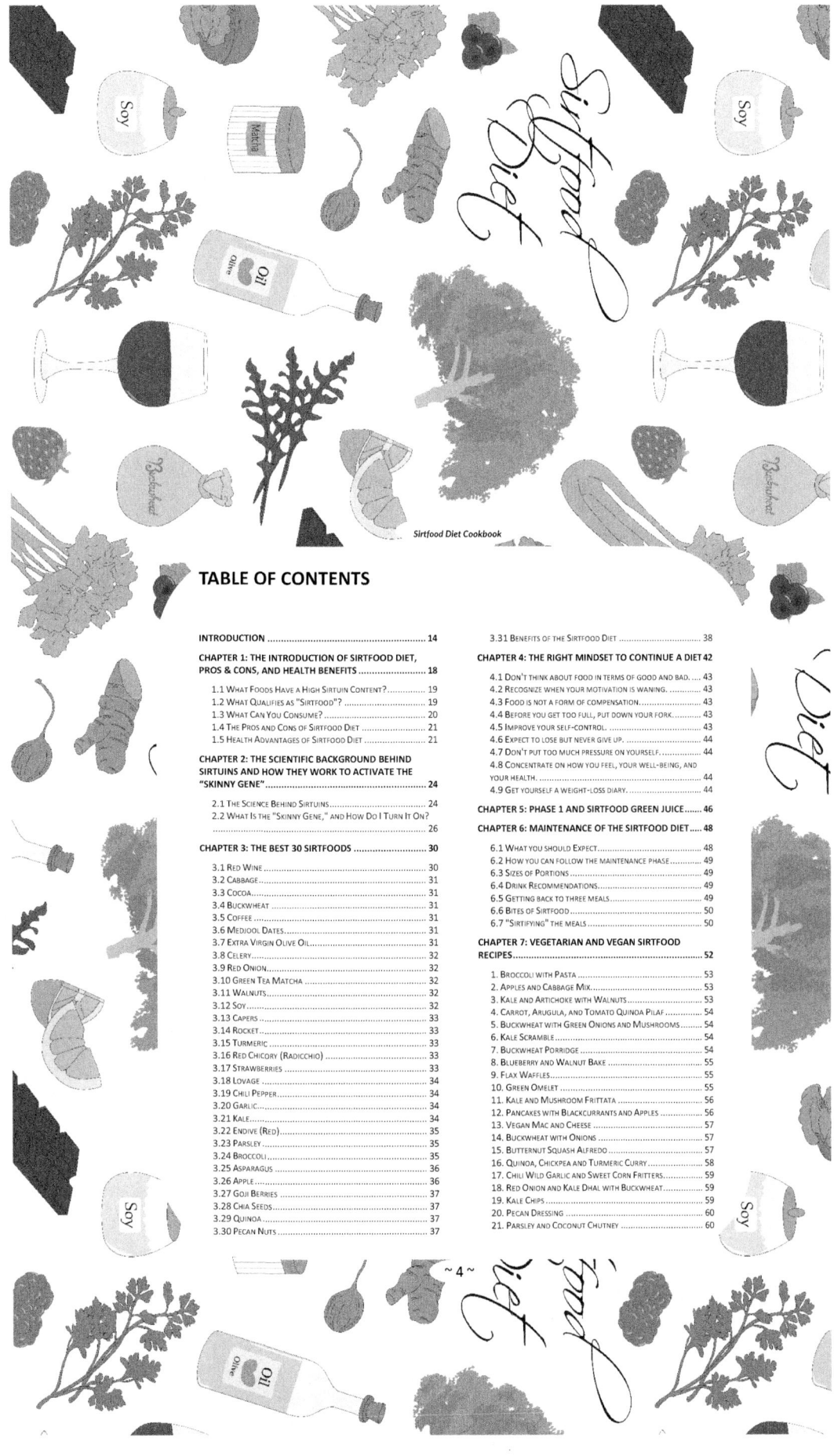

Sirtfood Diet Cookbook

TABLE OF CONTENTS

INTRODUCTION 14

CHAPTER 1: THE INTRODUCTION OF SIRTFOOD DIET, PROS & CONS, AND HEALTH BENEFITS 18

1.1 WHAT FOODS HAVE A HIGH SIRTUIN CONTENT?.............. 19
1.2 WHAT QUALIFIES AS "SIRTFOOD"? 19
1.3 WHAT CAN YOU CONSUME? 20
1.4 THE PROS AND CONS OF SIRTFOOD DIET 21
1.5 HEALTH ADVANTAGES OF SIRTFOOD DIET 21

CHAPTER 2: THE SCIENTIFIC BACKGROUND BEHIND SIRTUINS AND HOW THEY WORK TO ACTIVATE THE "SKINNY GENE" 24

2.1 THE SCIENCE BEHIND SIRTUINS.................................... 24
2.2 WHAT IS THE "SKINNY GENE," AND HOW DO I TURN IT ON?
.... 26

CHAPTER 3: THE BEST 30 SIRTFOODS 30

3.1 RED WINE 30
3.2 CABBAGE 31
3.3 COCOA.. 31
3.4 BUCKWHEAT 31
3.5 COFFEE.. 31
3.6 MEDJOOL DATES.. 31
3.7 EXTRA VIRGIN OLIVE OIL 31
3.8 CELERY.. 32
3.9 RED ONION 32
3.10 GREEN TEA MATCHA 32
3.11 WALNUTS 32
3.12 SOY.. 32
3.13 CAPERS 33
3.14 ROCKET 33
3.15 TURMERIC 33
3.16 RED CHICORY (RADICCHIO) 33
3.17 STRAWBERRIES 33
3.18 LOVAGE 34
3.19 CHILI PEPPER.. 34
3.20 GARLIC.. 34
3.21 KALE 34
3.22 ENDIVE (RED).. 35
3.23 PARSLEY.. 35
3.24 BROCCOLI.. 35
3.25 ASPARAGUS.. 36
3.26 APPLE.. 36
3.27 GOJI BERRIES.. 37
3.28 CHIA SEEDS.. 37
3.29 QUINOA 37
3.30 PECAN NUTS 37

3.31 BENEFITS OF THE SIRTFOOD DIET 38

CHAPTER 4: THE RIGHT MINDSET TO CONTINUE A DIET 42

4.1 DON'T THINK ABOUT FOOD IN TERMS OF GOOD AND BAD. 43
4.2 RECOGNIZE WHEN YOUR MOTIVATION IS WANING. 43
4.3 FOOD IS NOT A FORM OF COMPENSATION...................... 43
4.4 BEFORE YOU GET TOO FULL, PUT DOWN YOUR FORK. 43
4.5 IMPROVE YOUR SELF-CONTROL. 43
4.6 EXPECT TO LOSE BUT NEVER GIVE UP. 44
4.7 DON'T PUT TOO MUCH PRESSURE ON YOURSELF. 44
4.8 CONCENTRATE ON HOW YOU FEEL, YOUR WELL-BEING, AND YOUR HEALTH. 44
4.9 GET YOURSELF A WEIGHT-LOSS DIARY. 44

CHAPTER 5: PHASE 1 AND SIRTFOOD GREEN JUICE 46

CHAPTER 6: MAINTENANCE OF THE SIRTFOOD DIET 48

6.1 WHAT YOU SHOULD EXPECT...................................... 48
6.2 HOW YOU CAN FOLLOW THE MAINTENANCE PHASE............ 49
6.3 SIZES OF PORTIONS 49
6.4 DRINK RECOMMENDATIONS 49
6.5 GETTING BACK TO THREE MEALS 49
6.6 BITES OF SIRTFOOD 50
6.7 "SIRTIFYING" THE MEALS 50

CHAPTER 7: VEGETARIAN AND VEGAN SIRTFOOD RECIPES 52

1. BROCCOLI WITH PASTA 53
2. APPLES AND CABBAGE MIX... 53
3. KALE AND ARTICHOKE WITH WALNUTS 53
4. CARROT, ARUGULA, AND TOMATO QUINOA PILAF 54
5. BUCKWHEAT WITH GREEN ONIONS AND MUSHROOMS........ 54
6. KALE SCRAMBLE 54
7. BUCKWHEAT PORRIDGE 54
8. BLUEBERRY AND WALNUT BAKE 55
9. FLAX WAFFLES 55
10. GREEN OMELET 55
11. KALE AND MUSHROOM FRITTATA 56
12. PANCAKES WITH BLACKCURRANTS AND APPLES 56
13. VEGAN MAC AND CHEESE 57
14. BUCKWHEAT WITH ONIONS 57
15. BUTTERNUT SQUASH ALFREDO 57
16. QUINOA, CHICKPEA AND TURMERIC CURRY 58
17. CHILI WILD GARLIC AND SWEET CORN FRITTERS............ 59
18. RED ONION AND KALE DHAL WITH BUCKWHEAT............. 59
19. KALE CHIPS 59
20. PECAN DRESSING 60
21. PARSLEY AND COCONUT CHUTNEY 60

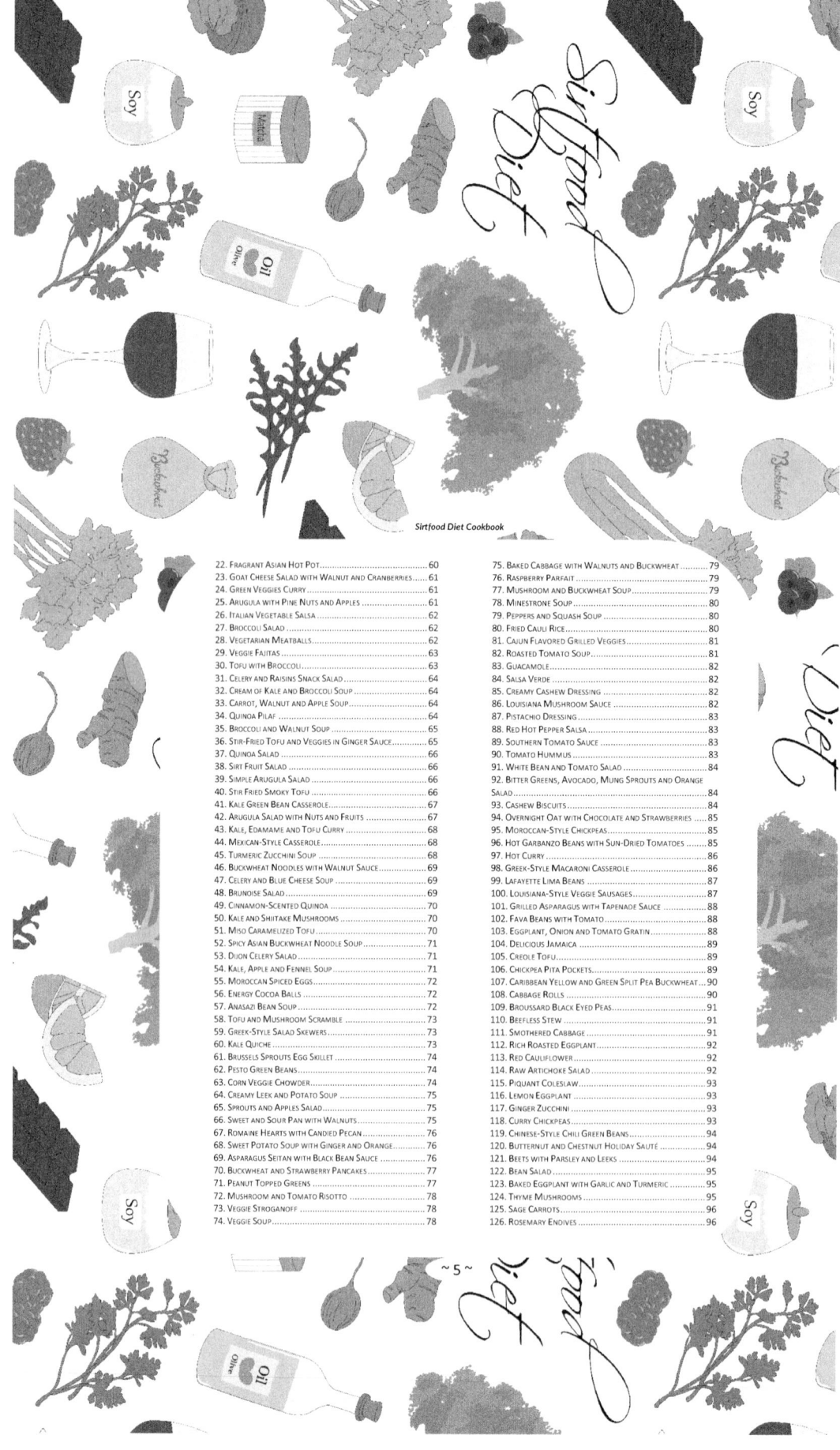

Sirtfood Diet Cookbook

22. Fragrant Asian Hot Pot..60
23. Goat Cheese Salad with Walnut and Cranberries......61
24. Green Veggies Curry...61
25. Arugula with Pine Nuts and Apples 61
26. Italian Vegetable Salsa..62
27. Broccoli Salad 62
28. Vegetarian Meatballs..62
29. Veggie Fajitas 63
30. Tofu with Broccoli...63
31. Celery and Raisins Snack Salad.............................64
32. Cream of Kale and Broccoli Soup 64
33. Carrot, Walnut and Apple Soup.............................64
34. Quinoa Pilaf 64
35. Broccoli and Walnut Soup 65
36. Stir-Fried Tofu and Veggies in Ginger Sauce...........65
37. Quinoa Salad 66
38. Sirt Fruit Salad 66
39. Simple Arugula Salad 66
40. Stir Fried Smoky Tofu 66
41. Kale Green Bean Casserole....................................67
42. Arugula Salad with Nuts and Fruits 67
43. Kale, Edamame and Tofu Curry 68
44. Mexican-Style Casserole..68
45. Turmeric Zucchini Soup 68
46. Buckwheat Noodles with Walnut Sauce..................69
47. Celery and Blue Cheese Soup 69
48. Brunoise Salad...69
49. Cinnamon-Scented Quinoa 70
50. Kale and Shiitake Mushrooms 70
51. Miso Caramelized Tofu..70
52. Spicy Asian Buckwheat Noodle Soup......................71
53. Dijon Celery Salad 71
54. Kale, Apple and Fennel Soup 71
55. Moroccan Spiced Eggs...72
56. Energy Cocoa Balls 72
57. Anasazi Bean Soup 72
58. Tofu and Mushroom Scramble 73
59. Greek-Style Salad Skewers.....................................73
60. Kale Quiche 73
61. Brussels Sprouts Egg Skillet 74
62. Pesto Green Beans 74
63. Corn Veggie Chowder..74
64. Creamy Leek and Potato Soup 75
65. Sprouts and Apples Salad......................................75
66. Sweet and Sour Pan with Walnuts.........................75
67. Romaine Hearts with Candied Pecan 76
68. Sweet Potato Soup with Ginger and Orange............76
69. Asparagus Seitan with Black Bean Sauce 76
70. Buckwheat and Strawberry Pancakes.....................77
71. Peanut Topped Greens 77
72. Mushroom and Tomato Risotto 78
73. Veggie Stroganoff 78
74. Veggie Soup...78

75. Baked Cabbage with Walnuts and Buckwheat 79
76. Raspberry Parfait 79
77. Mushroom and Buckwheat Soup.............................79
78. Minestrone Soup 80
79. Peppers and Squash Soup 80
80. Fried Cauli Rice..80
81. Cajun Flavored Grilled Veggies..............................81
82. Roasted Tomato Soup..81
83. Guacamole...82
84. Salsa Verde..82
85. Creamy Cashew Dressing 82
86. Louisiana Mushroom Sauce 82
87. Pistachio Dressing...83
88. Red Hot Pepper Salsa 83
89. Southern Tomato Sauce 83
90. Tomato Hummus 83
91. White Bean and Tomato Salad 84
92. Bitter Greens, Avocado, Mung Sprouts and Orange
Salad...84
93. Cashew Biscuits 84
94. Overnight Oat with Chocolate and Strawberries 85
95. Moroccan-Style Chickpeas.....................................85
96. Hot Garbanzo Beans with Sun-Dried Tomatoes 85
97. Hot Curry 86
98. Greek-Style Macaroni Casserole.............................86
99. Lafayette Lima Beans 87
100. Louisiana-Style Veggie Sausages..........................87
101. Grilled Asparagus with Tapenade Sauce 88
102. Fava Beans with Tomato 88
103. Eggplant, Onion and Tomato Gratin......................88
104. Delicious Jamaica 89
105. Creole Tofu...89
106. Chickpea Pita Pockets...89
107. Caribbean Yellow and Green Split Pea Buckwheat ...90
108. Cabbage Rolls 90
109. Broussard Black Eyed Peas..................................91
110. Beefless Stew 91
111. Smothered Cabbage 91
112. Rich Roasted Eggplant...92
113. Red Cauliflower 92
114. Raw Artichoke Salad 92
115. Piquant Coleslaw..93
116. Lemon Eggplant 93
117. Ginger Zucchini 93
118. Curry Chickpeas 93
119. Chinese-Style Chili Green Beans...........................94
120. Butternut and Chestnut Holiday Sauté 94
121. Beets with Parsley and Leeks 94
122. Bean Salad 95
123. Baked Eggplant with Garlic and Turmeric 95
124. Thyme Mushrooms 95
125. Sage Carrots 96
126. Rosemary Endives 96

~5~

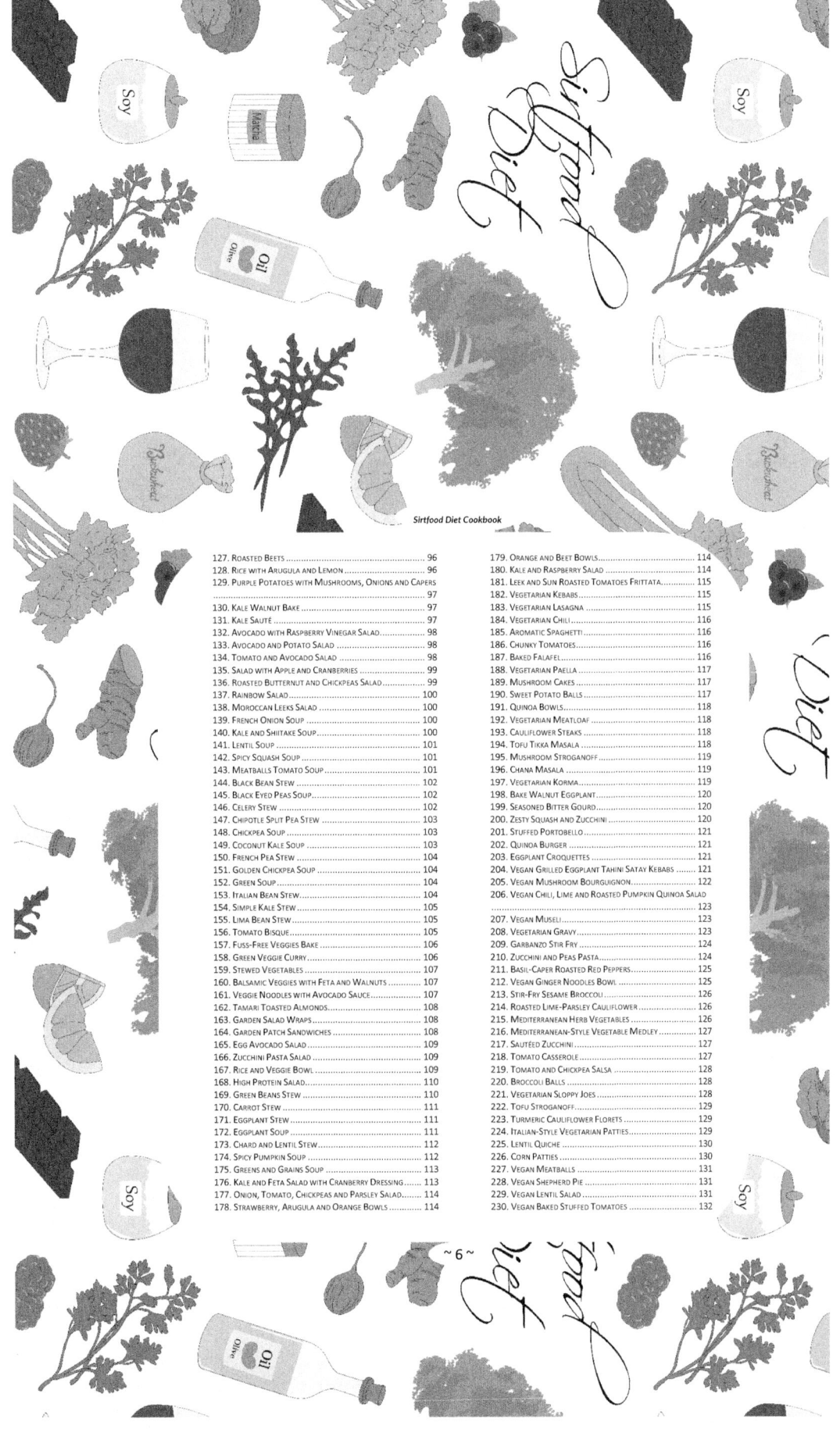

Sirtfood Diet Cookbook

127. ROASTED BEETS 96
128. RICE WITH ARUGULA AND LEMON 96
129. PURPLE POTATOES WITH MUSHROOMS, ONIONS AND CAPERS
.... 97
130. KALE WALNUT BAKE 97
131. KALE SAUTÉ 97
132. AVOCADO WITH RASPBERRY VINEGAR SALAD 98
133. AVOCADO AND POTATO SALAD 98
134. TOMATO AND AVOCADO SALAD 98
135. SALAD WITH APPLE AND CRANBERRIES 99
136. ROASTED BUTTERNUT AND CHICKPEAS SALAD 99
137. RAINBOW SALAD 100
138. MOROCCAN LEEKS SALAD 100
139. FRENCH ONION SOUP 100
140. KALE AND SHIITAKE SOUP 100
141. LENTIL SOUP 101
142. SPICY SQUASH SOUP 101
143. MEATBALLS TOMATO SOUP 101
144. BLACK BEAN STEW 102
145. BLACK EYED PEAS SOUP 102
146. CELERY STEW 102
147. CHIPOTLE SPLIT PEA STEW 103
148. CHICKPEA SOUP 103
149. COCONUT KALE SOUP 103
150. FRENCH PEA STEW 104
151. GOLDEN CHICKPEA SOUP 104
152. GREEN SOUP 104
153. ITALIAN BEAN STEW 104
154. SIMPLE KALE STEW 105
155. LIMA BEAN STEW 105
156. TOMATO BISQUE 105
157. FUSS-FREE VEGGIES BAKE 106
158. GREEN VEGGIE CURRY 106
159. STEWED VEGETABLES 107
160. BALSAMIC VEGGIES WITH FETA AND WALNUTS 107
161. VEGGIE NOODLES WITH AVOCADO SAUCE 107
162. TAMARI TOASTED ALMONDS 108
163. GARDEN SALAD WRAPS 108
164. GARDEN PATCH SANDWICHES 108
165. EGG AVOCADO SALAD 109
166. ZUCCHINI PASTA SALAD 109
167. RICE AND VEGGIE BOWL 109
168. HIGH PROTEIN SALAD 110
169. GREEN BEANS STEW 110
170. CARROT STEW 111
171. EGGPLANT STEW 111
172. EGGPLANT SOUP 111
173. CHARD AND LENTIL STEW 112
174. SPICY PUMPKIN SOUP 112
175. GREENS AND GRAINS SOUP 113
176. KALE AND FETA SALAD WITH CRANBERRY DRESSING 113
177. ONION, TOMATO, CHICKPEAS AND PARSLEY SALAD 114
178. STRAWBERRY, ARUGULA AND ORANGE BOWLS 114

179. ORANGE AND BEET BOWLS 114
180. KALE AND RASPBERRY SALAD 114
181. LEEK AND SUN ROASTED TOMATOES FRITTATA 115
182. VEGETARIAN KEBABS 115
183. VEGETARIAN LASAGNA 115
184. VEGETARIAN CHILI 116
185. AROMATIC SPAGHETTI 116
186. CHUNKY TOMATOES 116
187. BAKED FALAFEL 116
188. VEGETARIAN PAELLA 117
189. MUSHROOM CAKES 117
190. SWEET POTATO BALLS 117
191. QUINOA BOWLS 118
192. VEGETARIAN MEATLOAF 118
193. CAULIFLOWER STEAKS 118
194. TOFU TIKKA MASALA 118
195. MUSHROOM STROGANOFF 119
196. CHANA MASALA 119
197. VEGETARIAN KORMA 119
198. BAKE WALNUT EGGPLANT 120
199. SEASONED BITTER GOURD 120
200. ZESTY SQUASH AND ZUCCHINI 120
201. STUFFED PORTOBELLO 121
202. QUINOA BURGER 121
203. EGGPLANT CROQUETTES 121
204. VEGAN GRILLED EGGPLANT TAHINI SATAY KEBABS 121
205. VEGAN MUSHROOM BOURGUIGNON 122
206. VEGAN CHILI, LIME AND ROASTED PUMPKIN QUINOA SALAD
.... 123
207. VEGAN MUSELI 123
208. VEGETARIAN GRAVY 123
209. GARBANZO STIR FRY 124
210. ZUCCHINI AND PEAS PASTA 124
211. BASIL-CAPER ROASTED RED PEPPERS 125
212. VEGAN GINGER NOODLES BOWL 125
213. STIR-FRY SESAME BROCCOLI 126
214. ROASTED LIME-PARSLEY CAULIFLOWER 126
215. MEDITERRANEAN HERB VEGETABLES 126
216. MEDITERRANEAN-STYLE VEGETABLE MEDLEY 127
217. SAUTÉED ZUCCHINI 127
218. TOMATO CASSEROLE 127
219. TOMATO AND CHICKPEA SALSA 128
220. BROCCOLI BALLS 128
221. VEGETARIAN SLOPPY JOES 128
222. TOFU STROGANOFF 129
223. TURMERIC CAULIFLOWER FLORETS 129
224. ITALIAN-STYLE VEGETARIAN PATTIES 129
225. LENTIL QUICHE 130
226. CORN PATTIES 130
227. VEGAN MEATBALLS 131
228. VEGAN SHEPHERD PIE 131
229. VEGAN LENTIL SALAD 131
230. VEGAN BAKED STUFFED TOMATOES 132

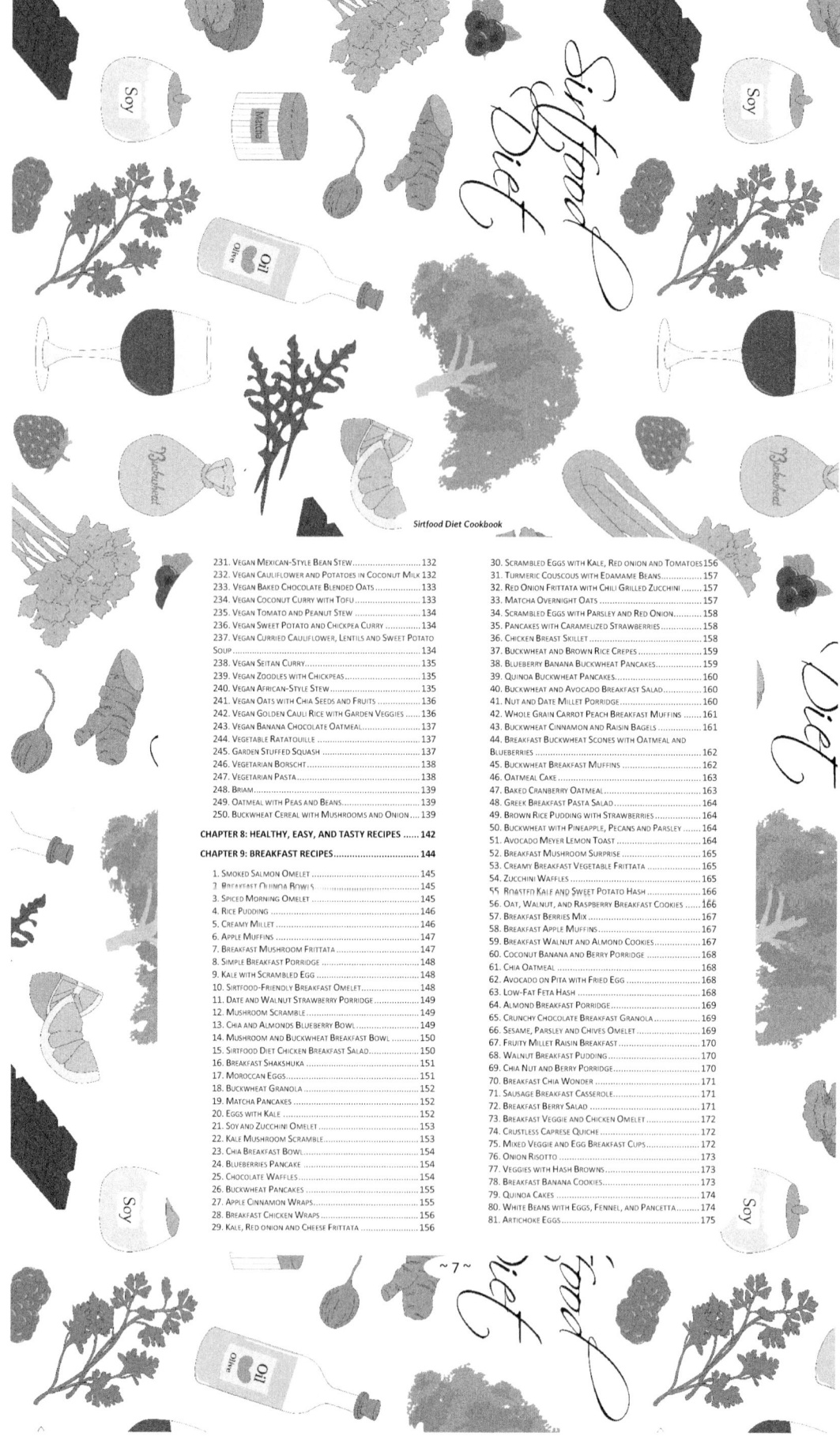

231. Vegan Mexican-Style Bean Stew...........................132
232. Vegan Cauliflower and Potatoes in Coconut Milk 132
233. Vegan Baked Chocolate Blended Oats 133
234. Vegan Coconut Curry with Tofu.........................133
235. Vegan Tomato and Peanut Stew.........................134
236. Vegan Sweet Potato and Chickpea Curry 134
237. Vegan Curried Cauliflower, Lentils and Sweet Potato
Soup 134
238. Vegan Seitan Curry..135
239. Vegan Zoodles with Chickpeas..........................135
240. Vegan African-Style Stew...................................135
241. Vegan Oats with Chia Seeds and Fruits 136
242. Vegan Golden Cauli Rice with Garden Veggies 136
243. Vegan Banana Chocolate Oatmeal......................137
244. Vegetable Ratatouille 137
245. Garden Stuffed Squash 137
246. Vegetarian Borscht..138
247. Vegetarian Pasta...138
248. Briam...139
249. Oatmeal with Peas and Beans.............................139
250. Buckwheat Cereal with Mushrooms and Onion.... 139

CHAPTER 8: HEALTHY, EASY, AND TASTY RECIPES 142

CHAPTER 9: BREAKFAST RECIPES.................................144

1. Smoked Salmon Omelet 145
2. Breakfast Quinoa Bowls 145
3. Spiced Morning Omelet 145
4. Rice Pudding 146
5. Creamy Millet 146
6. Apple Muffins..147
7. Breakfast Mushroom Frittata 147
8. Simple Breakfast Porridge 148
9. Kale with Scrambled Egg 148
10. Sirtfood-Friendly Breakfast Omelet........................148
11. Date and Walnut Strawberry Porridge 149
12. Mushroom Scramble..149
13. Chia and Almonds Blueberry Bowl 149
14. Mushroom and Buckwheat Breakfast Bowl 150
15. Sirtfood Diet Chicken Breakfast Salad....................150
16. Breakfast Shakshuka 151
17. Moroccan Eggs...151
18. Buckwheat Granola 152
19. Matcha Pancakes 152
20. Eggs with Kale 152
21. Soy and Zucchini Omelet 153
22. Kale Mushroom Scramble.....................................153
23. Chia Breakfast Bowl 154
24. Blueberries Pancake 154
25. Chocolate Waffles...154
26. Buckwheat Pancakes..155
27. Apple Cinnamon Wraps..155
28. Breakfast Chicken Wraps......................................156
29. Kale, Red onion and Cheese Frittata 156

30. Scrambled Eggs with Kale, Red onion and Tomatoes156
31. Turmeric Couscous with Edamame Beans...............157
32. Red Onion Frittata with Chili Grilled Zucchini 157
33. Matcha Overnight Oats..157
34. Scrambled Eggs with Parsley and Red Onion..........158
35. Pancakes with Caramelized Strawberries...............158
36. Chicken Breast Skillet 158
37. Buckwheat and Brown Rice Crepes 159
38. Blueberry Banana Buckwheat Pancakes................159
39. Quinoa Buckwheat Pancakes...............................160
40. Buckwheat and Avocado Breakfast Salad...............160
41. Nut and Date Millet Porridge................................160
42. Whole Grain Carrot Peach Breakfast Muffins 161
43. Buckwheat Cinnamon and Raisin Bagels 161
44. Breakfast Buckwheat Scones with Oatmeal and
Blueberries 162
45. Buckwheat Breakfast Muffins 162
46. Oatmeal Cake..163
47. Baked Cranberry Oatmeal 163
48. Greek Breakfast Pasta Salad.................................164
49. Brown Rice Pudding with Strawberries..................164
50. Buckwheat with Pineapple, Pecans and Parsley 164
51. Avocado Meyer Lemon Toast 164
52. Breakfast Mushroom Surprise 165
53. Creamy Breakfast Vegetable Frittata 165
54. Zucchini Waffles...165
55. Roasted Kale and Sweet Potato Hash 166
56. Oat, Walnut, and Raspberry Breakfast Cookies 166
57. Breakfast Berries Mix 167
58. Breakfast Apple Muffins.......................................167
59. Breakfast Walnut and Almond Cookies..................167
60. Coconut Banana and Berry Porridge 168
61. Chia Oatmeal 168
62. Avocado on Pita with Fried Egg 168
63. Low-Fat Feta Hash 168
64. Almond Breakfast Porridge...................................169
65. Crunchy Chocolate Breakfast Granola 169
66. Sesame, Parsley and Chives Omelet 169
67. Fruity Millet Raisin Breakfast 170
68. Walnut Breakfast Pudding....................................170
69. Chia Nut and Berry Porridge 170
70. Breakfast Chia Wonder 171
71. Sausage Breakfast Casserole.................................171
72. Breakfast Berry Salad 171
73. Breakfast Veggie and Chicken Omelet....................172
74. Crustless Caprese Quiche 172
75. Mixed Veggie and Egg Breakfast Cups 172
76. Onion Risotto 173
77. Veggies with Hash Browns....................................173
78. Breakfast Banana Cookies.....................................173
79. Quinoa Cakes 174
80. White Beans with Eggs, Fennel, and Pancetta........174
81. Artichoke Eggs...175

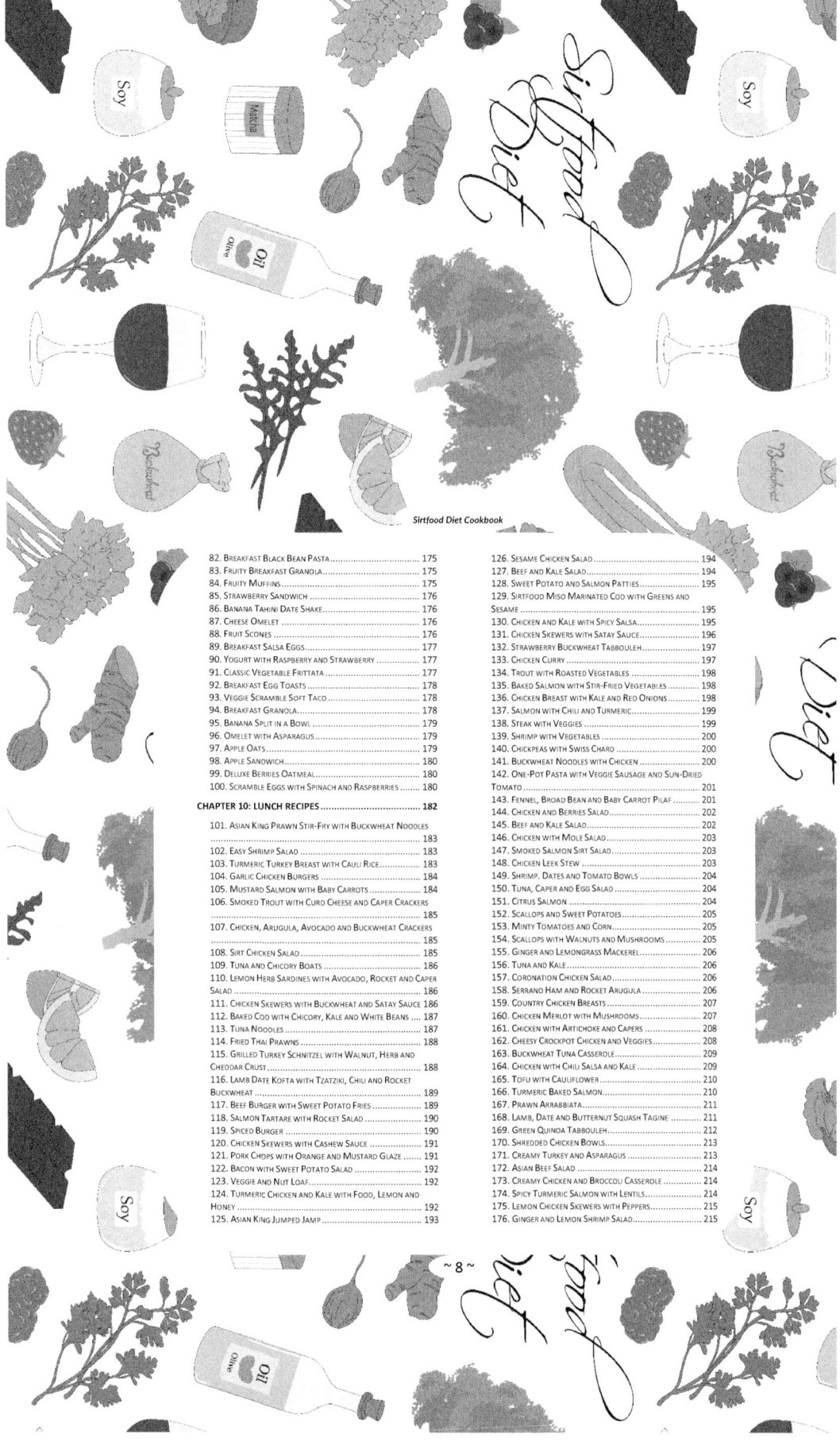

82. Breakfast Black Bean Pasta 175
83. Fruity Breakfast Granola 175
84. Fruity Muffins 175
85. Strawberry Sandwich 176
86. Banana Tahini Date Shake 176
87. Cheese Omelet 176
88. Fruit Scones 176
89. Breakfast Salsa Eggs 177
90. Yogurt with Raspberry and Strawberry 177
91. Classic Vegetable Frittata 177
92. Breakfast Egg Toasts 178
93. Veggie Scramble Soft Taco 178
94. Breakfast Granola 178
95. Banana Split in a Bowl 179
96. Omelet with Asparagus 179
97. Apple Oats 179
98. Apple Sandwich 180
99. Deluxe Berries Oatmeal 180
100. Scramble Eggs with Spinach and Raspberries 180

CHAPTER 10: LUNCH RECIPES 182

101. Asian King Prawn Stir-Fry with Buckwheat Noodles
.... 183
102. Easy Shrimp Salad 183
103. Turmeric Turkey Breast with Cauli Rice 183
104. Garlic Chicken Burgers 184
105. Mustard Salmon with Baby Carrots 184
106. Smoked Trout with Curd Cheese and Caper Crackers
.... 185
107. Chicken, Arugula, Avocado and Buckwheat Crackers
.... 185
108. Sirt Chicken Salad 185
109. Tuna and Chicory Boats 186
110. Lemon Herb Sardines with Avocado, Rocket and Caper
Salad 186
111. Chicken Skewers with Buckwheat and Satay Sauce 186
112. Baked Cod with Chicory, Kale and White Beans 187
113. Tuna Noodles 187
114. Fried Thai Prawns 188
115. Grilled Turkey Schnitzel with Walnut, Herb and
Cheddar Crust 188
116. Lamb Date Kofta with Tzatziki, Chili and Rocket
Buckwheat 189
117. Beef Burger with Sweet Potato Fries 189
118. Salmon Tartare with Rocket Salad 190
119. Spiced Burger 190
120. Chicken Skewers with Cashew Sauce 191
121. Pork Chops with Orange and Mustard Glaze 191
122. Bacon with Sweet Potato Salad 192
123. Veggie and Nut Loaf 192
124. Turmeric Chicken and Kale with Food, Lemon and
Honey 192
125. Asian King Jumped Jamp 193

126. Sesame Chicken Salad 194
127. Beef and Kale Salad 194
128. Sweet Potato and Salmon Patties 195
129. Sirtfood Miso Marinated Cod with Greens and
Sesame 195
130. Chicken and Kale with Spicy Salsa 195
131. Chicken Skewers with Satay Sauce 196
132. Strawberry Buckwheat Tabbouleh 197
133. Chicken Curry 197
134. Trout with Roasted Vegetables 198
135. Baked Salmon with Stir-Fried Vegetables 198
136. Chicken Breast with Kale and Red Onions 198
137. Salmon with Chili and Turmeric 199
138. Steak with Veggies 199
139. Shrimp with Vegetables 200
140. Chickpeas with Swiss Chard 200
141. Buckwheat Noodles with Chicken 200
142. One-Pot Pasta with Veggie Sausage and Sun-Dried
Tomato 201
143. Fennel, Broad Bean and Baby Carrot Pilaf 201
144. Chicken and Berries Salad 202
145. Beef and Kale Salad 202
146. Chicken with Mole Salad 203
147. Smoked Salmon Sirt Salad 203
148. Chicken Leek Stew 203
149. Shrimp, Dates and Tomato Bowls 204
150. Tuna, Caper and Egg Salad 204
151. Citrus Salmon 204
152. Scallops and Sweet Potatoes 205
153. Minty Tomatoes and Corn 205
154. Scallops with Walnuts and Mushrooms 205
155. Ginger and Lemongrass Mackerel 206
156. Tuna and Kale 206
157. Coronation Chicken Salad 206
158. Serrano Ham and Rocket Arugula 206
159. Country Chicken Breasts 207
160. Chicken Merlot with Mushrooms 207
161. Chicken with Artichoke and Capers 208
162. Cheesy Crockpot Chicken and Veggies 208
163. Buckwheat Tuna Casserole 209
164. Chicken with Chili Salsa and Kale 209
165. Tofu with Cauliflower 210
166. Turmeric Baked Salmon 210
167. Prawn Arrabbiata 211
168. Lamb, Date and Butternut Squash Tagine 211
169. Green Quinoa Tabbouleh 212
170. Shredded Chicken Bowls 213
171. Creamy Turkey and Asparagus 213
172. Asian Beef Salad 214
173. Creamy Chicken and Broccoli Casserole 214
174. Spicy Turmeric Salmon with Lentils 214
175. Lemon Chicken Skewers with Peppers 215
176. Ginger and Lemon Shrimp Salad 215

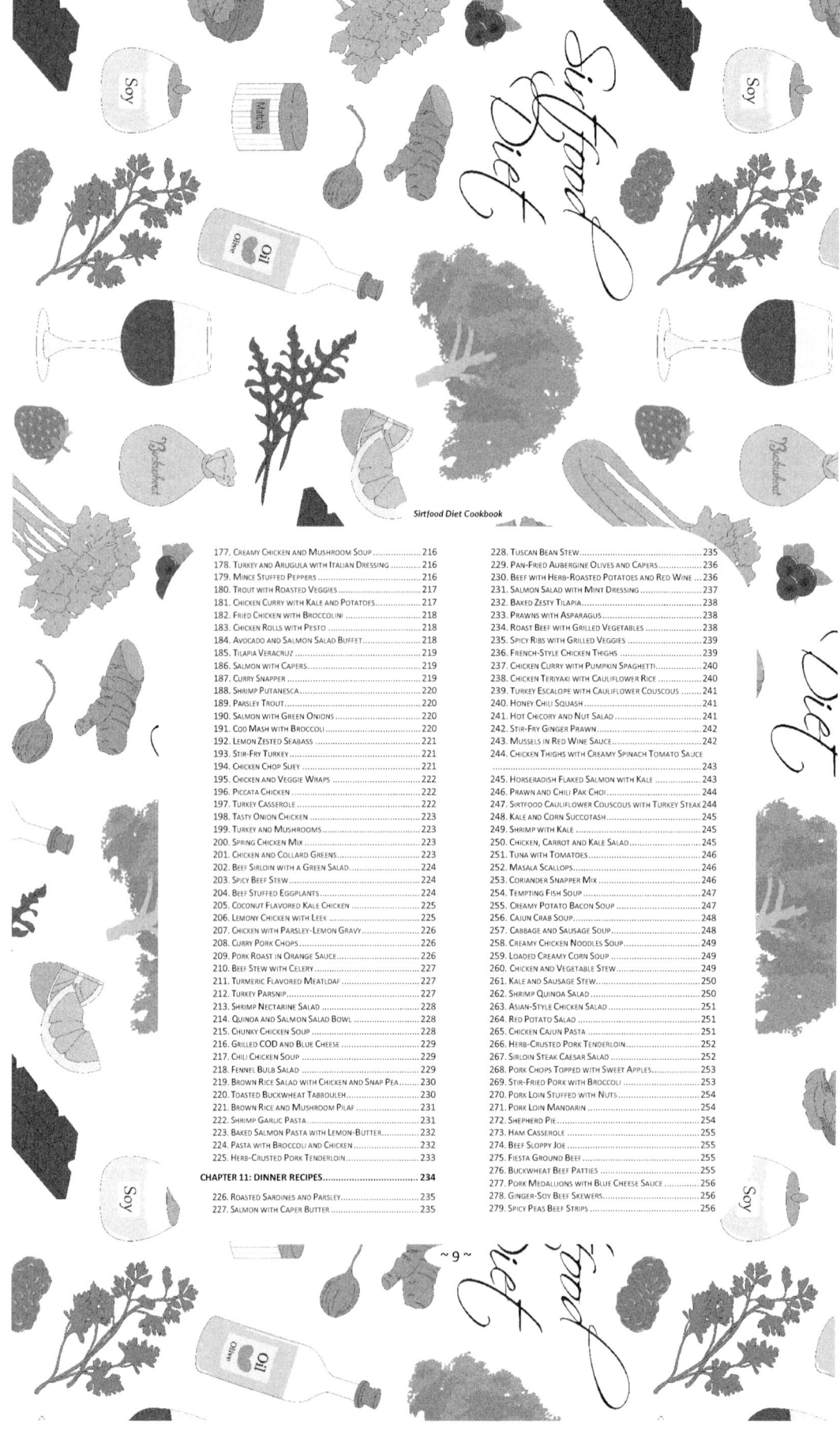

Sirtfood Diet Cookbook

177. Creamy Chicken and Mushroom Soup 216
178. Turkey and Arugula with Italian Dressing 216
179. Mince Stuffed Peppers 216
180. Trout with Roasted Veggies 217
181. Chicken Curry with Kale and Potatoes................. 217
182. Fried Chicken with Broccolini 218
183. Chicken Rolls with Pesto 218
184. Avocado and Salmon Salad Buffet 218
185. Tilapia Veracruz 219
186. Salmon with Capers 219
187. Curry Snapper 219
188. Shrimp Putanesca 220
189. Parsley Trout 220
190. Salmon with Green Onions 220
191. Cod Mash with Broccoli 220
192. Lemon Zested Seabass 221
193. Stir-Fry Turkey 221
194. Chicken Chop Suey 221
195. Chicken and Veggie Wraps 222
196. Piccata Chicken 222
197. Turkey Casserole 222
198. Tasty Onion Chicken 223
199. Turkey and Mushrooms 223
200. Spring Chicken Mix 223
201. Chicken and Collard Greens 223
202. Beef Sirloin with a Green Salad 224
203. Spicy Beef Stew 224
204. Beef Stuffed Eggplants 224
205. Coconut Flavored Kale Chicken 225
206. Lemony Chicken with Leek 225
207. Chicken with Parsley-Lemon Gravy...................... 226
208. Curry Pork Chops 226
209. Pork Roast in Orange Sauce 226
210. Beef Stew with Celery 227
211. Turmeric Flavored Meatloaf 227
212. Turkey Parsnip 227
213. Shrimp Nectarine Salad 228
214. Quinoa and Salmon Salad Bowl 228
215. Chunky Chicken Soup 228
216. Grilled Cod and Blue Cheese 229
217. Chili Chicken Soup 229
218. Fennel Bulb Salad 229
219. Brown Rice Salad with Chicken and Snap Pea........ 230
220. Toasted Buckwheat Tabbouleh............................ 230
221. Brown Rice and Mushroom Pilaf 231
222. Shrimp Garlic Pasta 231
223. Baked Salmon Pasta with Lemon-Butter................ 232
224. Pasta with Broccoli and Chicken 232
225. Herb-Crusted Pork Tenderloin............................ 233

CHAPTER 11: DINNER RECIPES..................................234

226. Roasted Sardines and Parsley............................. 235
227. Salmon with Caper Butter 235

228. Tuscan Bean Stew.. 235
229. Pan-Fried Aubergine Olives and Capers................. 236
230. Beef with Herb-Roasted Potatoes and Red Wine ... 236
231. Salmon Salad with Mint Dressing 237
232. Baked Zesty Tilapia.. 238
233. Prawns with Asparagus..................................... 238
234. Roast Beef with Grilled Vegetables 238
235. Spicy Ribs with Grilled Veggies 239
236. French-Style Chicken Thighs 239
237. Chicken Curry with Pumpkin Spaghetti................. 240
238. Chicken Teriyaki with Cauliflower Rice 240
239. Turkey Escalope with Cauliflower Couscous 241
240. Honey Chili Squash 241
241. Hot Chicory and Nut Salad 241
242. Stir-Fry Ginger Prawn....................................... 242
243. Mussels in Red Wine Sauce 242
244. Chicken Thighs with Creamy Spinach Tomato Sauce
.... 243
245. Horseradish Flaked Salmon with Kale 243
246. Prawn and Chili Pak Choi 244
247. Sirtfood Cauliflower Couscous with Turkey Steak 244
248. Kale and Corn Succotash 245
249. Shrimp with Kale 245
250. Chicken, Carrot and Kale Salad.......................... 245
251. Tuna with Tomatoes... 246
252. Masala Scallops 246
253. Coriander Snapper Mix 246
254. Tempting Fish Soup 247
255. Creamy Potato Bacon Soup 247
256. Cajun Crab Soup... 248
257. Cabbage and Sausage Soup................................ 248
258. Creamy Chicken Noodles Soup........................... 249
259. Loaded Creamy Corn Soup 249
260. Chicken and Vegetable Stew 249
261. Kale and Sausage Stew 250
262. Shrimp Quinoa Salad 250
263. Asian-Style Chicken Salad 251
264. Red Potato Salad 251
265. Chicken Cajun Pasta 251
266. Herb-Crusted Pork Tenderloin............................ 252
267. Sirloin Steak Caesar Salad 252
268. Pork Chops Topped with Sweet Apples.................. 253
269. Stir-Fried Pork with Broccoli 253
270. Pork Loin Stuffed with Nuts 254
271. Pork Loin Mandarin 254
272. Shepherd Pie 254
273. Ham Casserole 255
274. Beef Sloppy Joe 255
275. Fiesta Ground Beef 255
276. Buckwheat Beef Patties 255
277. Pork Medallions with Blue Cheese Sauce 256
278. Ginger-Soy Beef Skewers................................... 256
279. Spicy Peas Beef Strips 256

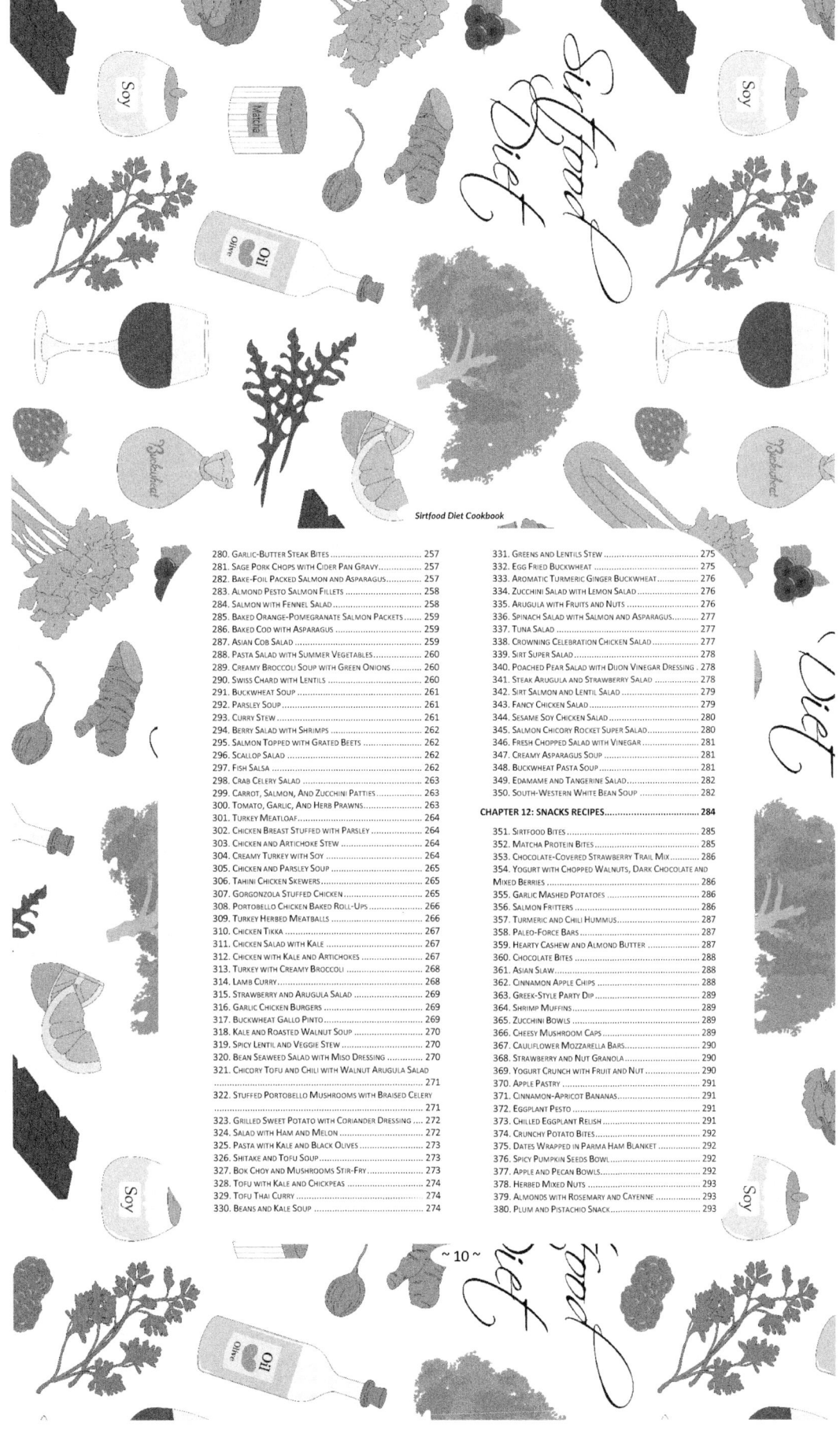

280. Garlic-Butter Steak Bites 257
281. Sage Pork Chops with Cider Pan Gravy 257
282. Bake-Foil Packed Salmon and Asparagus 257
283. Almond Pesto Salmon Fillets 258
284. Salmon with Fennel Salad 258
285. Baked Orange-Pomegranate Salmon Packets 259
286. Baked Cod with Asparagus 259
287. Asian Cob Salad 259
288. Pasta Salad with Summer Vegetables................. 260
289. Creamy Broccoli Soup with Green Onions 260
290. Swiss Chard with Lentils 260
291. Buckwheat Soup 261
292. Parsley Soup 261
293. Curry Stew 261
294. Berry Salad with Shrimps 262
295. Salmon Topped with Grated Beets 262
296. Scallop Salad 262
297. Fish Salsa 262
298. Crab Celery Salad 263
299. Carrot, Salmon, And Zucchini Patties 263
300. Tomato, Garlic, And Herb Prawns 263
301. Turkey Meatloaf 264
302. Chicken Breast Stuffed with Parsley 264
303. Chicken and Artichoke Stew 264
304. Creamy Turkey with Soy 264
305. Chicken and Parsley Soup 265
306. Tahini Chicken Skewers 265
307. Gorgonzola Stuffed Chicken 265
308. Portobello Chicken Baked Roll-Ups 266
309. Turkey Herbed Meatballs 266
310. Chicken Tikka 267
311. Chicken Salad with Kale 267
312. Chicken with Kale and Artichokes 267
313. Turkey with Creamy Broccoli 268
314. Lamb Curry 268
315. Strawberry and Arugula Salad 269
316. Garlic Chicken Burgers 269
317. Buckwheat Gallo Pinto 269
318. Kale and Roasted Walnut Soup 270
319. Spicy Lentil and Veggie Stew 270
320. Bean Seaweed Salad with Miso Dressing 270
321. Chicory Tofu and Chili with Walnut Arugula Salad
.... 271
322. Stuffed Portobello Mushrooms with Braised Celery
.... 271
323. Grilled Sweet Potato with Coriander Dressing 272
324. Salad with Ham and Melon 272
325. Pasta with Kale and Black Olives 273
326. Shitake and Tofu Soup 273
327. Bok Choy and Mushrooms Stir-Fry 273
328. Tofu with Kale and Chickpeas 274
329. Tofu Thai Curry 274
330. Beans and Kale Soup 274

331. Greens and Lentils Stew 275
332. Egg Fried Buckwheat 275
333. Aromatic Turmeric Ginger Buckwheat 276
334. Zucchini Salad with Lemon Salad 276
335. Arugula with Fruits and Nuts 276
336. Spinach Salad with Salmon and Asparagus 277
337. Tuna Salad 277
338. Crowning Celebration Chicken Salad 277
339. Sirt Super Salad 278
340. Poached Pear Salad with Dijon Vinegar Dressing . 278
341. Steak Arugula and Strawberry Salad 278
342. Sirt Salmon and Lentil Salad 279
343. Fancy Chicken Salad 279
344. Sesame Soy Chicken Salad 280
345. Salmon Chicory Rocket Super Salad 280
346. Fresh Chopped Salad with Vinegar 281
347. Creamy Asparagus Soup 281
348. Buckwheat Pasta Soup 281
349. Edamame and Tangerine Salad 282
350. South-Western White Bean Soup 282

CHAPTER 12: SNACKS RECIPES 284

351. Sirtfood Bites 285
352. Matcha Protein Bites 285
353. Chocolate-Covered Strawberry Trail Mix 286
354. Yogurt with Chopped Walnuts, Dark Chocolate and
Mixed Berries 286
355. Garlic Mashed Potatoes 286
356. Salmon Fritters 286
357. Turmeric and Chili Hummus 287
358. Paleo-Force Bars 287
359. Hearty Cashew and Almond Butter 287
360. Chocolate Bites 288
361. Asian Slaw 288
362. Cinnamon Apple Chips 288
363. Greek-Style Party Dip 289
364. Shrimp Muffins 289
365. Zucchini Bowls 289
366. Cheesy Mushroom Caps 289
367. Cauliflower Mozzarella Bars 290
368. Strawberry and Nut Granola 290
369. Yogurt Crunch with Fruit and Nut 290
370. Apple Pastry 291
371. Cinnamon-Apricot Bananas 291
372. Eggplant Pesto 291
373. Chilled Eggplant Relish 291
374. Crunchy Potato Bites 292
375. Dates Wrapped in Parma Ham Blanket 292
376. Spicy Pumpkin Seeds Bowl 292
377. Apple and Pecan Bowls 292
378. Herbed Mixed Nuts 293
379. Almonds with Rosemary and Cayenne 293
380. Plum and Pistachio Snack 293

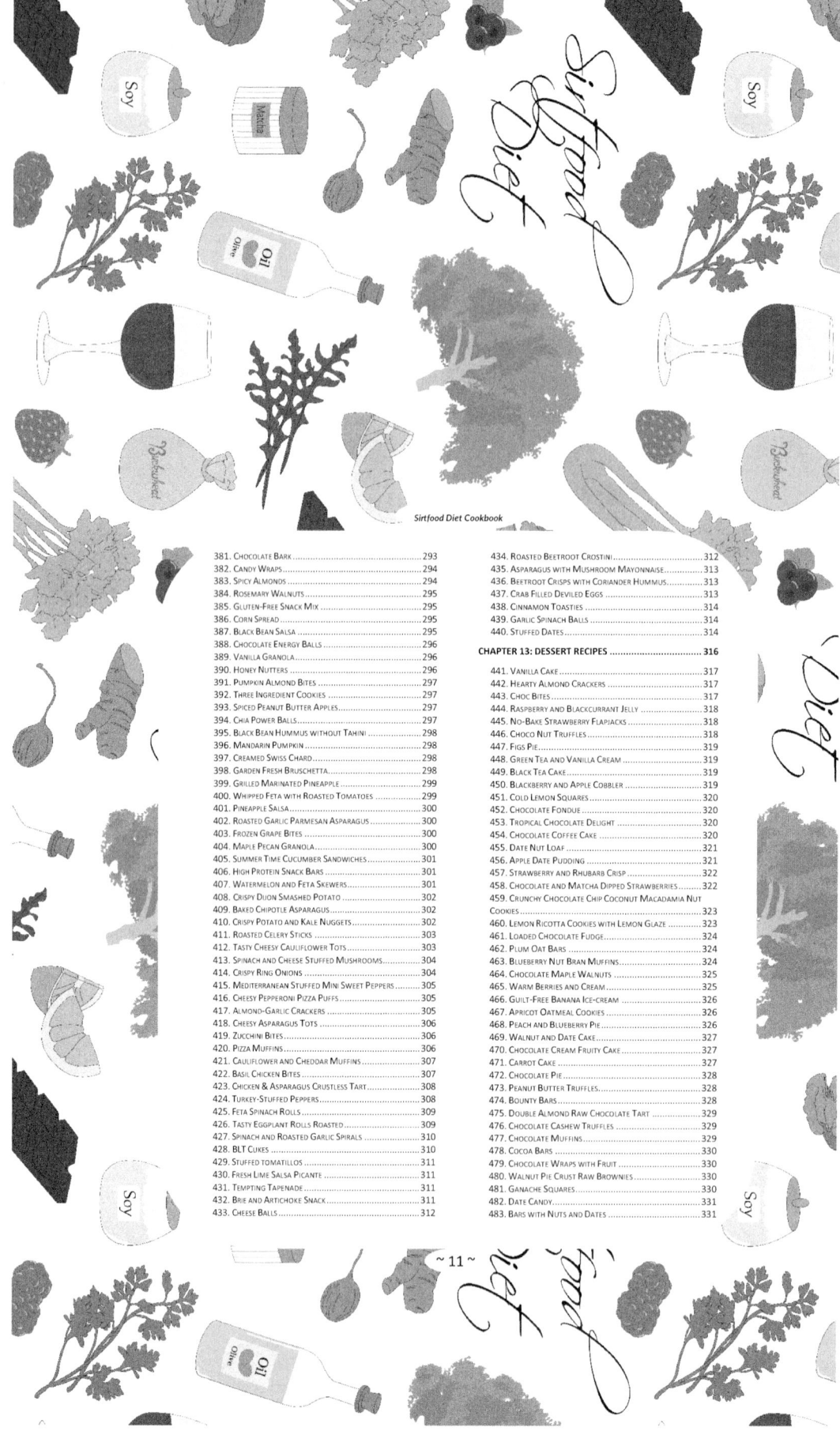

381. Chocolate Bark 293
382. Candy Wraps 294
383. Spicy Almonds 294
384. Rosemary Walnuts 295
385. Gluten-Free Snack Mix 295
386. Corn Spread 295
387. Black Bean Salsa 295
388. Chocolate Energy Balls 296
389. Vanilla Granola 296
390. Honey Nutters 296
391. Pumpkin Almond Bites 297
392. Three Ingredient Cookies 297
393. Spiced Peanut Butter Apples 297
394. Chia Power Balls 297
395. Black Bean Hummus without Tahini 298
396. Mandarin Pumpkin 298
397. Creamed Swiss Chard 298
398. Garden Fresh Bruschetta 298
399. Grilled Marinated Pineapple 299
400. Whipped Feta with Roasted Tomatoes 299
401. Pineapple Salsa 300
402. Roasted Garlic Parmesan Asparagus 300
403. Frozen Grape Bites 300
404. Maple Pecan Granola 300
405. Summer Time Cucumber Sandwiches 301
406. High Protein Snack Bars 301
407. Watermelon and Feta Skewers 301
408. Crispy Dijon Smashed Potato 302
409. Baked Chipotle Asparagus 302
410. Crispy Potato and Kale Nuggets 302
411. Roasted Celery Sticks 303
412. Tasty Cheesy Cauliflower Tots 303
413. Spinach and Cheese Stuffed Mushrooms 304
414. Crispy Ring Onions 304
415. Mediterranean Stuffed Mini Sweet Peppers 305
416. Cheesy Pepperoni Pizza Puffs 305
417. Almond-Garlic Crackers 305
418. Cheesy Asparagus Tots 306
419. Zucchini Bites 306
420. Pizza Muffins 306
421. Cauliflower and Cheddar Muffins 307
422. Basil Chicken Bites 307
423. Chicken & Asparagus Crustless Tart 308
424. Turkey-Stuffed Peppers 308
425. Feta Spinach Rolls 309
426. Tasty Eggplant Rolls Roasted 309
427. Spinach and Roasted Garlic Spirals 310
428. BLT Cukes 310
429. Stuffed tomatillos 311
430. Fresh Lime Salsa Picante 311
431. Tempting Tapenade 311
432. Brie and Artichoke Snack 311
433. Cheese Balls 312

434. Roasted Beetroot Crostini 312
435. Asparagus with Mushroom Mayonnaise............ 313
436. Beetroot Crisps with Coriander Hummus 313
437. Crab Filled Deviled Eggs 313
438. Cinnamon Toasties 314
439. Garlic Spinach Balls 314
440. Stuffed Dates 314

CHAPTER 13: DESSERT RECIPES 316

441. Vanilla Cake 317
442. Hearty Almond Crackers 317
443. Choc Bites 317
444. Raspberry and Blackcurrant Jelly 318
445. No-Bake Strawberry Flapjacks 318
446. Choco Nut Truffles 318
447. Figs Pie 319
448. Green Tea and Vanilla Cream 319
449. Black Tea Cake 319
450. Blackberry and Apple Cobbler 319
451. Cold Lemon Squares 320
452. Chocolate Fondue 320
453. Tropical Chocolate Delight 320
454. Chocolate Coffee Cake 320
455. Date Nut Loaf 321
456. Apple Date Pudding 321
457. Strawberry and Rhubarb Crisp 322
458. Chocolate and Matcha Dipped Strawberries......... 322
459. Crunchy Chocolate Chip Coconut Macadamia Nut Cookies 323
460. Lemon Ricotta Cookies with Lemon Glaze 323
461. Loaded Chocolate Fudge 324
462. Plum Oat Bars 324
463. Blueberry Nut Bran Muffins 324
464. Chocolate Maple Walnuts 325
465. Warm Berries and Cream 325
466. Guilt-Free Banana Ice-cream 326
467. Apricot Oatmeal Cookies 326
468. Peach and Blueberry Pie 326
469. Walnut and Date Cake 327
470. Chocolate Cream Fruity Cake 327
471. Carrot Cake 327
472. Chocolate Pie 328
473. Peanut Butter Truffles 328
474. Bounty Bars 328
475. Double Almond Raw Chocolate Tart 329
476. Chocolate Cashew Truffles 329
477. Chocolate Muffins 329
478. Cocoa Bars 330
479. Chocolate Wraps with Fruit 330
480. Walnut Pie Crust Raw Brownies 330
481. Ganache Squares 330
482. Date Candy... 331
483. Bars with Nuts and Dates 331

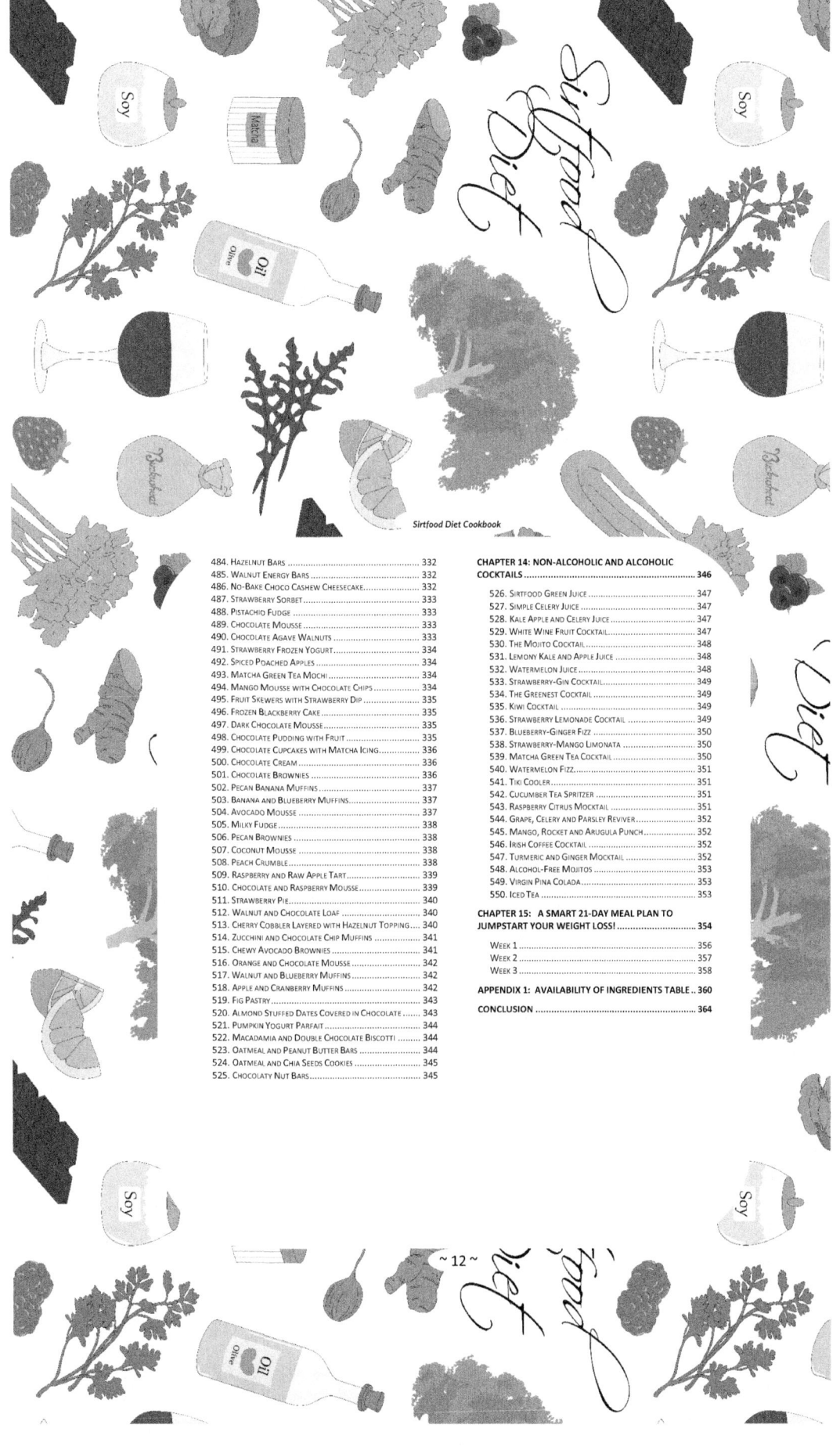

Sirtfood Diet Cookbook

484. HAZELNUT BARS 332
485. WALNUT ENERGY BARS 332
486. NO-BAKE CHOCO CASHEW CHEESECAKE................... 332
487. STRAWBERRY SORBET 333
488. PISTACHIO FUDGE 333
489. CHOCOLATE MOUSSE 333
490. CHOCOLATE AGAVE WALNUTS 333
491. STRAWBERRY FROZEN YOGURT 334
492. SPICED POACHED APPLES 334
493. MATCHA GREEN TEA MOCHI 334
494. MANGO MOUSSE WITH CHOCOLATE CHIPS 334
495. FRUIT SKEWERS WITH STRAWBERRY DIP 335
496. FROZEN BLACKBERRY CAKE 335
497. DARK CHOCOLATE MOUSSE 335
498. CHOCOLATE PUDDING WITH FRUIT 335
499. CHOCOLATE CUPCAKES WITH MATCHA ICING 336
500. CHOCOLATE CREAM 336
501. CHOCOLATE BROWNIES 336
502. PECAN BANANA MUFFINS 337
503. BANANA AND BLUEBERRY MUFFINS 337
504. AVOCADO MOUSSE 337
505. MILKY FUDGE 338
506. PECAN BROWNIES 338
507. COCONUT MOUSSE 338
508. PEACH CRUMBLE 338
509. RASPBERRY AND RAW APPLE TART 339
510. CHOCOLATE AND RASPBERRY MOUSSE 339
511. STRAWBERRY PIE 340
512. WALNUT AND CHOCOLATE LOAF 340
513. CHERRY COBBLER LAYERED WITH HAZELNUT TOPPING ... 340
514. ZUCCHINI AND CHOCOLATE CHIP MUFFINS 341
515. CHEWY AVOCADO BROWNIES 341
516. ORANGE AND CHOCOLATE MOUSSE 342
517. WALNUT AND BLUEBERRY MUFFINS 342
518. APPLE AND CRANBERRY MUFFINS 342
519. FIG PASTRY 343
520. ALMOND STUFFED DATES COVERED IN CHOCOLATE 343
521. PUMPKIN YOGURT PARFAIT 344
522. MACADAMIA AND DOUBLE CHOCOLATE BISCOTTI 344
523. OATMEAL AND PEANUT BUTTER BARS 344
524. OATMEAL AND CHIA SEEDS COOKIES 345
525. CHOCOLATY NUT BARS 345

CHAPTER 14: NON-ALCOHOLIC AND ALCOHOLIC
COCKTAILS 346

526. SIRTFOOD GREEN JUICE 347
527. SIMPLE CELERY JUICE 347
528. KALE APPLE AND CELERY JUICE 347
529. WHITE WINE FRUIT COCKTAIL 347
530. THE MOJITO COCKTAIL 348
531. LEMONY KALE AND APPLE JUICE 348
532. WATERMELON JUICE 348
533. STRAWBERRY-GIN COCKTAIL 349
534. THE GREENEST COCKTAIL 349
535. KIWI COCKTAIL 349
536. STRAWBERRY LEMONADE COCKTAIL 349
537. BLUEBERRY-GINGER FIZZ 350
538. STRAWBERRY-MANGO LIMONATA 350
539. MATCHA GREEN TEA COCKTAIL 350
540. WATERMELON FIZZ 351
541. TIKI COOLER 351
542. CUCUMBER TEA SPRITZER 351
543. RASPBERRY CITRUS MOCKTAIL 351
544. GRAPE, CELERY AND PARSLEY REVIVER 352
545. MANGO, ROCKET AND ARUGULA PUNCH 352
546. IRISH COFFEE COCKTAIL 352
547. TURMERIC AND GINGER MOCKTAIL 352
548. ALCOHOL-FREE MOJITOS 353
549. VIRGIN PINA COLADA 353
550. ICED TEA 353

CHAPTER 15: A SMART 21-DAY MEAL PLAN TO
JUMPSTART YOUR WEIGHT LOSS! 354

WEEK 1 356
WEEK 2 357
WEEK 3 358

APPENDIX 1: AVAILABILITY OF INGREDIENTS TABLE .. 360

CONCLUSION 364

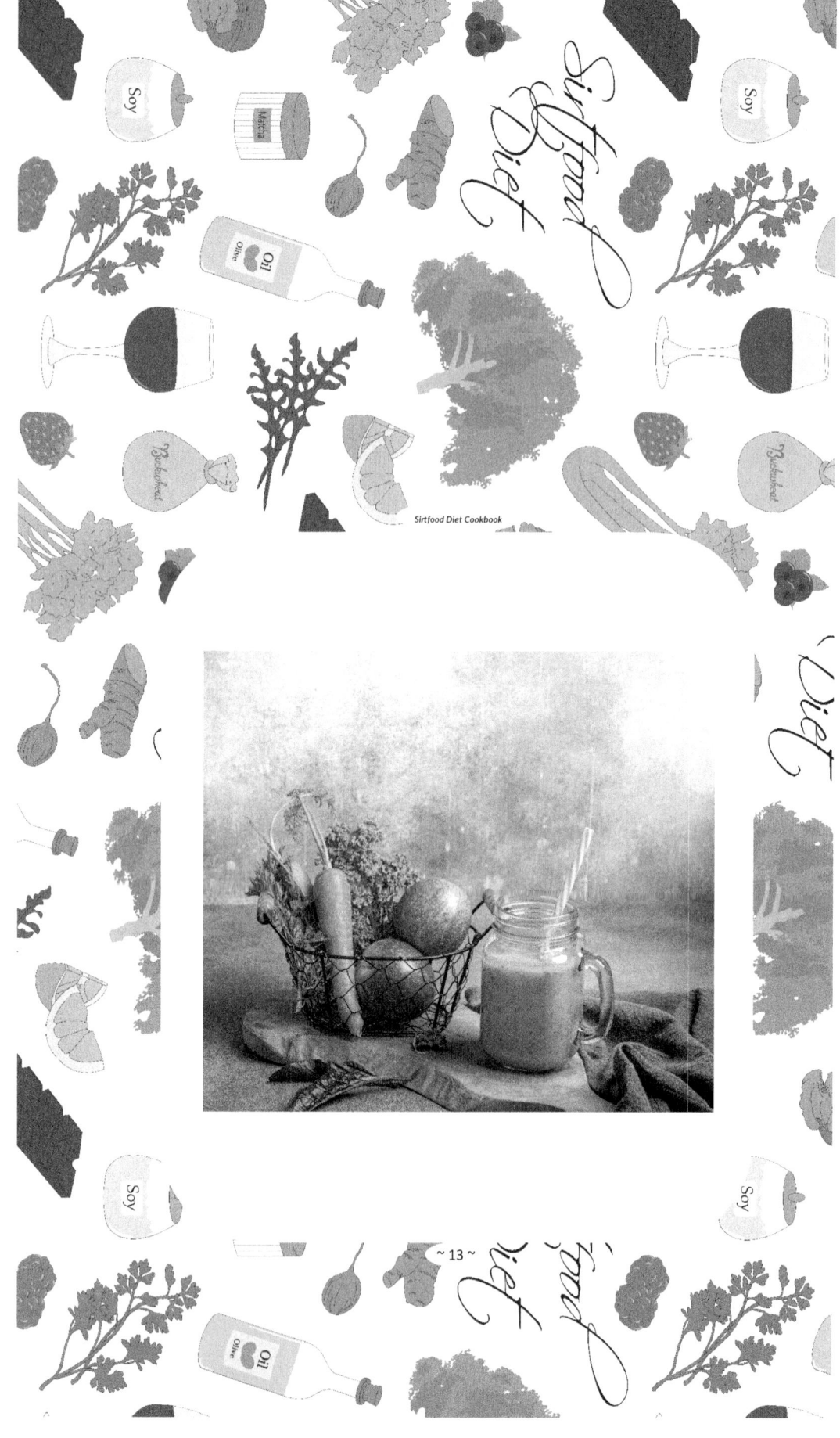

Sirtfood Diet Cookbook

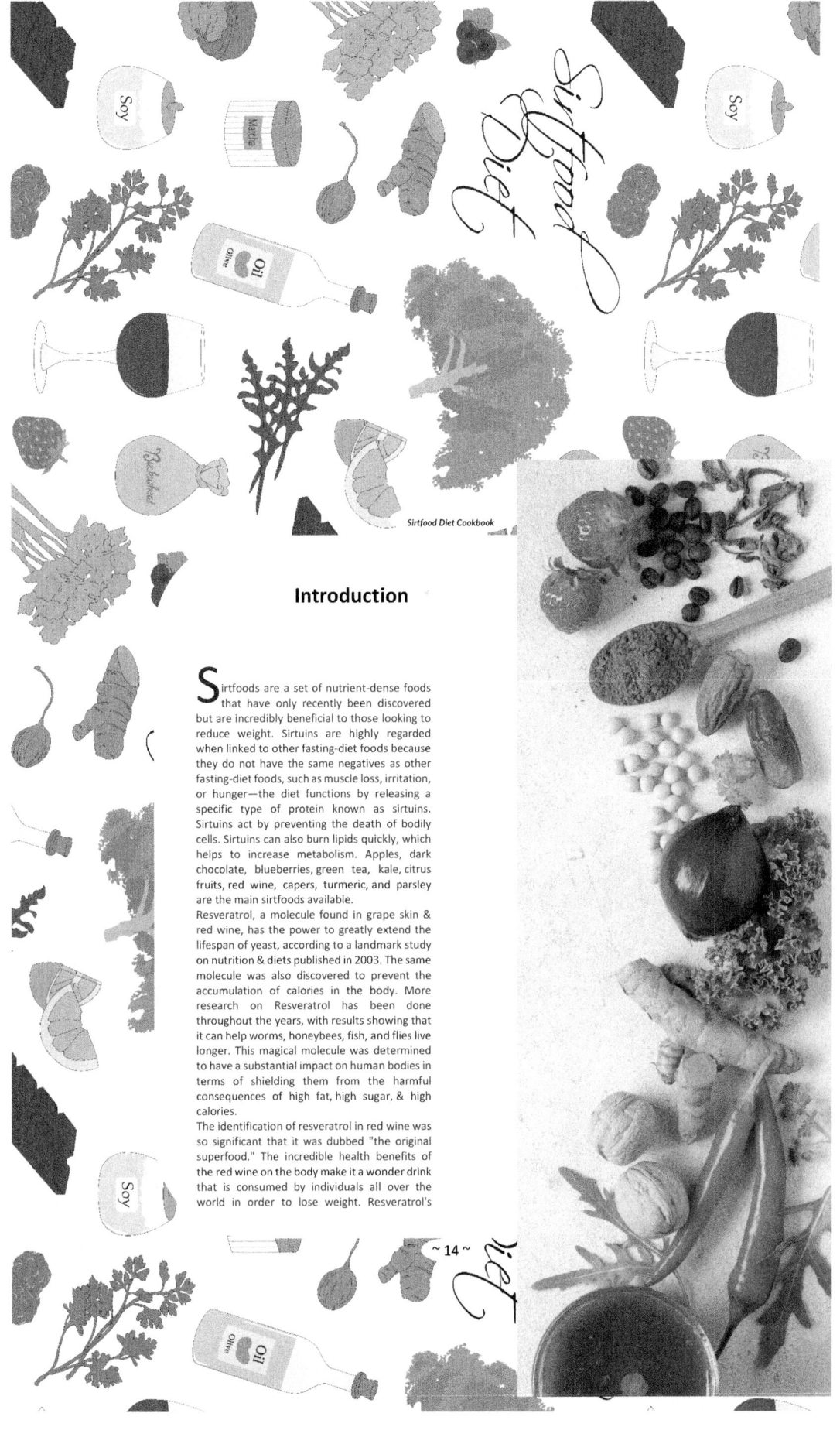

Sirtfood Diet Cookbook

Introduction

Sirtfoods are a set of nutrient-dense foods that have only recently been discovered but are incredibly beneficial to those looking to reduce weight. Sirtuins are highly regarded when linked to other fasting-diet foods because they do not have the same negatives as other fasting-diet foods, such as muscle loss, irritation, or hunger—the diet functions by releasing a specific type of protein known as sirtuins. Sirtuins act by preventing the death of bodily cells. Sirtuins can also burn lipids quickly, which helps to increase metabolism. Apples, dark chocolate, blueberries, green tea, kale, citrus fruits, red wine, capers, turmeric, and parsley are the main sirtfoods available.

Resveratrol, a molecule found in grape skin & red wine, has the power to greatly extend the lifespan of yeast, according to a landmark study on nutrition & diets published in 2003. The same molecule was also discovered to prevent the accumulation of calories in the body. More research on Resveratrol has been done throughout the years, with results showing that it can help worms, honeybees, fish, and flies live longer. This magical molecule was determined to have a substantial impact on human bodies in terms of shielding them from the harmful consequences of high fat, high sugar, & high calories.

The identification of resveratrol in red wine was so significant that it was dubbed "the original superfood." The incredible health benefits of the red wine on the body make it a wonder drink that is consumed by individuals all over the world in order to lose weight. Resveratrol's

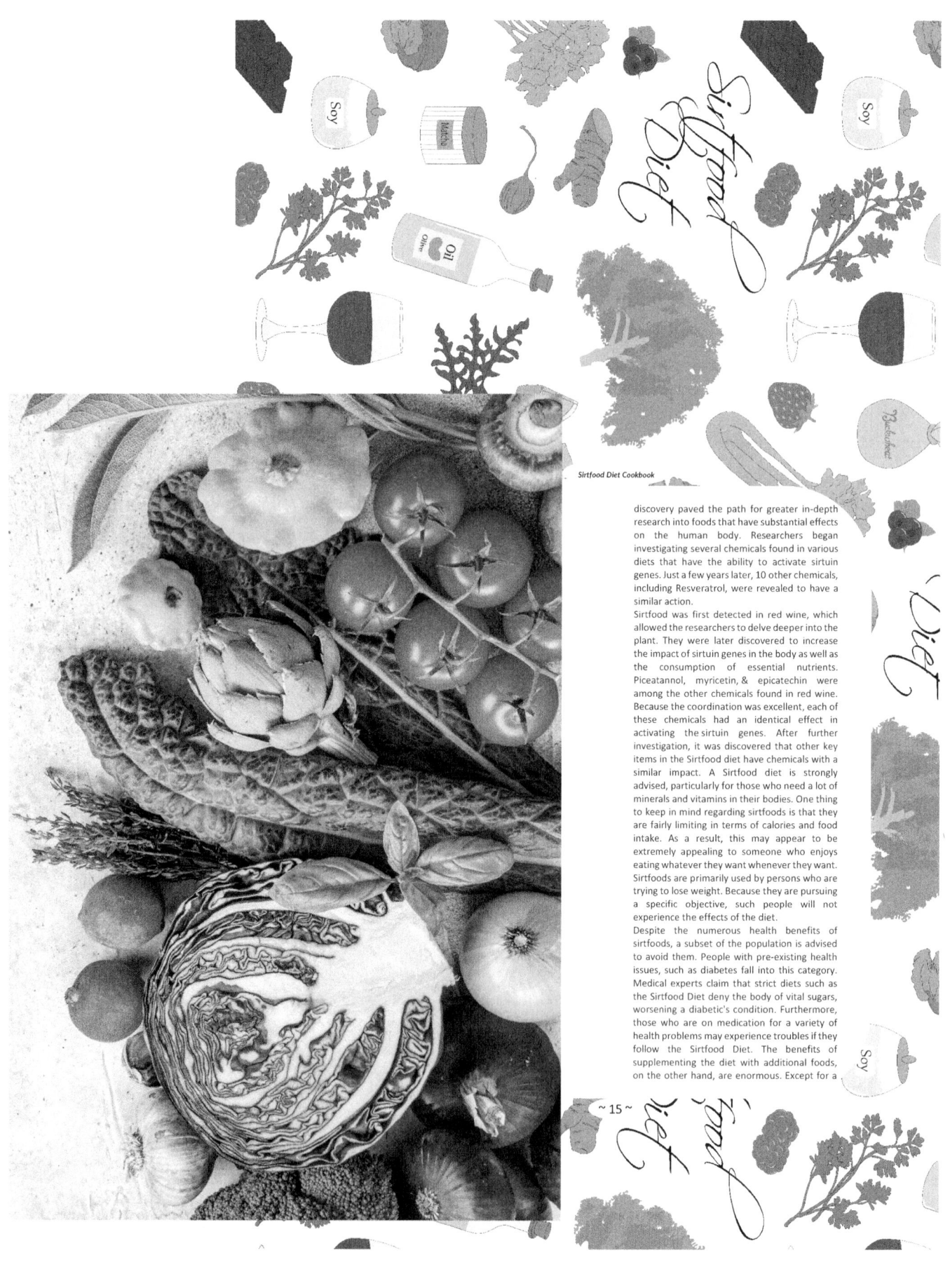

discovery paved the path for greater in-depth research into foods that have substantial effects on the human body. Researchers began investigating several chemicals found in various diets that have the ability to activate sirtuin genes. Just a few years later, 10 other chemicals, including Resveratrol, were revealed to have a similar action.

Sirtfood was first detected in red wine, which allowed the researchers to delve deeper into the plant. They were later discovered to increase the impact of sirtuin genes in the body as well as the consumption of essential nutrients. Piceatannol, myricetin, & epicatechin were among the other chemicals found in red wine. Because the coordination was excellent, each of these chemicals had an identical effect in activating the sirtuin genes. After further investigation, it was discovered that other key items in the Sirtfood diet have chemicals with a similar impact. A Sirtfood diet is strongly advised, particularly for those who need a lot of minerals and vitamins in their bodies. One thing to keep in mind regarding sirtfoods is that they are fairly limiting in terms of calories and food intake. As a result, this may appear to be extremely appealing to someone who enjoys eating whatever they want whenever they want. Sirtfoods are primarily used by persons who are trying to lose weight. Because they are pursuing a specific objective, such people will not experience the effects of the diet.

Despite the numerous health benefits of sirtfoods, a subset of the population is advised to avoid them. People with pre-existing health issues, such as diabetes fall into this category. Medical experts claim that strict diets such as the Sirtfood Diet deny the body of vital sugars, worsening a diabetic's condition. Furthermore, those who are on medication for a variety of health problems may experience troubles if they follow the Sirtfood Diet. The benefits of supplementing the diet with additional foods, on the other hand, are enormous. Except for a

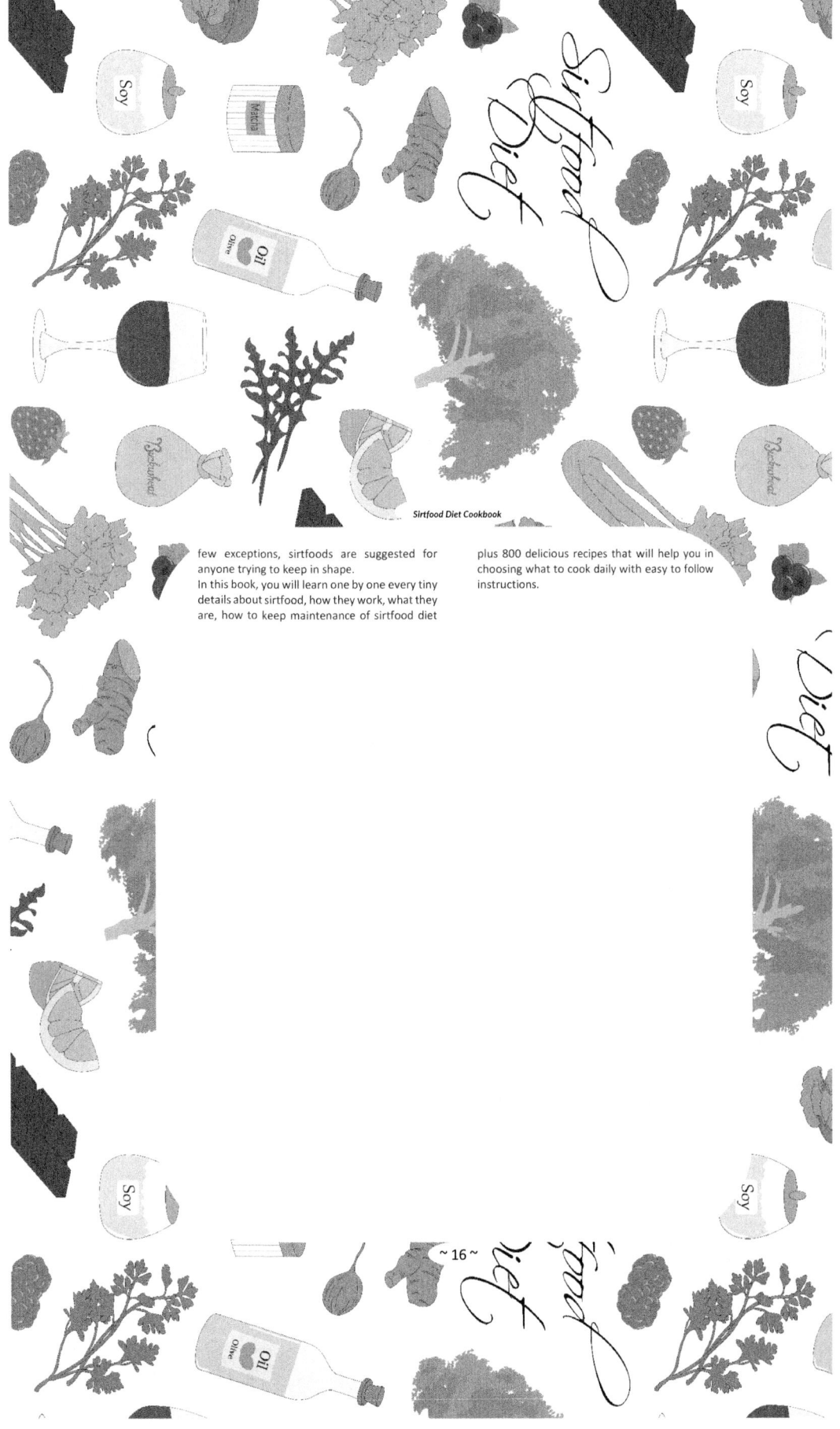

Sirtfood Diet Cookbook

few exceptions, sirtfoods are suggested for anyone trying to keep in shape.

In this book, you will learn one by one every tiny details about sirtfood, how they work, what they are, how to keep maintenance of sirtfood diet plus 800 delicious recipes that will help you in choosing what to cook daily with easy to follow instructions.

Sirtfood Diet Cookbook

CHAPTER 1:

The Introduction of Sirtfood Diet, Pros & Cons, and Health Benefits

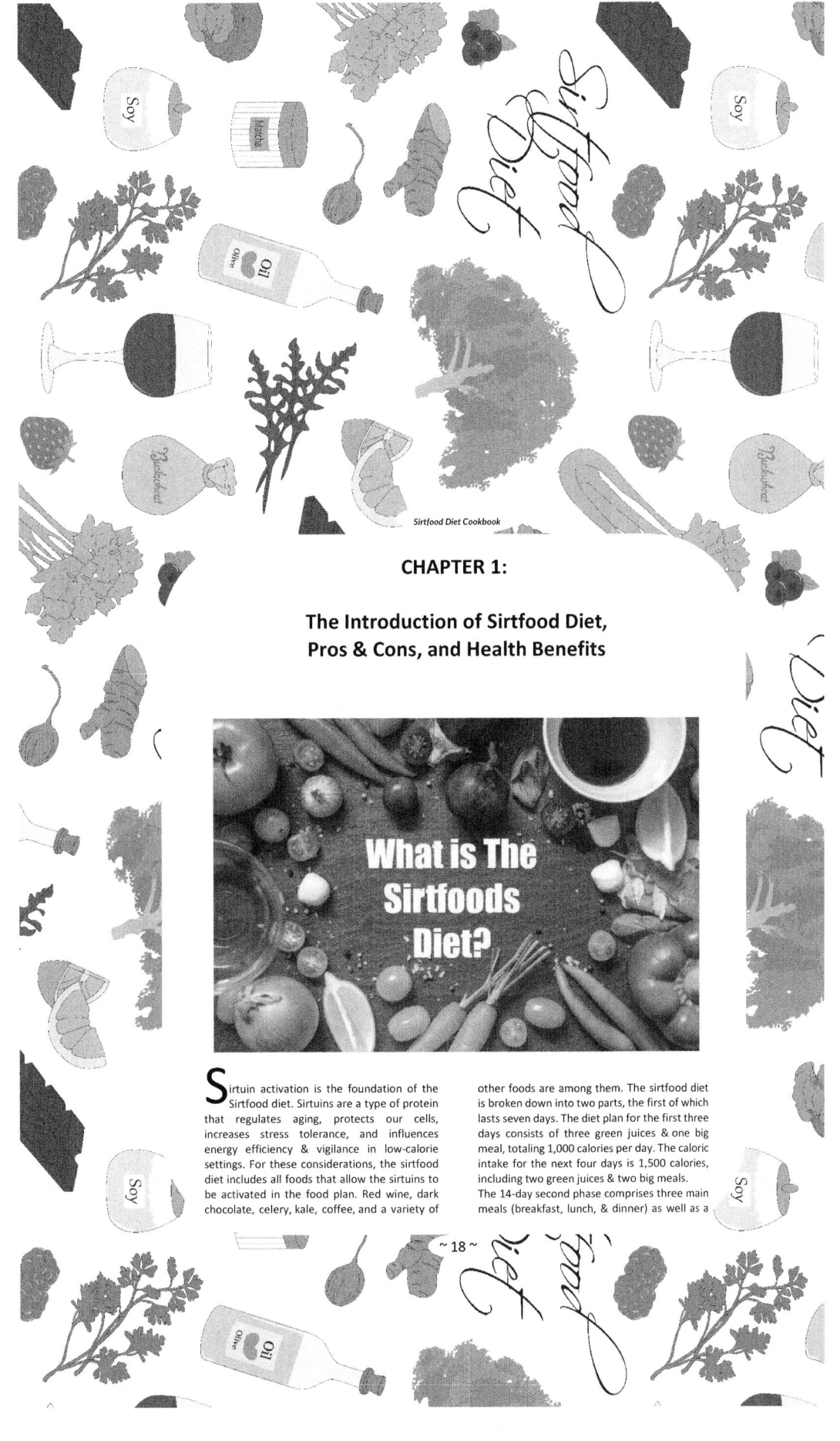

What is The Sirtfoods Diet?

Sirtuin activation is the foundation of the Sirtfood diet. Sirtuins are a type of protein that regulates aging, protects our cells, increases stress tolerance, and influences energy efficiency & vigilance in low-calorie settings. For these considerations, the sirtfood diet includes all foods that allow the sirtuins to be activated in the food plan. Red wine, dark chocolate, celery, kale, coffee, and a variety of other foods are among them. The sirtfood diet is broken down into two parts, the first of which lasts seven days. The diet plan for the first three days consists of three green juices & one big meal, totaling 1,000 calories per day. The caloric intake for the next four days is 1,500 calories, including two green juices & two big meals. The 14-day second phase comprises three main meals (breakfast, lunch, & dinner) as well as a

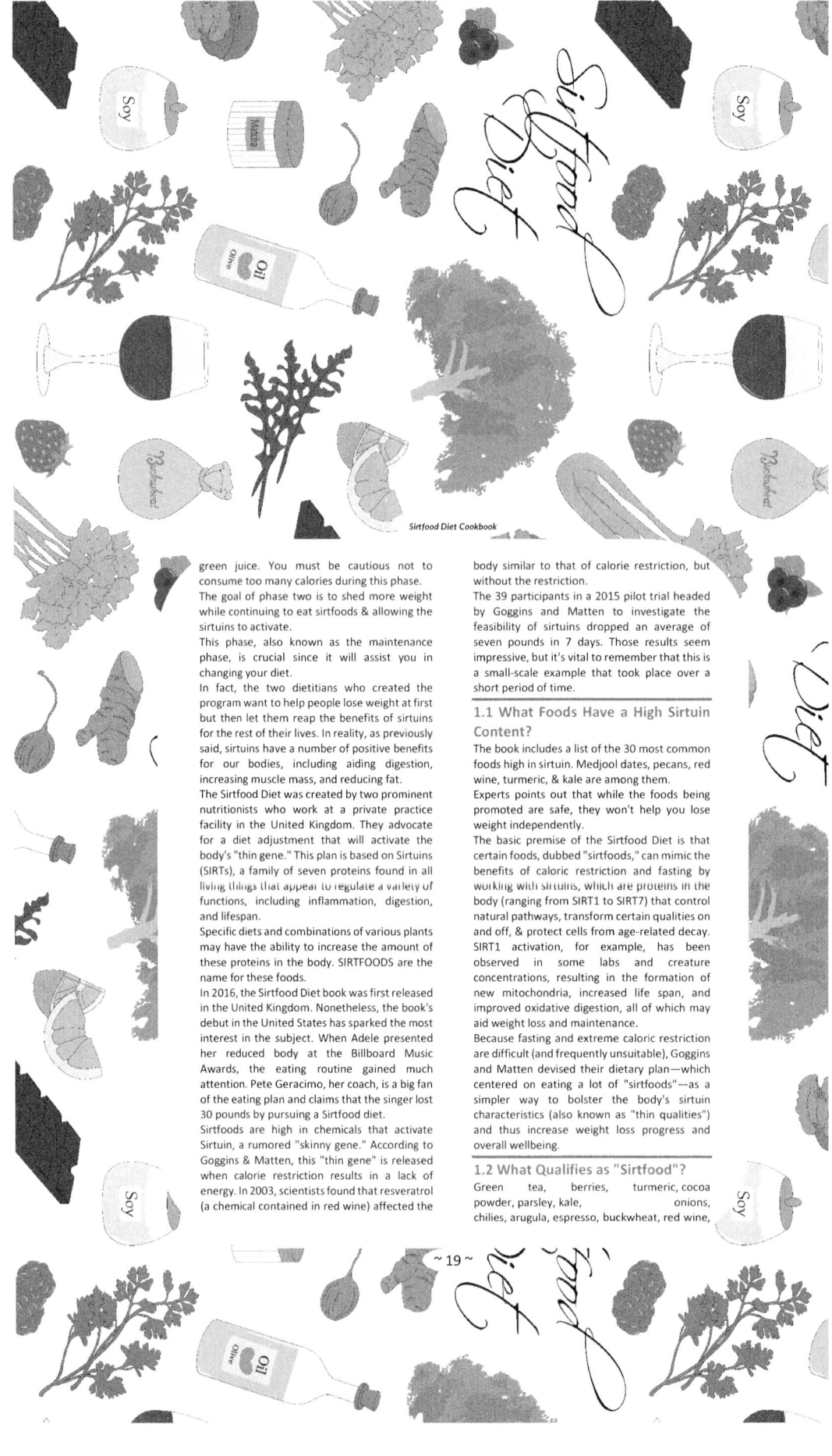

Sirtfood Diet Cookbook

green juice. You must be cautious not to consume too many calories during this phase.

The goal of phase two is to shed more weight while continuing to eat sirtfoods & allowing the sirtuins to activate.

This phase, also known as the maintenance phase, is crucial since it will assist you in changing your diet.

In fact, the two dietitians who created the program want to help people lose weight at first but then let them reap the benefits of sirtuins for the rest of their lives. In reality, as previously said, sirtuins have a number of positive benefits for our bodies, including aiding digestion, increasing muscle mass, and reducing fat.

The Sirtfood Diet was created by two prominent nutritionists who work at a private practice facility in the United Kingdom. They advocate for a diet adjustment that will activate the body's "thin gene." This plan is based on Sirtuins (SIRTs), a family of seven proteins found in all living things that appear to regulate a variety of functions, including inflammation, digestion, and lifespan.

Specific diets and combinations of various plants may have the ability to increase the amount of these proteins in the body. SIRTFOODS are the name for these foods.

In 2016, the Sirtfood Diet book was first released in the United Kingdom. Nonetheless, the book's debut in the United States has sparked the most interest in the subject. When Adele presented her reduced body at the Billboard Music Awards, the eating routine gained much attention. Pete Geracimo, her coach, is a big fan of the eating plan and claims that the singer lost 30 pounds by pursuing a Sirtfood diet.

Sirtfoods are high in chemicals that activate Sirtuin, a rumored "skinny gene." According to Goggins & Matten, this "thin gene" is released when calorie restriction results in a lack of energy. In 2003, scientists found that resveratrol (a chemical contained in red wine) affected the body similar to that of calorie restriction, but without the restriction.

The 39 participants in a 2015 pilot trial headed by Goggins and Matten to investigate the feasibility of sirtuins dropped an average of seven pounds in 7 days. Those results seem impressive, but it's vital to remember that this is a small-scale example that took place over a short period of time.

1.1 What Foods Have a High Sirtuin Content?

The book includes a list of the 30 most common foods high in sirtuin. Medjool dates, pecans, red wine, turmeric, & kale are among them.

Experts points out that while the foods being promoted are safe, they won't help you lose weight independently.

The basic premise of the Sirtfood Diet is that certain foods, dubbed "sirtfoods," can mimic the benefits of caloric restriction and fasting by working with sirtuins, which are proteins in the body (ranging from SIRT1 to SIRT7) that control natural pathways, transform certain qualities on and off, & protect cells from age-related decay. SIRT1 activation, for example, has been observed in some labs and creature concentrations, resulting in the formation of new mitochondria, increased life span, and improved oxidative digestion, all of which may aid weight loss and maintenance.

Because fasting and extreme caloric restriction are difficult (and frequently unsuitable), Goggins and Matten devised their dietary plan—which centered on eating a lot of "sirtfoods"—as a simpler way to bolster the body's sirtuin characteristics (also known as "thin qualities") and thus increase weight loss progress and overall wellbeing.

1.2 What Qualifies as "Sirtfood"?

Green tea, berries, turmeric, cocoa powder, parsley, kale, onions, chilies, arugula, espresso, buckwheat, red wine,

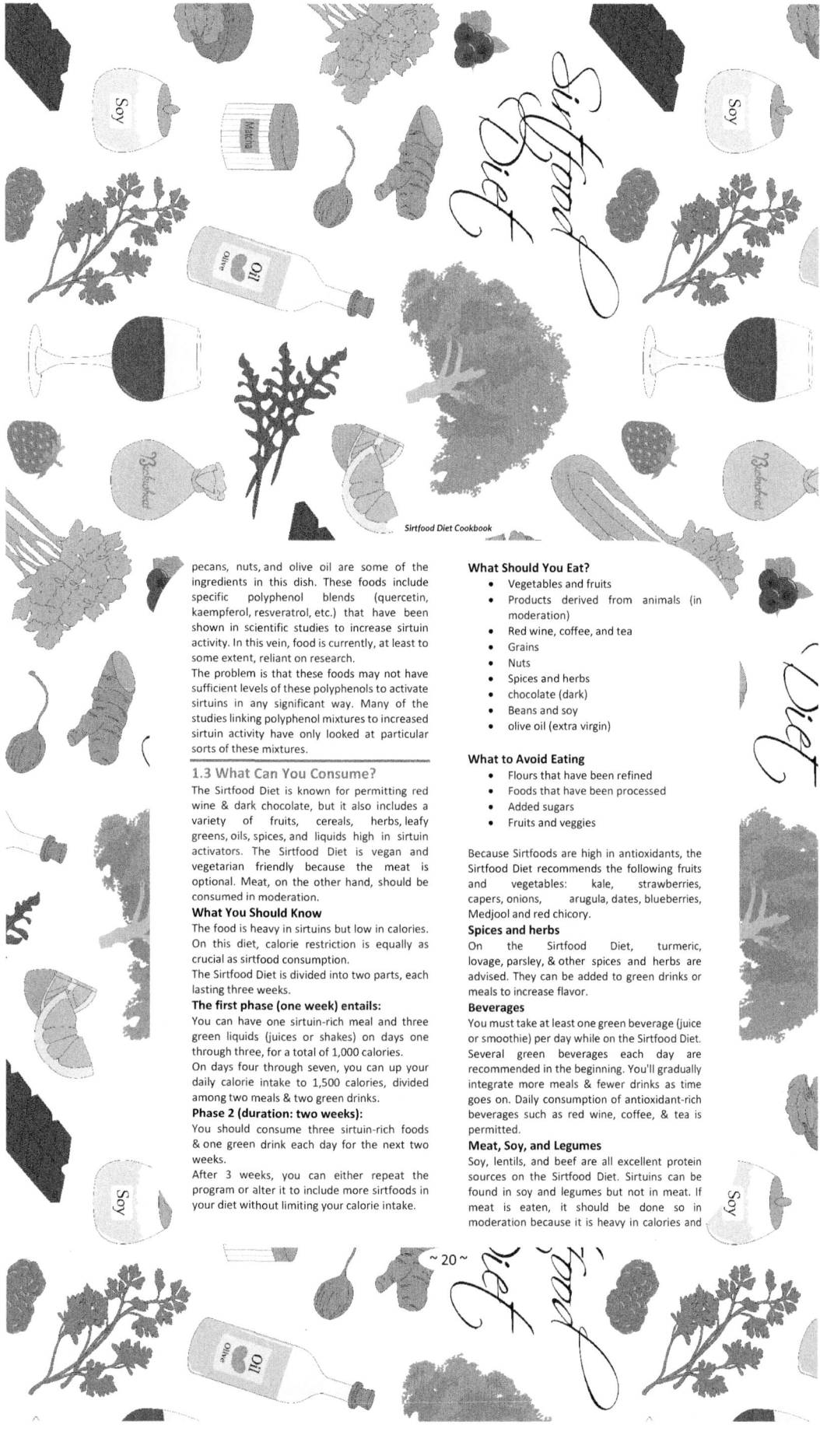

Sirtfood Diet Cookbook

pecans, nuts, and olive oil are some of the ingredients in this dish. These foods include specific polyphenol blends (quercetin, kaempferol, resveratrol, etc.) that have been shown in scientific studies to increase sirtuin activity. In this vein, food is currently, at least to some extent, reliant on research.

The problem is that these foods may not have sufficient levels of these polyphenols to activate sirtuins in any significant way. Many of the studies linking polyphenol mixtures to increased sirtuin activity have only looked at particular sorts of these mixtures.

1.3 What Can You Consume?

The Sirtfood Diet is known for permitting red wine & dark chocolate, but it also includes a variety of fruits, cereals, herbs, leafy greens, oils, spices, and liquids high in sirtuin activators. The Sirtfood Diet is vegan and vegetarian friendly because the meat is optional. Meat, on the other hand, should be consumed in moderation.

What You Should Know

The food is heavy in sirtuins but low in calories. On this diet, calorie restriction is equally as crucial as sirtfood consumption.

The Sirtfood Diet is divided into two parts, each lasting three weeks.

The first phase (one week) entails:

You can have one sirtuin-rich meal and three green liquids (juices or shakes) on days one through three, for a total of 1,000 calories.

On days four through seven, you can up your daily calorie intake to 1,500 calories, divided among two meals & two green drinks.

Phase 2 (duration: two weeks):

You should consume three sirtuin-rich foods & one green drink each day for the next two weeks.

After 3 weeks, you can either repeat the program or alter it to include more sirtfoods in your diet without limiting your calorie intake.

What Should You Eat?

- Vegetables and fruits
- Products derived from animals (in moderation)
- Red wine, coffee, and tea
- Grains
- Nuts
- Spices and herbs
- chocolate (dark)
- Beans and soy
- olive oil (extra virgin)

What to Avoid Eating

- Flours that have been refined
- Foods that have been processed
- Added sugars
- Fruits and veggies

Because Sirtfoods are high in antioxidants, the Sirtfood Diet recommends the following fruits and vegetables: kale, strawberries, capers, onions, arugula, dates, blueberries, Medjool and red chicory.

Spices and herbs

On the Sirtfood Diet, turmeric, lovage, parsley, & other spices and herbs are advised. They can be added to green drinks or meals to increase flavor.

Beverages

You must take at least one green beverage (juice or smoothie) per day while on the Sirtfood Diet. Several green beverages each day are recommended in the beginning. You'll gradually integrate more meals & fewer drinks as time goes on. Daily consumption of antioxidant-rich beverages such as red wine, coffee, & tea is permitted.

Meat, Soy, and Legumes

Soy, lentils, and beef are all excellent protein sources on the Sirtfood Diet. Sirtuins can be found in soy and legumes but not in meat. If meat is eaten, it should be done so in moderation because it is heavy in calories and

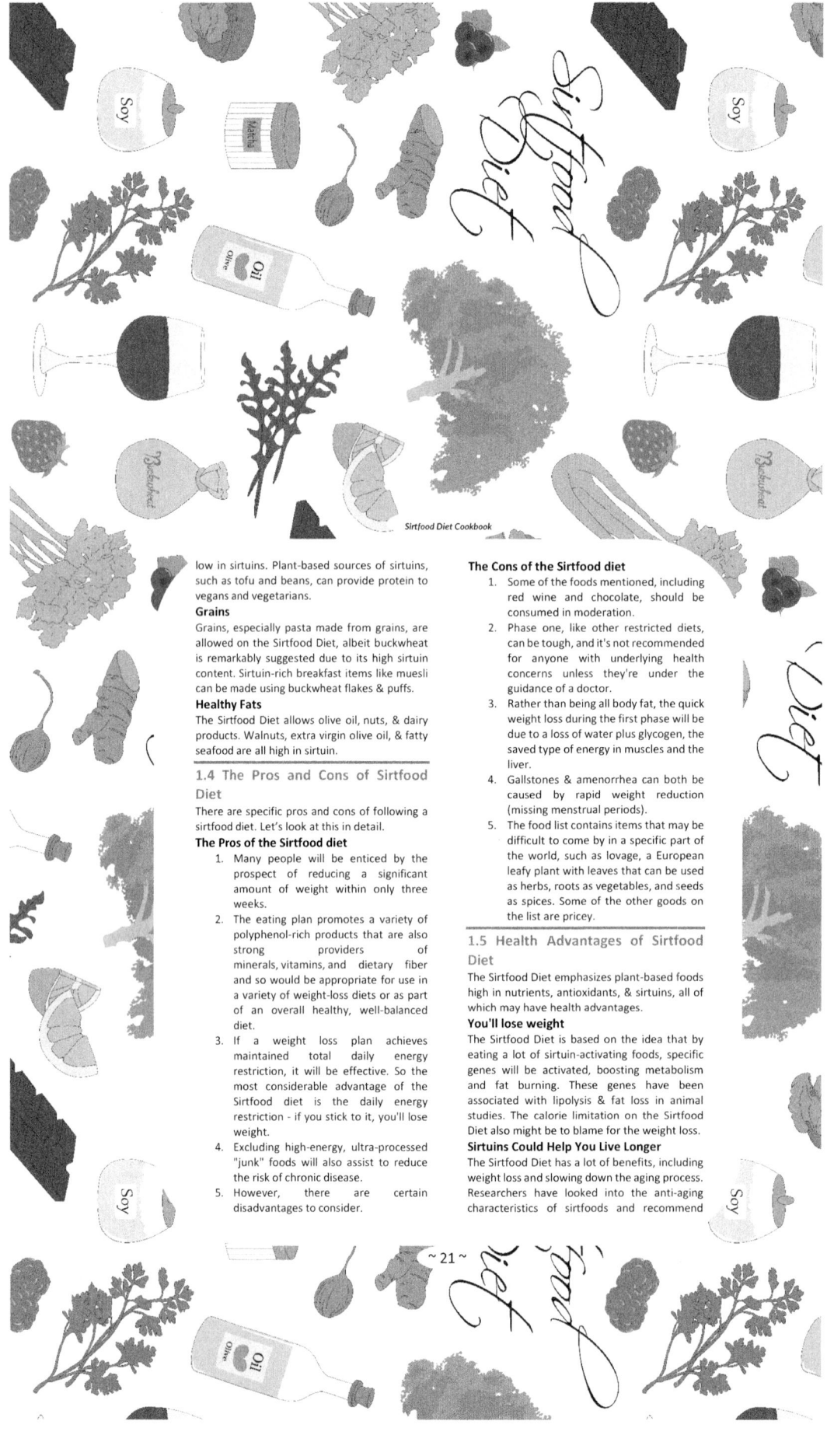

Sirtfood Diet Cookbook

low in sirtuins. Plant-based sources of sirtuins, such as tofu and beans, can provide protein to vegans and vegetarians.

Grains

Grains, especially pasta made from grains, are allowed on the Sirtfood Diet, albeit buckwheat is remarkably suggested due to its high sirtuin content. Sirtuin-rich breakfast items like muesli can be made using buckwheat flakes & puffs.

Healthy Fats

The Sirtfood Diet allows olive oil, nuts, & dairy products. Walnuts, extra virgin olive oil, & fatty seafood are all high in sirtuin.

1.4 The Pros and Cons of Sirtfood Diet

There are specific pros and cons of following a sirtfood diet. Let's look at this in detail.

The Pros of the Sirtfood diet

1. Many people will be enticed by the prospect of reducing a significant amount of weight within only three weeks.
2. The eating plan promotes a variety of polyphenol-rich products that are also strong providers of minerals, vitamins, and dietary fiber and so would be appropriate for use in a variety of weight-loss diets or as part of an overall healthy, well-balanced diet.
3. If a weight loss plan achieves maintained total daily energy restriction, it will be effective. So the most considerable advantage of the Sirtfood diet is the daily energy restriction - if you stick to it, you'll lose weight.
4. Excluding high-energy, ultra-processed "junk" foods will also assist to reduce the risk of chronic disease.
5. However, there are certain disadvantages to consider.

The Cons of the Sirtfood diet

1. Some of the foods mentioned, including red wine and chocolate, should be consumed in moderation.
2. Phase one, like other restricted diets, can be tough, and it's not recommended for anyone with underlying health concerns unless they're under the guidance of a doctor.
3. Rather than being all body fat, the quick weight loss during the first phase will be due to a loss of water plus glycogen, the saved type of energy in muscles and the liver.
4. Gallstones & amenorrhea can both be caused by rapid weight reduction (missing menstrual periods).
5. The food list contains items that may be difficult to come by in a specific part of the world, such as lovage, a European leafy plant with leaves that can be used as herbs, roots as vegetables, and seeds as spices. Some of the other goods on the list are pricey.

1.5 Health Advantages of Sirtfood Diet

The Sirtfood Diet emphasizes plant-based foods high in nutrients, antioxidants, & sirtuins, all of which may have health advantages.

You'll lose weight

The Sirtfood Diet is based on the idea that by eating a lot of sirtuin-activating foods, specific genes will be activated, boosting metabolism and fat burning. These genes have been associated with lipolysis & fat loss in animal studies. The calorie limitation on the Sirtfood Diet also might be to blame for the weight loss.

Sirtuins Could Help You Live Longer

The Sirtfood Diet has a lot of benefits, including weight loss and slowing down the aging process. Researchers have looked into the anti-aging characteristics of sirtfoods and recommend

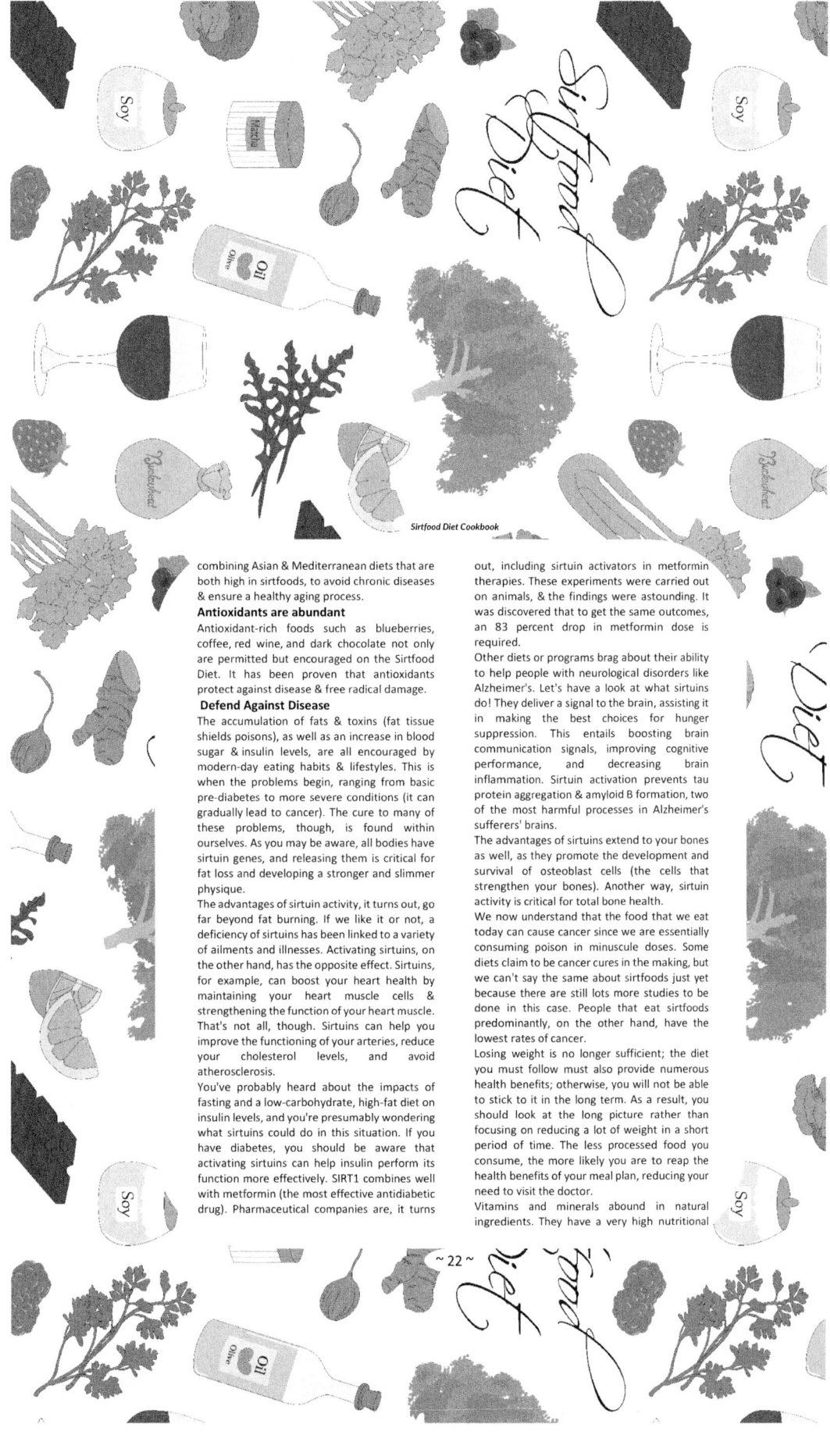

Sirtfood Diet Cookbook

combining Asian & Mediterranean diets that are both high in sirtfoods, to avoid chronic diseases & ensure a healthy aging process.

Antioxidants are abundant

Antioxidant-rich foods such as blueberries, coffee, red wine, and dark chocolate not only are permitted but encouraged on the Sirtfood Diet. It has been proven that antioxidants protect against disease & free radical damage.

Defend Against Disease

The accumulation of fats & toxins (fat tissue shields poisons), as well as an increase in blood sugar & insulin levels, are all encouraged by modern-day eating habits & lifestyles. This is when the problems begin, ranging from basic pre-diabetes to more severe conditions (it can gradually lead to cancer). The cure to many of these problems, though, is found within ourselves. As you may be aware, all bodies have sirtuin genes, and releasing them is critical for fat loss and developing a stronger and slimmer physique.

The advantages of sirtuin activity, it turns out, go far beyond fat burning. If we like it or not, a deficiency of sirtuins has been linked to a variety of ailments and illnesses. Activating sirtuins, on the other hand, has the opposite effect. Sirtuins, for example, can boost your heart health by maintaining your heart muscle cells & strengthening the function of your heart muscle. That's not all, though. Sirtuins can help you improve the functioning of your arteries, reduce your cholesterol levels, and avoid atherosclerosis.

You've probably heard about the impacts of fasting and a low-carbohydrate, high-fat diet on insulin levels, and you're presumably wondering what sirtuins could do in this situation. If you have diabetes, you should be aware that activating sirtuins can help insulin perform its function more effectively. SIRT1 combines well with metformin (the most effective antidiabetic drug). Pharmaceutical companies are, it turns out, including sirtuin activators in metformin therapies. These experiments were carried out on animals, & the findings were astounding. It was discovered that to get the same outcomes, an 83 percent drop in metformin dose is required.

Other diets or programs brag about their ability to help people with neurological disorders like Alzheimer's. Let's have a look at what sirtuins do! They deliver a signal to the brain, assisting it in making the best choices for hunger suppression. This entails boosting brain communication signals, improving cognitive performance, and decreasing brain inflammation. Sirtuin activation prevents tau protein aggregation & amyloid B formation, two of the most harmful processes in Alzheimer's sufferers' brains.

The advantages of sirtuins extend to your bones as well, as they promote the development and survival of osteoblast cells (the cells that strengthen your bones). Another way, sirtuin activity is critical for total bone health.

We now understand that the food that we eat today can cause cancer since we are essentially consuming poison in minuscule doses. Some diets claim to be cancer cures in the making, but we can't say the same about sirtfoods just yet because there are still lots more studies to be done in this case. People that eat sirtfoods predominantly, on the other hand, have the lowest rates of cancer.

Losing weight is no longer sufficient; the diet you must follow must also provide numerous health benefits; otherwise, you will not be able to stick to it in the long term. As a result, you should look at the long picture rather than focusing on reducing a lot of weight in a short period of time. The less processed food you consume, the more likely you are to reap the health benefits of your meal plan, reducing your need to visit the doctor.

Vitamins and minerals abound in natural ingredients. They have a very high nutritional

value. Sirtuins are primarily found in such components, whether by chance or not (essentially fruits & veggies). As a result, you'll need to consume these incredible components on a daily basis to reap these benefits.

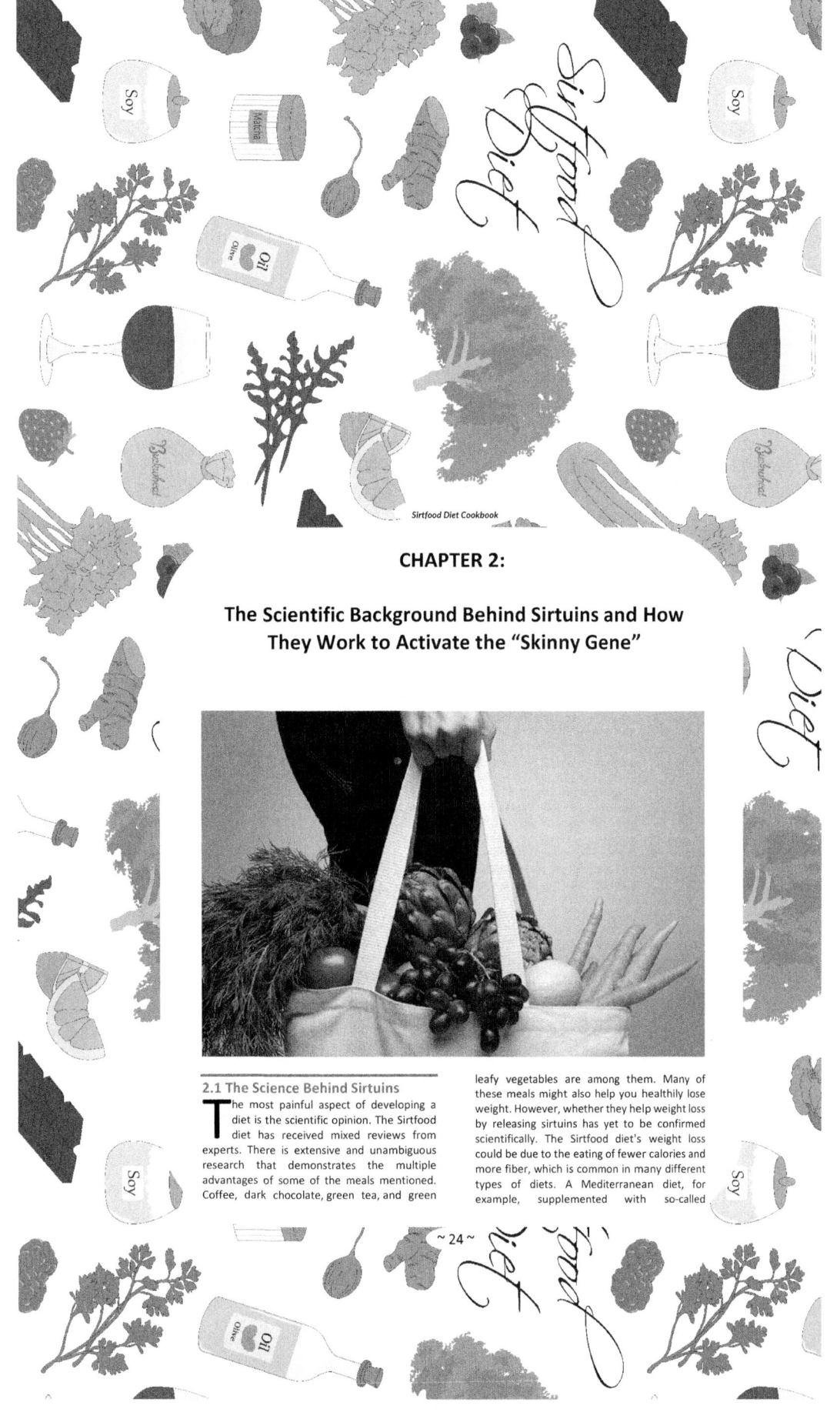

Sirtfood Diet Cookbook

CHAPTER 2:

The Scientific Background Behind Sirtuins and How They Work to Activate the "Skinny Gene"

2.1 The Science Behind Sirtuins

The most painful aspect of developing a diet is the scientific opinion. The Sirtfood diet has received mixed reviews from experts. There is extensive and unambiguous research that demonstrates the multiple advantages of some of the meals mentioned. Coffee, dark chocolate, green tea, and green leafy vegetables are among them. Many of these meals might also help you healthily lose weight. However, whether they help weight loss by releasing sirtuins has yet to be confirmed scientifically. The Sirtfood diet's weight loss could be due to the eating of fewer calories and more fiber, which is common in many different types of diets. A Mediterranean diet, for example, supplemented with so-called

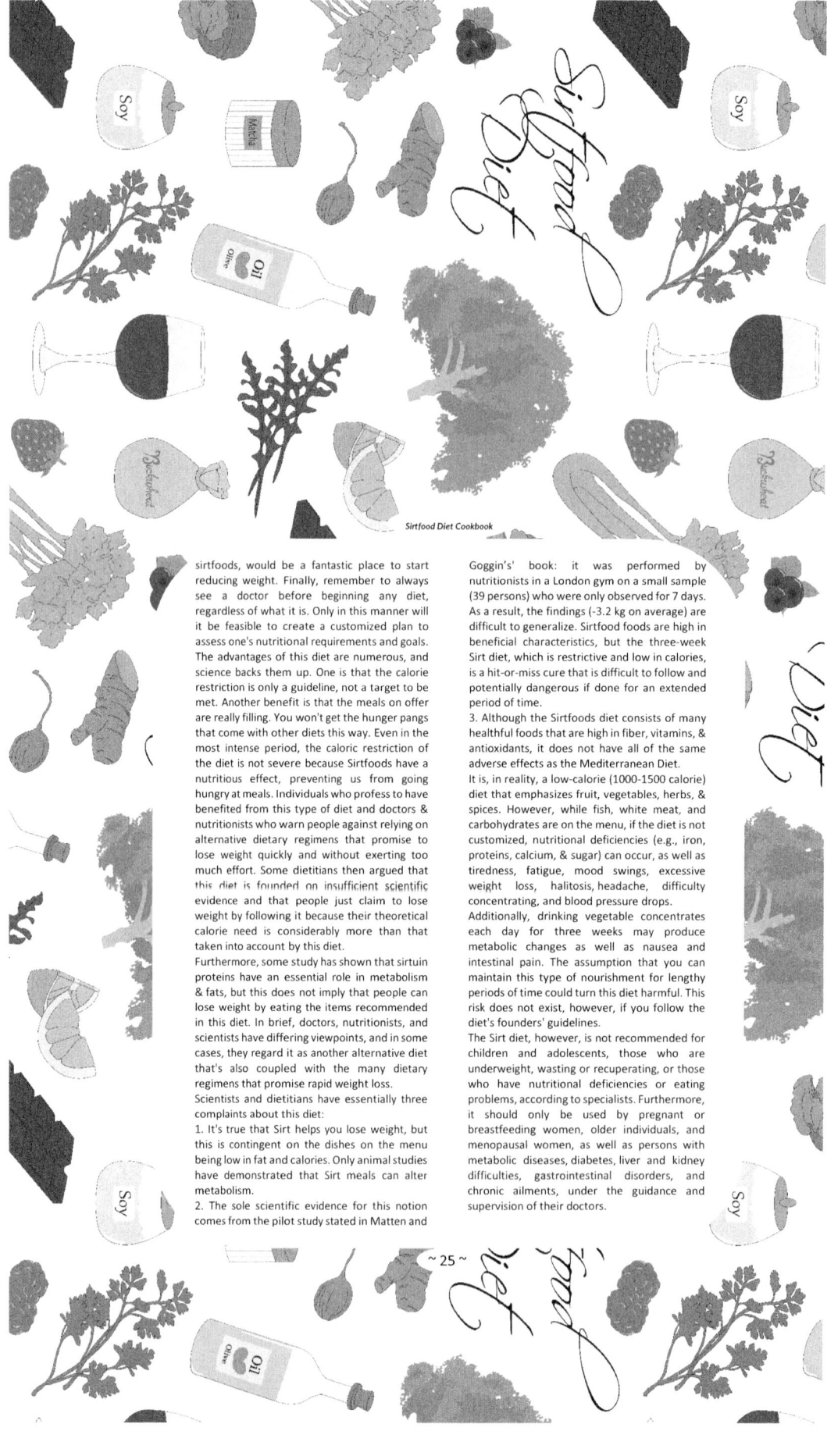

Sirtfood Diet Cookbook

sirtfoods, would be a fantastic place to start reducing weight. Finally, remember to always see a doctor before beginning any diet, regardless of what it is. Only in this manner will it be feasible to create a customized plan to assess one's nutritional requirements and goals. The advantages of this diet are numerous, and science backs them up. One is that the calorie restriction is only a guideline, not a target to be met. Another benefit is that the meals on offer are really filling. You won't get the hunger pangs that come with other diets this way. Even in the most intense period, the caloric restriction of the diet is not severe because Sirtfoods have a nutritious effect, preventing us from going hungry at meals. Individuals who profess to have benefited from this type of diet and doctors & nutritionists who warn people against relying on alternative dietary regimens that promise to lose weight quickly and without exerting too much effort. Some dietitians then argued that this diet is founded on insufficient scientific evidence and that people just claim to lose weight by following it because their theoretical calorie need is considerably more than that taken into account by this diet.

Furthermore, some study has shown that sirtuin proteins have an essential role in metabolism & fats, but this does not imply that people can lose weight by eating the items recommended in this diet. In brief, doctors, nutritionists, and scientists have differing viewpoints, and in some cases, they regard it as another alternative diet that's also coupled with the many dietary regimens that promise rapid weight loss.

Scientists and dietitians have essentially three complaints about this diet:

1. It's true that Sirt helps you lose weight, but this is contingent on the dishes on the menu being low in fat and calories. Only animal studies have demonstrated that Sirt meals can alter metabolism.

2. The sole scientific evidence for this notion comes from the pilot study stated in Matten and Goggin's' book: it was performed by nutritionists in a London gym on a small sample (39 persons) who were only observed for 7 days. As a result, the findings (-3.2 kg on average) are difficult to generalize. Sirtfood foods are high in beneficial characteristics, but the three-week Sirt diet, which is restrictive and low in calories, is a hit-or-miss cure that is difficult to follow and potentially dangerous if done for an extended period of time.

3. Although the Sirtfoods diet consists of many healthful foods that are high in fiber, vitamins, & antioxidants, it does not have all of the same adverse effects as the Mediterranean Diet.

It is, in reality, a low-calorie (1000-1500 calorie) diet that emphasizes fruit, vegetables, herbs, & spices. However, while fish, white meat, and carbohydrates are on the menu, if the diet is not customized, nutritional deficiencies (e.g., iron, proteins, calcium, & sugar) can occur, as well as tiredness, fatigue, mood swings, excessive weight loss, halitosis, headache, difficulty concentrating, and blood pressure drops.

Additionally, drinking vegetable concentrates each day for three weeks may produce metabolic changes as well as nausea and intestinal pain. The assumption that you can maintain this type of nourishment for lengthy periods of time could turn this diet harmful. This risk does not exist, however, if you follow the diet's founders' guidelines.

The Sirt diet, however, is not recommended for children and adolescents, those who are underweight, wasting or recuperating, or those who have nutritional deficiencies or eating problems, according to specialists. Furthermore, it should only be used by pregnant or breastfeeding women, older individuals, and menopausal women, as well as persons with metabolic diseases, diabetes, liver and kidney difficulties, gastrointestinal disorders, and chronic ailments, under the guidance and supervision of their doctors.

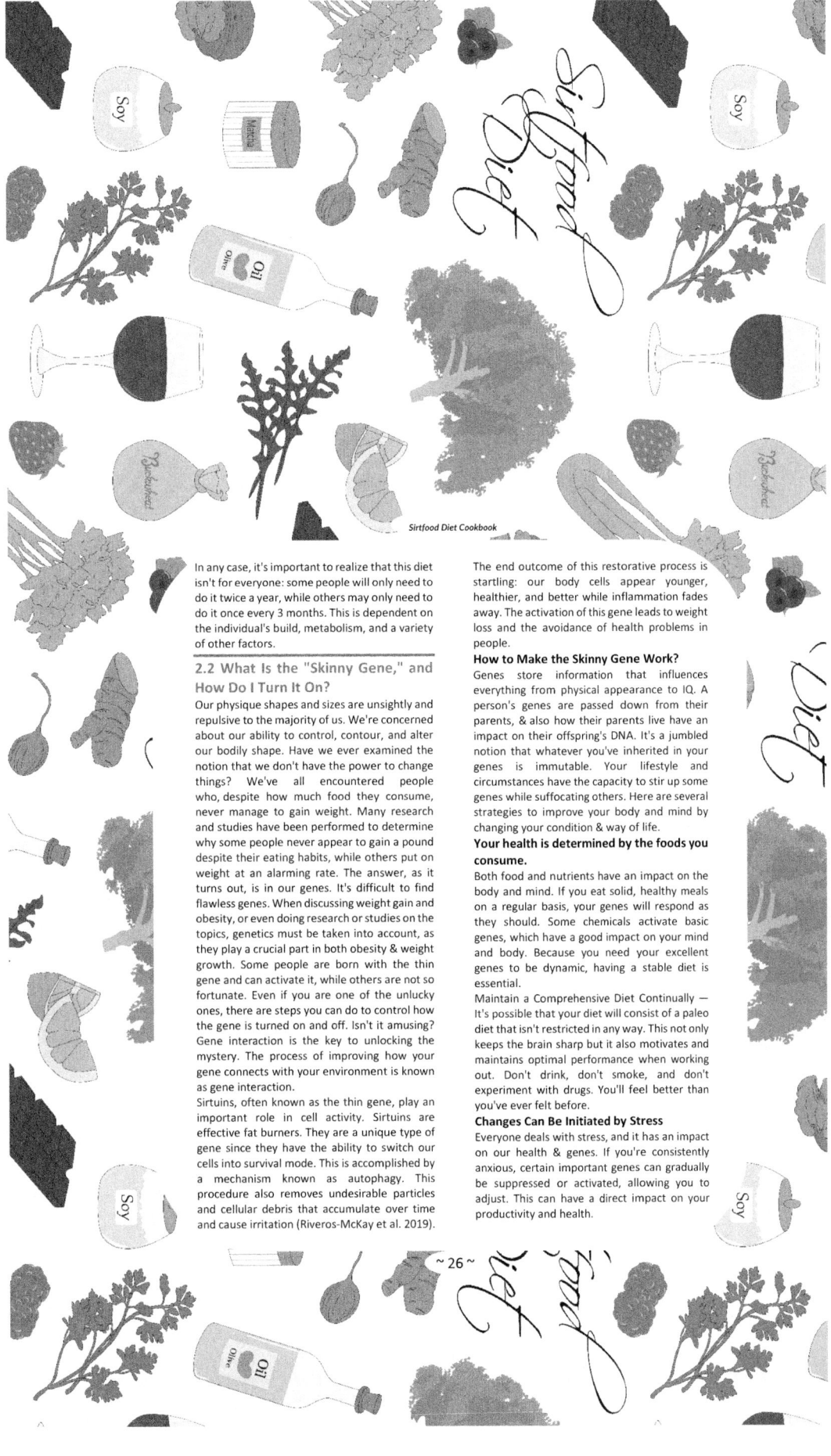

Sirtfood Diet Cookbook

In any case, it's important to realize that this diet isn't for everyone: some people will only need to do it twice a year, while others may only need to do it once every 3 months. This is dependent on the individual's build, metabolism, and a variety of other factors.

2.2 What Is the "Skinny Gene," and How Do I Turn It On?

Our physique shapes and sizes are unsightly and repulsive to the majority of us. We're concerned about our ability to control, contour, and alter our bodily shape. Have we ever examined the notion that we don't have the power to change things? We've all encountered people who, despite how much food they consume, never manage to gain weight. Many research and studies have been performed to determine why some people never appear to gain a pound despite their eating habits, while others put on weight at an alarming rate. The answer, as it turns out, is in our genes. It's difficult to find flawless genes. When discussing weight gain and obesity, or even doing research or studies on the topics, genetics must be taken into account, as they play a crucial part in both obesity & weight growth. Some people are born with the thin gene and can activate it, while others are not so fortunate. Even if you are one of the unlucky ones, there are steps you can do to control how the gene is turned on and off. Isn't it amusing? Gene interaction is the key to unlocking the mystery. The process of improving how your gene connects with your environment is known as gene interaction.

Sirtuins, often known as the thin gene, play an important role in cell activity. Sirtuins are effective fat burners. They are a unique type of gene since they have the ability to switch our cells into survival mode. This is accomplished by a mechanism known as autophagy. This procedure also removes undesirable particles and cellular debris that accumulate over time and cause irritation (Riveros-McKay et al. 2019).

The end outcome of this restorative process is startling: our body cells appear younger, healthier, and better while inflammation fades away. The activation of this gene leads to weight loss and the avoidance of health problems in people.

How to Make the Skinny Gene Work?

Genes store information that influences everything from physical appearance to IQ. A person's genes are passed down from their parents, & also how their parents live have an impact on their offspring's DNA. It's a jumbled notion that whatever you've inherited in your genes is immutable. Your lifestyle and circumstances have the capacity to stir up some genes while suffocating others. Here are several strategies to improve your body and mind by changing your condition & way of life.

Your health is determined by the foods you consume.

Both food and nutrients have an impact on the body and mind. If you eat solid, healthy meals on a regular basis, your genes will respond as they should. Some chemicals activate basic genes, which have a good impact on your mind and body. Because you need your excellent genes to be dynamic, having a stable diet is essential.

Maintain a Comprehensive Diet Continually — It's possible that your diet will consist of a paleo diet that isn't restricted in any way. This not only keeps the brain sharp but it also motivates and maintains optimal performance when working out. Don't drink, don't smoke, and don't experiment with drugs. You'll feel better than you've ever felt before.

Changes Can Be Initiated by Stress

Everyone deals with stress, and it has an impact on our health & genes. If you're consistently anxious, certain important genes can gradually be suppressed or activated, allowing you to adjust. This can have a direct impact on your productivity and health.

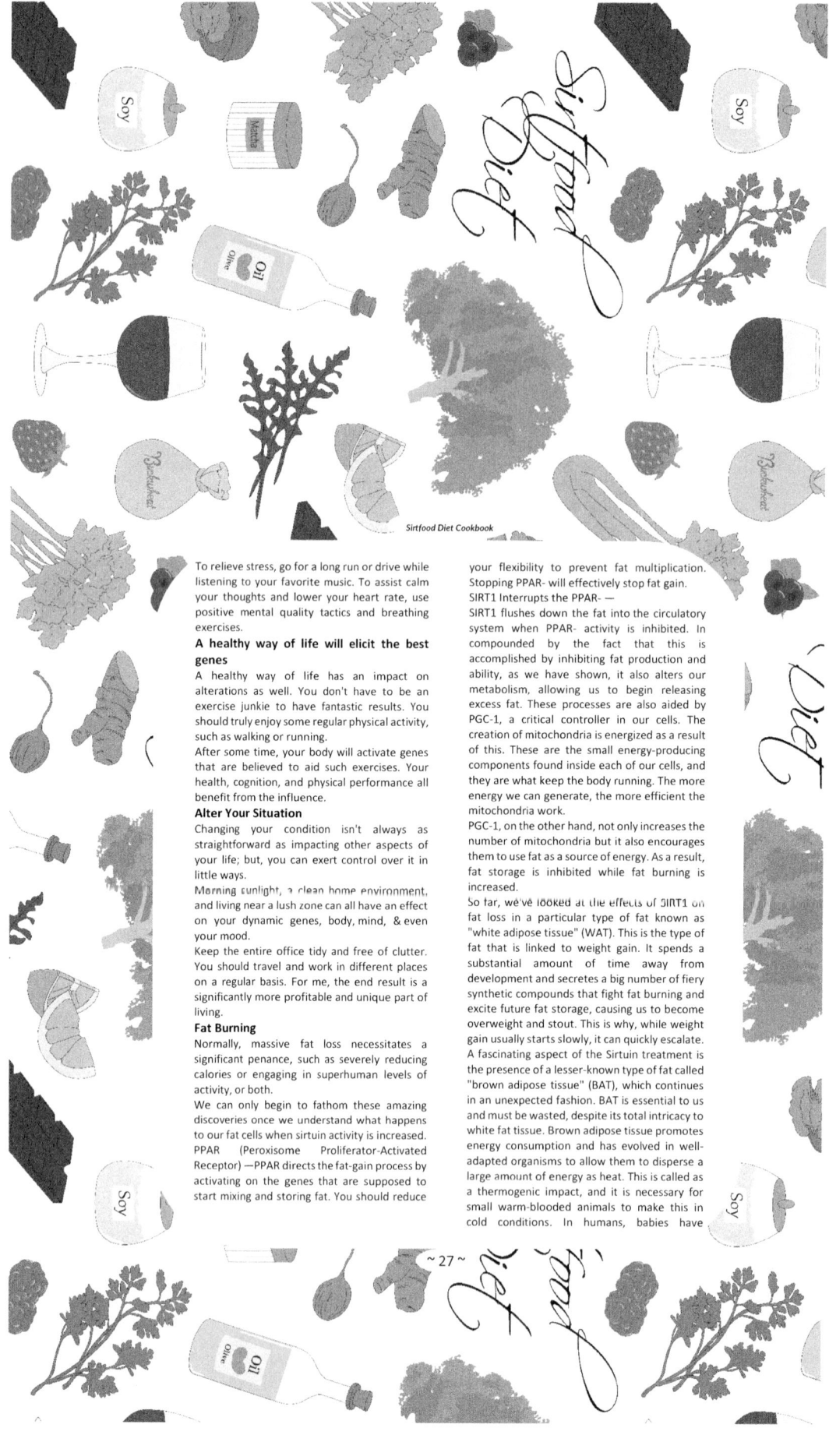

Sirtfood Diet Cookbook

To relieve stress, go for a long run or drive while listening to your favorite music. To assist calm your thoughts and lower your heart rate, use positive mental quality tactics and breathing exercises.

A healthy way of life will elicit the best genes

A healthy way of life has an impact on alterations as well. You don't have to be an exercise junkie to have fantastic results. You should truly enjoy some regular physical activity, such as walking or running.

After some time, your body will activate genes that are believed to aid such exercises. Your health, cognition, and physical performance all benefit from the influence.

Alter Your Situation

Changing your condition isn't always as straightforward as impacting other aspects of your life; but, you can exert control over it in little ways.

Morning sunlight, a clean home environment, and living near a lush zone can all have an effect on your dynamic genes, body, mind, & even your mood.

Keep the entire office tidy and free of clutter. You should travel and work in different places on a regular basis. For me, the end result is a significantly more profitable and unique part of living.

Fat Burning

Normally, massive fat loss necessitates a significant penance, such as severely reducing calories or engaging in superhuman levels of activity, or both.

We can only begin to fathom these amazing discoveries once we understand what happens to our fat cells when sirtuin activity is increased. PPAR (Peroxisome Proliferator-Activated Receptor) —PPAR directs the fat-gain process by activating on the genes that are supposed to start mixing and storing fat. You should reduce your flexibility to prevent fat multiplication. Stopping PPAR- will effectively stop fat gain. SIRT1 Interrupts the PPAR- —

SIRT1 flushes down the fat into the circulatory system when PPAR- activity is inhibited. In compounded by the fact that this is accomplished by inhibiting fat production and ability, as we have shown, it also alters our metabolism, allowing us to begin releasing excess fat. These processes are also aided by PGC-1, a critical controller in our cells. The creation of mitochondria is energized as a result of this. These are the small energy-producing components found inside each of our cells, and they are what keep the body running. The more energy we can generate, the more efficient the mitochondria work.

PGC-1, on the other hand, not only increases the number of mitochondria but it also encourages them to use fat as a source of energy. As a result, fat storage is inhibited while fat burning is increased.

So far, we've looked at the effects of SIRT1 on fat loss in a particular type of fat known as "white adipose tissue" (WAT). This is the type of fat that is linked to weight gain. It spends a substantial amount of time away from development and secretes a big number of fiery synthetic compounds that fight fat burning and excite future fat storage, causing us to become overweight and stout. This is why, while weight gain usually starts slowly, it can quickly escalate. A fascinating aspect of the Sirtuin treatment is the presence of a lesser-known type of fat called "brown adipose tissue" (BAT), which continues in an unexpected fashion. BAT is essential to us and must be wasted, despite its total intricacy to white fat tissue. Brown adipose tissue promotes energy consumption and has evolved in well-adapted organisms to allow them to disperse a large amount of energy as heat. This is called as a thermogenic impact, and it is necessary for small warm-blooded animals to make this in cold conditions. In humans, babies have

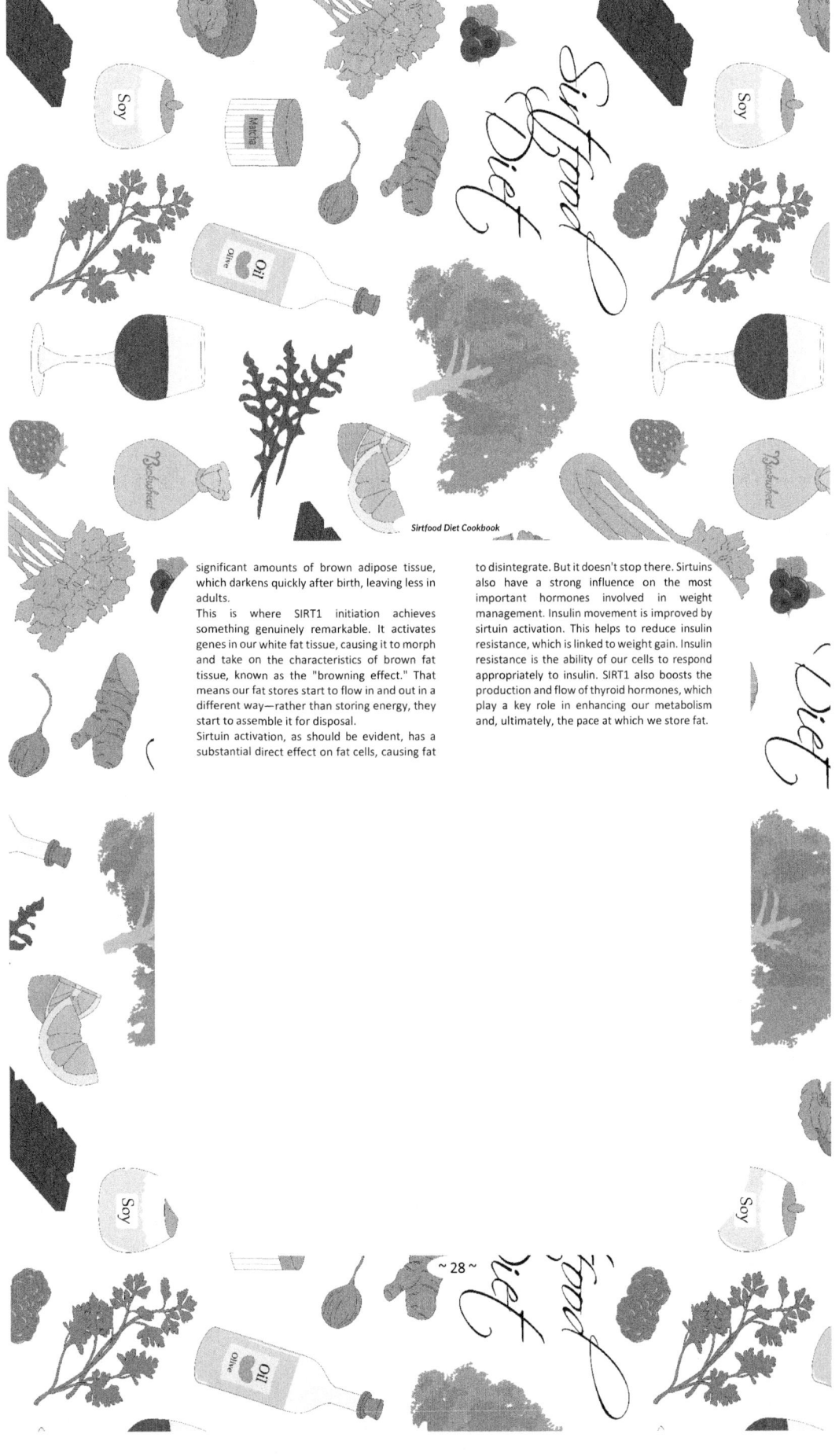

Sirtfood Diet Cookbook

significant amounts of brown adipose tissue, which darkens quickly after birth, leaving less in adults.

This is where SIRT1 initiation achieves something genuinely remarkable. It activates genes in our white fat tissue, causing it to morph and take on the characteristics of brown fat tissue, known as the "browning effect." That means our fat stores start to flow in and out in a different way—rather than storing energy, they start to assemble it for disposal.

Sirtuin activation, as should be evident, has a substantial direct effect on fat cells, causing fat to disintegrate. But it doesn't stop there. Sirtuins also have a strong influence on the most important hormones involved in weight management. Insulin movement is improved by sirtuin activation. This helps to reduce insulin resistance, which is linked to weight gain. Insulin resistance is the ability of our cells to respond appropriately to insulin. SIRT1 also boosts the production and flow of thyroid hormones, which play a key role in enhancing our metabolism and, ultimately, the pace at which we store fat.

Sirtfood Diet Cookbook

~ 29 ~

CHAPTER 3:

The Best 30 Sirtfoods

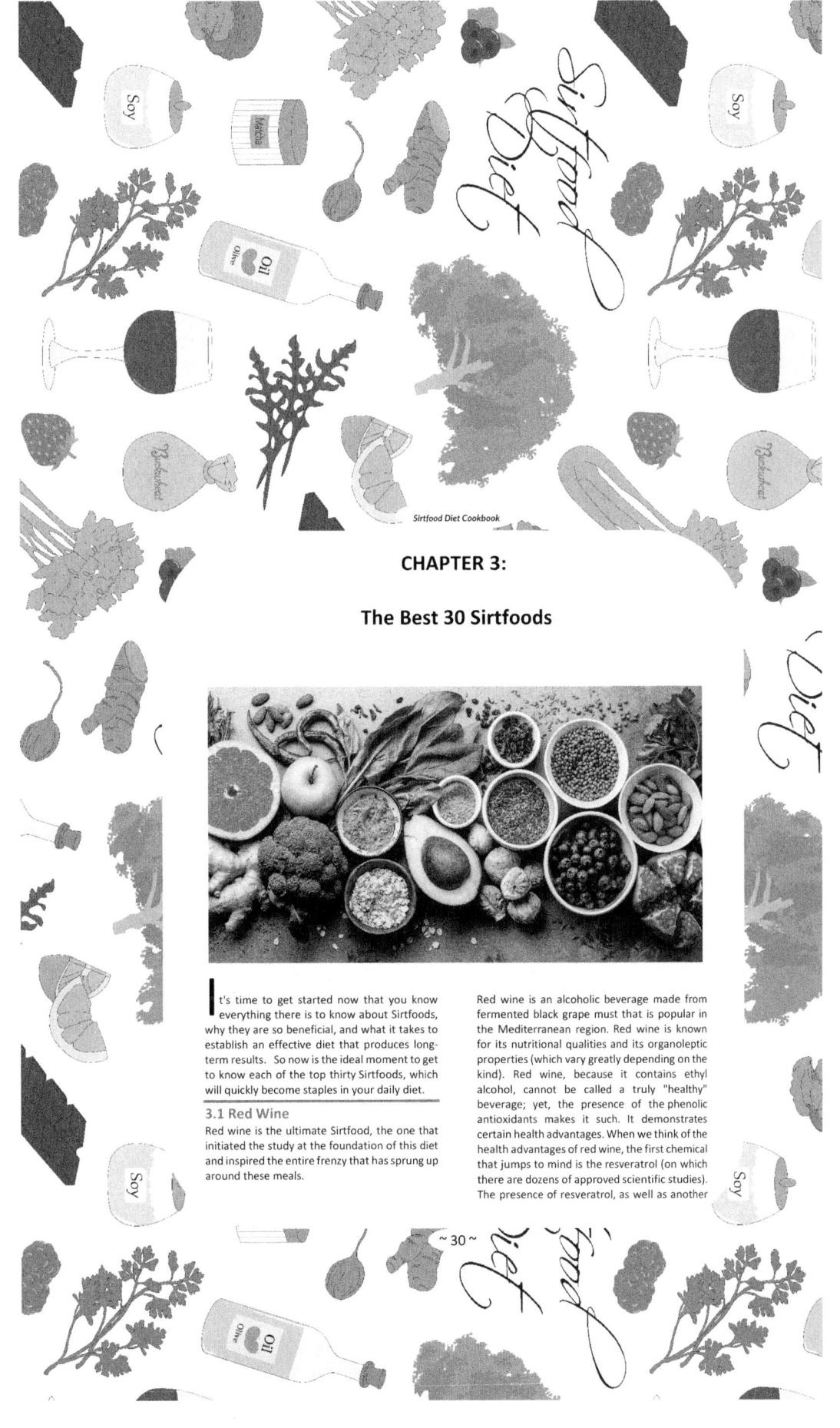

It's time to get started now that you know everything there is to know about Sirtfoods, why they are so beneficial, and what it takes to establish an effective diet that produces long-term results. So now is the ideal moment to get to know each of the top thirty Sirtfoods, which will quickly become staples in your daily diet.

3.1 Red Wine

Red wine is the ultimate Sirtfood, the one that initiated the study at the foundation of this diet and inspired the entire frenzy that has sprung up around these meals.

Red wine is an alcoholic beverage made from fermented black grape must that is popular in the Mediterranean region. Red wine is known for its nutritional qualities and its organoleptic properties (which vary greatly depending on the kind). Red wine, because it contains ethyl alcohol, cannot be called a truly "healthy" beverage; yet, the presence of the phenolic antioxidants makes it such. It demonstrates certain health advantages. When we think of the health advantages of red wine, the first chemical that jumps to mind is the resveratrol (on which there are dozens of approved scientific studies). The presence of resveratrol, as well as another

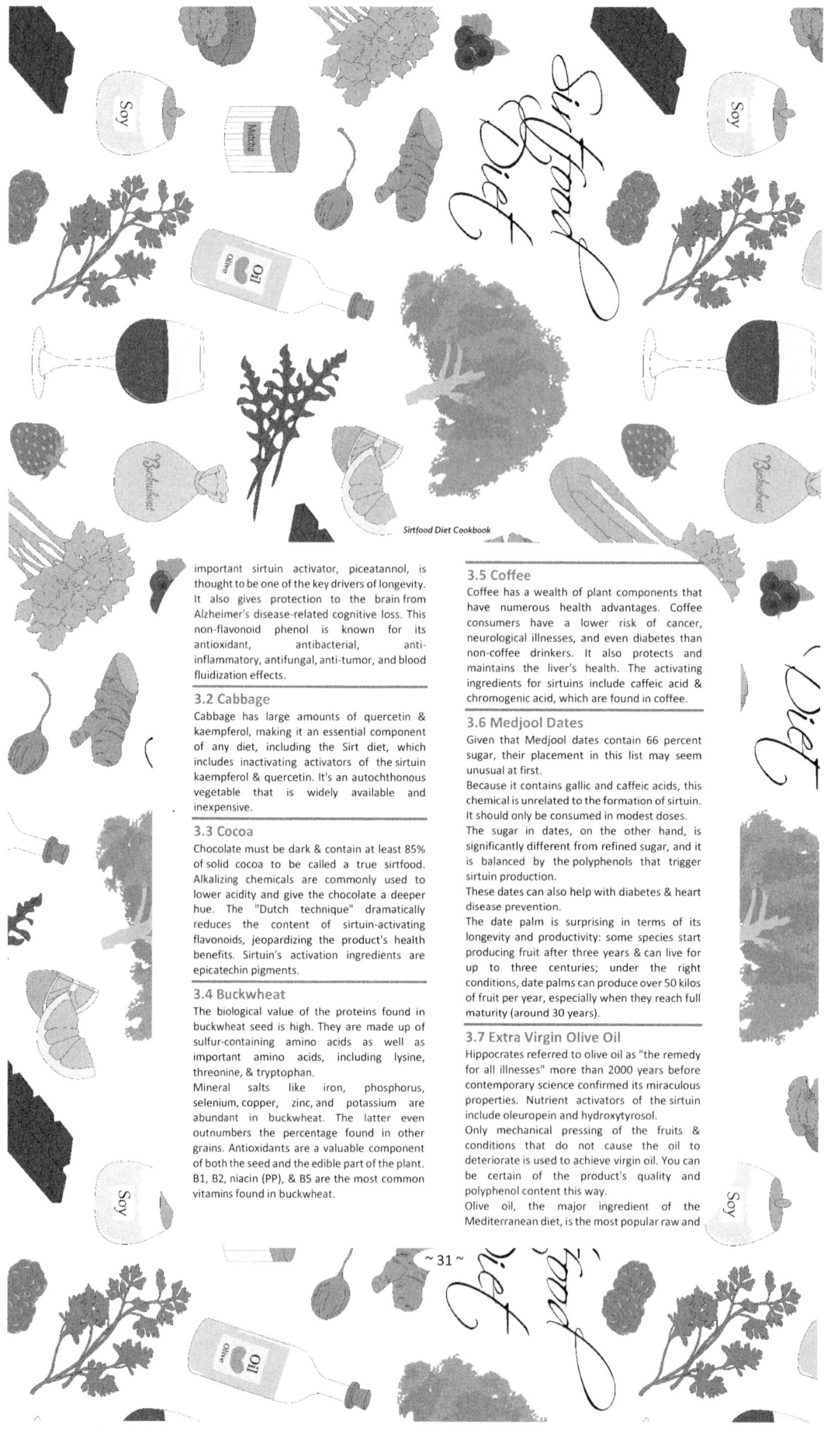

Sirtfood Diet Cookbook

important sirtuin activator, piceatannol, is thought to be one of the key drivers of longevity. It also gives protection to the brain from Alzheimer's disease-related cognitive loss. This non-flavonoid phenol is known for its antioxidant, antibacterial, anti-inflammatory, antifungal, anti-tumor, and blood fluidization effects.

3.2 Cabbage

Cabbage has large amounts of quercetin & kaempferol, making it an essential component of any diet, including the Sirt diet, which includes inactivating activators of the sirtuin kaempferol & quercetin. It's an autochthonous vegetable that is widely available and inexpensive.

3.3 Cocoa

Chocolate must be dark & contain at least 85% of solid cocoa to be called a true sirtfood. Alkalizing chemicals are commonly used to lower acidity and give the chocolate a deeper hue. The "Dutch technique" dramatically reduces the content of sirtuin-activating flavonoids, jeopardizing the product's health benefits. Sirtuin's activation ingredients are epicatechin pigments.

3.4 Buckwheat

The biological value of the proteins found in buckwheat seed is high. They are made up of sulfur-containing amino acids as well as important amino acids, including lysine, threonine, & tryptophan.

Mineral salts like iron, phosphorus, selenium, copper, zinc, and potassium are abundant in buckwheat. The latter even outnumbers the percentage found in other grains. Antioxidants are a valuable component of both the seed and the edible part of the plant. B1, B2, niacin (PP), & B5 are the most common vitamins found in buckwheat.

3.5 Coffee

Coffee has a wealth of plant components that have numerous health advantages. Coffee consumers have a lower risk of cancer, neurological illnesses, and even diabetes than non-coffee drinkers. It also protects and maintains the liver's health. The activating ingredients for sirtuins include caffeic acid & chromogenic acid, which are found in coffee.

3.6 Medjool Dates

Given that Medjool dates contain 66 percent sugar, their placement in this list may seem unusual at first.

Because it contains gallic and caffeic acids, this chemical is unrelated to the formation of sirtuin. It should only be consumed in modest doses.

The sugar in dates, on the other hand, is significantly different from refined sugar, and it is balanced by the polyphenols that trigger sirtuin production.

These dates can also help with diabetes & heart disease prevention.

The date palm is surprising in terms of its longevity and productivity: some species start producing fruit after three years & can live for up to three centuries; under the right conditions, date palms can produce over 50 kilos of fruit per year, especially when they reach full maturity (around 30 years).

3.7 Extra Virgin Olive Oil

Hippocrates referred to olive oil as "the remedy for all illnesses" more than 2000 years before contemporary science confirmed its miraculous properties. Nutrient activators of the sirtuin include oleuropein and hydroxytyrosol.

Only mechanical pressing of the fruits & conditions that do not cause the oil to deteriorate is used to achieve virgin oil. You can be certain of the product's quality and polyphenol content this way.

Olive oil, the major ingredient of the Mediterranean diet, is the most popular raw and

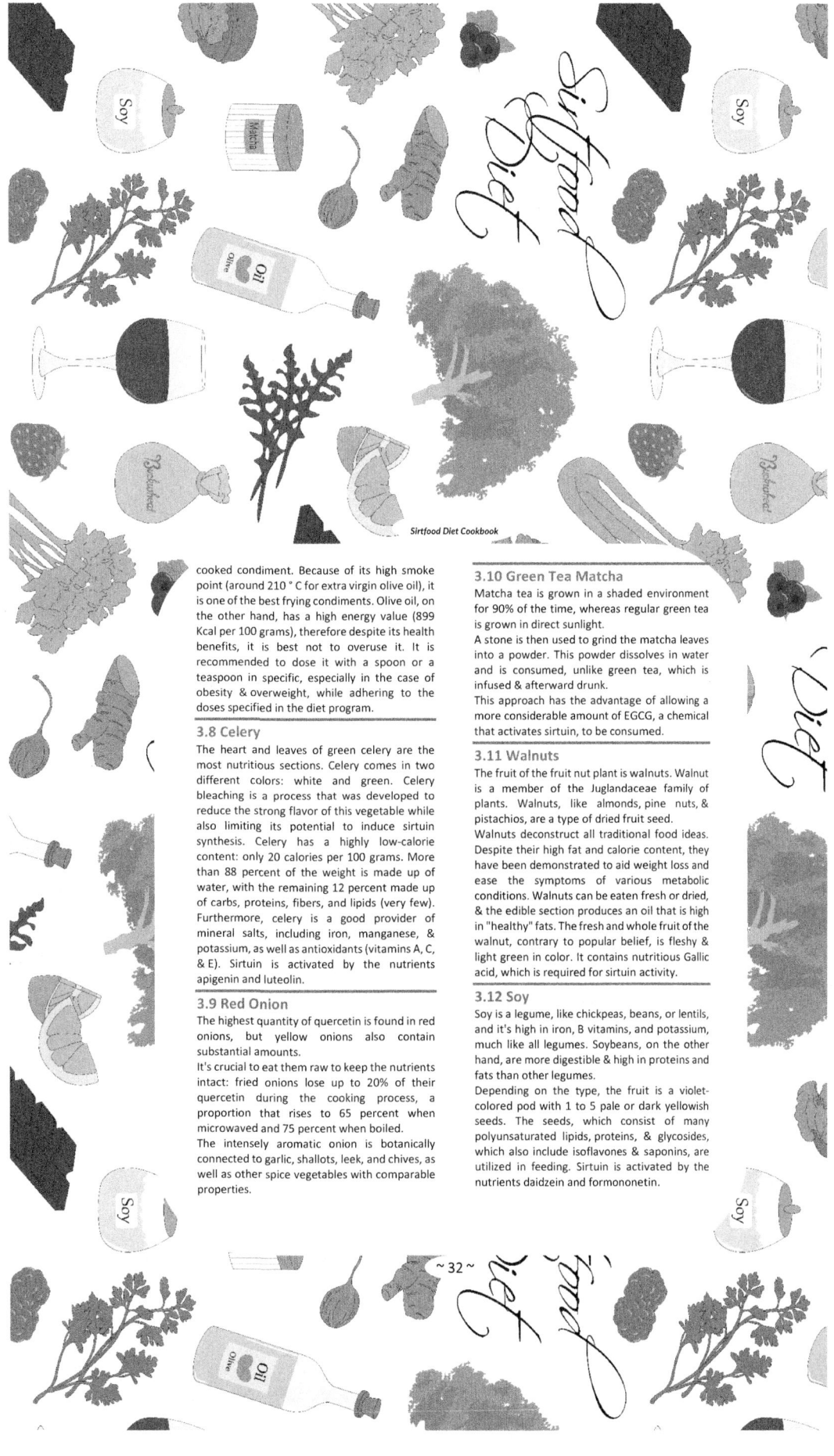

cooked condiment. Because of its high smoke point (around 210 ° C for extra virgin olive oil), it is one of the best frying condiments. Olive oil, on the other hand, has a high energy value (899 Kcal per 100 grams), therefore despite its health benefits, it is best not to overuse it. It is recommended to dose it with a spoon or a teaspoon in specific, especially in the case of obesity & overweight, while adhering to the doses specified in the diet program.

3.8 Celery

The heart and leaves of green celery are the most nutritious sections. Celery comes in two different colors: white and green. Celery bleaching is a process that was developed to reduce the strong flavor of this vegetable while also limiting its potential to induce sirtuin synthesis. Celery has a highly low-calorie content: only 20 calories per 100 grams. More than 88 percent of the weight is made up of water, with the remaining 12 percent made up of carbs, proteins, fibers, and lipids (very few). Furthermore, celery is a good provider of mineral salts, including iron, manganese, & potassium, as well as antioxidants (vitamins A, C, & E). Sirtuin is activated by the nutrients apigenin and luteolin.

3.9 Red Onion

The highest quantity of quercetin is found in red onions, but yellow onions also contain substantial amounts.

It's crucial to eat them raw to keep the nutrients intact: fried onions lose up to 20% of their quercetin during the cooking process, a proportion that rises to 65 percent when microwaved and 75 percent when boiled.

The intensely aromatic onion is botanically connected to garlic, shallots, leek, and chives, as well as other spice vegetables with comparable properties.

3.10 Green Tea Matcha

Matcha tea is grown in a shaded environment for 90% of the time, whereas regular green tea is grown in direct sunlight.

A stone is then used to grind the matcha leaves into a powder. This powder dissolves in water and is consumed, unlike green tea, which is infused & afterward drunk.

This approach has the advantage of allowing a more considerable amount of EGCG, a chemical that activates sirtuin, to be consumed.

3.11 Walnuts

The fruit of the fruit nut plant is walnuts. Walnut is a member of the Juglandaceae family of plants. Walnuts, like almonds, pine nuts, & pistachios, are a type of dried fruit seed.

Walnuts deconstruct all traditional food ideas. Despite their high fat and calorie content, they have been demonstrated to aid weight loss and ease the symptoms of various metabolic conditions. Walnuts can be eaten fresh or dried, & the edible section produces an oil that is high in "healthy" fats. The fresh and whole fruit of the walnut, contrary to popular belief, is fleshy & light green in color. It contains nutritious Gallic acid, which is required for sirtuin activity.

3.12 Soy

Soy is a legume, like chickpeas, beans, or lentils, and it's high in iron, B vitamins, and potassium, much like all legumes. Soybeans, on the other hand, are more digestible & high in proteins and fats than other legumes.

Depending on the type, the fruit is a violet-colored pod with 1 to 5 pale or dark yellowish seeds. The seeds, which consist of many polyunsaturated lipids, proteins, & glycosides, which also include isoflavones & saponins, are utilized in feeding. Sirtuin is activated by the nutrients daidzein and formononetin.

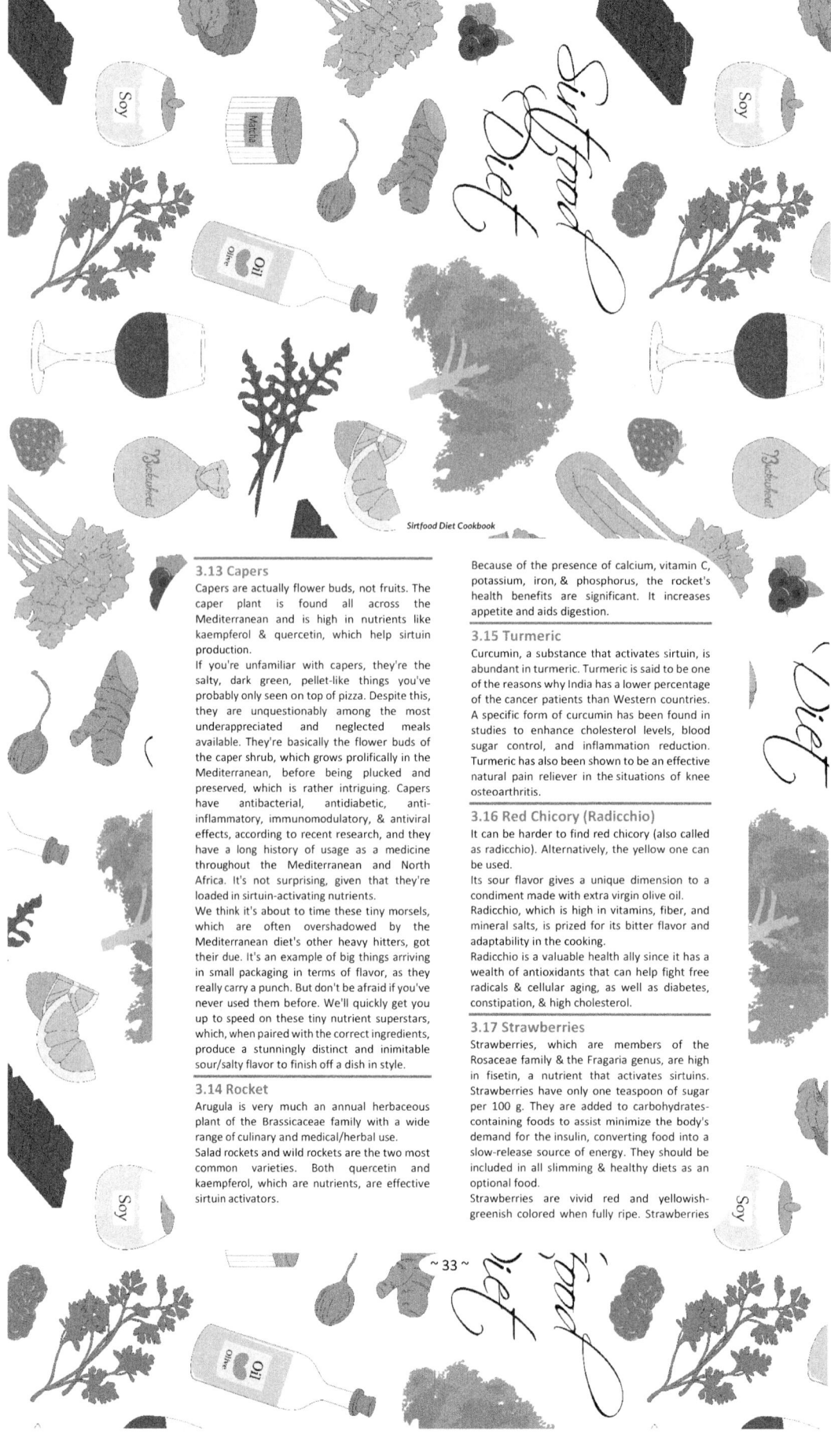

Sirtfood Diet Cookbook

3.13 Capers

Capers are actually flower buds, not fruits. The caper plant is found all across the Mediterranean and is high in nutrients like kaempferol & quercetin, which help sirtuin production.

If you're unfamiliar with capers, they're the salty, dark green, pellet-like things you've probably only seen on top of pizza. Despite this, they are unquestionably among the most underappreciated and neglected meals available. They're basically the flower buds of the caper shrub, which grows prolifically in the Mediterranean, before being plucked and preserved, which is rather intriguing. Capers have antibacterial, antidiabetic, anti-inflammatory, immunomodulatory, & antiviral effects, according to recent research, and they have a long history of usage as a medicine throughout the Mediterranean and North Africa. It's not surprising, given that they're loaded in sirtuin-activating nutrients.

We think it's about to time these tiny morsels, which are often overshadowed by the Mediterranean diet's other heavy hitters, got their due. It's an example of big things arriving in small packaging in terms of flavor, as they really carry a punch. But don't be afraid if you've never used them before. We'll quickly get you up to speed on these tiny nutrient superstars, which, when paired with the correct ingredients, produce a stunningly distinct and inimitable sour/salty flavor to finish off a dish in style.

3.14 Rocket

Arugula is very much an annual herbaceous plant of the Brassicaceae family with a wide range of culinary and medical/herbal use.

Salad rockets and wild rockets are the two most common varieties. Both quercetin and kaempferol, which are nutrients, are effective sirtuin activators.

Because of the presence of calcium, vitamin C, potassium, iron, & phosphorus, the rocket's health benefits are significant. It increases appetite and aids digestion.

3.15 Turmeric

Curcumin, a substance that activates sirtuin, is abundant in turmeric. Turmeric is said to be one of the reasons why India has a lower percentage of the cancer patients than Western countries. A specific form of curcumin has been found in studies to enhance cholesterol levels, blood sugar control, and inflammation reduction. Turmeric has also been shown to be an effective natural pain reliever in the situations of knee osteoarthritis.

3.16 Red Chicory (Radicchio)

It can be harder to find red chicory (also called as radicchio). Alternatively, the yellow one can be used.

Its sour flavor gives a unique dimension to a condiment made with extra virgin olive oil.

Radicchio, which is high in vitamins, fiber, and mineral salts, is prized for its bitter flavor and adaptability in the cooking.

Radicchio is a valuable health ally since it has a wealth of antioxidants that can help fight free radicals & cellular aging, as well as diabetes, constipation, & high cholesterol.

3.17 Strawberries

Strawberries, which are members of the Rosaceae family & the Fragaria genus, are high in fisetin, a nutrient that activates sirtuins. Strawberries have only one teaspoon of sugar per 100 g. They are added to carbohydrates-containing foods to assist minimize the body's demand for the insulin, converting food into a slow-release source of energy. They should be included in all slimming & healthy diets as an optional food.

Strawberries are vivid red and yellowish-greenish colored when fully ripe. Strawberries

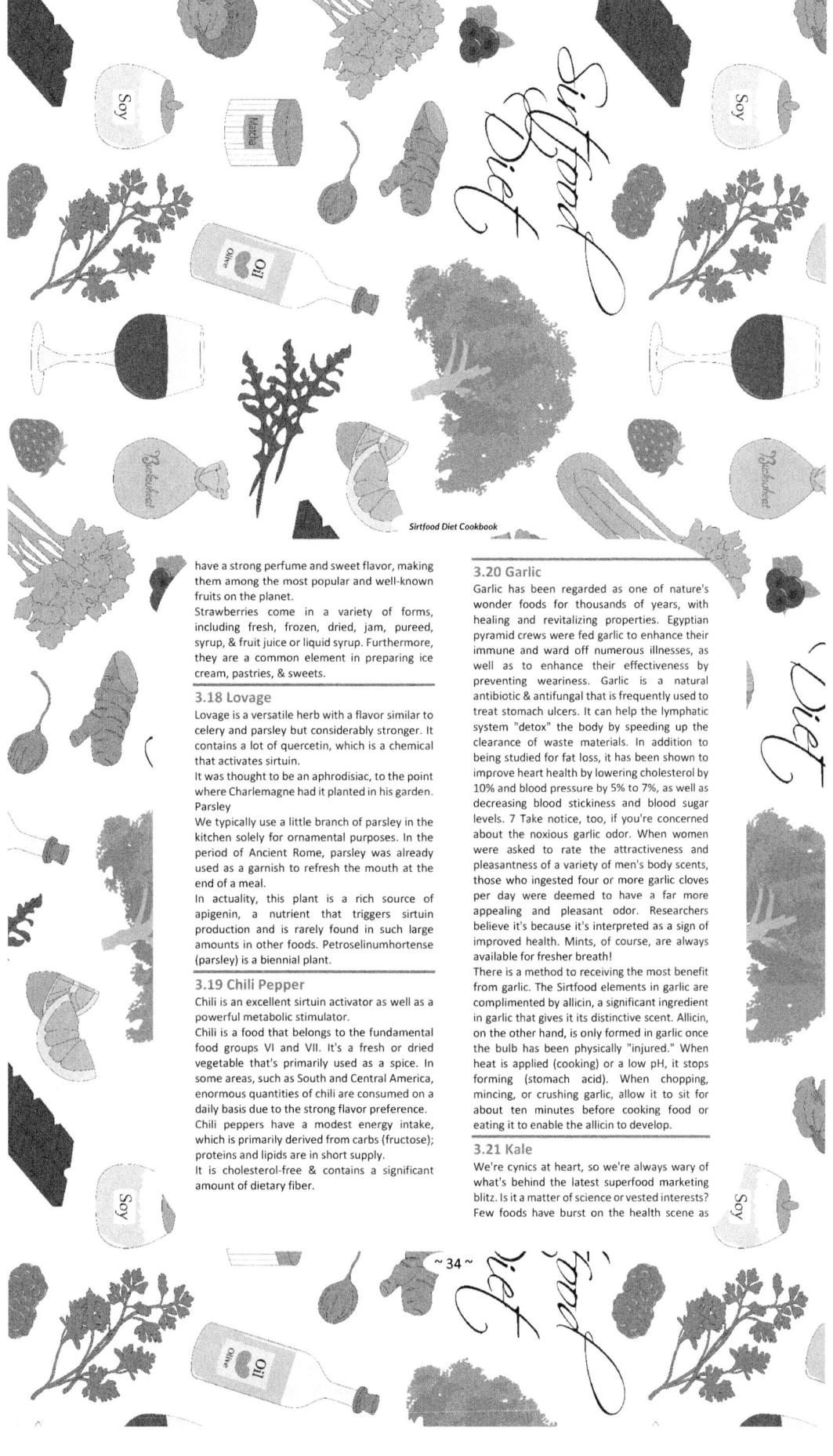

Sirtfood Diet Cookbook

have a strong perfume and sweet flavor, making them among the most popular and well-known fruits on the planet.

Strawberries come in a variety of forms, including fresh, frozen, dried, jam, pureed, syrup, & fruit juice or liquid syrup. Furthermore, they are a common element in preparing ice cream, pastries, & sweets.

3.18 Lovage

Lovage is a versatile herb with a flavor similar to celery and parsley but considerably stronger. It contains a lot of quercetin, which is a chemical that activates sirtuin.

It was thought to be an aphrodisiac, to the point where Charlemagne had it planted in his garden. Parsley

We typically use a little branch of parsley in the kitchen solely for ornamental purposes. In the period of Ancient Rome, parsley was already used as a garnish to refresh the mouth at the end of a meal.

In actuality, this plant is a rich source of apigenin, a nutrient that triggers sirtuin production and is rarely found in such large amounts in other foods. Petroselinumhortense (parsley) is a biennial plant.

3.19 Chili Pepper

Chili is an excellent sirtuin activator as well as a powerful metabolic stimulator.

Chili is a food that belongs to the fundamental food groups VI and VII. It's a fresh or dried vegetable that's primarily used as a spice. In some areas, such as South and Central America, enormous quantities of chili are consumed on a daily basis due to the strong flavor preference.

Chili peppers have a modest energy intake, which is primarily derived from carbs (fructose); proteins and lipids are in short supply.

It is cholesterol-free & contains a significant amount of dietary fiber.

3.20 Garlic

Garlic has been regarded as one of nature's wonder foods for thousands of years, with healing and revitalizing properties. Egyptian pyramid crews were fed garlic to enhance their immune and ward off numerous illnesses, as well as to enhance their effectiveness by preventing weariness. Garlic is a natural antibiotic & antifungal that is frequently used to treat stomach ulcers. It can help the lymphatic system "detox" the body by speeding up the clearance of waste materials. In addition to being studied for fat loss, it has been shown to improve heart health by lowering cholesterol by 10% and blood pressure by 5% to 7%, as well as decreasing blood stickiness and blood sugar levels. 7 Take notice, too, if you're concerned about the noxious garlic odor. When women were asked to rate the attractiveness and pleasantness of a variety of men's body scents, those who ingested four or more garlic cloves per day were deemed to have a far more appealing and pleasant odor. Researchers believe it's because it's interpreted as a sign of improved health. Mints, of course, are always available for fresher breath!

There is a method to receiving the most benefit from garlic. The Sirtfood elements in garlic are complimented by allicin, a significant ingredient in garlic that gives it its distinctive scent. Allicin, on the other hand, is only formed in garlic once the bulb has been physically "injured." When heat is applied (cooking) or a low pH, it stops forming (stomach acid). When chopping, mincing, or crushing garlic, allow it to sit for about ten minutes before cooking food or eating it to enable the allicin to develop.

3.21 Kale

We're cynics at heart, so we're always wary of what's behind the latest superfood marketing blitz. Is it a matter of science or vested interests? Few foods have burst on the health scene as

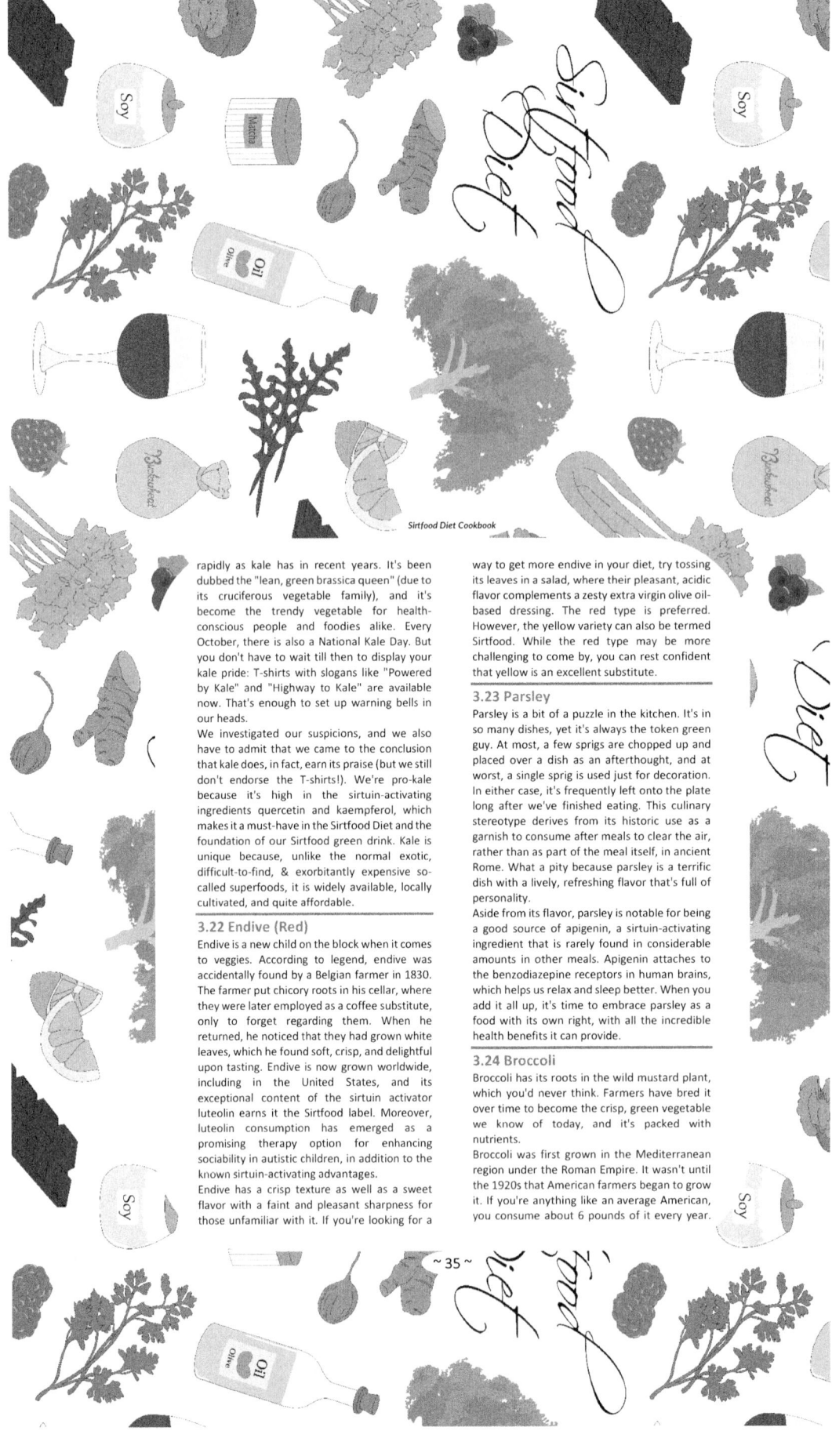

Sirtfood Diet Cookbook

rapidly as kale has in recent years. It's been dubbed the "lean, green brassica queen" (due to its cruciferous vegetable family), and it's become the trendy vegetable for health-conscious people and foodies alike. Every October, there is also a National Kale Day. But you don't have to wait till then to display your kale pride: T-shirts with slogans like "Powered by Kale" and "Highway to Kale" are available now. That's enough to set up warning bells in our heads.

We investigated our suspicions, and we also have to admit that we came to the conclusion that kale does, in fact, earn its praise (but we still don't endorse the T-shirts!). We're pro-kale because it's high in the sirtuin-activating ingredients quercetin and kaempferol, which makes it a must-have in the Sirtfood Diet and the foundation of our Sirtfood green drink. Kale is unique because, unlike the normal exotic, difficult-to-find, & exorbitantly expensive so-called superfoods, it is widely available, locally cultivated, and quite affordable.

3.22 Endive (Red)

Endive is a new child on the block when it comes to veggies. According to legend, endive was accidentally found by a Belgian farmer in 1830. The farmer put chicory roots in his cellar, where they were later employed as a coffee substitute, only to forget regarding them. When he returned, he noticed that they had grown white leaves, which he found soft, crisp, and delightful upon tasting. Endive is now grown worldwide, including in the United States, and its exceptional content of the sirtuin activator luteolin earns it the Sirtfood label. Moreover, luteolin consumption has emerged as a promising therapy option for enhancing sociability in autistic children, in addition to the known sirtuin-activating advantages.

Endive has a crisp texture as well as a sweet flavor with a faint and pleasant sharpness for those unfamiliar with it. If you're looking for a way to get more endive in your diet, try tossing its leaves in a salad, where their pleasant, acidic flavor complements a zesty extra virgin olive oil-based dressing. The red type is preferred. However, the yellow variety can also be termed Sirtfood. While the red type may be more challenging to come by, you can rest confident that yellow is an excellent substitute.

3.23 Parsley

Parsley is a bit of a puzzle in the kitchen. It's in so many dishes, yet it's always the token green guy. At most, a few sprigs are chopped up and placed over a dish as an afterthought, and at worst, a single sprig is used just for decoration. In either case, it's frequently left onto the plate long after we've finished eating. This culinary stereotype derives from its historic use as a garnish to consume after meals to clear the air, rather than as part of the meal itself, in ancient Rome. What a pity because parsley is a terrific dish with a lively, refreshing flavor that's full of personality.

Aside from its flavor, parsley is notable for being a good source of apigenin, a sirtuin-activating ingredient that is rarely found in considerable amounts in other meals. Apigenin attaches to the benzodiazepine receptors in human brains, which helps us relax and sleep better. When you add it all up, it's time to embrace parsley as a food with its own right, with all the incredible health benefits it can provide.

3.24 Broccoli

Broccoli has its roots in the wild mustard plant, which you'd never think. Farmers have bred it over time to become the crisp, green vegetable we know of today, and it's packed with nutrients.

Broccoli was first grown in the Mediterranean region under the Roman Empire. It wasn't until the 1920s that American farmers began to grow it. If you're anything like an average American, you consume about 6 pounds of it every year.

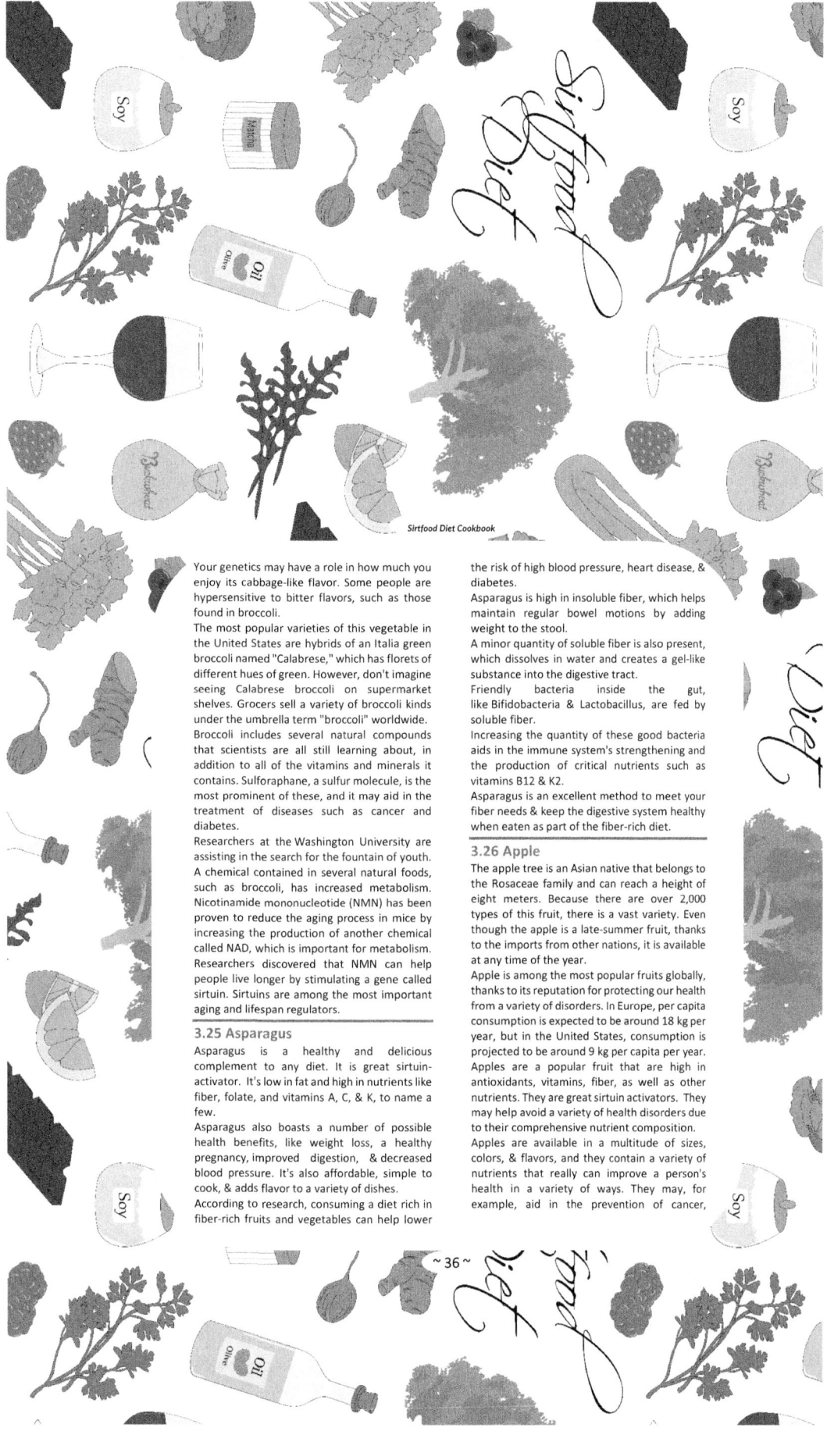

Sirtfood Diet Cookbook

Your genetics may have a role in how much you enjoy its cabbage-like flavor. Some people are hypersensitive to bitter flavors, such as those found in broccoli.

The most popular varieties of this vegetable in the United States are hybrids of an Italia green broccoli named "Calabrese," which has florets of different hues of green. However, don't imagine seeing Calabrese broccoli on supermarket shelves. Grocers sell a variety of broccoli kinds under the umbrella term "broccoli" worldwide.

Broccoli includes several natural compounds that scientists are all still learning about, in addition to all of the vitamins and minerals it contains. Sulforaphane, a sulfur molecule, is the most prominent of these, and it may aid in the treatment of diseases such as cancer and diabetes.

Researchers at the Washington University are assisting in the search for the fountain of youth. A chemical contained in several natural foods, such as broccoli, has increased metabolism. Nicotinamide mononucleotide (NMN) has been proven to reduce the aging process in mice by increasing the production of another chemical called NAD, which is important for metabolism. Researchers discovered that NMN can help people live longer by stimulating a gene called sirtuin. Sirtuins are among the most important aging and lifespan regulators.

3.25 Asparagus

Asparagus is a healthy and delicious complement to any diet. It is great sirtuin-activator. It's low in fat and high in nutrients like fiber, folate, and vitamins A, C, & K, to name a few.

Asparagus also boasts a number of possible health benefits, like weight loss, a healthy pregnancy, improved digestion, & decreased blood pressure. It's also affordable, simple to cook, & adds flavor to a variety of dishes.

According to research, consuming a diet rich in fiber-rich fruits and vegetables can help lower the risk of high blood pressure, heart disease, & diabetes.

Asparagus is high in insoluble fiber, which helps maintain regular bowel motions by adding weight to the stool.

A minor quantity of soluble fiber is also present, which dissolves in water and creates a gel-like substance into the digestive tract.

Friendly bacteria inside the gut, like Bifidobacteria & Lactobacillus, are fed by soluble fiber.

Increasing the quantity of these good bacteria aids in the immune system's strengthening and the production of critical nutrients such as vitamins B12 & K2.

Asparagus is an excellent method to meet your fiber needs & keep the digestive system healthy when eaten as part of the fiber-rich diet.

3.26 Apple

The apple tree is an Asian native that belongs to the Rosaceae family and can reach a height of eight meters. Because there are over 2,000 types of this fruit, there is a vast variety. Even though the apple is a late-summer fruit, thanks to the imports from other nations, it is available at any time of the year.

Apple is among the most popular fruits globally, thanks to its reputation for protecting our health from a variety of disorders. In Europe, per capita consumption is expected to be around 18 kg per year, but in the United States, consumption is projected to be around 9 kg per capita per year.

Apples are a popular fruit that are high in antioxidants, vitamins, fiber, as well as other nutrients. They are great sirtuin activators. They may help avoid a variety of health disorders due to their comprehensive nutrient composition.

Apples are available in a multitude of sizes, colors, & flavors, and they contain a variety of nutrients that really can improve a person's health in a variety of ways. They may, for example, aid in the prevention of cancer,

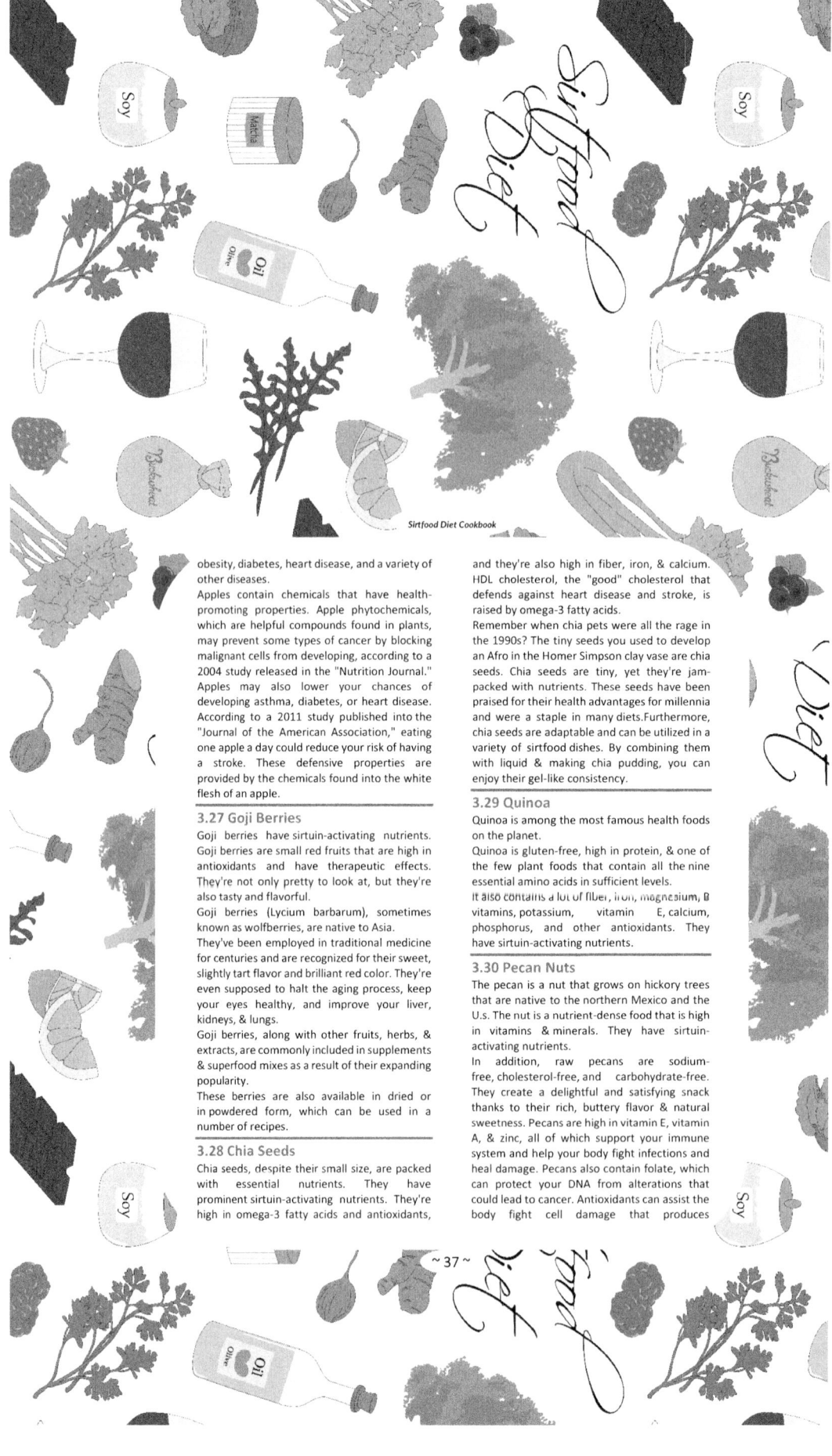

Sirtfood Diet Cookbook

obesity, diabetes, heart disease, and a variety of other diseases.

Apples contain chemicals that have health-promoting properties. Apple phytochemicals, which are helpful compounds found in plants, may prevent some types of cancer by blocking malignant cells from developing, according to a 2004 study released in the "Nutrition Journal." Apples may also lower your chances of developing asthma, diabetes, or heart disease. According to a 2011 study published into the "Journal of the American Association," eating one apple a day could reduce your risk of having a stroke. These defensive properties are provided by the chemicals found into the white flesh of an apple.

3.27 Goji Berries

Goji berries have sirtuin-activating nutrients. Goji berries are small red fruits that are high in antioxidants and have therapeutic effects. They're not only pretty to look at, but they're also tasty and flavorful.

Goji berries (Lycium barbarum), sometimes known as wolfberries, are native to Asia.

They've been employed in traditional medicine for centuries and are recognized for their sweet, slightly tart flavor and brilliant red color. They're even supposed to halt the aging process, keep your eyes healthy, and improve your liver, kidneys, & lungs.

Goji berries, along with other fruits, herbs, & extracts, are commonly included in supplements & superfood mixes as a result of their expanding popularity.

These berries are also available in dried or in powdered form, which can be used in a number of recipes.

3.28 Chia Seeds

Chia seeds, despite their small size, are packed with essential nutrients. They have prominent sirtuin-activating nutrients. They're high in omega-3 fatty acids and antioxidants, and they're also high in fiber, iron, & calcium. HDL cholesterol, the "good" cholesterol that defends against heart disease and stroke, is raised by omega-3 fatty acids.

Remember when chia pets were all the rage in the 1990s? The tiny seeds you used to develop an Afro in the Homer Simpson clay vase are chia seeds. Chia seeds are tiny, yet they're jam-packed with nutrients. These seeds have been praised for their health advantages for millennia and were a staple in many diets.Furthermore, chia seeds are adaptable and can be utilized in a variety of sirtfood dishes. By combining them with liquid & making chia pudding, you can enjoy their gel-like consistency.

3.29 Quinoa

Quinoa is among the most famous health foods on the planet.

Quinoa is gluten-free, high in protein, & one of the few plant foods that contain all the nine essential amino acids in sufficient levels.

It also contains a lot of fiber, iron, magnesium, B vitamins, potassium, vitamin E, calcium, phosphorus, and other antioxidants. They have sirtuin-activating nutrients.

3.30 Pecan Nuts

The pecan is a nut that grows on hickory trees that are native to the northern Mexico and the U.s. The nut is a nutrient-dense food that is high in vitamins & minerals. They have sirtuin-activating nutrients.

In addition, raw pecans are sodium-free, cholesterol-free, and carbohydrate-free. They create a delightful and satisfying snack thanks to their rich, buttery flavor & natural sweetness. Pecans are high in vitamin E, vitamin A, & zinc, all of which support your immune system and help your body fight infections and heal damage. Pecans also contain folate, which can protect your DNA from alterations that could lead to cancer. Antioxidants can assist the body fight cell damage that produces

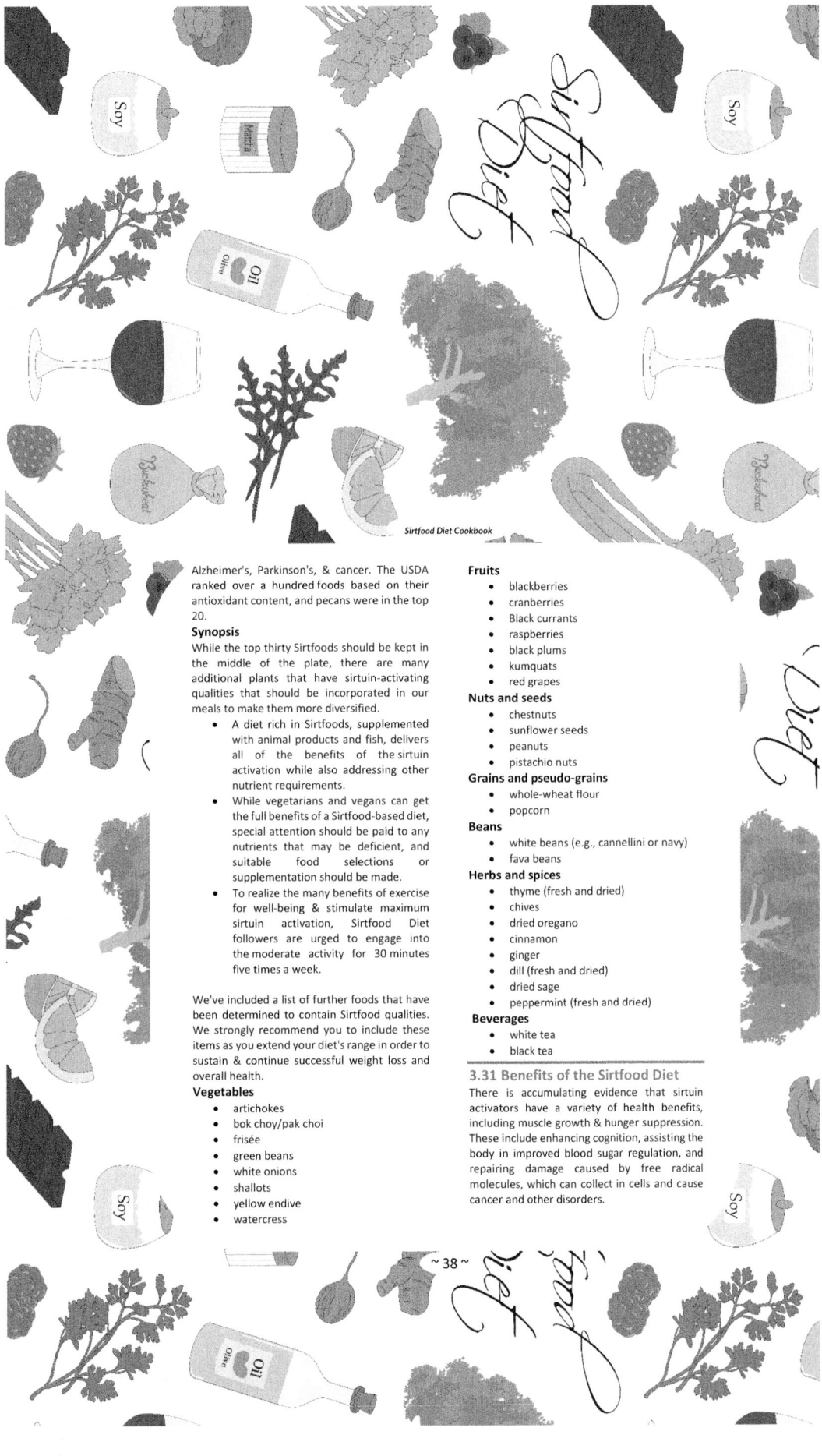

Sirtfood Diet Cookbook

Alzheimer's, Parkinson's, & cancer. The USDA ranked over a hundred foods based on their antioxidant content, and pecans were in the top 20.

Synopsis

While the top thirty Sirtfoods should be kept in the middle of the plate, there are many additional plants that have sirtuin-activating qualities that should be incorporated in our meals to make them more diversified.

- A diet rich in Sirtfoods, supplemented with animal products and fish, delivers all of the benefits of the sirtuin activation while also addressing other nutrient requirements.
- While vegetarians and vegans can get the full benefits of a Sirtfood-based diet, special attention should be paid to any nutrients that may be deficient, and suitable food selections or supplementation should be made.
- To realize the many benefits of exercise for well-being & stimulate maximum sirtuin activation, Sirtfood Diet followers are urged to engage into the moderate activity for 30 minutes five times a week.

We've included a list of further foods that have been determined to contain Sirtfood qualities. We strongly recommend you to include these items as you extend your diet's range in order to sustain & continue successful weight loss and overall health.

Vegetables

- artichokes
- bok choy/pak choi
- frisée
- green beans
- white onions
- shallots
- yellow endive
- watercress

Fruits

- blackberries
- cranberries
- Black currants
- raspberries
- black plums
- kumquats
- red grapes

Nuts and seeds

- chestnuts
- sunflower seeds
- peanuts
- pistachio nuts

Grains and pseudo-grains

- whole-wheat flour
- popcorn

Beans

- white beans (e.g., cannellini or navy)
- fava beans

Herbs and spices

- thyme (fresh and dried)
- chives
- dried oregano
- cinnamon
- ginger
- dill (fresh and dried)
- dried sage
- peppermint (fresh and dried)

Beverages

- white tea
- black tea

3.31 Benefits of the Sirtfood Diet

There is accumulating evidence that sirtuin activators have a variety of health benefits, including muscle growth & hunger suppression. These include enhancing cognition, assisting the body in improved blood sugar regulation, and repairing damage caused by free radical molecules, which can collect in cells and cause cancer and other disorders.

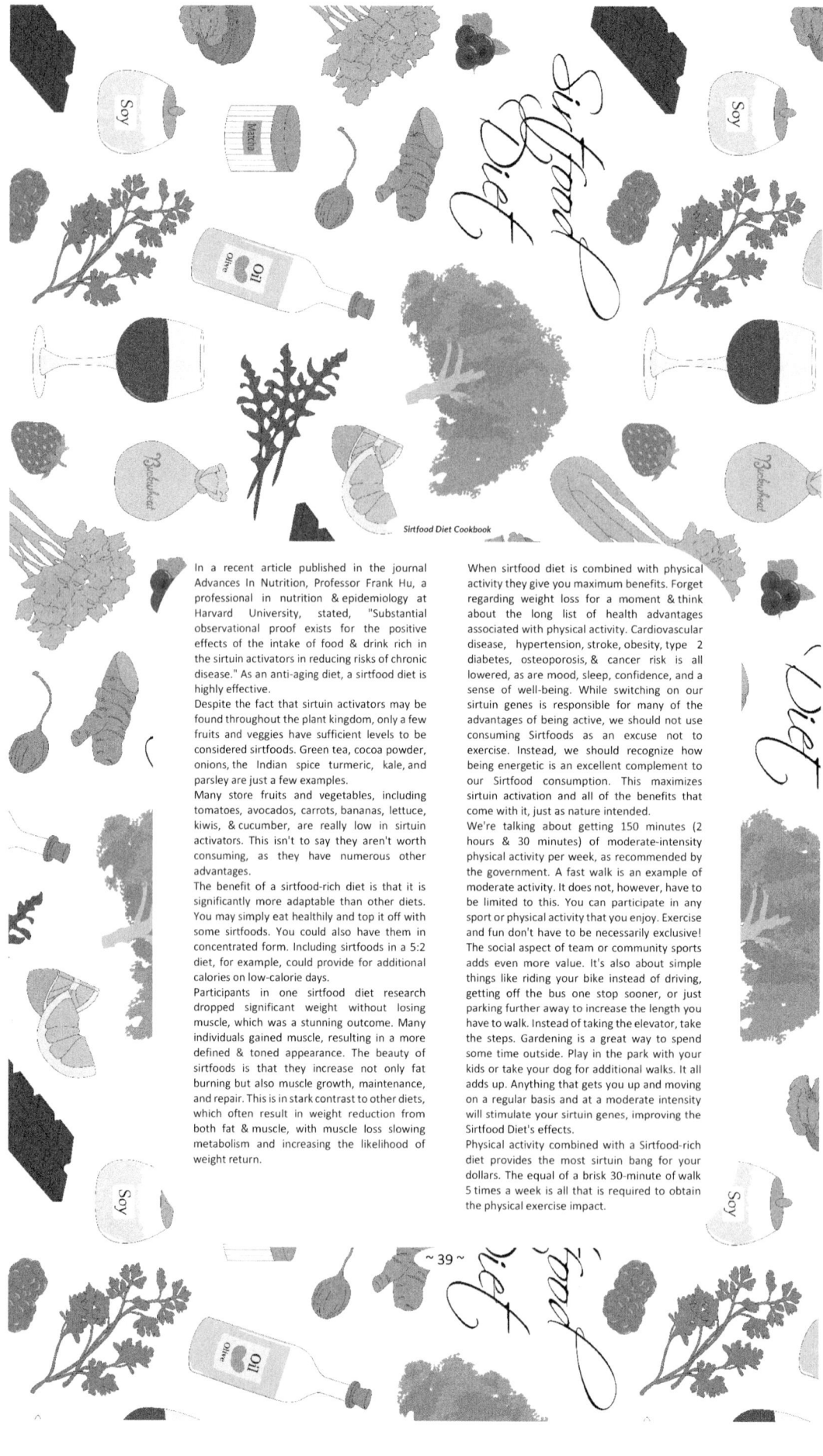

Sirtfood Diet Cookbook

In a recent article published in the journal Advances In Nutrition, Professor Frank Hu, a professional in nutrition & epidemiology at Harvard University, stated, "Substantial observational proof exists for the positive effects of the intake of food & drink rich in the sirtuin activators in reducing risks of chronic disease." As an anti-aging diet, a sirtfood diet is highly effective.

Despite the fact that sirtuin activators may be found throughout the plant kingdom, only a few fruits and veggies have sufficient levels to be considered sirtfoods. Green tea, cocoa powder, onions, the Indian spice turmeric, kale, and parsley are just a few examples.

Many store fruits and vegetables, including tomatoes, avocados, carrots, bananas, lettuce, kiwis, & cucumber, are really low in sirtuin activators. This isn't to say they aren't worth consuming, as they have numerous other advantages.

The benefit of a sirtfood-rich diet is that it is significantly more adaptable than other diets. You may simply eat healthily and top it off with some sirtfoods. You could also have them in concentrated form. Including sirtfoods in a 5:2 diet, for example, could provide for additional calories on low-calorie days.

Participants in one sirtfood diet research dropped significant weight without losing muscle, which was a stunning outcome. Many individuals gained muscle, resulting in a more defined & toned appearance. The beauty of sirtfoods is that they increase not only fat burning but also muscle growth, maintenance, and repair. This is in stark contrast to other diets, which often result in weight reduction from both fat & muscle, with muscle loss slowing metabolism and increasing the likelihood of weight return.

When sirtfood diet is combined with physical activity they give you maximum benefits. Forget regarding weight loss for a moment & think about the long list of health advantages associated with physical activity. Cardiovascular disease, hypertension, stroke, obesity, type 2 diabetes, osteoporosis, & cancer risk is all lowered, as are mood, sleep, confidence, and a sense of well-being. While switching on our sirtuin genes is responsible for many of the advantages of being active, we should not use consuming Sirtfoods as an excuse not to exercise. Instead, we should recognize how being energetic is an excellent complement to our Sirtfood consumption. This maximizes sirtuin activation and all of the benefits that come with it, just as nature intended.

We're talking about getting 150 minutes (2 hours & 30 minutes) of moderate-intensity physical activity per week, as recommended by the government. A fast walk is an example of moderate activity. It does not, however, have to be limited to this. You can participate in any sport or physical activity that you enjoy. Exercise and fun don't have to be necessarily exclusive! The social aspect of team or community sports adds even more value. It's also about simple things like riding your bike instead of driving, getting off the bus one stop sooner, or just parking further away to increase the length you have to walk. Instead of taking the elevator, take the steps. Gardening is a great way to spend some time outside. Play in the park with your kids or take your dog for additional walks. It all adds up. Anything that gets you up and moving on a regular basis and at a moderate intensity will stimulate your sirtuin genes, improving the Sirtfood Diet's effects.

Physical activity combined with a Sirtfood-rich diet provides the most sirtuin bang for your dollars. The equal of a brisk 30-minute of walk 5 times a week is all that is required to obtain the physical exercise impact.

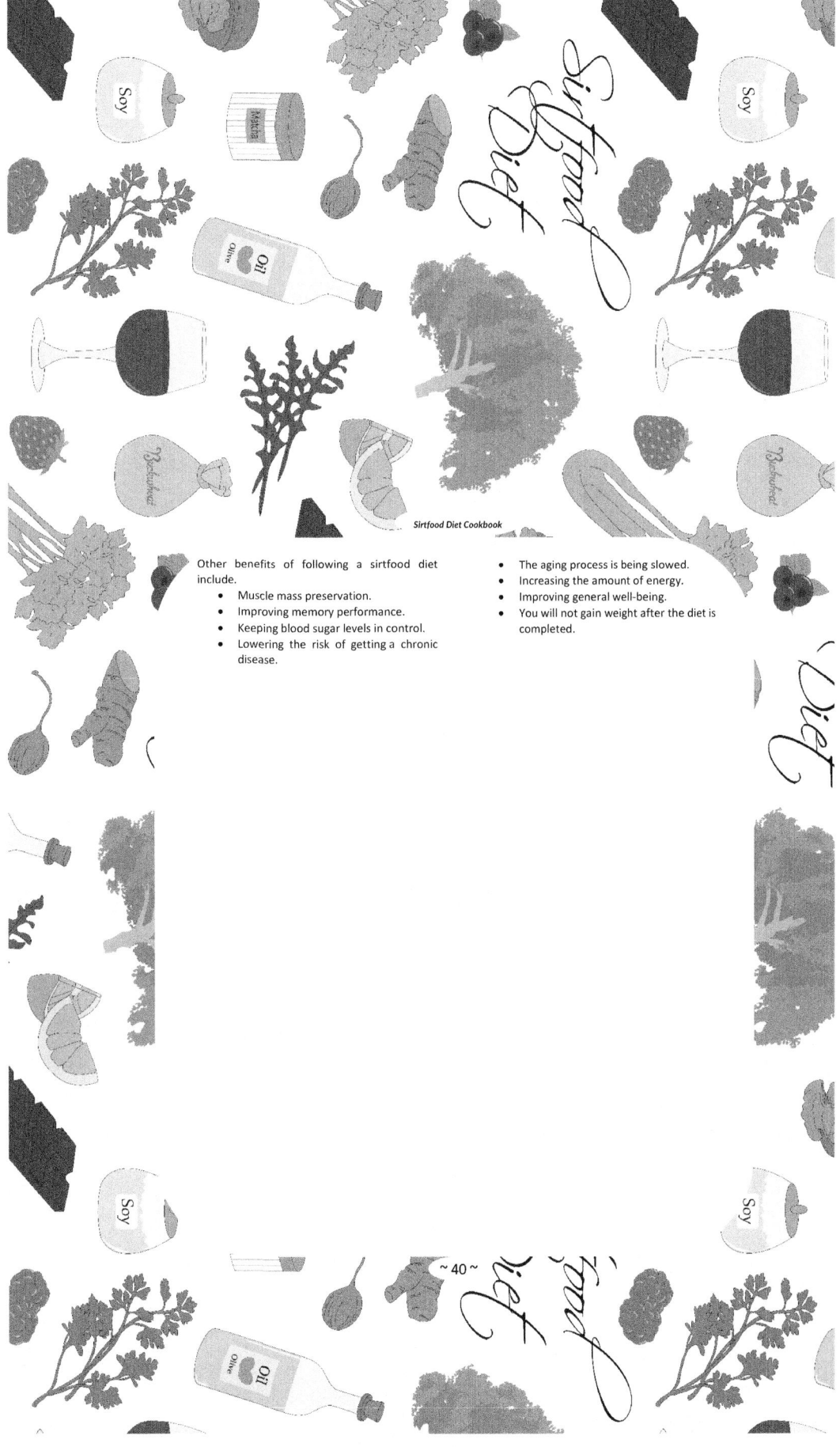

Sirtfood Diet Cookbook

Other benefits of following a sirtfood diet include.

- Muscle mass preservation.
- Improving memory performance.
- Keeping blood sugar levels in control.
- Lowering the risk of getting a chronic disease.

- The aging process is being slowed.
- Increasing the amount of energy.
- Improving general well-being.
- You will not gain weight after the diet is completed.

Sirtfood Diet Cookbook

CHAPTER 4:

The Right Mindset to Continue a Diet

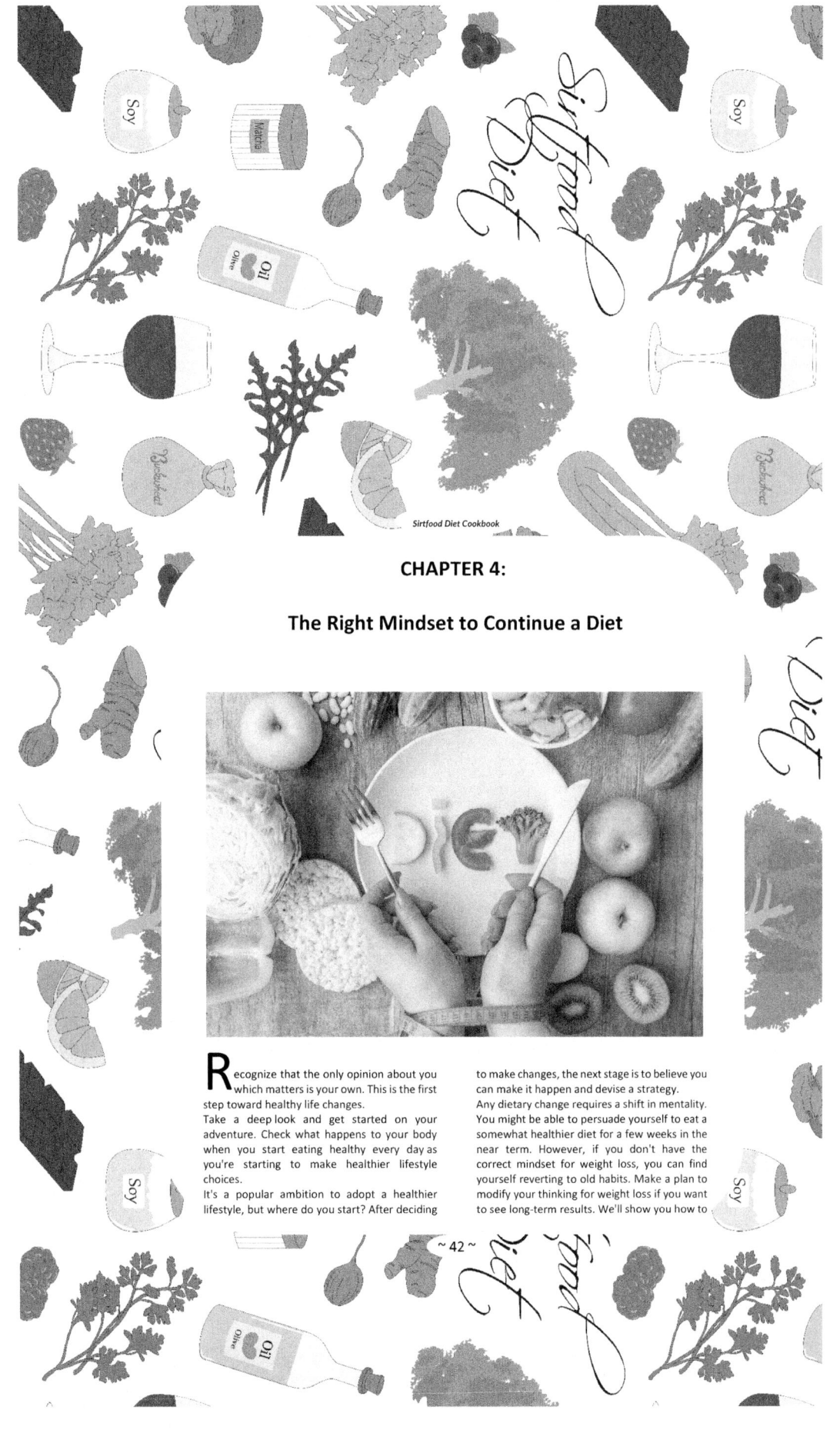

Recognize that the only opinion about you which matters is your own. This is the first step toward healthy life changes.

Take a deep look and get started on your adventure. Check what happens to your body when you start eating healthy every day as you're starting to make healthier lifestyle choices.

It's a popular ambition to adopt a healthier lifestyle, but where do you start? After deciding to make changes, the next stage is to believe you can make it happen and devise a strategy.

Any dietary change requires a shift in mentality. You might be able to persuade yourself to eat a somewhat healthier diet for a few weeks in the near term. However, if you don't have the correct mindset for weight loss, you can find yourself reverting to old habits. Make a plan to modify your thinking for weight loss if you want to see long-term results. We'll show you how to

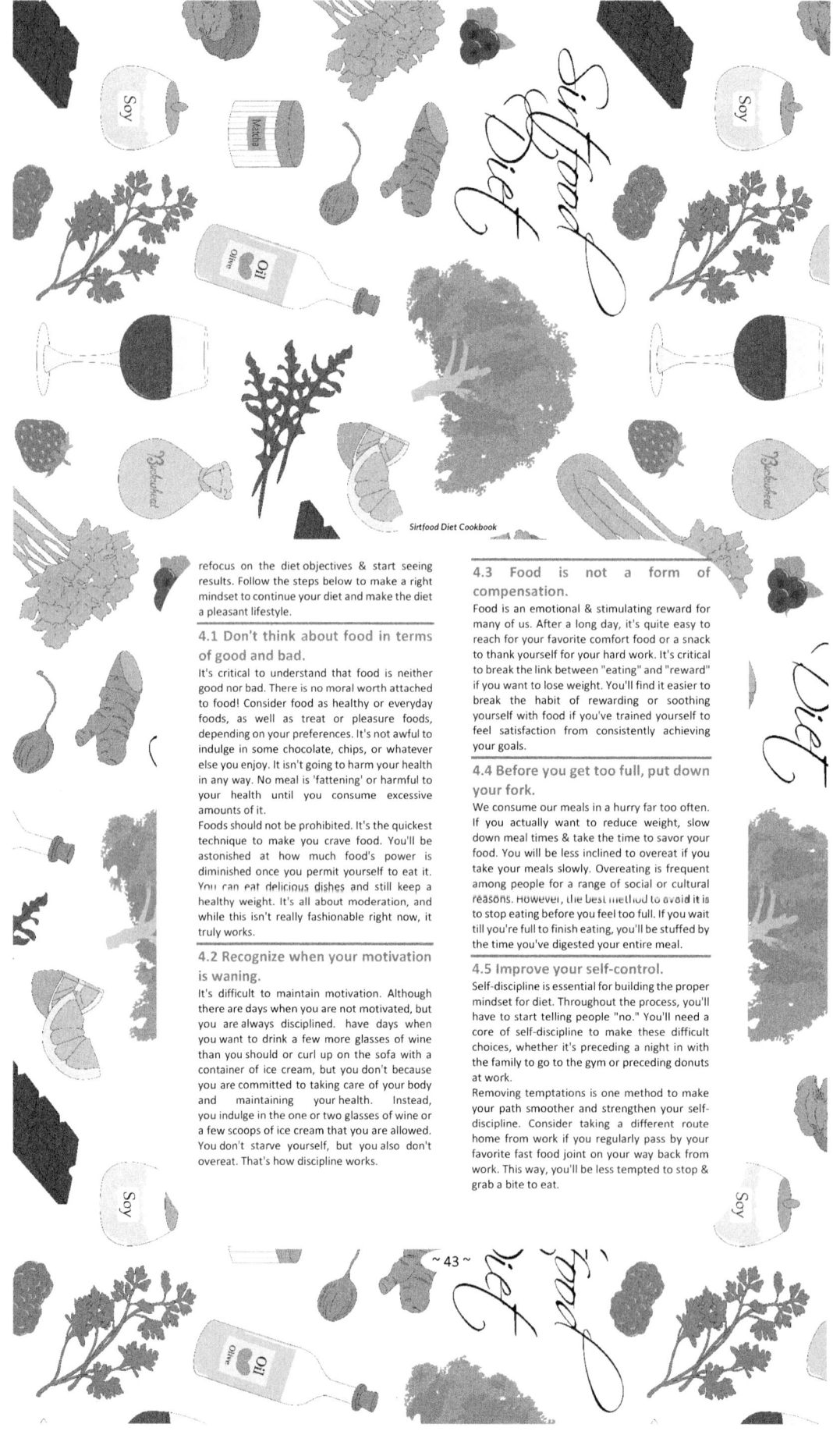

Sirtfood Diet Cookbook

refocus on the diet objectives & start seeing results. Follow the steps below to make a right mindset to continue your diet and make the diet a pleasant lifestyle.

4.1 Don't think about food in terms of good and bad.

It's critical to understand that food is neither good nor bad. There is no moral worth attached to food! Consider food as healthy or everyday foods, as well as treat or pleasure foods, depending on your preferences. It's not awful to indulge in some chocolate, chips, or whatever else you enjoy. It isn't going to harm your health in any way. No meal is 'fattening' or harmful to your health until you consume excessive amounts of it.

Foods should not be prohibited. It's the quickest technique to make you crave food. You'll be astonished at how much food's power is diminished once you permit yourself to eat it. You can eat delicious dishes and still keep a healthy weight. It's all about moderation, and while this isn't really fashionable right now, it truly works.

4.2 Recognize when your motivation is waning.

It's difficult to maintain motivation. Although there are days when you are not motivated, but you are always disciplined. have days when you want to drink a few more glasses of wine than you should or curl up on the sofa with a container of ice cream, but you don't because you are committed to taking care of your body and maintaining your health. Instead, you indulge in the one or two glasses of wine or a few scoops of ice cream that you are allowed. You don't starve yourself, but you also don't overeat. That's how discipline works.

4.3 Food is not a form of compensation.

Food is an emotional & stimulating reward for many of us. After a long day, it's quite easy to reach for your favorite comfort food or a snack to thank yourself for your hard work. It's critical to break the link between "eating" and "reward" if you want to lose weight. You'll find it easier to break the habit of rewarding or soothing yourself with food if you've trained yourself to feel satisfaction from consistently achieving your goals.

4.4 Before you get too full, put down your fork.

We consume our meals in a hurry far too often. If you actually want to reduce weight, slow down meal times & take the time to savor your food. You will be less inclined to overeat if you take your meals slowly. Overeating is frequent among people for a range of social or cultural reasons. However, the best method to avoid it is to stop eating before you feel too full. If you wait till you're full to finish eating, you'll be stuffed by the time you've digested your entire meal.

4.5 Improve your self-control.

Self-discipline is essential for building the proper mindset for diet. Throughout the process, you'll have to start telling people "no." You'll need a core of self-discipline to make these difficult choices, whether it's preceding a night in with the family to go to the gym or preceding donuts at work.

Removing temptations is one method to make your path smoother and strengthen your self-discipline. Consider taking a different route home from work if you regularly pass by your favorite fast food joint on your way back from work. This way, you'll be less tempted to stop & grab a bite to eat.

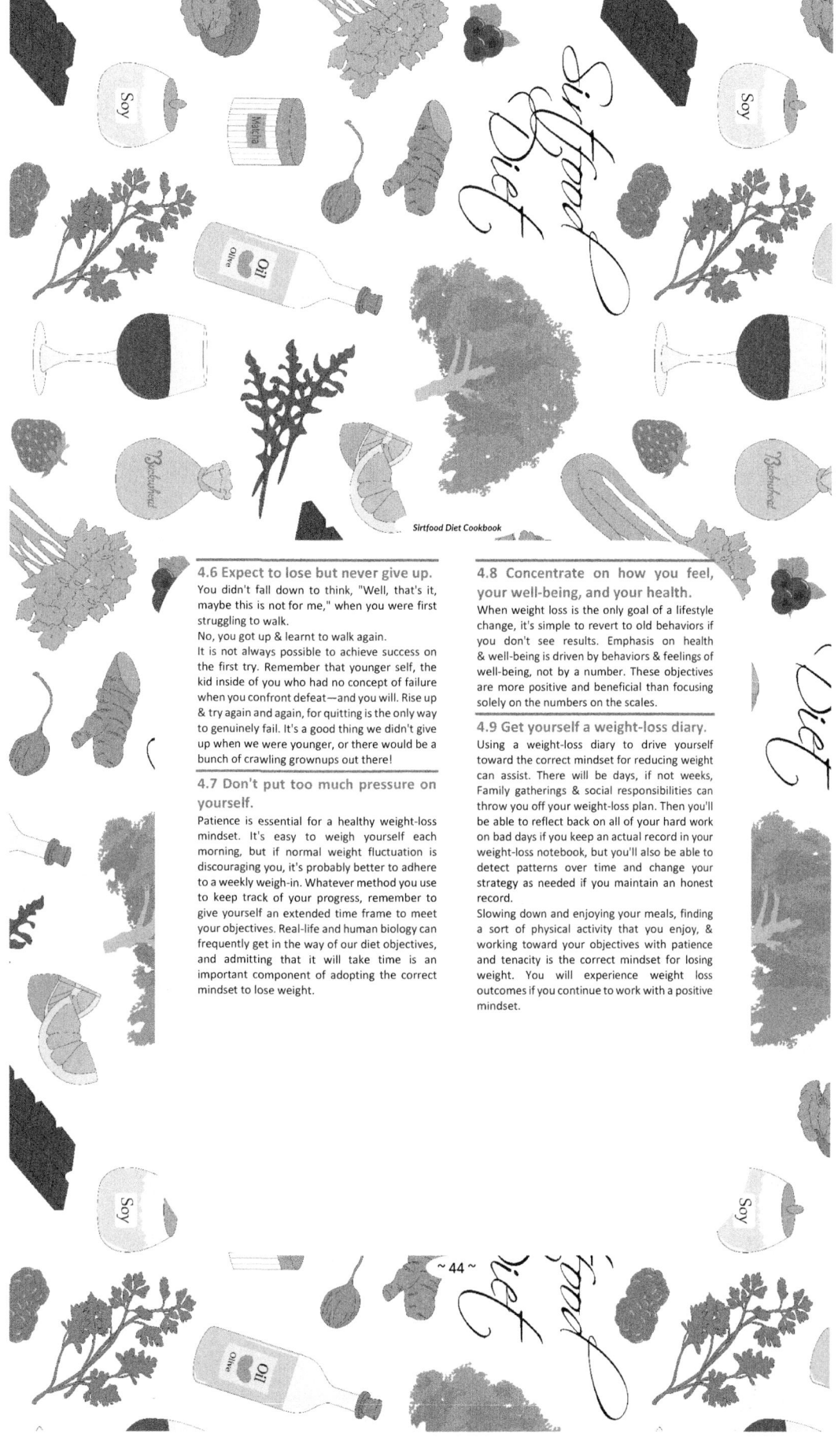

Sirtfood Diet Cookbook

4.6 Expect to lose but never give up.

You didn't fall down to think, "Well, that's it, maybe this is not for me," when you were first struggling to walk.

No, you got up & learnt to walk again.

It is not always possible to achieve success on the first try. Remember that younger self, the kid inside of you who had no concept of failure when you confront defeat—and you will. Rise up & try again and again, for quitting is the only way to genuinely fail. It's a good thing we didn't give up when we were younger, or there would be a bunch of crawling grownups out there!

4.7 Don't put too much pressure on yourself.

Patience is essential for a healthy weight-loss mindset. It's easy to weigh yourself each morning, but if normal weight fluctuation is discouraging you, it's probably better to adhere to a weekly weigh-in. Whatever method you use to keep track of your progress, remember to give yourself an extended time frame to meet your objectives. Real-life and human biology can frequently get in the way of our diet objectives, and admitting that it will take time is an important component of adopting the correct mindset to lose weight.

4.8 Concentrate on how you feel, your well-being, and your health.

When weight loss is the only goal of a lifestyle change, it's simple to revert to old behaviors if you don't see results. Emphasis on health & well-being is driven by behaviors & feelings of well-being, not by a number. These objectives are more positive and beneficial than focusing solely on the numbers on the scales.

4.9 Get yourself a weight-loss diary.

Using a weight-loss diary to drive yourself toward the correct mindset for reducing weight can assist. There will be days, if not weeks, Family gatherings & social responsibilities can throw you off your weight-loss plan. Then you'll be able to reflect back on all of your hard work on bad days if you keep an actual record in your weight-loss notebook, but you'll also be able to detect patterns over time and change your strategy as needed if you maintain an honest record.

Slowing down and enjoying your meals, finding a sort of physical activity that you enjoy, & working toward your objectives with patience and tenacity is the correct mindset for losing weight. You will experience weight loss outcomes if you continue to work with a positive mindset.

Sirtfood Diet Cookbook

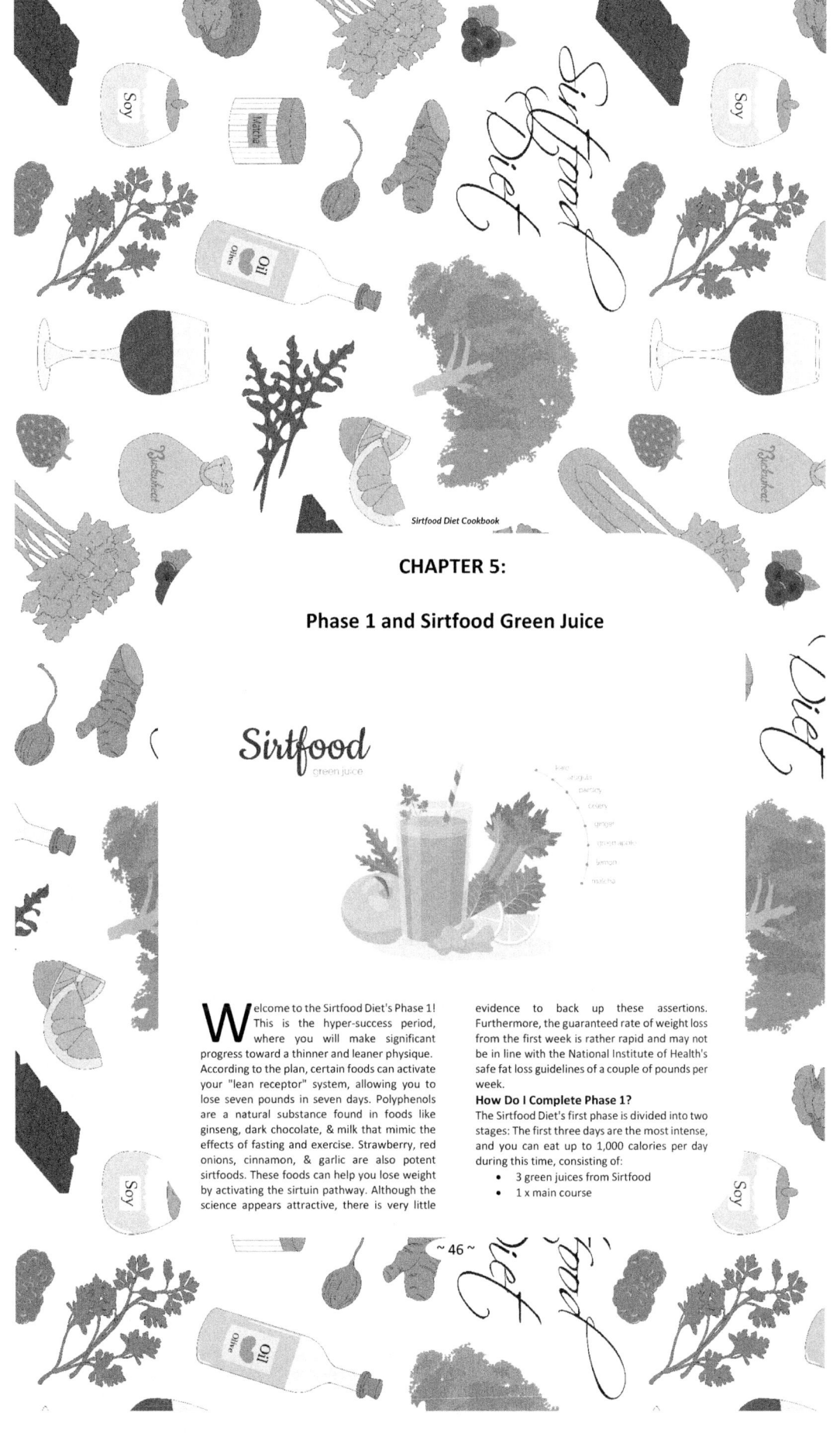

Sirtfood Diet Cookbook

CHAPTER 5:

Phase 1 and Sirtfood Green Juice

Welcome to the Sirtfood Diet's Phase 1! This is the hyper-success period, where you will make significant progress toward a thinner and leaner physique. According to the plan, certain foods can activate your "lean receptor" system, allowing you to lose seven pounds in seven days. Polyphenols are a natural substance found in foods like ginseng, dark chocolate, & milk that mimic the effects of fasting and exercise. Strawberry, red onions, cinnamon, & garlic are also potent sirtfoods. These foods can help you lose weight by activating the sirtuin pathway. Although the science appears attractive, there is very little evidence to back up these assertions. Furthermore, the guaranteed rate of weight loss from the first week is rather rapid and may not be in line with the National Institute of Health's safe fat loss guidelines of a couple of pounds per week.

How Do I Complete Phase 1?

The Sirtfood Diet's first phase is divided into two stages: The first three days are the most intense, and you can eat up to 1,000 calories per day during this time, consisting of:

- 3 green juices from Sirtfood
- 1 x main course

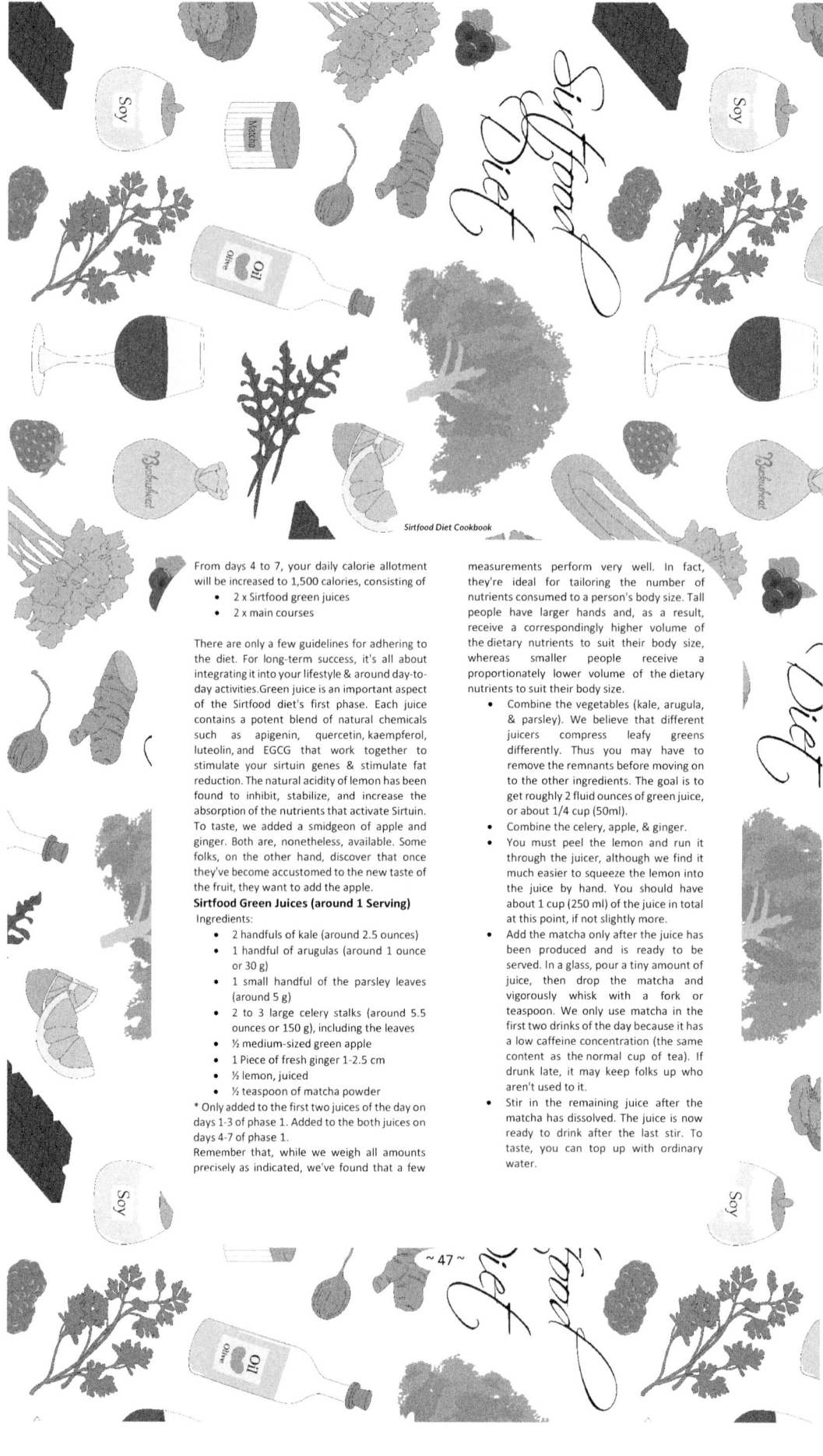

Sirtfood Diet Cookbook

From days 4 to 7, your daily calorie allotment will be increased to 1,500 calories, consisting of

- 2 x Sirtfood green juices
- 2 x main courses

There are only a few guidelines for adhering to the diet. For long-term success, it's all about integrating it into your lifestyle & around day-to-day activities. Green juice is an important aspect of the Sirtfood diet's first phase. Each juice contains a potent blend of natural chemicals such as apigenin, quercetin, kaempferol, luteolin, and EGCG that work together to stimulate your sirtuin genes & stimulate fat reduction. The natural acidity of lemon has been found to inhibit, stabilize, and increase the absorption of the nutrients that activate Sirtuin. To taste, we added a smidgeon of apple and ginger. Both are, nonetheless, available. Some folks, on the other hand, discover that once they've become accustomed to the new taste of the fruit, they want to add the apple.

Sirtfood Green Juices (around 1 Serving)
Ingredients:

- 2 handfuls of kale (around 2.5 ounces)
- 1 handful of arugulas (around 1 ounce or 30 g)
- 1 small handful of the parsley leaves (around 5 g)
- 2 to 3 large celery stalks (around 5.5 ounces or 150 g), including the leaves
- ½ medium-sized green apple
- 1 Piece of fresh ginger 1-2.5 cm
- ½ lemon, juiced
- ½ teaspoon of matcha powder

* Only added to the first two juices of the day on days 1-3 of phase 1. Added to the both juices on days 4-7 of phase 1.

Remember that, while we weigh all amounts precisely as indicated, we've found that a few measurements perform very well. In fact, they're ideal for tailoring the number of nutrients consumed to a person's body size. Tall people have larger hands and, as a result, receive a correspondingly higher volume of the dietary nutrients to suit their body size, whereas smaller people receive a proportionately lower volume of the dietary nutrients to suit their body size.

- Combine the vegetables (kale, arugula, & parsley). We believe that different juicers compress leafy greens differently. Thus you may have to remove the remnants before moving on to the other ingredients. The goal is to get roughly 2 fluid ounces of green juice, or about 1/4 cup (50ml).
- Combine the celery, apple, & ginger.
- You must peel the lemon and run it through the juicer, although we find it much easier to squeeze the lemon into the juice by hand. You should have about 1 cup (250 ml) of the juice in total at this point, if not slightly more.
- Add the matcha only after the juice has been produced and is ready to be served. In a glass, pour a tiny amount of juice, then drop the matcha and vigorously whisk with a fork or teaspoon. We only use matcha in the first two drinks of the day because it has a low caffeine concentration (the same content as the normal cup of tea). If drunk late, it may keep folks up who aren't used to it.
- Stir in the remaining juice after the matcha has dissolved. The juice is now ready to drink after the last stir. To taste, you can top up with ordinary water.

CHAPTER 6:

Maintenance of the Sirtfood diet

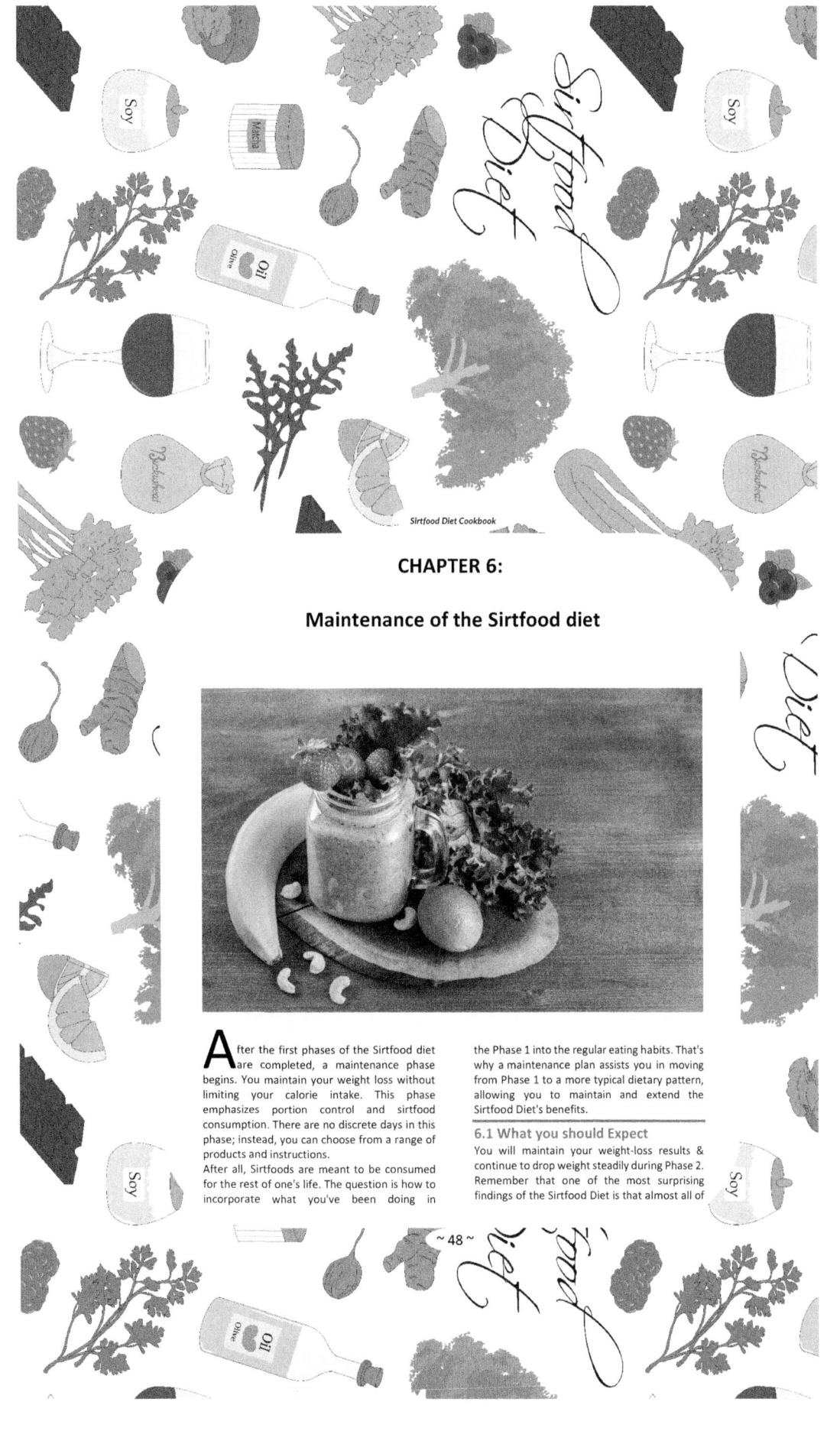

After the first phases of the Sirtfood diet are completed, a maintenance phase begins. You maintain your weight loss without limiting your calorie intake. This phase emphasizes portion control and sirtfood consumption. There are no discrete days in this phase; instead, you can choose from a range of products and instructions.

After all, Sirtfoods are meant to be consumed for the rest of one's life. The question is how to incorporate what you've been doing in the Phase 1 into the regular eating habits. That's why a maintenance plan assists you in moving from Phase 1 to a more typical dietary pattern, allowing you to maintain and extend the Sirtfood Diet's benefits.

6.1 What you should Expect
You will maintain your weight-loss results & continue to drop weight steadily during Phase 2. Remember that one of the most surprising findings of the Sirtfood Diet is that almost all of

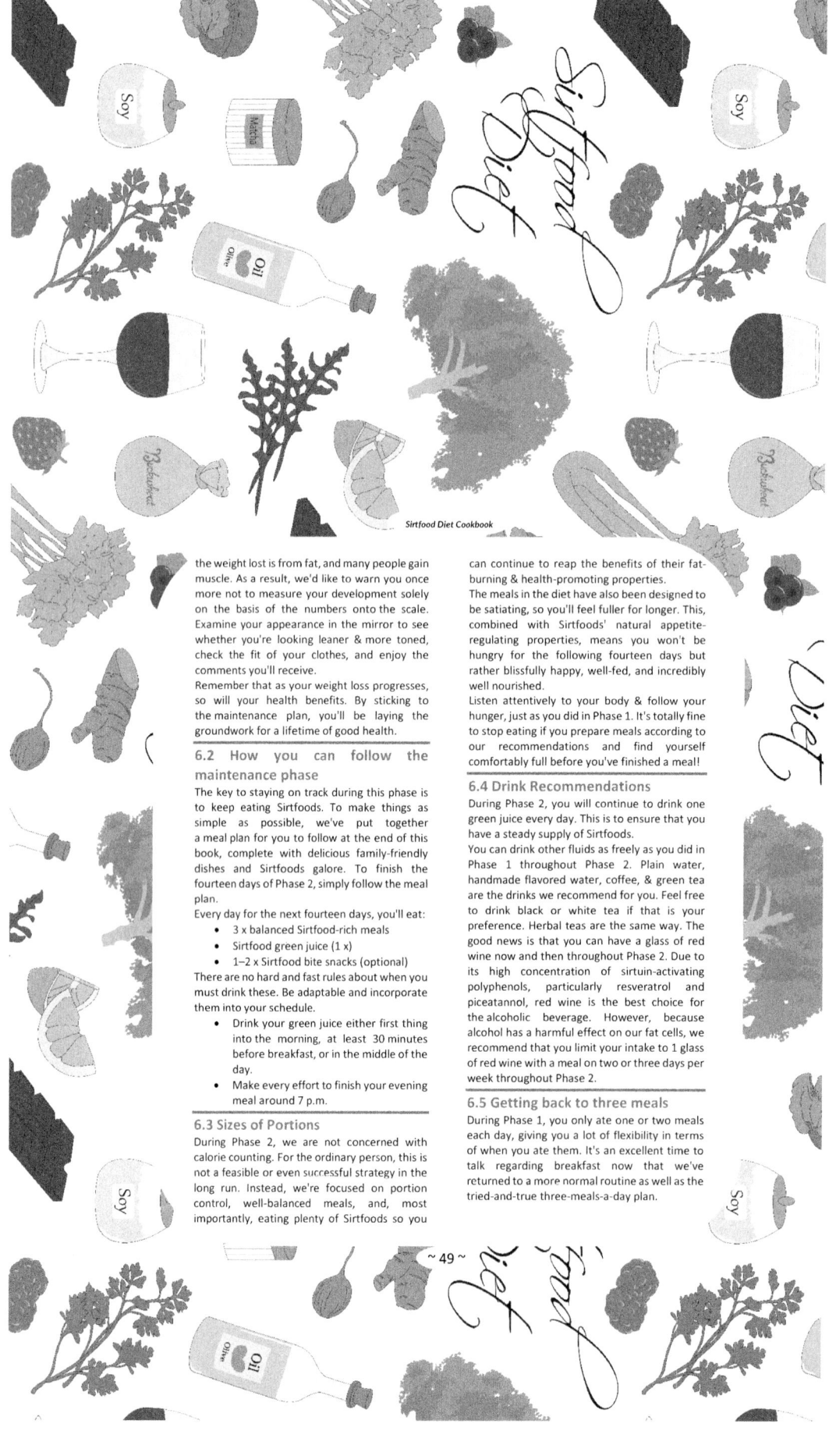

Sirtfood Diet Cookbook

the weight lost is from fat, and many people gain muscle. As a result, we'd like to warn you once more not to measure your development solely on the basis of the numbers onto the scale. Examine your appearance in the mirror to see whether you're looking leaner & more toned, check the fit of your clothes, and enjoy the comments you'll receive.

Remember that as your weight loss progresses, so will your health benefits. By sticking to the maintenance plan, you'll be laying the groundwork for a lifetime of good health.

6.2 How you can follow the maintenance phase

The key to staying on track during this phase is to keep eating Sirtfoods. To make things as simple as possible, we've put together a meal plan for you to follow at the end of this book, complete with delicious family-friendly dishes and Sirtfoods galore. To finish the fourteen days of Phase 2, simply follow the meal plan.

Every day for the next fourteen days, you'll eat:

- 3 x balanced Sirtfood-rich meals
- Sirtfood green juice (1 x)
- 1–2 x Sirtfood bite snacks (optional)

There are no hard and fast rules about when you must drink these. Be adaptable and incorporate them into your schedule.

- Drink your green juice either first thing into the morning, at least 30 minutes before breakfast, or in the middle of the day.
- Make every effort to finish your evening meal around 7 p.m.

6.3 Sizes of Portions

During Phase 2, we are not concerned with calorie counting. For the ordinary person, this is not a feasible or even successful strategy in the long run. Instead, we're focused on portion control, well-balanced meals, and, most importantly, eating plenty of Sirtfoods so you

can continue to reap the benefits of their fat-burning & health-promoting properties.

The meals in the diet have also been designed to be satiating, so you'll feel fuller for longer. This, combined with Sirtfoods' natural appetite-regulating properties, means you won't be hungry for the following fourteen days but rather blissfully happy, well-fed, and incredibly well nourished.

Listen attentively to your body & follow your hunger, just as you did in Phase 1. It's totally fine to stop eating if you prepare meals according to our recommendations and find yourself comfortably full before you've finished a meal!

6.4 Drink Recommendations

During Phase 2, you will continue to drink one green juice every day. This is to ensure that you have a steady supply of Sirtfoods.

You can drink other fluids as freely as you did in Phase 1 throughout Phase 2. Plain water, handmade flavored water, coffee, & green tea are the drinks we recommend for you. Feel free to drink black or white tea if that is your preference. Herbal teas are the same way. The good news is that you can have a glass of red wine now and then throughout Phase 2. Due to its high concentration of sirtuin-activating polyphenols, particularly resveratrol and piceatannol, red wine is the best choice for the alcoholic beverage. However, because alcohol has a harmful effect on our fat cells, we recommend that you limit your intake to 1 glass of red wine with a meal on two or three days per week throughout Phase 2.

6.5 Getting back to three meals

During Phase 1, you only ate one or two meals each day, giving you a lot of flexibility in terms of when you ate them. It's an excellent time to talk regarding breakfast now that we've returned to a more normal routine as well as the tried-and-true three-meals-a-day plan.

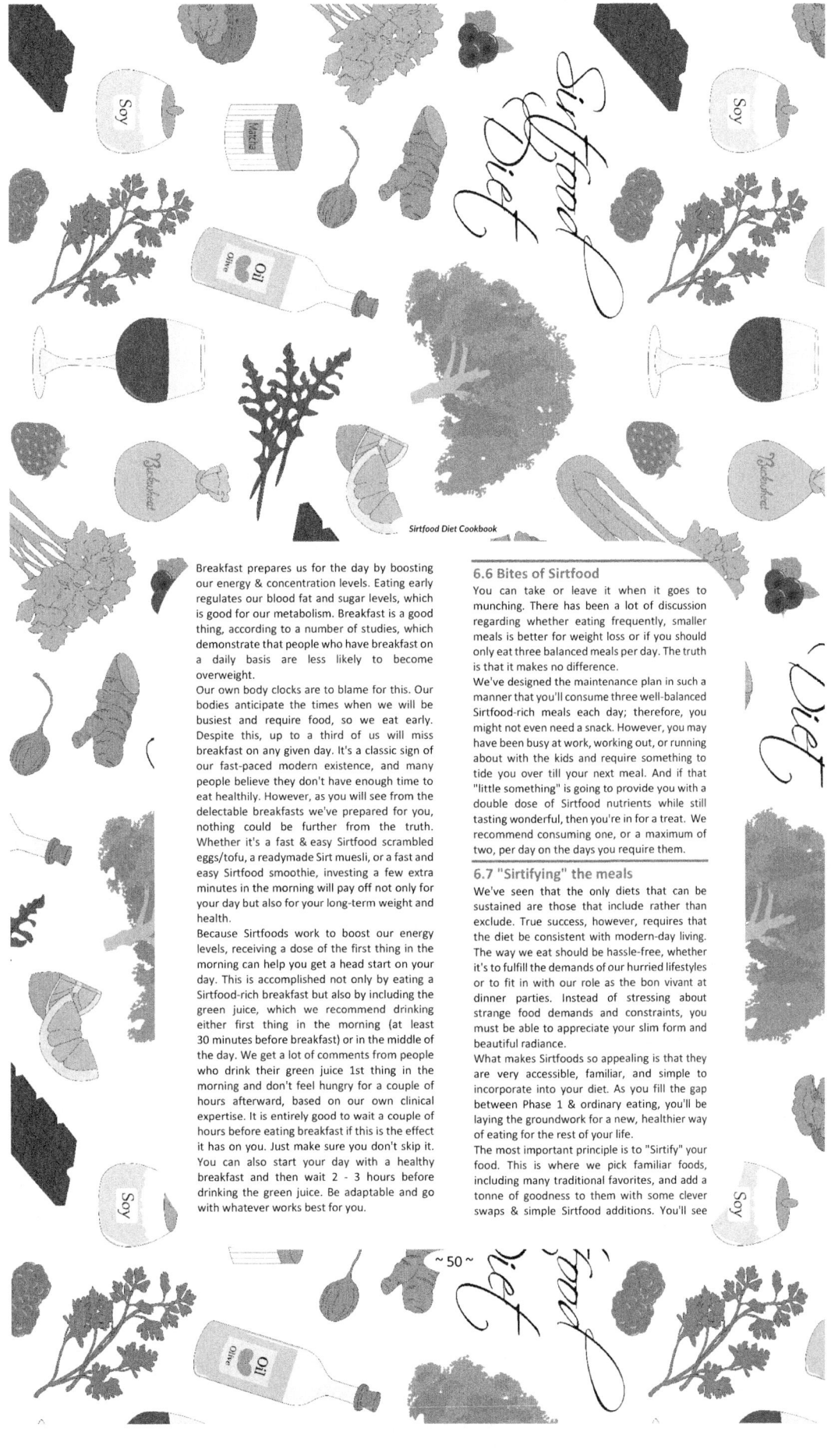

Sirtfood Diet Cookbook

Breakfast prepares us for the day by boosting our energy & concentration levels. Eating early regulates our blood fat and sugar levels, which is good for our metabolism. Breakfast is a good thing, according to a number of studies, which demonstrate that people who have breakfast on a daily basis are less likely to become overweight.

Our own body clocks are to blame for this. Our bodies anticipate the times when we will be busiest and require food, so we eat early. Despite this, up to a third of us will miss breakfast on any given day. It's a classic sign of our fast-paced modern existence, and many people believe they don't have enough time to eat healthily. However, as you will see from the delectable breakfasts we've prepared for you, nothing could be further from the truth. Whether it's a fast & easy Sirtfood scrambled eggs/tofu, a readymade Sirt muesli, or a fast and easy Sirtfood smoothie, investing a few extra minutes in the morning will pay off not only for your day but also for your long-term weight and health.

Because Sirtfoods work to boost our energy levels, receiving a dose of the first thing in the morning can help you get a head start on your day. This is accomplished not only by eating a Sirtfood-rich breakfast but also by including the green juice, which we recommend drinking either first thing in the morning (at least 30 minutes before breakfast) or in the middle of the day. We get a lot of comments from people who drink their green juice 1st thing in the morning and don't feel hungry for a couple of hours afterward, based on our own clinical expertise. It is entirely good to wait a couple of hours before eating breakfast if this is the effect it has on you. Just make sure you don't skip it. You can also start your day with a healthy breakfast and then wait 2 - 3 hours before drinking the green juice. Be adaptable and go with whatever works best for you.

6.6 Bites of Sirtfood

You can take or leave it when it goes to munching. There has been a lot of discussion regarding whether eating frequently, smaller meals is better for weight loss or if you should only eat three balanced meals per day. The truth is that it makes no difference.

We've designed the maintenance plan in such a manner that you'll consume three well-balanced Sirtfood-rich meals each day; therefore, you might not even need a snack. However, you may have been busy at work, working out, or running about with the kids and require something to tide you over till your next meal. And if that "little something" is going to provide you with a double dose of Sirtfood nutrients while still tasting wonderful, then you're in for a treat. We recommend consuming one, or a maximum of two, per day on the days you require them.

6.7 "Sirtifying" the meals

We've seen that the only diets that can be sustained are those that include rather than exclude. True success, however, requires that the diet be consistent with modern-day living. The way we eat should be hassle-free, whether it's to fulfill the demands of our hurried lifestyles or to fit in with our role as the bon vivant at dinner parties. Instead of stressing about strange food demands and constraints, you must be able to appreciate your slim form and beautiful radiance.

What makes Sirtfoods so appealing is that they are very accessible, familiar, and simple to incorporate into your diet. As you fill the gap between Phase 1 & ordinary eating, you'll be laying the groundwork for a new, healthier way of eating for the rest of your life.

The most important principle is to "Sirtify" your food. This is where we pick familiar foods, including many traditional favorites, and add a tonne of goodness to them with some clever swaps & simple Sirtfood additions. You'll see

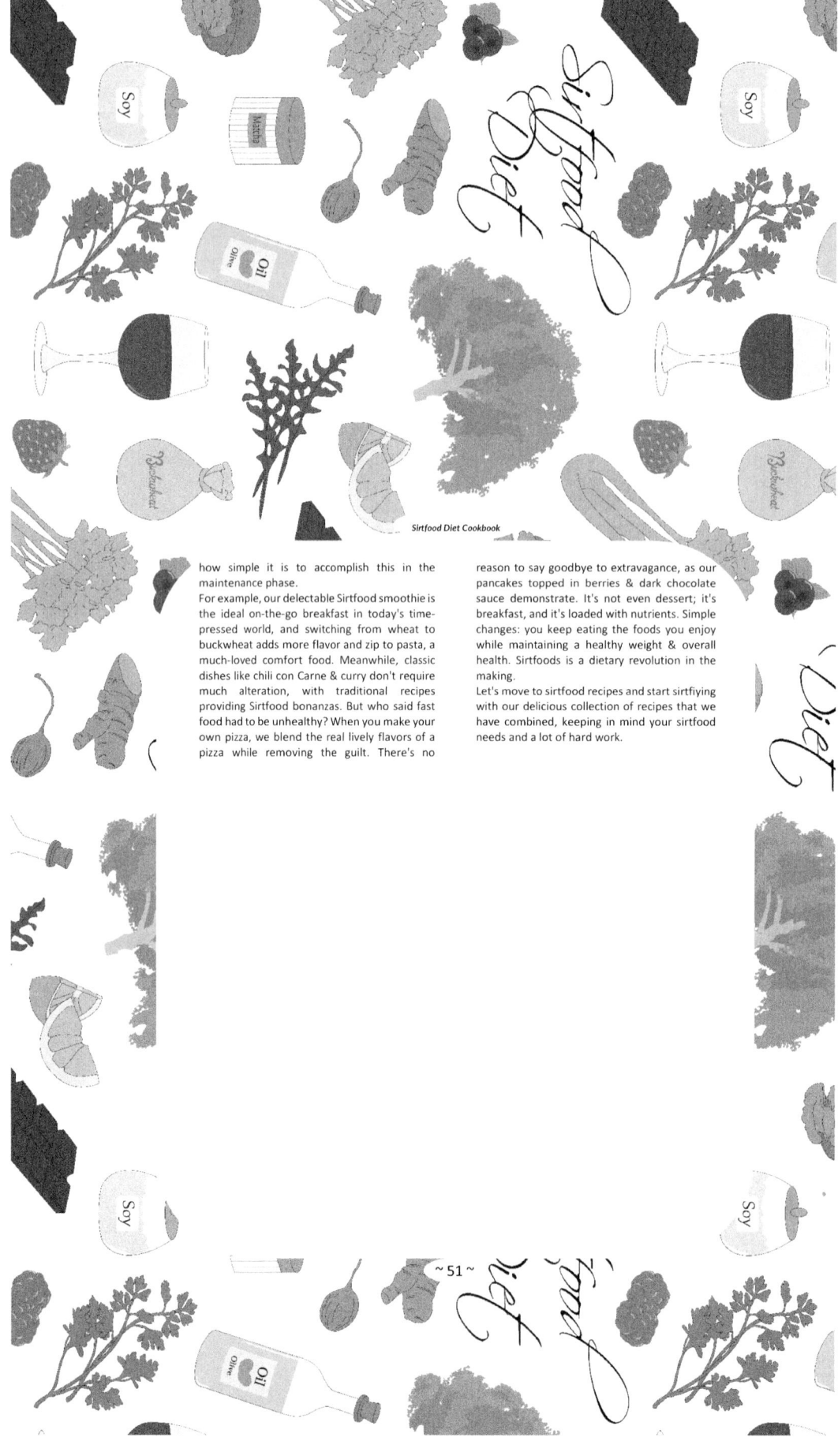

Sirtfood Diet Cookbook

how simple it is to accomplish this in the maintenance phase.

For example, our delectable Sirtfood smoothie is the ideal on-the-go breakfast in today's time-pressed world, and switching from wheat to buckwheat adds more flavor and zip to pasta, a much-loved comfort food. Meanwhile, classic dishes like chili con Carne & curry don't require much alteration, with traditional recipes providing Sirtfood bonanzas. But who said fast food had to be unhealthy? When you make your own pizza, we blend the real lively flavors of a pizza while removing the guilt. There's no reason to say goodbye to extravagance, as our pancakes topped in berries & dark chocolate sauce demonstrate. It's not even dessert; it's breakfast, and it's loaded with nutrients. Simple changes: you keep eating the foods you enjoy while maintaining a healthy weight & overall health. Sirtfoods is a dietary revolution in the making.

Let's move to sirtfood recipes and start sirtfiying with our delicious collection of recipes that we have combined, keeping in mind your sirtfood needs and a lot of hard work.

CHAPTER 7:

Vegetarian and Vegan Sirtfood Recipes

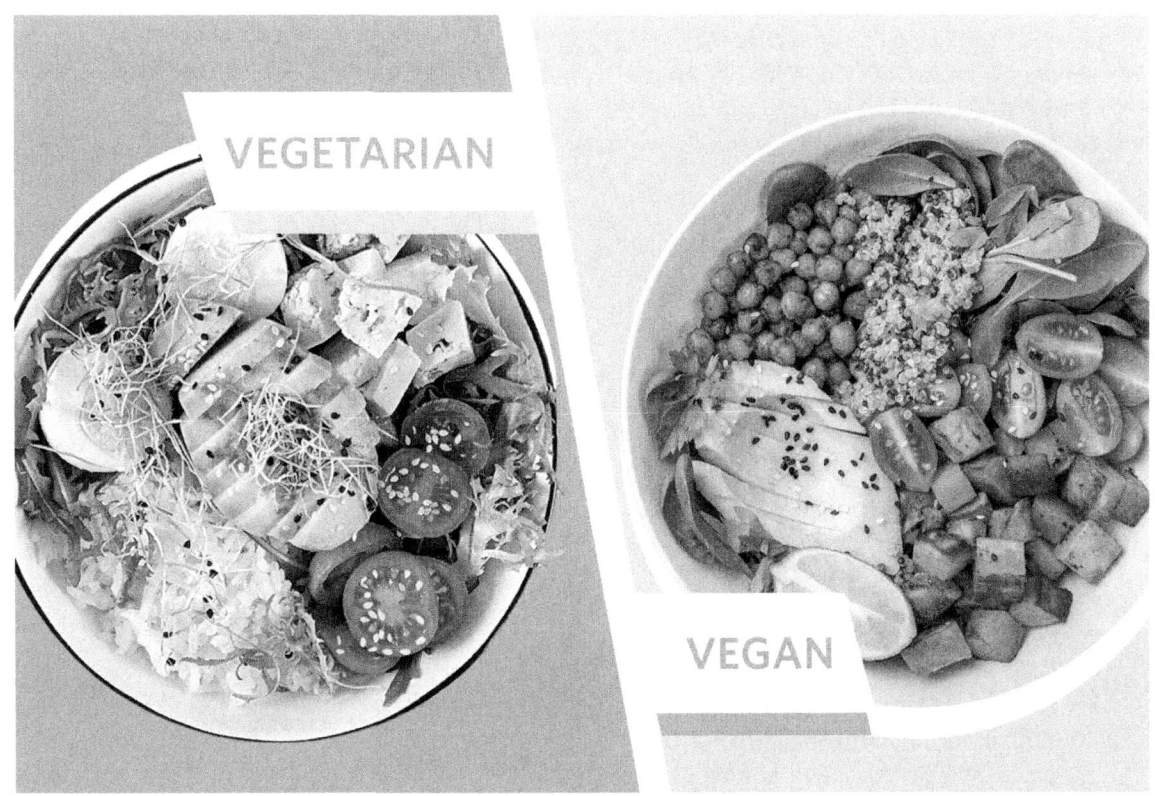

A vegetarian diet excludes all animal products, including meat and seafood. However, there are various variants on this: some vegetarians may eat eggs & dairy products, while others may forgo one or both.

A vegan diet is a type of vegetarianism in which only plant foods are consumed, and no animal products are consumed (meat, eggs, seafood, dairy & many times honey & gelatin).

Vegetarian diets have numerous health advantages. If properly prepared, they can deliver all of the required vitamins and minerals for long & healthy life.

In this chapter, you will find all the vegan and vegetarian recipes that include sirtfood. We have compiled these recipes especially for vegetarians so you can continue being vegetarian while on a sirtfood diet.

1. Broccoli with Pasta

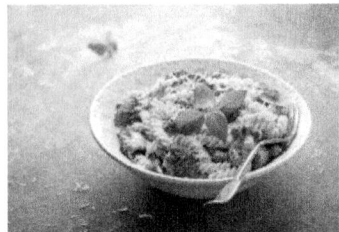

(Preparation time: 15 minutes | Cooking time: 25 minutes | Difficulty: Easy | Servings: 2)
Per serving: Calories 350, Total fat 8g, Protein 6g, Carbs 35g
Ingredients:

- ¼ teaspoon of crushed chilies
- 1 garlic clove, finely chopped
- 3 tablespoons of extra-virgin olive oil
- 2 scallions sliced - 1 cup of broccoli
- 12 sage shredded leaves
- Grated Parmesan (optional)
- 1 cup of buckwheat spaghetti

Instructions:

- Boil the broccoli for 5 minutes, then add the spaghetti and simmer till both the pasta and the broccoli are done (around 8 to 10 minutes).
- Meanwhile, into a frying pan, heat the oil, add the scallions & garlic.
- Cook for 5 minutes, or till golden brown.
- Add the chilies and sage to the pan and simmer for 1 minute on low flame. Drain pasta and broccoli and combine with scallion mixture in pan. Serve with a sprinkle of Parmesan cheese, if desired.

2. Apples and Cabbage Mix

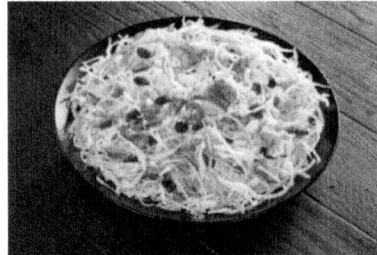

(Preparation time: 10 minutes | Cooking time: 0 minutes | Difficulty: Easy | Servings: 4)
Per serving: Calories 165, Total fat 8g, Protein 3g, Carbs 26g
Ingredients:

- Black pepper as required
- 2 tablespoons of Balsamic vinegar
- 2 tablespoons of Olive oil
- ½ teaspoon of caraway seeds
- 2 cored & cubed green apples
- 1 shredded red cabbage head

Instructions:

- Combine the cabbage, apples, and other ingredients into a mixing bowl, toss, & serve.

3. Kale and Artichoke with Walnuts

(Preparation time: 10 minutes | Cooking time: 30 minutes | Difficulty: Easy | Servings: 2)
Per serving: Calories 152, Total fat 32g, Protein 23g, Carbs 19g
Ingredients:

- Salt and black pepper, to taste
- 1 tablespoon of parsley, chopped
- ½ tablespoon of balsamic vinegar
- 1 tablespoon of olive oil
- 1 cup of artichoke hearts
- 1 cup of kale, torn
- 1 cup of Cheddar cheese, crumbled
- ½ cup of walnuts

Instructions:

- Preheat the oven at 250-270°F & roast the walnuts for around 10 minutes, or till lightly browned & crispy, before setting aside.
- In a pot, combine the artichoke hearts, kale, olive oil, salt, & black pepper and simmer for around 20 to 25 minutes till the artichoke hearts are tender.
- Stir in the cheese and balsamic vinegar. Serve the vegetables on two plates with toasted walnuts & parsley on top.

4. Carrot, Arugula, and Tomato Quinoa Pilaf

(Preparation time: 10 minutes | Cooking time: 30 minutes | Difficulty: Easy | Servings: 4)
Per serving: Calories 165, Total fat 4g, Protein 6g, Carbs 20g
Ingredients:

- 2 teaspoons of extra-virgin olive oil
- 1 tomato, chopped
- ½ red onion, chopped 1 carrot, chopped
- 2 cups of vegetable or chicken broth
- 1 cup of arugula - 1 cup of quinoa, raw
- 1 teaspoon of fresh lovage, chopped

Instructions:

- In a medium-sized saucepan, heat the olive oil and add the red onion. Cook and stir for 5 minutes, or till transparent. Reduce the flame to low, add the quinoa, then toast for 2 minutes, tossing constantly. Combine the broth, black pepper, & thyme.
- Bring them to a boil over high flame. Cover, reduce to low flame and cook for 5 minutes. Stir in the carrots, cover, & cook for another 10 minutes, or till all the water has been absorbed.
- Remove the pan from the heat and add the tomatoes, arugula, & lovage. Set aside for 5 minutes. Season to taste with salt and pepper.

5. Buckwheat with Green Onions and Mushrooms

(Preparation time: 10 minutes | Cooking time: 40 minutes | Difficulty: Easy | Servings: 4)
Per serving: Calories 340, Total fat 10g, Protein 11g, Carbs 31g
Ingredients:

- 2 teaspoons of extra-virgin olive oil
- 3 green onions, thinly sliced
- 2 cups of vegetable or chicken broth
- 1 cup of mushrooms, sliced

- 1 cup of buckwheat groats

Instructions:

- In a pot, combine all of the ingredients and cook on low flame for around 35 to 40 minutes, or till the broth is completely absorbed.
- Serve immediately by dividing the mixture between two dishes.

6. Kale Scramble

(Preparation time: 10 minutes | Cooking time: 20 minutes | Difficulty: Easy | Servings: 2)
Per serving: Calories 183, Total fat 14g, Protein 12g, Carbs 4g
Ingredients:

- 1 tablespoon of water
- 1/8 teaspoon of ground turmeric
- Salt & ground black pepper, to taste
- 2 teaspoons of olive oil - 4 eggs
- 1 cup of fresh kale, chopped

Instructions:

- In a mixing bowl, whisk together the eggs, turmeric, salt, black pepper, & water till frothy. Heat the oil in a pan on medium flame.
- Stir in the egg mixture till everything is well combined. Reduce the flame to medium-low and cook, constantly stirring, for 1 to 2 minutes. Cook, stirring regularly, for 3 to 4 minutes after adding the greens. Remove the pan out from the flame and serve right away.

7. Buckwheat Porridge

(Preparation time: 10 minutes | Cooking time: 15 minutes | Difficulty: Easy | Servings: 2)
Per serving: Calories 258, Total fat 5g, Protein 12g, Carbs 4g
Ingredients:

- 1 cup of water - ½ teaspoon of ground cinnamon
- 1 tablespoon of honey (optional)
- ½ teaspoon of vanilla extract
- ¼ cup fresh blueberries

- 1 cup of buckwheat, rinsed
- 1 cup of almond milk, unsweetened

Instructions:

- Bring all of the ingredients (save the honey and blueberries) to a boil in a saucepan on medium-high flame.
- Reduce the flame to low and cook for around 10 minutes, covered. Remove the pan from the flame and stir in the honey. Cover and set aside for around 5 minutes. Fluff the mixture with a fork before transferring it to serving bowls.
- Serve with blueberries on top.

8. Blueberry and Walnut Bake

(Preparation time: 10 minutes | Cooking time: 35 minutes | Difficulty: Easy | Servings: 2)

Per serving: Calories 208, Total fat 5g, Protein 15g, Carbs 4g

Ingredients:

- ½ teaspoon of vanilla extract
- 1 banana, ripe & mashed
- 1/2 cup of rolled oats
- To serve: ½ cup of plain yogurt
- 1 cup of blueberries - 1 1/2 cups of almond milk, unsweetened
- 2 tablespoons of walnuts, chopped

Instructions:

- Preheat the oven at 400°F.
- In a mixing dish, combine the oats, milk, blueberries, vanilla, banana, & walnuts. Cook for around 30 minutes on a baking tray coated using parchment paper.
- It can be consumed by itself or with 1/2 cup plain yogurt.

9. Flax Waffles

(Preparation time: 10 minutes | Cooking time: 15 minutes | Difficulty: Easy | Servings: 2)

Per serving: Calories 220, Total fat 4g, Protein 21g, Carbs 7g

Ingredients:

- ½ teaspoon of baking powder

- ¼ teaspoon of vanilla extract, unsweetened - 1 tablespoon of olive oil
- ½ tablespoon of flaxseed meal
- 2 tablespoons of honey, or a few stevia drops (optional)
- ½ cup of whole-wheat flour
- ½ cup of almond milk, unsweetened

Instructions:

- Preheat a tiny waffle machine for 5 minutes after turning it on. Meanwhile, in a mixing dish, combine all of the ingredients and blend with an immersion blender till smooth.
- Fill the waffle machine halfway with batter, close the top, and cook for 3 to 4 minutes, or till firm and golden brown.
- Serve immediately. Cool the waffles, then split them into two meal prep containers, evenly distribute the berries, and finish with agave syrup in mini-meal prep cups.
- Refrigerate for up to 5 days after covering each container with a lid.
- When you're ready to eat, leave them cold or reheat in the microwave for 40 to 60 seconds or till hot.

10. Green Omelet

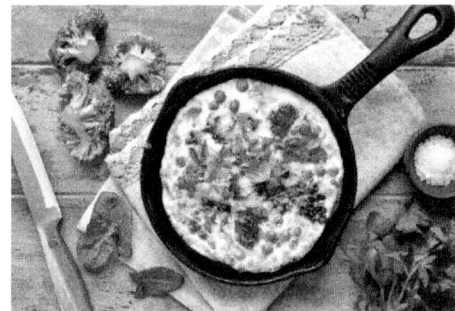

(Preparation time: 10 minutes | Cooking time: 10 minutes | Difficulty: Easy | Servings: 1)

Per serving: Calories 221, Total fat 28g, Protein 9g, Carbs 10g

Ingredients:

- Salt and freshly ground black pepper

- 1 teaspoon of olive oil
- 1 scallion peeled & finely chopped
- A handful of parsley, finely chopped
- A handful of arugula leaves - 2 eggs

Instructions:

- In a frying pan, heat the oil over medium-low heat. Add the scallion and cook for 5 minutes on low heat. Cook for another two minutes on high heat.
- Whisk the eggs in a cup or bowl, then spread the scallion in the pan before adding the eggs. By tipping the pan on all sides, evenly distribute the eggs.
- Cook for a minute before lifting the sides and letting the runny eggs to fall to the bottom of the pan.
- Season using pepper and salt to taste and top with arugula leaves and parsley.
- Tip the base onto a dish and serve immediately away when it begins to brown.

11. Kale and Mushroom Frittata

(Preparation time: 10 minutes | Cooking time: 30 minutes | Difficulty: Easy | Servings: 4)
Per serving: Calories 151, Total fat 10g, Protein 10g, Carbs 6g

Ingredients:

- Salt and ground black pepper, to taste
- 1 tablespoon of extra-virgin olive oil
- 1 garlic clove, minced
- 1 red onion, chopped - 8 eggs
- 1½ cups of fresh kale, chopped
- 1 cup of fresh mushrooms, chopped
- ½ cup of unsweetened almond milk

Instructions:

- Preheat the oven at 350ºF. In a mixing dish, whisk together the eggs, almond milk, salt, & black pepper. Remove from the equation. Heat the oil in an ovenproof pan over medium flame and sauté the onion and garlic for around 3–

4 minutes. Cook for 8–10 minutes after adding the kale salt and black pepper.

- Cook for 3–4 minutes after adding the mushrooms. Pour the egg mixture evenly over the top and simmer for 4 minutes without stirring. Place the pan in the oven and bake for around 12–15 minutes, or till done to your liking.
- Before serving, remove the pan from the oven and set it aside for 3–5 minutes.

12. Pancakes with Blackcurrants and Apples

(Preparation time: 10 minutes | Cooking time: 45 minutes | Difficulty: Easy | Servings: 4)
Per serving: Calories 270, Total fat 11g, Protein 29g, Carbs 6g

Ingredients:

- 3 tablespoons of water may use less
- 2 tablespoons of honey, or a few stevia drops (optional) - 2 egg whites
- 1 cup of whole-wheat flour
- 2 apples cut into small chunks
- 2 cups of quick-cooking oats
- 1 cup of blackcurrants, stalks removed
- 1 ¼ cups of almond milk, unsweetened
- Cooking spray

Instructions:

- In a small pot, combine the topping ingredients. Simmer. For about 10 minutes, often stir till it cooks down, and the juices are released. In a mixing dish, combine the dry ingredients.
- After that, add the apples and milk a little at a time till you have a batter (you may not need all of it). Whisk the egg whites till hard, then fold them into the pancake batter gently.
- Refrigerate till ready to use. When the pan is heated, spray it with cooking spray and spoon some of the batter into it in a pancake form. When the edges of

the pancakes begin to become golden brown, and air bubbles appear, they are ready to be flipped. Repeat with the remaining pancakes. Place a berry topping on top of each pancake.

13. Vegan Mac and Cheese
(Preparation time: 10 minutes | Cooking time: 45 minutes | Difficulty: Easy | Servings: 4)
Per serving: Calories 263, Total fat 14g, Protein 4g, Carbs 26g
Ingredients:
- 2 tablespoons of olive oil
- ½ teaspoon of chili flakes
- 1 ½ teaspoon of apple cider vinegar
- 3 cloves of garlic
- ½ teaspoon of garlic powder
- ½ teaspoon of mustard powder
- ½ teaspoon of onion powder
- ½ cup of nutritional yeast
- 1 white onion - 1 russet potato
- 1 head broccoli - 1 cup of cashews
- 2 cups of buckwheat macaroni

Instructions:
- Potatoes should be peeled and grated. Garlic should be finely diced. Over medium flame, heat the oil in a saucepan. Cook the onion in the pot with a pinch of salt till tender.
- In a large-sized pot, combine the potato, chili flakes, garlic, mustard, onion, & garlic powders. Stir well to unleash their flavors before adding one cup of water and the cashews. Continue to stir over a low flame till the potatoes are tender.ombine the entire mixture with the apple cider vinegar, nutritional yeast, salt, & pepper in a blender. The consistency should be thick but runny, like a cheese sauce. If it's too thick, thin it out with more water. If it needs extra salt, garlic powder, chili flakes, or vinegar, season it now to your liking.

- In a pot of salted water, cook the pasta. Boil the broccoli in bite-sized florets in a separate saucepan till cooked. When they're both done, combine them into one.

14. Buckwheat with Onions
(Preparation time: 10 minutes | Cooking time: 45 minutes | Difficulty: Easy | Servings: 4)
Per serving: Calories 132, Total fat 32g, Protein 22g, Carbs 24g
Ingredients:
- 3 cups of water
- Salt and pepper, to taste
- 1/4 cup of extra-virgin olive oil
- 1 white onion, chopped
- 4 red onions, chopped
- 3 cups of buckwheat, rinsed

Instructions:
- Soak the buckwheat for 10 minutes in warm water. Then, in your pot, add the buckwheat. Stir in the water, salt, & pepper thoroughly.
- Close the lid and cook till the buckwheat is done around 30-35 minutes. Meanwhile, heat the extra-virgin olive oil in a skillet and sauté the chopped onions for 15 minutes, or till they are transparent and caramelized.
- Mix with a pinch of salt and pepper. The buckwheat should be divided into four dishes or mugs. The onions should then be dolloped into each bowl. It's important to remember that this dish should be served hot.

15. Butternut Squash Alfredo
(Preparation time: 10 minutes | Cooking time: 30 minutes | Difficulty: Easy | Servings: 4)
Per serving: Calories 232, Total fat 14g, Protein 34g, Carbs 26g
Ingredients:
- 2 tablespoons of olive oil
- 1 teaspoon of paprika

- 2 cloves garlic
- 2 cups of vegetable broth
- 1 white onion
- 2 tablespoons of sage
- 1 cup of green peas
- 1 zucchini
- 3 cups of butternut squash, diced
- 1 1/4 cups of buckwheat linguine

Instructions:

1. In a medium-sized fry pan, heat the oil. While it's heating up, make sure the sage leaves are clean & dry before placing them in the oil to fry, moving them about so they don't burn.
2. Remove them and place them onto a paper towel.
3. Put the peeled and chopped squash, paprika, diced onion, & black pepper in a frying pan.
4. Cook till the onion has softened, then pour the broth and season using salt & pepper to taste.
5. Bring to the boil, then reduce to a low flame and allow the squash to finish cooking. Cook the linguine into the water with a pinch of salt in a separate saucepan.
6. Place the squash, along with all of the liquid & other ingredients, in a blender when it is tender. Blend till creamy, then taste to determine if you need additional salt, pepper, or spice.
7. Return it to the frying pan and keep it heated over low flame.
8. Grate the zucchini lengthwise with a grater to produce long noodles. To mix in with the linguine, make quite so many long ones as possible.
9. Add them to the sauce along with the green peas & simmer for five minutes in the butternut squash.
10. Before draining the pasta, save one cup of the cooking liquid. Toss in the linguine and toss thoroughly to coat the linguine.
11. Add a little pasta water if the sauce is too thick. Serve the spaghetti with sautéed sage leaves & a pinch of black pepper on top.

16. Quinoa, Chickpea and Turmeric Curry

(Preparation time: 10 minutes | Cooking time: 55 minutes | Difficulty: Easy | Servings: 4)
Per serving: Calories 309, Total fat 12g, Protein 23g, Carbs 26g
Ingredients:

- 3 teaspoons of ground turmeric
- 1 teaspoon of ground ginger
- 3 garlic cloves, crushed
- 1 tablespoon of tomato purée
- 1 can of tomatoes
- 1 lb. potatoes
- 2 cups of spinach
- 1 teaspoon of mild curry
- 1 can of chickpeas, drained
- 6 oz. quinoa
- 2 cups of coconut milk, unsweetened

Instructions:

- Place the potatoes in a pan, cover with cold water, and bring to the boil. Cook for around 25 minutes, or till tender (always check with a stick). Drain them thoroughly, then peel off the skin and set them aside.
- In a skillet, combine the garlic, turmeric, tomato purée, bean stew, ginger, coconut milk, and tomatoes. Bring to the boil, season using salt and pepper, and then add the quinoa and another cup of water.
- Reduce to a low flame, cover, and cook for 30 minutes, stirring regularly. Add the chickpeas halfway through the cooking process. Add the kale and

potatoes, coarsely chopped, when there are only 5 minutes left.

- Serve immediately after dividing into 4 servings.

17. Chili Wild Garlic and Sweet Corn Fritters

(Preparation time: 10 minutes | Cooking time: 15 minutes | Difficulty: Easy | Servings: 4)
Per serving: Calories 198, Total fat 7g, Protein 3g, Carbs 25g
Ingredients:

- Fry-light extra-virgin olive oil spray
- 1 Bird's Eye chili, finely chopped
- ¾ cup of wild garlic leaves and bulbs, finely diced - 3 eggs
- 2 cups of blettuce, chopped
- ¾ cup of whole-wheat flour
- 2 cups of tinned or frozen sweetcorn

Instructions:

- In a mixing dish, combine the eggs, flour, chili, sliced wild garlic, & sweetcorn; season using pepper and salt.
- Spray a nonstick frypan using cooking spray and heat on medium.
- Spoon the egg mixture into the frypan in batches with a spoon. Each individual will get two large fritters or four tiny fritters from the mixture.
- Fry the pancakes for 4 minutes on one side, then gently flip & fry for another 3 minutes till golden brown.
- Serve with a salad right away.

18. Red Onion and Kale Dhal with Buckwheat

(Preparation time: 10 minutes | Cooking time: 35 minutes | Difficulty: Easy | Servings: 2)
Per serving: Calories 273, Total fat 3g, Protein 8g, Carbs 21g
Ingredients:

- 2 teaspoons of turmeric

- 1 teaspoon of extra-virgin olive oil
- 1 clove of garlic, very finely chopped
- 1 teaspoon of very finely chopped ginger
- 1 teaspoon of mustard seeds
- 1 Thai chili, very finely chopped
- 1 teaspoon of curry powder
- 3 tablespoons of red onions, finely chopped
- 1 1/2 cups of vegetable broth
- 4 tablespoons of kale, chopped
- 4 tablespoons of red lentils
- 1/2 cup of buckwheat
- 4 tablespoons of coconut milk

Instructions:

1. In a medium-sized pan, heat the oil and add the mustard seeds. Add the onion, ginger, garlic, and chili when the seeds start to crack. Heat until all of the ingredients are tender.
2. Mix in the curry powder & turmeric well. Bring the vegetable stock to a boil, then remove it from the flame.
3. Cook the lentils for around 25 to 30 minutes, or till they are done. Simmer for 5 minutes after adding the greens and coconut milk. Prepare the buckwheat while the lentils are cooking. With the dahl, serve buckwheat.

19. Kale Chips

(Preparation time: 10 minutes | Cooking time: 15 minutes | Difficulty: Easy | Servings: 2)
Per serving: Calories 159, Total fat 8g, Protein 7g, Carbs 10g
Ingredients:

- 2 teaspoons of turmeric
- 1/2 tablespoon of garlic
- 2 tablespoons of extra-virgin olive oil
- 6 cups kale leaves, chopped
- 1 tablespoon of sesame seeds
- 1 tablespoon of soy sauce
- 1/4 tablespoon of poppy seeds

Instructions:

- Kale leaves should be washed and dried. Put them in a dish after cutting them into 2-inch pieces. To coat the kale, combine the olive oil & soy sauce and massage it in with clean hands. Mix in the sesame seeds, salt, garlic, poppy seeds, and pepper to taste.
- Cook the kale in the batches at 375°F for 5–6 minutes, or till crisp.

20. Pecan Dressing

(Preparation time: 10 minutes | Cooking time: 15 minutes | Difficulty: Easy | Servings: 6)
Per serving: Calories 199, Total fat 5g, Protein 18g, Carbs 15g
Ingredients:

- 1 1/2 teaspoon of salt
- 2 teaspoons of paprika
- 1/3 cup of olive oil
- 1 red onion diced
- 1 teaspoon of ground cumin
- 1/8 teaspoon of cayenne
- 1/2 teaspoon of thyme
- 1/2 teaspoon of oregano
- 1 green pepper diced
- 3 green onions diced
- 3 stalks celery diced
- 2 cups of pecans, chopped

Instructions:

- Green onions, celery, red onions, & bell pepper should be sautéed for 15 minutes in a saucepan with oil.
- Blend in the paprika, cumin, thyme, oregano, salt, cayenne, and pecans till smooth.
- With steamed rice, this dish is ideal.

21. Parsley and Coconut Chutney

(Preparation time: 10 minutes | Cooking time: 20 minutes | Difficulty: Easy | Servings: 4)
Per serving: Calories 199, Total fat 5g, Protein 18g, Carbs 16g

Ingredients:

- 2 tablespoons of lemon juice
- 1 teaspoon of extra-virgin olive oil
- 1-inch ginger, grated
- 1/ green chili, chopped
- 1 teaspoon of ground cumin
- 1 cup of parsley
- 1 cup of shredded coconut
- 1/3 cup of firm tofu, chopped

Instructions:

- In a blender, combine the 1/2 cup of water, lemon juice, tofu, coconut, cumin, parsley, ginger, green chili, & salt.
- Pulse till the mixture is reduced to a thick puree; if required, add a little more water.
- Fill a small-sized bowl halfway with the mixture.

22. Fragrant Asian Hot Pot

(Preparation time: 10 minutes | Cooking time: 20 minutes | Difficulty: Easy | Servings: 2)
Per serving: Calories 297, Total fat 15g, Protein 19g, Carbs 23g
Ingredients:

- 2 inch. ginger, sliced
- 1 teaspoon of tomato purée
- Juice of 1/2 lime
- 2 cups of vegetable stock
- 1-star anise, crushed
- 2 tablespoons of parsley, finely chopped
- ½ carrot, cut into matchsticks
- ½ cup of broccoli
- 1 tablespoon of miso paste
- 1/4 cup of bean sprouts
- 1/2 cup of tofu
- 4 tablespoons of buckwheat noodles
- 4 tablespoons chestnuts, cooked

Instructions:

- Into a saucepan, combine the tomato purée, star anise, parsley stalks, lime juice, & stock. Simmer for 10 minutes.

- Simmer gently till the beansprouts, broccoli, carrot, tofu, noodles, & chestnuts are done.
- Take the pan off the flame and mix in the miso paste. Serve with a garnish of parsley leaves.

23. Goat Cheese Salad with Walnut and Cranberries

(Preparation time: 10 minutes | Cooking time: 15 minutes | Difficulty: Easy | Servings: 2)
Per serving: Calories 250, Total fat 21g, Protein 20g, Carbs 3g
Ingredients:
- Salt and pepper to taste
- 2 teaspoons of extra-virgin olive oil
- 1 tablespoon of balsamic vinegar
- 1 teaspoon of mustard
- ½ cup of arugula
- ½ cup of baby spinach
- 1 cup of lettuce
- ½ cup of goat cheese
- 10 walnuts, chopped

Instructions:
- In a bowl, combine lettuce, arugula, & baby spinach. Combine the oil, mustard, salt, black pepper, & vinegar, then pour the dressing over the salad and toss thoroughly.
- Place on a serving platter. Top with crumbled goat cheese.
- Serve with cranberries & walnuts on top.

24. Green Veggies Curry

(Preparation time: 10 minutes | Cooking time: 35 minutes | Difficulty: Easy | Servings: 2)
Per serving: Calories 224, Total fat 24g, Protein 17g, Carbs 8g
Ingredients:
- 2 teaspoons of olive oil
- 1 teaspoon of garlic, minced
- 1 teaspoon of fresh ginger, minced

- 1 tablespoon of red curry paste or powder
- ½ bird's eye chili
- 1 teaspoon of fresh parsley, chopped finely
- 2 teaspoons of low-sodium soy sauce
- ¼ red onion, chopped
- 1 cup of broccoli florets
- 2 cups of spinach
- ½ cup of coconut cream

Instructions:
- In a skillet over medium flame, melt the olive oil & sauté the onion for 5 minutes. Stir in the garlic, chili, curry, and ginger until everything is well combined. Reduce the flame to low and simmer the broccoli for 5 minutes. Simmer for 10 minutes with the soy sauce & coconut cream. Cook, occasionally stirring, till the curry has reached the desired thickness, around 8 to 10 minutes. Remove from the flame and garnish with parsley before serving.

25. Arugula with Pine Nuts and Apples

(Preparation time: 10 minutes | Cooking time: 10 minutes | Difficulty: Easy | Servings: 4)
Per serving: Calories 121, Total fat 9g, Protein 3g, Carbs 8g
Ingredients:
- Salt and pepper to taste
- 2 cloves of garlic, slivered
- 2 tablespoons of extra-virgin olive oil
- 1 apple, peeled, cored, & chopped
- 2 tablespoons of pine nuts
- 1 1/4 cups of arugula

Instructions:
- In a skillet or wok, heat the olive oil over a low flame. Combine the pine nuts, garlic, and apple. Cook for 3 to 5 minutes, or till the nuts & garlic are brown, and the apple is just beginning

to soften. Raise the flame to medium-high and toss in the arugula. Cook for another 2 to 3 minutes, stirring occasionally. To taste, season using salt and pepper.

26. Italian Vegetable Salsa

(Preparation time: 10 minutes | Cooking time: 15 minutes | Difficulty: Easy | Servings: 4)
Per serving: Calories 132, Total fat 3g, Protein 4g, Carbs 7g
Ingredients:

- A pinch of black pepper
- ½ cup of garlic, minced
- 2 tablespoons of olive oil
- 1 teaspoon of Italian seasoning
- 2 red bell peppers, chopped
- 3 zucchinis, sliced

Instructions:

- Over medium-high flame, heat the oil in a pan, then add the bell peppers & zucchini, mix, & cook for around 5 minutes.
- Toss in the garlic, black pepper, & Italian seasoning, and simmer for another 5 minutes.
- In a food processor, blitz till completely smooth.

27. Broccoli Salad

(Preparation time: 10 minutes | Cooking time: 20 minutes | Difficulty: Easy | Servings: 2)
Per serving: Calories 230, Total fat 18g, Protein 10g, Carbs 25g
Ingredients:

- 1 tablespoon of Water
- 1 pinch of salt
- 1 teaspoon of mustard
- 1 / 2 red onion
- 2 carrots, grated
- 1 head of broccoli
- ¼ cup of red grapes
- 2 1 / 2 tablespoons of Coconut yogurt

Instructions:

- Cook for around 8 minutes after cutting the broccoli into florets. Thinly slice the red onion into half-rings. Cut the grapes in half. To prepare the dressing, combine coconut yogurt, water, & mustard with a touch of salt.
- To halt the cooking process, drain the broccoli, then rinse it with ice-cold water.
- In a bowl, combine the broccoli, carrot, onion, & red grapes. The dressing should be served separately on the side.

28. Vegetarian Meatballs

(Preparation time: 10 minutes | Cooking time: 40 minutes | Difficulty: Easy | Servings: 2)
Per serving: Calories 312, Total fat 8g, Protein 18g, Carbs 29g
Ingredients:

- ½ teaspoon of turmeric
- 1 teaspoon of ginger
- 2 cloves of garlic crushed
- 1 teaspoon of extra-virgin olive oil
- 1 egg
- 1 tablespoon of extra-virgin olive oil
- 1 tablespoon of parsley, chopped
- 1 red onion-diced
- 1 ½ tablespoons of garam masala
- 1 teaspoon of smoked paprika
- Broth (if needed)
- 1 cup of broccoli
- 1 cup of brown rice
- 1 cup of tomato sauce
- ¼ cup of whole-wheat breadcrumbs
- 1/3 cup of full-fat coconut milk

Instructions:

- After 5 minutes of steaming, puree the broccoli with the rice. To produce a result comparable to mince, use the pulse button. In a large mixing bowl, combine the egg, breadcrumbs, 1 garlic clove, paprika, salt, pepper, turmeric, & finely chopped parsley.

- Mix thoroughly till meatballs can be formed. Add 1 tablespoon of egg white & mix if it's too dry. If it's too runny, stir in 1 tablespoon of breadcrumbs. Coat a pan using cooking spray, heat it, and cook the meatballs gently for 5 minutes, or till browned. When turning them, be careful not to break them. Set them aside. Put oil, onion, salt, ginger, garlic, & pepper in a separate pan and simmer on low heat till the onion is done. Stir in the tomato sauce & coconut milk, and cook for around 15 minutes, or till the sauce has thickened. Cook for another 5 minutes before serving the meatballs in the sauce.

29. Veggie Fajitas

(Preparation time: 10 minutes | Cooking time: 20 minutes | Difficulty: Easy | Servings: 2)
Per serving: Calories 253, Total fat 5g, Protein 28g, Carbs 25g
Ingredients:

- 1 teaspoon of extra-virgin olive oil
- 2 tablespoons of black olives, finely chopped - 1 handful of parsley, chopped
- 1 carrot, grated
- ½ cup of cherry tomatoes halved
- 1 red onion - 2 whole-wheat tortillas
- 6 tablespoons of hummus
- 1/2 cup of tofu, sliced

Instructions:

- On medium flame, sauté the onion for 5 minutes with the olive oil, then add the tofu & heat for another 4 to 5 minutes.
- Heat the tortillas briefly in a pan (to keep them soft), then spread the hummus & top with the tofu and onions. Serve immediately with cherry tomatoes, carrots, parsley, & olives on top.

30. Tofu with Broccoli

(Preparation time: 10 minutes | Cooking time: 45 minutes | Difficulty: Easy | Servings: 2)
Per serving: Calories 298, Total fat 5g, Protein 27g, Carbs 35g
Ingredients:

- 1 teaspoon of olive oil
- Juice of ½ lemon
- 2 cloves of garlic
- 1 pinch of cumin
- 1 teaspoon of finely chopped ginger
- 2 teaspoons of turmeric
- 1 pinch of parsley
- 1 Thai chili, seeded
- 2 tablespoons of parsley, chopped
- 4 tablespoons of red onions, finely chopped
- ¼ cup of red pepper, seeded
- 2 tablespoons of sun-dried tomatoes, chopped - 1 cup of broccoli, chopped
- 1 cup of tofu

Instructions:

- Preheat the oven at 400°F. Slice the peppers and combine them with the chili and garlic in an ovenproof dish.
- Drizzle some olive oil over it, toss in the dried herbs, and bake for about 20 minutes, or till the peppers are tender.
- Allow cooling before combining the peppers with the lemon juice in a blender and blending till smooth.
- To make the triangles, cut the tofu in half and then in half again.
- Place the tofu in a casserole dish & top with the paprika mixture. Bake for around 20 minutes.
- Chop the broccoli into small pieces, about the size of a grain of rice. Then, in a saucepan with olive oil, heat the chili, garlic, onions, and ginger till they are transparent. Return to a high flame and stir in the turmeric and

cauliflower. Remove the pan from the flame and stir in the parsley and tomatoes. Mix thoroughly. Toss the tofu in the sauce before serving.

31. Celery and Raisins Snack Salad

(Preparation time: 10 minutes | Cooking time: 0 minutes | Difficulty: Easy | Servings: 2)
Per serving: Calories 120, Total fat 1g, Protein 5g, Carbs 6g
Ingredients:
- Salt and black pepper to taste
- 2 tablespoons of olive oil
- Juice of ½ lemon
- ¼ cup of parsley, chopped
- 4 cups of celery, sliced
- ½ cup of raisins
- ½ cup of walnuts, chopped

Instructions:
- Stir celery with parsley, raisins, walnuts, oil, lemon juice, and black pepper into a salad bowl, toss, and serve as a snack in tiny cups.

32. Cream of Kale and Broccoli Soup

(Preparation time: 10 minutes | Cooking time: 30 minutes | Difficulty: Easy | Servings: 4)
Per serving: Calories 207, Total fat 12g, Protein 9g, Carbs 15g
Ingredients:
- 1 tablespoon of olive oil
- 1 red onion, chopped
- 1 potato, peeled and chopped
- 1-pint of vegetable stock
- 1 cup of broccoli
- 1 cup of kale
- ½ pint of almond milk

Instructions:
- In a saucepan, heat the olive oil, then add the onion & simmer for 5 minutes. Cook for 5 minutes after adding the potato, kale, & broccoli.

- Simmer for around 20 minutes after adding the stock and milk.
- Blitz the soup in a food processor till it's smooth and creamy. Add salt & pepper to taste. Serve right away.

33. Carrot, Walnut and Apple Soup

(Preparation time: 10 minutes | Cooking time: 35 minutes | Difficulty: Easy | Servings: 4)
Per serving: Calories 194, Total fat 4g, Protein 16g, Carbs 18g
Ingredients:
- 2 tablespoons of extra-virgin olive oil
- 1 white onion, chopped
- 1 potato, diced
- 1 apple, diced
- 1 lb. of carrots, chopped
- 2 pints of vegetable stock
- 4 tablespoons of walnuts, chopped

Instructions:
- In a pot with oil, sauté the vegetables for around 5 minutes, stirring regularly.
- Season using salt and pepper and add the stock. Bring to the boil, then reduce to a low flame and cook for around 30 minutes, or till the veggies are tender. Blend till smooth in a food processor, then serve.

34. Quinoa Pilaf

(Preparation time: 10 minutes | Cooking time: 30 minutes | Difficulty: Easy | Servings: 4)
Per serving: Calories 165, Total fat 4g, Protein 6g, Carbs 20g
Ingredients:
- 2 teaspoons of extra-virgin olive oil
- A pinch of cinnamon
- 1 teaspoon of fresh lovage, chopped
- ½ red onion, chopped
- 1 tomato, chopped
- 1 carrot, chopped
- 1 cup of arugula
- 1 cup of quinoa, raw

- 2 cups of vegetable or chicken broth

Instructions:
- In a medium-sized saucepan, heat the olive oil, then add the red onion. Cook and stir for 5 minutes, or till transparent.
- Reduce the flame to low, add the quinoa, and toast for 2 minutes, tossing constantly. Combine the broth, black pepper, & thyme.
- Bring everything to the boil over high flame. Cover, reduce to low flame and cook for 5 minutes.
- Toss in the carrots, cover, & cook for another 10 minutes, or till all the water has been absorbed.
- Remove the pan from the flame and add the tomatoes, arugula, and lovage. Set aside for 5 minutes. Season to taste with salt and pepper. Sprinkle with a pinch of cinnamon.

35. Broccoli and Walnut Soup

(Preparation time: 10 minutes | Cooking time: 20 minutes | Difficulty: Easy | Servings: 4)
Per serving: Calories 240, Total fat 5g, Protein 3g, Carbs 2g
Ingredients:
- ½ teaspoon of turmeric
- 1 tablespoon of olive oil
- 1 red onion, chopped
- 2 cups of vegetable stock
- 1 lb. of broccoli, chopped
- 1/2 cup of double heavy cream
- 8 walnut halves, chopped

Instructions:
- Into a saucepan, heat the oil, then add the broccoli & red onion and cook, constantly stirring, for around 4 minutes. Bring the stock to the boil, then reduce to a low flame and simmer for 15 minutes. Combine the double heavy cream & the turmeric.

- Blitz the soup in a food processor till it's smooth and creamy.
- Serve in dishes with a sprinkle of chopped walnuts on top.

36. Stir-Fried Tofu and Veggies in Ginger Sauce

(Preparation time: 15 minutes | Cooking time: 30 minutes | Difficulty: Medium | Servings: 4)
Per serving: Calories 258, Total fat 7g, Protein 28g, Carbs 18g
Ingredients:
- 1-2 teaspoon of ginger, grated
- 2 tablespoons of olive oil
- 1 red onion, chopped
- 3/4 cup of lemon juice
- 3/4 cup of soy sauce
- 1 green pepper, chopped
- 2 green onions, chopped
- 3 carrots, chopped
- 1 cup of broccoli florets
- 1 cup of cauliflower florets
- 1 cup of snow peas
- 1 cup of mushrooms, chopped
- 1 lb. of extra firm tofu
- 2 cups of cooked brown rice

Instructions:
- Combine the soy sauce, lemon juice, & ginger in a bowl and pour over the tofu.
- Allow 45 minutes for marinating. Save the marinade after draining the tofu. In a skillet, heat the oil and add the cauliflower, green pepper, broccoli, carrots, onion, and tofu, stirring to combine.
- Cooking evenly requires constant stirring. Mix the snow peas, mushrooms, & green onions.
- Stir constantly till the vegetables are cooked but still crisp, about 5 minutes.
- Serve over rice with the marinade on top.

37. Quinoa Salad

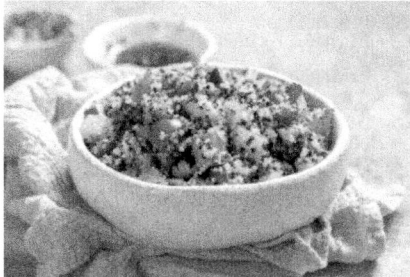

(Preparation time: 10 minutes | Cooking time: 25 minutes | Difficulty: Easy | Servings: 4)
Per serving: Calories 199, Total fat 5g, Protein 18g, Carbs 15g
Ingredients:

- 1 pinch of cumin
- 2 tablespoons of extra-virgin olive oil
- 2 sprigs of fresh basil, chopped
- 1/2 red pepper, finely diced
- 1 tomato, diced
- 2 stems of green onions, finely chopped
- 1/4 cup of parsley, chopped
- 1/8 cup of red wine vinegar
- 1/4 cup of corn - 1 cup of quinoa

Instructions:

- Rinse quinoa completely in cold water. Cook quinoa for around 25 minutes in 2 cups of salted water. Set them aside.
- Avoid over stirring the quinoa since it will get mushy. Toss in the chopped veggies. Combine the remaining ingredients and stir lightly.

38. Sirt Fruit Salad

(Preparation time: 10 minutes | Cooking time: 0 minutes | Difficulty: Easy | Servings: 1)
Per serving: Calories 110, Total fat 1g, Protein 2g, Carbs 15g
Ingredients:

- 1 teaspoon of honey
- 1 apple, cored and roughly chopped
- 1 orange, halved
- 1/2 cup of matcha green tea
- 10 red seedless grapes - 10 blueberries

Instructions:

- Allow 1/2 cup of green tea to cool before adding the honey.
- Add half an orange juice once it's cold.
- Slice the remaining half and combine with the chopped blueberries, apple, and grapes in a bowl. Cover with tea and chill for at least 30 minutes before serving.

39. Simple Arugula Salad

(Preparation time: 10 minutes | Cooking time: 0 minutes | Difficulty: Easy | Servings: 4)
Per serving: Calories 200, Total fat 2g, Protein 7g, Carbs 5g
Ingredients:

- 1 tablespoon of lemon juice
- 2 garlic cloves, peeled and minced
- 2 tablespoons of extra-virgin olive oil
- 2 tablespoons of parsley, chopped
- 1 tablespoon of red wine vinegar
- 1 red onion, chopped - 2 cups of arugula
- ¼ cup of walnuts, chopped

Instructions:

- Mix the water & vinegar in a dish, then add the onion and set it aside for 5 minutes before draining well. Blend the arugula, walnuts, & onion in a salad bowl and swirl to combine.
- Toss thoroughly with the garlic, salt, parsley, pepper, lemon juice, and oil, and serve.

40. Stir Fried Smoky Tofu

(Preparation time: 10 minutes | Cooking time: 30 minutes | Difficulty: Easy | Servings: 4)
Per serving: Calories 372, Total fat 8g, Protein 26g, Carbs 20g
Ingredients:

- 2 tablespoons of extra-virgin olive oil
- 2 chilies - 6 garlic cloves, chopped
- 1-inch ginger, peeled and diced
- 1 dash of liquid smoke - 2 green onions

- 1 red bell pepper, chopped
- 1 zucchini, chopped
- 1/2 cup of buckwheat noodles
- 2 cups of baby corn
- 2 broccolis, chopped
- 3 celery stalks, chopped
- 4 carrots peeled and chopped
- 1 lb. of extra-firm tofu, cubed
- 1 cup of snow peas, trimmed

Instructions:

- A kettle of water should be brought to a boil. Stir in the bean threads, remove from the flame, and leave aside to soak till the stir-fry is finished.
- Green onions, white & light green portions should be sliced into 3/4-inch thick slices. Green portions should be thinly sliced. In a skillet, heat a few tablespoons of oil. In a wok, combine the chilies, garlic, and ginger. Allow 1 minute of stir-frying Cook for around 3 minutes after adding the carrots. Stir in the celery & green onions for another 2 minutes.
- Cook the tofu in a heated pot with oil & liquid smoke for around 6 to 8 minutes, till it begins to brown.
- In a sauté pan or wok, combine the zucchini, baby corn, snow peas, and bell pepper. Mix in the broccoli and cook for 2 minutes, or till the florets begin to turn green.
- In a pot of salted water, boil the noodles for 5 minutes. Drain and toss with the stir fry before serving.

41. Kale Green Bean Casserole

(Preparation time: 10 minutes | Cooking time: 35 minutes | Difficulty: Easy | Servings: 4)
Per serving: Calories 130, Total fat 6g, Protein 2g, Carbs 12g
Ingredients:

- 2 cups of green beans, chopped

- ¼ cup of capers, drained
- 1 cup of mushrooms, chopped
- 2 cups of kale, chopped
- 1 cup of sour cream
- ¼ cup of walnuts, crushed
- 1 ½ cups of almond milk

Instructions:

- Preheat the oven at 375°F and butter a casserole dish lightly.
- In a mixing bowl, combine the milk & sour cream.
- Combine the mushrooms, green beans, kale, & capers. Spoon into the casserole dish & top with walnuts that have been smashed. Bake for around 40 minutes, uncovered, in a preheated oven till bubbling and browned on top.

42. Arugula Salad with Nuts and Fruits

(Preparation time: 10 minutes | Cooking time: 0 minutes | Difficulty: Easy | Servings: 1)
Per serving: Calories 160, Total fat 7g, Protein 3g, Carbs 20g
Ingredients:

- 1 tablespoon of extra-virgin olive oil
- 1 spring of fresh basi
- ½ red onion
- 2 tablespoons of red wine vinegar
- ½ cup of arugula
- ½ peach
- ¼ cup of blueberries
- 5 walnuts, chopped

Instructions:

- Remove the seed from the peach and cut it in half. Preheat a grill pan & grill it from both sides for a few minutes. Thinly slice the red onion into half-rings. Chop the pecans coarsely.
- Warm a pan and toast the pecans in it till fragrant. Spread peaches, blueberries, red onions, and roasted pecans over the arugula on a platter.

- In a food processor, combine all of the dressing ingredients and blend till smooth. Drizzle the dressing over the salad and toss to combine.

43. Kale, Edamame and Tofu Curry

(Preparation time: 10 minutes | Cooking time: 1 hour | Difficulty: Medium | Servings: 4)

Per serving: Calories 225, Total fat 6g, Protein 28g, Carbs 47g

Ingredients:

- 1 teaspoon of salt - Juice of 1 lime
- 1 tablespoon of extra-virgin olive oil
- 1 Bird's Eye chili, thinly sliced
- 4 cloves of garlic, peeled and grated
- 1 3-inch fresh ginger, peeled and grated
- 1/2 teaspoon of ground turmeric
- 1 teaspoon of paprika
- 1/2 teaspoon of ground cumin
- 1/4 teaspoon of cayenne pepper
- ½ cup of parsley stalks removed
- 1 big onion, chopped
- 2 tomatoes, roughly chopped
- 1 cup of dried red lentils
- 1/4 cup of soya edamame beans
- 1 cup of firm tofu, cubed

Instructions:

- In a medium-sized pan, heat the oil. Add the onion to the boiling oil & cook for around 5 minutes. Cook for another 2 minutes after adding the ginger, garlic, & chili.
- Combine the turmeric, cumin, cayenne, paprika, and salt. Then stir and mix the soya edamame beans, red lentils, and tomatoes. Pour in 4 cups of boiling water and bring to a simmer for around 10 minutes, then reduce to a low flame and cook for another 40 minutes, or till the curry thickens and all flavors are combined.
- Stir in the lime juice & parsley before serving.

44. Mexican-Style Casserole

(Preparation time: 10 minutes | Cooking time: 40 minutes | Difficulty: Easy | Servings: 2)

Per serving: Calories 253, Total fat 5g, Protein 28g, Carbs 22g

Ingredients:

- 1 garlic clove
- ½ bird's eye chili
- ½ red onion
- 1 tablespoon of paprika
- 1/2 cup of black beans, rinsed
- 2 cups of spinach
- ½ cup of buckwheat
- 1 cup of soy mince, ready to cook
- 1 cup of shredded cheddar

Instructions:

- Buckwheat should be boiled for around 25 minutes before being rinsed and set aside.
- Oil should be heated in a pan. Cook for 5 minutes after adding the onion, garlic, & chili. Cook for around 10 minutes, frequently stirring, after adding the soy mince and spices. Cook for another 3 minutes after adding the spinach.
- Fill a baking dish halfway with buckwheat, then halfway with soy mince.
- Spread the cheese over the top & bake for around 10 minutes, or till melted.

45. Turmeric Zucchini Soup

(Preparation time: 10 minutes | Cooking time: 20 minutes | Difficulty: Easy | Servings: 2)

Per serving: Calories 141, Total fat 11g, Protein 4g, Carbs 7g

Ingredients:

- 1 tablespoon of extra-virgin olive oil
- 2 teaspoons of turmeric powder
- 2 tablespoons of lime juice
- 1 tablespoon of mild curry powder
- 3 cloves of garlic, diced
- 1 tablespoon of fresh parsley

- ¼ teaspoon of white pepper
- 1 teaspoon of fish sauce
- 1 red onion, diced
- 3 zucchinis, cubed
- 1 cup of vegetable stock
- 1 cup of coconut milk

Instructions:

- Melt the olive oil in a saucepan over medium flame. When the pan is hot, add the onion & cook for around 5 minutes, stirring regularly, till golden and tender.
- Combine the garlic, zucchini, & salt. To combine with the onion, stir.
- Stir in the pepper, curry powder, & turmeric for a few seconds to release the flavors. Stir in the fish sauce, coconut milk, & vegetable stock till thoroughly combined.
- Allow it to boil, then turn the flame down to low. Simmer for around 10 minutes with the lid on.
- Stir in the lime juice till it is completely dissolved. Add a few fresh parsley leaves as a finishing touch.

46. Buckwheat Noodles with Walnut Sauce

(Preparation time: 10 minutes | Cooking time: 20 minutes | Difficulty: Easy | Servings: 4)
Per serving: Calories 316, Total fat 6g, Protein 7g, Carbs 13g

Ingredients:

- 1 dash cayenne - 1-inch ginger, grated
- 1 tsp. chili powder
- 2 tbsp. rice vinegar
- 4 tbsp. soy sauce
- 1/2 lb. cooked buckwheat spaghetti
- 1/2 cup walnuts

Instructions:

- Bring a pot with salted water to a boil, then add the spaghetti and cook till it is al dente (around 8 minutes).

- Blend the walnuts with 1/2 cup of lukewarm water in a blender till smooth. Mix in the soy sauce, chili powder, ginger, rice vinegar, and cayenne pepper.
- Drain the spaghetti and place it in a bowl when it's done. Mix in the walnut sauce & toss well till the pasta is fully coated.

47. Celery and Blue Cheese Soup

(Preparation time: 10 minutes | Cooking time: 30 minutes | Difficulty: Easy | Servings: 3)
Per serving: Calories 240, Total fat 16g, Protein 31g, Carbs 21g

Ingredients:

- 2 tablespoons of butter
- 1 red onion, chopped
- 1 head of celery
- 1½ pints of chicken stock
- 1/2 cup of blue cheese
- 1/2 cup of single cream

Instructions:

- In a saucepan, melt the butter and add the onion & celery, cooking till the veggies are softened.
- Bring the stock to a boil, then reduce to a low flame & simmer for 15 minutes.
- Add in the cream & continue to stir till the cheese has melted.
- Serve and eat as soon as possible.

48. Brunoise Salad

(Preparation time: 10 minutes | Cooking time: 0 minutes | Difficulty: Easy | Servings: 2)
Per serving: Calories 84, Total fat 3g, Protein 1g, Carbs 3g

Ingredients:

- ½ lemon - 2 tablespoons of olive oil
- 1 tomato - 1 zucchini - ½ red onion
- 3 sprigs of fresh parsley
- ½ red bell pepper
- ½ yellow bell pepper

Instructions:

- To make a brunoise, finely dice the tomatoes, peppers, zucchini, and red onions. In a mixing bowl, combine all of the cubes.
- Chop the parsley and toss it in with the salad. Pour the olive oil over the salad & squeeze the lemon over it. Add salt & pepper to taste.

49. Cinnamon-Scented Quinoa

(Preparation time: 10 minutes | Cooking time: 20 minutes | Difficulty: Easy | Servings: 4)
Per serving: Calories 160, Total fat 3g, Protein 6g, Carbs 24g

Ingredients:

- 1 ½ cup of water
- 2 cinnamon sticks - Agave syrup
- Chopped walnuts
- 1 cup of quinoa

Instructions:

- Wash the quinoa in a dish till the water runs clear. Drain it using a fine-mesh strainer.
- Use a trivet and a steaming basket to prepare your pressure cooker. Pour the water over the quinoa and cinnamon sticks in the basket.
- Close the lid and secure it. Cook for 6 minutes on high pressure. Once the cooking time is up, use the quick-release method to relieve the pressure.
- Remove the cinnamon sticks and fluff the quinoa using a fork. Serve the cooked quinoa with agave syrup & chopped walnuts in serving bowls.

50. Kale and Shiitake Mushrooms

(Preparation time: 10 minutes | Cooking time: 40 minutes | Difficulty: Easy | Servings: 4)
Per serving: Calories 124, Total fat 2g, Protein 9g, Carbs 15g

Ingredients:

- 3 tablespoons of extra-virgin olive oil
- 3 garlic cloves, minced
- 2 cups of red onions, chopped
- 1 cup of kale
- 4 cups of vegetable broth
- 2 lbs. of dry shiitake mushrooms

Instructions:

- Put the oil, garlic, onion, & kale in a pan over medium flame and cook for a few minutes to soften.
- Sauté the mushrooms for 2 minutes. Bring the stock to a boil, then reduce to a low flame and leave to simmer for 30 minutes.
- Serve right away.

51. Miso Caramelized Tofu

(Preparation time: 10 minutes | Cooking time: 40 minutes | Difficulty: Easy | Servings: 2)
Per serving: Calories 101, Total fat 5g, Protein 4g, Carbs 12g

Ingredients:

- 1 garlic clove, finely chopped
- 1 teaspoon of ground turmeric
- 1 Bird's Eye chili
- 1 teaspoon of fresh ginger, finely chopped
- 2 teaspoons of extra-virgin olive oil
- 2 teaspoons of sesame seeds
- 1 tablespoon of mirin
- 1 tablespoon of miso paste
- 1 teaspoon of tamari (or soy sauce)
- 4 tablespoons of red onion
- 1/4 cup of celery, trimmed
- 1/2 cup of kale, chopped
- 1 1/4 cups of firm tofu
- 1/2 cup of zucchini
- 1/4 cup of buckwheat

Instructions:

- Preheat the oven at 400°F. Using parchment paper, cover a tray. Combine the mirin & miso in a mixing bowl. Toss the tofu in the mirin-miso mixture and let it marinade. To make lengthy slices, cut the vegetables (excluding the kale) at a diagonal angle.

- Cook the kale for 5 minutes in a steamer and set aside. Sprinkle sesame seeds over the tofu and spread them out on the prepared tray. Cook for 20 minutes, or till the sugars have caramelized. Using a sieve and running water, rinse the buckwheat.
- Cook the buckwheat as per the packet instructions in a pan of boiling water with turmeric.
- In a skillet, heat the oil over a high flame. Fry for 2 to 3 minutes after tossing in the vegetables, herbs, & spices. Reduce the flame to medium and cook for another 5 minutes, or till the chicken is done but still crisp.

52. Spicy Asian Buckwheat Noodle Soup

(Preparation time: 10 minutes | Cooking time: 30 minutes | Difficulty: Easy | Servings: 2)
Per serving: Calories 220, Total fat 3g, Protein 25g, Carbs 20g
Ingredients:

- Juice of ½ lime
- 1 teaspoon of extra-virgin olive oil
- 1 clove of garlic, minced
- 1 chunk of ginger, diced
- ½ Bird's Eye chili pepper
- 1 teaspoon of sesame seeds
- 1 tablespoon of soy sauce
- 1 red onion
- 2 stalks of celery, chopped
- 1 cup of arugula
- 5 cups of vegetable stock
- ¼ cup of basil leaves, chopped
- 1 package of buckwheat noodles
- ¼ cup of walnuts

Instructions:

- Cook the noodles according to the package directions and set them aside.

Sauté all of the vegetables, garlic, ginger, chili, & almonds in a skillet over very low flame for around 10 minutes.

- Simmer for additional 5 minutes after adding the stock.
- Cut the noodles into small enough pieces to comfortably consume in a soup. Remove the soup from the flame, stir in the sesame seeds and lime juice. Serve the dish warm.

53. Dijon Celery Salad

(Preparation time: 10 minutes | Cooking time: 0 minutes | Difficulty: Easy | Servings: 4)
Per serving: Calories 125, Total fat 2g, Protein 7g, Carbs 7g
Ingredients:

- Black pepper to taste
- ½ cup of lemon juice
- 2/3 cup of olive oil
- 1 bunch of celery roughly chopped
- 2 apples, cored, peeled, & cubed
- 1/3 cup of Dijon mustard
- ¾ cup of walnuts, chopped

Instructions:

- Mix celery & its leaves with apple slices and walnuts in a salad bowl.
- Whisk together the black pepper, mustard, lemon juice, and olive oil, then add to your salad, toss, and serve in tiny cups.

54. Kale, Apple and Fennel Soup

(Preparation time: 10 minutes | Cooking time: 20 minutes | Difficulty: Easy | Servings: 4)
Per serving: Calories 165, Total fat 9g, Protein 3g, Carbs 20g
Ingredients:

- 1 tablespoon of olive oil
- 2 tablespoons of fresh parsley, chopped
- 2 apples, chopped
- 1 cup of fennel, chopped

- 1 lb. of kale, chopped

Instructions:

- In a saucepan, heat the oil, then add the kale & fennel. Cook for around 5 minutes or till the fennel has softened. Combine the apples & parsley. Cover with the hot water, once come to the boil, and then reduce to a low flame for 10 minutes.
- In a food processor, puree the soup till it is smooth. Add s alt & pepper to taste.

55. Moroccan Spiced Eggs

(Preparation time: 10 minutes | Cooking time: 45 minutes | Difficulty: Easy | Servings: 2)

Per serving: Calories 316, Total fat 6g, Protein 7g, Carbs 13g

Ingredients:

- ½ teaspoon of salt
- 1 teaspoon of extra-virgin olive oil
- ¼ teaspoon of ground cinnamon
- ¼ teaspoon of ground cumin
- 1 garlic clove, finely chopped
- 1 tablespoon of parsley
- 1 tablespoon of tomato paste
- 4 eggs
- 1 scallion, finely chopped
- ½ teaspoon of mild curry
- 1 red bell pepper, finely chopped
- 1 zucchini, finely chopped
- 1 can of tomatoes
- 1 can of chickpeas, drained

Instructions:

- In a pan, heat the oil; add the scallion & red bell pepper and cook for around 5 minutes on low flame. Cook for 2 minutes after adding the garlic and zucchini. Stir in the tomato paste, spices, & salt.
- Bring the tomatoes and chickpeas to a simmer over medium flame. Cover and cook for 30 minutes, or till the sauce has thickened.

- Remove the pan from the flame and stir in the chopped parsley. Preheat the grill at 350°F.
- In a baking dish, spread the tomato sauce and crack the eggs in the center. Serve after putting the tray underneath the grill for around 10 minutes.

56. Energy Cocoa Balls

(Preparation time: 10 minutes | Cooking time: 0 minutes | Difficulty: Easy | Servings: 2)

Per serving: Calories 132, Total fat 5g, Protein 4g, Carbs 20g

Ingredients:

- 1 tablespoon of peanut butter
- 4 Medjool dates, pitted
- 20 almonds
- Cocoa powder for coating

Instructions:

- Combine all of the ingredients in a blender, then chill for 30 minutes. Coat the balls in cocoa powder once they've been formed. Return them to the refrigerator for another 4 hours before eating.

57. Anasazi Bean Soup

(Preparation time: 10 minutes | Cooking time: 2 hours | Difficulty: Easy | Servings: 4)

Per serving: Calories 199, Total fat 5g, Protein 18g, Carbs 20g

Ingredients:

- 1 Bird's Eye chili, finely chopped
- 1/4 teaspoon of parsley
- 1/2 teaspoon of cumin
- 2 garlic cloves - pressed or diced
- 1 red onion - chopped
- 1 handful of parsley, chopped
- 1 cup of Anasazi beans, dry–soaked overnight
- 6 cups of vegetable stock

Instructions:
- Bring the stock to the boil in a pot with the cumin, beans, onion, garlic, and chili. Simmer for 2 hours on low flame or till beans are soft.
- Season to taste using salt and pepper, and serve immediately with parsley on top.

58. Tofu and Mushroom Scramble

(Preparation time: 10 minutes | Cooking time: 20 minutes | Difficulty: Easy | Servings: 1)
Per serving: Calories 333, Total fat 23g, Protein 21g, Carbs 15g
Ingredients:
- 1 teaspoon of ground turmeric
- 1 teaspoon of extra-virgin olive oil
- 1 teaspoon of mild curry powder
- A few parsley leaves, finely chopped
- 2 tablespoons of red onion, thinly sliced
- 1/2 cup of tofu, extra firm
- 1/2 cup of kale, roughly chopped
- 1/2 cup of mushrooms, thinly sliced

Instructions:
- Place 2 sheets of the kitchen towel under & on top of the tofu, then place a heavy object, such as a saucepan, on top of the tofu to ensure the liquid drains away. To make a paste, combine the curry powder, turmeric, & 1 to 2 teaspoons of water. Cook kale for around 3 to 4 minutes into a steamer.
- Warm the oil in a skillet over medium flame. Cook for several minutes, or till chilies, mushrooms, & onion are golden and soft. Toss the tofu in the skillet after breaking it up into small pieces. Stir in the spice paste to ensure that everything is uniformly coated.
- Cook for 5 minutes, or till the tofu is golden brown. Cook for another 2 minutes after adding the kale. Before serving, garnish with parsley.

59. Greek-Style Salad Skewers

(Preparation time: 10 minutes | Cooking time: 0 minutes | Difficulty: Easy | Servings: 2)
Per serving: Calories 236, Total fat 21g, Protein 7g, Carbs 14g
Ingredients:
- Juice of 1/2 lemon
- 1/2 teaspoon of garlic, crushed
- 1 tablespoon of extra-virgin olive oil
- 1 teaspoon of balsamic vinegar
- ½ red onion, split into 8 wedges
- 8 cherry tomatoes
- 1 yellow pepper, cut into 8 squares
- 1 cucumber, cut into 8 pieces
- 8 big black olives
- 1/2 cup of feta, cut into 8 cubes

Instructions:
- On the skewers, arrange the salad components as follows: cherry tomato, yellow pepper, cucumber, red onion, feta, and black olive.
- Place each skewer on a serving platter and repeat.
- Put olive oil, balsamic vinegar, a pinch of salt and pepper, lemon juice, & crushed garlic in a bowl as a dressing. Drizzle over the skewers after whisking thoroughly.

60. Kale Quiche

(Preparation time: 10 minutes | Cooking time: 40 minutes | Difficulty: Easy | Servings: 2)
Per serving: Calories 353, Total fat 5g, Protein 28g, Carbs 20g
Ingredients:
- ½ cup of water
- 1 small pinch of baking soda
- 2 tablespoons of extra-virgin olive oil
- 3 eggs
- 1 tablespoon of parmesan
- 1/2 cup of whole-wheat flour
- 4 tablespoons of buckwheat flour

- 6 tablespoons of almond flour
- 1 cup of ricotta cheese
- 3 cups of kale

Instructions:

- Combine the flours, salt, & baking soda in a mixing bowl. Mix in the water till you have a dough. Add more water if necessary. Allow 30 minutes for the dough to rest.
- Preheat the oven at 350°F. Heat the oil in a skillet, add the kale and salt, and simmer for 5 minutes over low flame. Set them aside.
- When the dough is finished, roll it out to a thickness of 1/8 inch and place it in a baking pan. Fill the tin with a mixture of ricotta, pepper, eggs, salt, & kale.
- With a knife, cut away any excess dough. Bake for around 35 minutes in the oven. Allow 10 minutes for cooling before serving.
- In an airtight container, store the remaining dough in the fridge or freezer.

61. Brussels Sprouts Egg Skillet

(Preparation time: 10 minutes | Cooking time: 15 minutes | Difficulty: Easy | Servings: 2)
Per serving: Calories 194, Total fat 11g, Protein 7g, Carbs 15g
Ingredients:

- 1 teaspoon of extra-virgin olive oil
- 1 red onion, chopped
- 4 eggs
- 10 cherry tomatoes, halved
- ½ lb. of Brussels sprouts halved

Instructions:

- Heat olive oil in an 8-inch cast-iron pan on medium flame.
- Sauté for around 1-2 minutes after adding the onion.

- Season using salt and pepper to taste after adding the Brussels sprouts and tomatoes.
- Cook for around 3-4 minutes, then break the eggs, cover, & continue to cook till the egg whites have set and the egg yolk has reached the desired consistency.

62. Pesto Green Beans

(Preparation time: 10 minutes | Cooking time: 15 minutes | Difficulty: Easy | Servings: 2)
Per serving: Calories 280, Total fat 10g, Protein 5g, Carbs 14g
Ingredients:

- ¼ teaspoon of black pepper
- Juice of 1 lemon
- 2 tablespoons of Extra-virgin olive oil
- 2 teaspoons of sweet paprika
- 1 sliced red onion
- 2 tablespoons of basil pesto
- 1 lb. of trimmed and halved green beans

Instructions:

- Over medium-high flame, heat the oil in a pan; add the onion, stir, & cook for 5 minutes. Toss in the beans & the remaining ingredients, cook for 10 minutes over medium flame, then divide across plates and serve.

63. Corn Veggie Chowder

(Preparation time: 10 minutes | Cooking time: 35 minutes | Difficulty: Easy | Servings: 4)
Per serving: Calories 204, Total fat 3g, Protein 3g, Carbs 20g
Ingredients:

- 1 cup of water
- 2 tablespoons of olive oil
- 1 red onion, diced
- 1 teaspoon of paprika
- 1/4 teaspoon of cayenne
- 2 stalks of celery, diced
- 1 red bell pepper, diced

- 2 potatoes, diced - 4 cups of corn
- 3 cups of soy milk

Instructions:

- Blend two cups of corn with soy milk and set them aside. For 10 minutes, sauté onion, bell pepper, and celery in oil.
- Cook, frequently stirring, for around 15 minutes after adding the potatoes.
- Reduce the flame to low and cook for 10 minutes, adding the corn mixture, the remaining 2 cups of corn, cayenne, & paprika.

64. Creamy Leek and Potato Soup

(Preparation time: 10 minutes | Cooking time: 25 minutes | Difficulty: Easy | Servings: 4)

Per serving: Calories 197, Total fat 5g, Protein 18g, Carbs 15g

Ingredients:

- 8 cups of water
- 2 tablespoons of extra-virgin olive oil
- 4 cups of potatoes, diced
- 2 to 3 leeks, diced
- ½ stalk celery, finely chopped
- 1/4 lb. of mushrooms, chopped
- 1 1/2 cups of firm tofu

Instructions:

- Cook the potatoes into salted water for around 14 minutes or till they are tender. Heat the oil in a skillet and sauté the mushrooms & leeks for around 5 minutes, then pour 1/4 cup of water and cook for another 6 to 8 minutes, till tender.
- Return the tofu to the pot and cook for 3 minutes over medium flame. To taste, season using salt and pepper.

65. Sprouts and Apples Salad

(Preparation time: 10 minutes | Cooking time: 0 minutes | Difficulty: Easy | Servings: 4)

Per serving: Calories 120, Total fat 2g, Protein 6g, Carbs 8g

Ingredients:

- Black pepper to the taste
- 1 garlic clove, crushed
- 1 red onion, chopped
- ½ cup of olive oil
- 3 tablespoons of red wine vinegar
- 1 tablespoon of mustard
- 1 apple, cored and cubed
- 1 lb. of Brussels sprouts, shredded
- 1 cup of walnuts, chopped

Instructions:

- Combine sprouts, onion, apple, and walnuts in a salad bowl.
- In a separate dish, whisk together the vinegar, garlic, mustard, oil, & pepper. Pour this into your salad, toss well, and serve.

66. Sweet and Sour Pan with Walnuts

(Preparation time: 10 minutes | Cooking time: 25 minutes | Difficulty: Easy | Servings: 4)

Per serving: Calories 373, Total fat 28g, Protein 15g, Carbs 40g

Ingredients:

- ¼ cup of water 2 tablespoons of olive oil
- 1 1/2 tablespoon of tomato paste
- ¼ cup of apple cider vinegar
- 2 red onions - 2 yellow bell pepper
- 1 1/2 cups of white cabbage
- 1/2 cup of bok choy
- 4 tablespoons of mung bean sprouts
- 4 pineapple slices
- 4 tablespoons of walnuts
- 4 tablespoons of coconut sugar
- 1 teaspoon of coconut-aminos
- 2 teaspoons of arrowroot powder

Instructions:

- Cut the vegetables into rough pieces. Make a paste with the arrowroot & five tablespoons of cold water. Then, in a saucepan, combine all of the sauce's other components, along with the arrowroot paste for the binding.

- In a pan, melt the olive oil and cook the onion. Stir in the bell pepper, bok choy, cabbage, and bean sprouts till the veggies have softened somewhat.
- Stir in the pineapple & cashew nuts a few times more. Serve with a dollop of sauce on top of the wok dish.

67. Romaine Hearts with Candied Pecan

(Preparation time: 10 minutes | Cooking time: 15 minutes | Difficulty: Easy | Servings: 4)
Per serving: Calories 210, Total fat 7g, Protein 13g, Carbs 20g
Ingredients:

- 1 teaspoon of extra-virgin olive oil
- 3/4 tablespoon of balsamic vinegar
- 1 teaspoon of Dijon mustard
- 1 teaspoon of each chopped fresh parsley and basil - 1/2 cup of pecans
- 3 tablespoons of olive oil 2 teaspoons of agave syrup 2 romaine hearts, chopped
- 1/2 cup of tofu

Instructions:

- Combine the pecans, agave syrup, and 1 tablespoon of oil in a preheated 375°F oven for around 10 minutes, or till lightly toasted. Allow cooling at room temperature before serving. In a salad bowl, whisk together the vinegar, pepper, mustard, salt, & parsley. Mix in the olive oil in a slow, steady stream. Toss in the romaine and coat well. Pecans and crumbled tofu are sprinkled on top.
- Serve right away.

68. Sweet Potato Soup with Ginger and Orange

(Preparation time: 10 minutes | Cooking time: 35 minutes | Difficulty: Easy | Servings: 6)
Per serving: Calories 168, Total fat 4g, Protein 5g, Carbs 20g

Ingredients:

- 1/2 teaspoon of salt - 1/4 teaspoon of pepper - 1 tablespoon of extra-virgin olive oil - 2 cloves of garlic, diced
- 1-1/2 tablespoons of ginger, grated
- 1 teaspoon of ground cumin
- Fresh parsley, chopped. - 1 tablespoon of orange zest 1-1/2 cups of red onions, chopped 5 cups of vegetable broth
- 6 cups of sweet potato, diced

Instructions:

- A shallow baking pan should be greased. Combine the yams, olive oil, onions, and garlic. Stir everything together thoroughly. Roast for around 25 minutes at 425°F, uncovered. Halfway through the cooking time, stir one more.
- Shift into a soup pot. Combine the broth, salt, orange zest, clove, ginger root, cumin, and pepper. Bring them to the boil. Reduce flame to medium-low & cook for 10 minutes, covered. Transfer the soup to a blender or food processor in stages and puree till smooth. Garnish with fresh parsley & serve immediately.

69. Asparagus Seitan with Black Bean Sauce

(Preparation time: 10 minutes | Cooking time: 30 minutes | Difficulty: Easy | Servings: 5)
Per serving: Calories 340, Total fat 5g, Protein 18g, Carbs 20g
Ingredients:

- 1 teaspoon of water
- 1 tablespoon of extra-virgin oil
- 2 cloves garlic, diced or crushed
- 1 tablespoon of soy sauce
- 1 teaspoon of cornstarch
- 1/2 cup of veggie broth
- 2 teaspoons of black beans, mashed
- 1 lb. of asparagus into 1-inch pieces

- 2 cups of seitan, sliced
- 2 teaspoons of red wine

Instructions:

- In a mixing dish, combine the seitan slices, red wine, 1 teaspoon of water, 1 teaspoon of cornstarch, and 1 teaspoon of soy sauce.
- When the oil is hot, add onion, garlic, & crushed black beans to the skillet. Over a high flame, sauté for 1 minute. Cook for another 4 minutes, or till the seitan is golden on all sides.
- Stir-fry the asparagus for 5 minutes in the pan. Reduce the flame to low, add 4 tablespoons of water, and then let the sauce thicken for 2 to 3 minutes due to the cornstarch. Serve immediately.

70. Buckwheat and Strawberry Pancakes

(Preparation time: 10 minutes | Cooking time: 25 minutes | Difficulty: Easy | Servings: 4)
Per serving: Calories 180, Total fat 8g, Protein 7g, Carbs 21g
Ingredients:

- 1 egg
- 1 teaspoon of olive oil
- 1 teaspoon of olive oil for frying
- 1 orange, juiced
- 1/2 cup of strawberries, chopped
- 1/2 cup of buckwheat flour
- 1 cup of almond milk

Instructions:

- In a mixing bowl, combine the milk, egg, and a teaspoon of olive oil. In a separate bowl, sift the flour into the liquid mixture till it is smooth and creamy.
- Allow 15 minutes for it to rest. In a pan with a little oil, heat a quarter of the mix or the size you desire.
- Into the batter, add a quarter of the strawberries. Cook each side for around 2 minutes.

- Serve immediately with a squeeze of orange juice.
- Other berries, including blueberries and blackberries, can be used in this recipe.

71. Peanut Topped Greens

(Preparation time: 10 minutes | Cooking time: 20 minutes | Difficulty: Easy | Servings: 6)
Per serving: Calories 230, Total fat 8g, Protein 14g, Carbs 22g
Ingredients:

- 1/4 teaspoon of salt
- 1/8 teaspoon of black pepper
- 2 tablespoons of extra-virgin olive oil
- 1/4 teaspoon of turmeric
- 2 teaspoons of ground cumin
- 1 tablespoon of ginger, diced
- 1 whole dried red chili
- 1 teaspoon of green chili, chopped
- 1 bay leaf
- 6 cups of mixed greens: kale, spinach, chard, collard, etc.
- 1/2 cup of soy milk
- ¼ cup of peanuts
- 1/4 cup of walnuts, chopped

Instructions:

- Greens should be steamed till tender, then pureed in a blender. Set them aside. In a skillet, heat the oil over medium-low flame. Fry the bay leaf & red chili till they are tender.
- Add the red chili flakes. Green chili, ginger, cumin, turmeric, black pepper, and salt should all be added at this point. Cook, frequently stirring, till the soymilk has reduced to roughly half its original volume, cook for around 3 to 5 minutes. Add the greens that have been pureed. Cover and cook on low flame for around 3 to 5 minutes to heat through and stir in the flavors. Remove the pan from the flame.
- Top with a sprinkling of peanuts.

72. Mushroom and Tomato Risotto

(Preparation time: 10 minutes | Cooking time: 30 minutes | Difficulty: Easy | Servings: 4)
Per serving: Calories 304, Total fat 5g, Protein 14g, Carbs 20g
Ingredients:

- 4 teaspoons of extra-virgin olive oil
- 2 cloves of garlic, crushed
- 1 teaspoon of thyme - 1 red onion, chopped - 1 teaspoon of oregano
- 7 cups of boiling broth
- 1 lb. of tomatoes, peeled and chopped
- 4 cups of mushrooms, chopped
- 2 1/2 cups of long-grain brown rice

Instructions:

- Half the onion should be sautéed for 5 minutes in a pot with 2 teaspoons of oil. Add the rice & toast it over high flame for around 2 to 3 minutes. Cook for around 5 minutes after adding the mushrooms. Stir in half of the boiling liquid and cook for around 50 minutes (time will based on the variety of the brown rice). When the previous ladle of broth has been absorbed, add another ladle. The rice will not overcook & will not be runny as a result of this method.
- Sauté the remaining garlic and onions in a separate pan. Season using salt and pepper to taste, then reduce to a low flame and cook for at least 25 minutes, or till sauce thickens.
- Just before removing the sauce from the flame, add the thyme and oregano, then toss with the rice. Mix thoroughly, then set aside for a few minutes to allow the flavors to meld.

73. Veggie Stroganoff

(Preparation time: 10 minutes | Cooking time: 25 minutes | Difficulty: Easy | Servings: 4)
Per serving: Calories 59, Total fat 1g, Protein 5g, Carbs 10g

Ingredients:

- 2 cups of boiling water
- 1 teaspoon of extra-virgin olive oil
- 1 teaspoon of dry mustard
- 2 tablespoons of tomato paste
- 1 red onion, thinly chopped
- 1/2 lb. of white button mushrooms, chopped
- 2 cups of Portobello mushrooms, sliced and grilled
- 1/3 cup of dry red wine

Instructions:

- In a skillet with oil, cook the onion & white mushrooms till the onion begins to soften.
- Stir in the grilled mushrooms and cook for 5 minutes. Along with the wine, add the tomato paste. Allow for evaporation. Add the boiling water to the pan along with the mustard.
- Simmer for 5 minutes over medium-low flame. Serve right away.

74. Veggie Soup

(Preparation time: 10 minutes | Cooking time: 45 minutes | Difficulty: Easy | Servings: 6)
Per serving: Calories 89, Total fat 2g, Protein 3g, Carbs 10g

Ingredients:

- Salt and black pepper to taste
- 1 celery stalk - 1 handful of parsley
- 1 bay leaf
- 1 cup of yellow split peas, dried
- 1/2 cup of parsnips, grated
- 1/2 cup of carrots, grated

Instructions:

- Cook the split peas for around 40 minutes in 4 cups water.
- Add the parsnips, salt, carrots, & bay leaf halfway through the cooking time. Simmer with the lid slightly closed.
- Before serving, remove the bay leaf. Serve after blending till smooth.

75. Baked Cabbage with Walnuts and Buckwheat

(Preparation time: 10 minutes | Cooking time: 25 minutes | Difficulty: Easy | Servings: 4)
Per serving: Calories 199, Total fat 5g, Protein 18g, Carbs 15g
Ingredients:

- 1 cup of boiling water
- 2 tablespoons of extra-virgin olive oil
- 1 onion, finely chopped
- 1 cup of vegetable stock
- 1 lb. of white or green cabbage, finely chopped
- 2 cups of buckwheat, cooked
- 4 tablespoons of walnuts
- 4 tablespoons of raisins

Instructions:

- In a small amount of olive oil, cook the finely chopped onion till it is transparent. Stir the cabbage, then the stock, seasoning to taste with salt and black pepper.
- Simmer on low flame for around 20 minutes, or till the cabbage is still crunchy.
- Transfer the cabbage to an oven-safe baking dish. Cook the buckwheat in salted water while the cabbage is cooking, then drain and add in the walnuts and raisins.
- Cook for around 20 minutes at 350°F with the buckwheat spread over the cabbage.

76. Raspberry Parfait

(Preparation time: 10 minutes | Cooking time: 20 minutes | Difficulty: Easy | Servings: 2)
Per serving: Calories 239, Total fat 10g, Protein 34g, Carbs 10g
Ingredients:

- ½ teaspoon of vanilla extract, unsweetened

- 3 tablespoons of agave syrup
- 3 tablespoons of chia seeds
- 2 ½ tablespoons of shredded coconut
- 1/2 cup of raspberries
- 1 cup of almond milk, unsweetened

Instructions:

- Place the chia and coconut in a medium-sized mixing bowl; add the agave syrup & vanilla, then pour in the milk and stir till thoroughly combined. Allow 30 minutes for the mixture to rest before stirring it and chilling it for at least 3 hours or overnight.
- To make the parfait, pour 1/2 of the chia mixture into the bottom of a serving glass, then top with three-quarters of the raspberries evenly.
- Cover the berries with the remaining chia seed mixture, then top with the remaining berries. Serve immediately.
- Layer parfait in wide-mouth pint jars, cover tightly using lids, and preserve in the refrigerator for up to 7 days.
- Once you're ready to eat, serve it chilled.

77. Mushroom and Buckwheat Soup

(Preparation time: 10 minutes | Cooking time: 30 minutes | Difficulty: Easy | Servings: 6)
Per serving: Calories 139, Total fat 3g, Protein 16g, Carbs 18g
Ingredients:

- 3 tablespoons of extra-virgin olive oil
- 1 onion, chopped
- 3 bay leaves
- 1 leek, chopped
- 1 carrot, chopped
- 8 cups of vegetable broth
- 1 lb. of white potatoes, peeled and diced
- 2 cups of buckwheat, cooked

Instructions:

- Separate the mushroom tops from the stems. Remove the caps and set them aside. Remove the stems.
- In a saucepan, heat extra-virgin olive oil on medium-high flame. Sauté the mushroom stems, onion, & leek for around 8 minutes, or till soft. Combine the vegetable broth, barley, potatoes, carrots, and bay leaves.
- Cover and cook for around 10 minutes, stirring occasionally. Remove the lid from the soup and add the cut mushroom caps & buckwheat. Cook for around 10 minutes before serving, seasoning using salt and pepper.

78. Minestrone Soup

(Preparation time: 10 minutes | Cooking time: 40 minutes | Difficulty: Easy | Servings: 4)
Per serving: Calories 147, Total fat 4g, Protein 6g, Carbs 20g
Ingredients:

- 2 tablespoons of extra-virgin olive oil
- 1 garlic clove, chopped
- 1 tablespoon of basil
- 2 tablespoons of parsley, chopped
- 1 tomato, chopped
- 1 cup of red onion
- 3 carrots, chopped
- 1 head of cabbage chopped
- 1/2 cup of celery, chopped
- 2 white turnips, chopped
- 2 cups of white beans, cooked
- 1 lb. can of tomatoes
- 1 cup of buckwheat short pasta

Instructions:

- Fry the garlic, cabbage, & onion in the oil in a soup pot.
- Add the beans, carrots, celery, turnips, tomatoes with 4 cups of water. Bring to the boil, then reduce the flame to low

and simmer for 30 minutes, or till vegetables are tender.
- After that, add the beans and pasta and cook for another 8 minutes, or till the pasta is done.

79. Peppers and Squash Soup

(Preparation time: 10 minutes | Cooking time: 35 minutes | Difficulty: Easy | Servings: 6)
Per serving: Calories 44, Total fat 30g, Protein 8g, Carbs 2g
Ingredients:

- ½-gallon water
- 1 tablespoon of extra-virgin olive oil
- 1 teaspoon of oregano
- 1 teaspoon of red cayenne pepper
- 1 teaspoon of basil
- 1 teaspoon of dill - 1 red onion, chopped
- 2 Roma tomatoes, diced
- 1/2 cup of chopped green peppers
- 1/2 cup of chopped red peppers
- 1/2 lb. of chickpeas, cooked
- 2 cups of butternut squash, chopped
- 2 cups of mushrooms, chopped
- 1/2 cup of buckwheat, cooked

Instructions:

- Bring the bring to the boil in a large pot. Simmer for 30 minutes with mushrooms, onion, peppers, salt, tomatoes, butternut squash, and pepper. Heat through the chickpeas, buckwheat, oregano, cayenne, and basil. Serve with a drizzle of olive oil on top.

80. Fried Cauli Rice

(Preparation time: 10 minutes | Cooking time: 25 minutes | Difficulty: Easy | Servings: 2)
Per serving: Calories 230, Total fat 17g, Protein 5g, Carbs 17g
Ingredients:

- 1⁄2 lemon, juiced
- 2 tablespoons of olive oil

- 1 teaspoon of chili flakes
- 4 cloves of garlic
- 2-inch ginger
- 2 tablespoons of fresh parsley
- 1 red onion
- 1 cauliflower
- 1/2 carrot
- 1/2 red bell pepper
- ¼ cup of vegetable broth
- 2 tablespoons of pumpkin seeds

Instructions:

- Using a food processor, shred the cauliflower into rice grains.
- Chop the carrot into thin strips, dice the bell pepper, & finely chop the herbs. Finely slice the onion, garlic, & ginger. In a pan, melt 1 tablespoon of olive oil, put 1/2 of the garlic and onions, and sauté till transparent.
- Season using salt and cauliflower rice. Pour in the stock and cook, constantly stirring, till the liquid has evaporated & the cauliflower rice is soft.
- Remove the rice from the pan and place it aside. In the same pan, melt the remaining olive oil & add the remaining onions, garlic, carrots, ginger, & peppers. Cook for a few minutes, or till the vegetables are cooked through. Season using a pinch of salt.
- Return the cauliflower rice to the pan, reheat the entire meal, and squeeze in the lemon juice.
- Before serving, garnish with pumpkin seeds & parsley.

81. Cajun Flavored Grilled Veggies

(Preparation time: 10 minutes | Cooking time: 35 minutes | Difficulty: Easy | Servings: 4)
Per serving: Calories 95, Total fat 7g, Protein 2g, Carbs 8g
Ingredients:

- ¼ cup of extra-virgin olive oil

- 1/2 teaspoon of cayenne pepper
- 1 teaspoon of Cajun seasoning
- 1 tablespoon of Worcestershire sauce
- 2 red onions, sliced into ½" wedges
- 2 zucchini cut into 1/2-inch slices
- 2 yellow squash, cut into 1/2-inch slices

Instructions:

- Combine olive oil, cayenne pepper, Cajun seasoning, & Worcestershire sauce into a mixing bowl. Add the zucchinis, onions, & yellow squash. Drizzle with the olive oil combination. Season using salt to taste.
- Refrigerate the vegetables for at least 30 minutes after covering the bowl. Preheat an outside grill to high heat and brush the grate gently using oil. Using skewers or direct on to the grill, place marinated vegetable pieces. Cook for another 5 minutes or till done.

82. Roasted Tomato Soup

(Preparation time: 10 minutes | Cooking time: 1 hour 10 minutes | Difficulty: Easy | Servings: 4)
Per serving: Calories 149, Total fat 5g, Protein 6g, Carbs 15g
Ingredients:

- 6 cups of water
- 6 tablespoons of extra-virgin olive oil
- 2 garlic cloves - 1 tablespoon of paprika
- 1 cup of parsley leaves
- 3 red peppers, halved and seeded
- 4 leeks, chopped
- 3 sun-dried tomatoes, puréed
- 2 lbs. of tomatoes, halved
- 2 cups of tomato juice
- 4 tablespoons of soy milk
- 1 cup of red wine

Instructions:

- Preheat the oven at 450°F. Toss tomatoes, 3 tablespoons of olive oil, garlic, leeks, peppers, and salt to taste in a mixing dish.

- Spread them out on a baking sheet in a single thin layer and roast for around 45 minutes, or till tender and charred.
- Allow cooling. In a soup saucepan, combine the vegetables, water, wine, sun-dried tomatoes, tomato juice, and paprika. Bring to the boil, then reduce to a low flame and cook for around 30 minutes. Add the milk and puree till fully smooth in a food processor. Season using salt and black pepper to taste, then garnish with parsley.

83. Guacamole

(Preparation time: 15 minutes | Cooking time: 0 minutes | Difficulty: Easy | Servings: 4)
Per serving: Calories 244, Total fat 25g, Protein 3g, Carbs 35g
Ingredients:
- ½ lime, juiced
- 1 garlic clove
- 3 tablespoons of olive oil
- 5 1/3 tablespoons of fresh parsley
- ½ white onion - 1 tomato, diced
- 2 ripe avocados

Instructions:
- Avocados should be peeled and mashed using a fork. Add the onion to the mashed potatoes, grated or finely chopped. Add the lime juice after squeezing it.
- Toss in the tomato, olive oil, & parsley, finely chopped. Mix well after seasoning using salt and black pepper.
- Refrigerate the sauce for at least 10 minutes to allow the flavors to blend.

84. Salsa Verde

(Preparation time: 10 minutes | Cooking time: 0 minutes | Difficulty: Easy | Servings: 4)
Per serving: Calories 323, Total fat 37g, Protein 1g, Carbs 2g
Ingredients:
- ½ teaspoon of ground black pepper

- 1 teaspoon of sea salt
- ½ lemon, juiced
- ¾ cup of olive oil
- 2 cloves of garlic, crushed
- 3 tablespoons of fresh basil, finely chopped
- 2 tablespoons of capers
- ½ cup of fresh parsley, finely chopped

Instructions:
- In a large-sized mixing bowl, combine all of the ingredients and blend with an immersion blender till the sauce reaches the desired consistency.
- The sauce can be kept in the refrigerator for up to 4-5 days or frozen.

85. Creamy Cashew Dressing

(Preparation time: 10 minutes | Cooking time: 0 minutes | Difficulty: Easy | Servings: 6)
Per serving: Calories 199, Total fat 5g, Protein 18g, Carbs 20g
Ingredients:
- 2 tablespoons of lemon juice
- 1 clove of garlic 1/2 cup of green onions
- 1 cup of walnuts, soaked for 4 hours
- 2 cups of cashews, soaked for 4 hours

Instructions:
- Cashews, walnuts, lemon juice, garlic, green onions, & salt should all be blended together till smooth. To use the sauce in salads, thin it with water. To season pasta dishes, keep it thick.

86. Louisiana Mushroom Sauce

(Preparation time: 10 minutes | Cooking time: 10 minutes | Difficulty: Easy | Servings: 2)
Per serving: Calories 199, Total fat 5g, Protein 18g, Carbs 20g
Ingredients:
- 2 tablespoons of extra-virgin olive oil
- 1 onion, diced - 1 pinch of cayenne
- 2 tablespoons of tamari
- 2 cups of mushrooms, chopped

- 3 tablespoons of almond butter
- 1/2 cup of walnuts, soaked

Instructions:

- For 10 minutes, sauté the onion & mushrooms in oil. Mix in the almond butter, tamari, cayenne pepper, and walnuts, then blend till smooth. To make a thinner sauce, add a little water.

87. Pistachio Dressing

(Preparation time: 10 minutes | Cooking time: 0 minutes | Difficulty: Easy | Servings: 2)
Per serving: Calories 199, Total fat 6g, Protein 15g, Carbs 18g
Ingredients:

- 1 garlic clove
- 3 tablespoons of extra-virgin olive oil
- 2 tablespoons of parsley
- 2 tablespoons of basil
- 1 tablespoon of soy sauce
- 1 scallion
- 2 soft Medjool dates, pitted
- 2 tablespoons of pistachio nuts shelled
- 1 tablespoon of red wine vinegar

Instructions:

- Combine all ingredients in a blender & serve!

88. Red Hot Pepper Salsa

(Preparation time: 10 minutes | Cooking time: 15 minutes | Difficulty: Easy | Servings: 2)
Per serving: Calories 199, Total fat 6g, Protein 18g, Carbs 19g
Ingredients:

- 1 tablespoon of extra-virgin olive oil
- 1 Bird's Eye chili
- 1 red onion, chopped
- 1 red bell pepper, diced

Instructions:

- When the oil is hot, add the chili, onion, & bell pepper to the pan. Cook for around 4 minutes, or till the onion is completely translucent. Season to taste

using salt and pepper, then add 1/2 cup water and turn the flame down to low.

- Cook for around 10 minutes with the lid on.
- 2 minutes in a food processor, puree until smooth. Warm the dish before serving.

89. Southern Tomato Sauce

(Preparation time: 10 minutes | Cooking time: 30 minutes | Difficulty: Easy | Servings: 6)
Per serving: Calories 100, Total fat 5g, Protein 3g, Carbs 15g
Ingredients:

- 2 teaspoons of olive oil
- 1 pinch of cayenne
- 1/2 teaspoon of thyme
- 1 teaspoon of basil
- 1 tablespoon of paprika
- 6 cloves of garlic, crushed
- 1 red onion, diced
- 3 stalks of celery, diced
- 2 bell peppers, thinly chopped
- 12 tomatoes, diced

Instructions:

- For around 10 minutes, sauté the celery, garlic, onion, & bell peppers in the oil.
- Cook, often stirring, for 20 minutes on low flame with the tomatoes, paprika, thyme, basil, & cayenne.
- Serve with rice or noodles as a side dish.

90. Tomato Hummus

(Preparation time: 10 minutes | Cooking time: 35 minutes | Difficulty: Easy | Servings: 4)
Per serving: Calories 195, Total fat 5g, Protein 18g, Carbs 15g
Ingredients:

- 1 garlic clove, crushed
- 4 tablespoons of extra-virgin olive oil
- 1 tablespoon of tomato paste
- 4 red onions, chopped

- 1 lb. of green beans, trimmed
- 1 cup of chickpeas, soaked overnight

Instructions:

- In a saucepan, heat the oil and sauté the onion and garlic for 5 minutes, or till golden. Cook for around 10 minutes with chickpeas and green beans.
- Season to taste using salt and pepper, then blend in the tomato paste till smooth.

91. White Bean and Tomato Salad

(Preparation time: 10 minutes | Cooking time: 0 minutes | Difficulty: Easy | Servings: 4)
Per serving: Calories 209, Total fat 4g, Protein 11g, Carbs 19g
Ingredients:

- 1 tablespoon of fresh lemon juice
- 2 tablespoons of olive oil
- 1 handful of parsley
- 4 scallions thinly chopped
- 2 cups of cherry tomatoes, halved
- 2 cups of cannellini beans, cooked

Instructions:

- In a mixing dish, combine cherry tomatoes, cannellini, & scallions. Season to taste with olive oil, salt, lemon juice, and pepper. Chop the parsley finely. Mix it up with the beans and serve.

92. Bitter Greens, Avocado, Mung Sprouts and Orange Salad

(Preparation time: 10 minutes | Cooking time: 0 minutes | Difficulty: Easy | Servings: 4)
Per serving: Calories 173, Total fat 4g, Protein 9g, Carbs 15g
Ingredients:

- Fresh cracked black pepper to taste
- 1 tablespoon of lemon juice
- 1 teaspoon of lemon zest
- 2 tablespoons of extra-virgin olive oil
- 1/2 teaspoon of diced fresh ginger

- 1 tablespoon of tahini
- 1 orange, into wedges
- 1 cup of baby spinach leaves
- 1 stir bitter greens (arugula, dandelion, watercress, etc.) 1 cup of Mung sprouts
- 1/2 cup of diced avocado
- ¼ cup of walnuts, soaked

Instructions:

- In a bowl, combine bitter greens, spinach leaves, & Mung sprouts. Mix the orange & avocado. Whisk together the lemon juice, lemon zest, olive oil, salt, ginger, pepper, & tahini in a separate bowl.
- Toss the salad in the dressing to evenly coat it. Garnish with chopped walnuts & serve right away.

93. Cashew Biscuits

(Preparation time: 10 minutes | Cooking time: 30 minutes | Difficulty: Easy | Servings: 8)
Per serving: Calories 166, Total fat 4g, Protein 4g, Carbs 25g
Ingredients:

- ½ teaspoon of fine sea salt
- 1½ teaspoons of baking powder
- 1 tablespoon of olive oil
- ½ cup of unsweetened plain yogurt
- 1¼ cups of whole-wheat flour
- ⅓ cup of toasted whole cashews, unsalted
- 3 tablespoons of natural smooth cashew butter

Instructions:

- Preheat the oven at 425°F. Using parchment paper, line a baking sheet. In a food processor, combine the flour with nuts.
- Pulse the nuts till almost all of them are finely chopped; a few larger parts are fine and lend texture to the cookies. Pulse a couple of times to incorporate the salt & baking powder.

- Pulse in the oil & nut butter to blend. Pulse in the yogurt till a crumbly (but not dry) dough forms.
- On a piece of parchment, gather the dough and pat it together to form a 6-inch square.
- Cut each biscuit into nine 2-inch squares. Place the cookies on the prepared baking sheet. Bake for around 12 to 14 minutes, or till golden brown around the edges. Allow cooling on the wire rack before serving.

94. Overnight Oat with Chocolate and Strawberries

(Preparation time: 10 minutes | Cooking time: 0 minutes | Difficulty: Easy | Servings: 2)
Per serving: Calories 258, Total fat 3g, Protein 14g, Carbs 25g
Ingredients:
- 1 teaspoon of honey
- 2 tablespoons of plain yogurt
- 1 cup of strawberries
- 4 tablespoons of rolled oats
- 1/2 cup of almond milk, unsweetened
- 1 square of 85% chocolate

Instructions:
- In a container, combine the oats & milk and set aside for overnight. Top the jar with yogurt, honey, strawberries, and little pieces of chocolate in the morning.
- It can be made ahead of time and stored in the refrigerator for up to three days.

95. Moroccan-Style Chickpeas

(Preparation time: 10 minutes | Cooking time: 40 minutes | Difficulty: Easy | Servings: 4)
Per serving: Calories 316, Total fat 6g, Protein 7g, Carbs 13g
Ingredients:
- 1 handful of parsley, chopped
- 2-inches ginger, peeled
- 1 teaspoon of turmeric

- ½ teaspoon of cayenne
- 1 cinnamon stick
- 1 red onion, chopped
- 1 carrot, chopped
- 1 celery stalk, chopped
- 2 ripe tomatoes
- 2 cups of chickpeas, soaked overnight
- 1 pinch of saffron

Instructions:
- Wash the chickpeas and combine them with 6 cups of fresh water in a pot. Combine the carrots & onion. Bring to the boil, then reduce to a low flame for around 65 minutes.
- Cook for 30 minutes with the parsley stalks, ginger, tomatoes, turmeric, cayenne, and saffron. Cook for another 20 minutes after adding salt and black pepper. 1/2 cup chickpeas, blended till smooth, returned to the pot to thicken the sauce. Remove the cinnamon, ginger, & parsley stalks and discard.
- Serve garnished with chopped parsley leaves.
- Serve alone or with couscous, steamed rice, or buckwheat.

96. Hot Garbanzo Beans with Sun-Dried Tomatoes

(Preparation time: 10 minutes | Cooking time: 35 minutes | Difficulty: Easy | Servings: 2)
Per serving: Calories 268, Total fat 5g, Protein 12g, Carbs 25g
Ingredients:
- 1 teaspoon of chili flakes
- 2 tablespoons of olive oil
- 2 garlic cloves, thinly chopped
- ½ red onion, thinly chopped
- 4 sun-dried tomatoes, thinly chopped
- 2 cups of garbanzo beans, cooked

Instructions:

- In a heated skillet with oil, sauté the onion, garlic, chili flakes, & sun-dried tomatoes.
- Cook for around 5 minutes after adding the garbanzo beans. Simmer for around 10 minutes, or till the liquid is virtually gone, after adding 1 cup of water.
- Season using salt & black pepper to taste, and serve right away.

97. Hot Curry

(Preparation time: 10 minutes | Cooking time: 45 minutes | Difficulty: Easy | Servings: 6)
Per serving: Calories 200, Total fat 5g, Protein 20g, Carbs 18g
Ingredients:

- 1 cup of water
- 3 tablespoons of extra-virgin olive oil
- 1/4 teaspoon of ground ginger
- 1 Bird's Eye chili, diced
- 1 teaspoon of turmeric
- 2 garlic cloves, diced
- 2 teaspoons of ground cumin
- 1 tablespoon of paprika
- 1 teaspoon of ground parsley
- 3 onions, diced
- 1 yellow bell pepper, chopped
- 2 carrots, chopped
- 1 1/4 cups of frozen spinach
- 2 1/2 cups of chickpeas, cooked
- 3 cups of buckwheat
- 1/2 cup of almonds
- 1/2 cup of golden raisins
- 1 cup of coconut milk

Instructions:

- Boil buckwheat for around 35 minutes in salted water, then drain & set aside.
- Allow 10 minutes for the spinach to defrost in a saucepan over medium flame. Set them aside. Add the oil to the same pan, and when it's heated, add the

chili, garlic, & onions, and cook for 3 minutes. Cook for 5 minutes after adding the carrots.

- Stir in the almonds, golden raisins, and garbanzo beans till thoroughly combined. Do 1 minute of sautéing Sauté for 1 minute with the turmeric, ginger, cumin, & paprika. Cook for 5 minutes after adding the spinach. Reduce flame to low and simmer for around 15 minutes with the coconut milk and bell pepper.
- Serve with buckwheat on the side.

98. Greek-Style Macaroni Casserole

(Preparation time: 10 minutes | Cooking time: 55 minutes | Difficulty: Medium | Servings: 6)
Per serving: Calories 210, Total fat 8g, Protein 22g, Carbs 20g
Ingredients:

- 1 1/2 cups of water
- 3 tablespoons of olive oil
- 1 1/2 teaspoons of soy sauce
- 1 tablespoon of tahini
- 1 1/2 tablespoons of arrowroot
- 2 tablespoons of black olives, pitted and chopped - 2 tablespoons of capers
- 2 cups of buckwheat macaroni
- 1 cup of buckwheat breadcrumbs
- 1 lb. of seitan
- 1 1/2 cups of plain soymilk

Instructions:

- To crumble the seitan, pulse it in a blender.
- Preheat the oven at 400°F.
- Cook the pasta al dente for around 8 minutes in salted boiling water, then drain and place in a bowl.
- Heat the oil in a skillet, then add the seitan & cook for around 3 to 4 minutes before adding the soy sauce. Set aside the seitan in the spaghetti bowl after thoroughly mixing it in.

- Using a few spoons of water, dissolve the arrowroot. Warm the soymilk, 1/2 cup of water, salt, tahini, olives, capers, & pepper to taste in a saucepan.
- Cook around 2 to 3 minutes, till the sauce thickens, with the arrowroot dissolved in a few spoons of water.
- To make the casserole, grease a baking dish using 1 teaspoon of oil and put the ingredients in two layers.
- Spread half of the pasta-seitan mixture on the dish first. Pour half of the sauce on top of that. Cover with the remaining sauce and top with the pasta. On top, strew breadcrumbs.
- Bake for around 35–40 minutes, or till the crust is golden brown and crisp. Serve immediately.

99. Lafayette Lima Beans

(Preparation time: 10 minutes | Cooking time: 1 hour 25 minutes | Difficulty: Easy | Servings: 4)
Per serving: Calories 298, Total fat 5g, Protein 12g, Carbs 21g
Ingredients:
- 8 cups of water
- 2 tablespoons of extra-virgin olive oil
- 1/4 teaspoon of cayenne
- 4 cloves of garlic, diced
- 1 red onion diced - 1 bell pepper diced
- 2 cups of dry lima beans, soaked overnight

Instructions:
- In a pan with oil, sauté the onion for around 10 minutes on low flame. Add the bell pepper, beans, garlic, cayenne pepper, and water to the pot.
- Bring to the boil, then reduce to a low flame and simmer for around 75 minutes. Cook for another 15 minutes after seasoning using salt and black pepper.
- Serve alongside cornbread.

100. Louisiana-Style Veggie Sausages

(Preparation time: 10 minutes | Cooking time: 1 hour | Difficulty: Medium | Servings: 4)
Per serving: Calories 368, Total fat 5g, Protein 15g, Carbs 25g
Ingredients:
- 3/4 cups of extra-virgin olive oil
- 2 garlic cloves, crushed
- 1/2 teaspoon of salt
- 2 teaspoons of garlic powder
- 2 teaspoons of oregano
- 1 teaspoon of fennel seeds
- 1/4 cup of soy sauce
- 1 cup of nutritional yeast flakes
- 2 cups of flour
- 1 cup of rolled oats
- 3 cups of chickpeas, soaked overnight
- 1 cup of soymilk

Instructions:
- Drain the chickpeas, rinse them under running water, and afterward crush them till extremely fine in a food processor.
- Combine flour, nutritional yeast, rolled oats, salt, oregano, garlic powder, and fennel seed in a mixing bowl. Combine soy sauce, soy milk, & chickpeas in a separate bowl. Combine the ingredients, then add to the flour. To make a dough, mix everything together thoroughly. Cut four 14 × 12 inch pieces of aluminum foil. Divide the ingredients into four equal portions and roll each one into a sausage.
- Roll the ends of the foil packages to seal them. Allow cooling after steaming for around 55 minutes.
- It can be served as is, with arugula salad on the side, or chopped & sautéed in 1 teaspoon of oil till brown.

101. Grilled Asparagus with Tapenade Sauce

(Preparation time: 10 minutes | Cooking time: 40 minutes | Difficulty: Easy | Servings: 4)
Per serving: Calories 200, Total fat 6g, Protein 19g, Carbs 20g
Ingredients:

- 4 teaspoons of extra-virgin olive oil
- 1 ½ teaspoon of balsamic vinegar
- ½ teaspoon of red wine vinegar
- 1 scallion - 2 blood oranges
- 4 slices of buckwheat or whole wheat bread - 1 garlic clove
- 1 ½ lb. of asparagus (25 –30 spears)
- 2 cups of black olives

Instructions:

- To make the tapenade, combine the olives, garlic, & olive oil in a blender.
- Peel and finely chop the scallion, then macerate for around 30 minutes in a mixture of 1/2 orange juice, balsamic vinegar, & red wine vinegar. To make a vinaigrette, whisk together the olive oil, salt, and pepper to taste.
- 1 orange's zest should be grated and added to the vinaigrette.
- Oranges should be peeled and sliced. Cut the bottom ends off the asparagus spears, spray with olive oil, and grill for 5 minutes, or till uniformly browned.
- Toast the bread, slice it diagonally, and top it with the tapenade. Arrange the asparagus spears on a dish with the orange slices on top and tapenade toasts on the side.
- Serve with vinaigrette drizzled over the top.

102. Fava Beans with Tomato

(Preparation time: 10 minutes | Cooking time: 1 hour | Difficulty: Medium | Servings: 4)
Per serving: Calories 189, Total fat 5g, Protein 14g, Carbs 18g

Ingredients:

- 2 cloves of garlic, crushed
- 4 tablespoons of extra-virgin olive oil
- 1/4 teaspoon of chili flakes
- 1/2 teaspoon of cumin
- 2 tablespoons of parsley, chopped
- 2 onions, finely chopped
- 2 cups of tomatoes, diced
- 2 cups of fava beans, shelled

Instructions:

- In a pot with oil, stir cook garlic and onions till they begin to brown, around 5 minutes. Cook for another 5 minutes after adding the fava beans & parsley.
- Bring to the boil with the tomatoes, chili, cumin, & enough water to cover the beans. Reduce to a low flame and cook for about an hour, or till the fava beans are soft.
- Serve warm or chilled.

103. Eggplant, Onion and Tomato Gratin

(Preparation time: 10 minutes | Cooking time: 30 minutes | Difficulty: Easy | Servings: 6)
Per serving: Calories 316, Total fat 6g, Protein 7g, Carbs 13g
Ingredients:

- 3 cloves of garlic, crushed
- 3 tablespoons of extra-virgin olive oil
- 3 sprigs of thyme
- 3 red onions, chopped
- 3 ripe tomatoes, sliced
- 3 eggplants, sliced

Instructions:

- Five minutes over medium flame, fry onion and garlic in 1 tablespoon of oil till tender, then season using salt, thyme, and pepper to taste.
- Preheat the oven to 40°F. Grease a gratin dish using 1 tablespoon of oil & spread the onions on top.

- Salt and black pepper and alternate tomato & eggplant slices, overlapping them by 2/3.
- Drizzle the remaining 1 tablespoon of olive oil on top and cook, covered with tin foil, for around 30 minutes, or till the eggplant is soft enough to cut with a fork.
- Uncover and continue to cook for another 15 minutes or till all of the liquid has been absorbed. The length of time depends on the vegetables & the juices that they produce.

104. Delicious Jamaica

(Preparation time: 10 minutes | Cooking time: 30 minutes | Difficulty: Easy | Servings: 4)
Per serving: Calories 220, Total fat 8g, Protein 7g, Carbs 13g
Ingredients:

- 2 cloves of garlic, crushed and chopped
- 1 teaspoon of hot pepper, seeded and chopped - 1 sprig of fresh thyme
- 1 tablespoon of sweet pepper, seeded and chopped
- 1 stick of celery, diced
- 1 red onion, chopped
- 3 tomatoes, chopped
- 6 pimento grains
- 2 medium carrots - 1 lb. of yams
- 1 cup of coconut milk

Instructions:

- Preheat the oven at 350°F. Cut the yams & carrots into small pieces. Bring the yams to a boil till they are firm and tender. Combine the onion, celery, salt, thyme, sweet pepper, hot pepper, and garlic.
- Alternate layers of yams, carrots, tomatoes, & seasoning mix in a dish that has been greased.
- Cover with coconut milk & bake till the dish is done (around 25 minutes).

105. Creole Tofu

(Preparation time: 10 minutes | Cooking time: 25 minutes | Difficulty: Easy | Servings: 6)
Per serving: Calories 199, Total fat 5g, Protein 18g, Carbs 20g
Ingredients:

- 1/2 lemon, thinly chopped
- 2 tablespoons of extra-virgin olive oil
- 3 cloves of garlic, crushed
- 1/4 tablespoon of chili powder
- 1/4 teaspoon of cayenne
- 1/4 cup of garlic powder
- 1 red onion diced
- 2 stalks of celery, diced
- 1 bell pepper diced
- 1/4 cup of parsley, chopped
- 6 tomatoes, diced
- 2 lbs. of tofu, chopped 1/4 inch thick

Instructions:

- Take 1 tablespoon of oil and heat in a saucepan; sauté the tofu till browned. Set them aside. In the remaining oil, sauté the garlic, onion, celery, chili, bell pepper, cayenne, and garlic powder for around 5 minutes.
- Cook for around 15 minutes after adding the tomatoes and a splash of water. Heat through the tofu, lemon, & parsley.
- When served over hot rice or steamed buckwheat, it's delicious.

106. Chickpea Pita Pockets

(Preparation time: 10 minutes | Cooking time: 15 minutes | Difficulty: Easy | Servings: 4)
Per serving: Calories 205, Total fat 10g, Protein 20g, Carbs 15g
Ingredients:

- 1 tablespoon of red onion, chopped
- Dash of garlic powder
- 1 teaspoon of mustard
- 1 tomato, sliced
- 1 carrot, grated

- 1/3 cup of celery, chopped
- 2 tablespoons of vegan mayonnaise
- 4 leaves lettuce
- 2 tablespoons of pickle relish
- 2 cups of chickpeas, cooked
- 4 whole-wheat pitas

Instructions:

- Use a potato masher to mash the chickpeas or a blender to swiftly puree them without leaving them too smooth.
- Toss the mashed potatoes with celery, mustard, onion, relish, mayonnaise, and garlic powder. Season using salt and pepper to taste after stirring thoroughly.
- Serve immediately by cutting the pitas in half and filling them with 1/4 of the chickpea spread, lettuce, tomato, & carrot.

107. Caribbean Yellow and Green Split Pea Buckwheat

(Preparation time: 10 minutes | Cooking time: 40 minutes | Difficulty: Easy | Servings: 4)
Per serving: Calories 199, Total fat 10g, Protein 18g, Carbs 12g

Ingredients:

- 2 tablespoons of extra-virgin olive oil
- 1 handful of parsley, chopped
- 2 garlic cloves, chopped
- 1 red onion, chopped
- 1/2 a green pepper, diced
- 1/2 a red pepper, diced
- 1 vegetable stock cube
- 1/2 cup of green split peas
- 1/2 cup of yellow split peas
- 1 1/2 pints of vegetable stock
- 3 cups of buckwheat
- 3 cardamom pods
- 1 pinch of saffron

Instructions:

- For around 3 minutes in a pot with oil, sauté the garlic and onion. Continue to sauté for the next few minutes after adding the buckwheat, split peas, & peppers.
- Stir in the stock & add salt and black pepper to taste, as well as the cardamom pods and a pinch of saffron for color. Cook for around 35 minutes on medium, then remove the cardamom pods and fluff the rice with a fork to make it light and fluffy.
- Using bowls loaded with rice to put onto plates or serving dishes is a lovely option for serving. Parsley leaves can be used as a finishing touch.
- Serve immediately.

108. Cabbage Rolls

(Preparation time: 10 minutes | Cooking time: 55 minutes | Difficulty: Medium | Servings: 4)
Per serving: Calories 350, Total fat 7g, Protein 18g, Carbs 20g

Ingredients:

- 2 teaspoons of salt
- ½ teaspoon of turmeric
- 1/4 teaspoon of cayenne
- 2 teaspoons of paprika
- 2 tablespoons of extra-virgin olive oil
- 2 cloves of garlic, diced
- 1/2 red onion, diced
- 1/3 cup of fresh parsley, chopped
- 3 green onions, diced
- 6 tomatoes, diced
- 1 head of cabbage, shredded
- 4 cups of brown rice, cooked
- 1 cup of tofu, crumbled

Instructions:

- Cook for 30 minutes after sautéing tomatoes with onions with 1 cup of boiling water. Remove the core from the cabbage, then steam the whole head for around 20 minutes with the core side down in a saucepan. Allow cooling. When the skillet is heated, add the onion and cook for 5 minutes. Simmer for 15 minutes on low flame with the salt, paprika, tofu, cayenne, green onions, garlic, and water. Stir in the rice thoroughly. Preheat the oven at 350°F. Separate cabbage leaves with care, paying special attention to keep them intact. Place a little amount of the rice stir-fry on each leaf, leaving enough room to fold the sides inward to form a roll. Arrange the cabbage rolls onto a baking sheet and pour the tomato sauce over them.

- Bake them for around 30 minutes.

109. Broussard Black Eyed Peas

(Preparation time: 10 minutes | Cooking time: 25 minutes | Difficulty: Easy | Servings: 4)
Per serving: Calories 210, Total fat 7g, Protein 15g, Carbs 18g
Ingredients:

- 8 cups of water
- 3/4 teaspoon of salt
- 1/4 teaspoon of cayenne
- 1 tablespoon of extra-virgin olive oil
- 1 red onion, diced
- 1 bell pepper, diced
- 2 stalks of celery, diced
- 1/3 cup of green onions, diced
- 1/3 cup of fresh parsley, chopped
- 2 cups of black-eyed peas, cooked

Instructions:

- In a pot with the oil, sauté the onion, celery, and bell peppers. Bring the water, black-eyed peas, pepper, green onions, salt, and cayenne to a boil, then reduce to a low flame and keep it simmering.
- Cook for around 45 minutes, or till the liquid has thickened. Serve immediately.

110. Beefless Stew

(Preparation time: 10 minutes | Cooking time: 40 minutes | Difficulty: Easy | Servings: 4)
Per serving: Calories 250, Total fat 10g, Protein 20g, Carbs 20g
Ingredients:

- 4 cups of water - 1 garlic clove, diced
- 1 teaspoon of lemon juice
- 1 bay leaf
- 1 tablespoon of extra-virgin olive oil
- 1 teaspoon of Worcestershire sauce
- 2 tablespoons of cornstarch
- 1 stalk of celery - 1 red onion, chopped
- 3 potatoes, chopped into bite-sized pieces - 6 carrots, chopped
- 1 1/2 cups of tomatoes
- 1 1/4 cups of peas
- 1 1/2 cups of dry soy "beef" protein chunks

Instructions:

- Place the soy pieces in a pot of boiling water with the lemon juice. Allow 15 minutes before squeezing out all of the water with your hands. Sauté the garlic and onions in the oil in a pan.
- Cook for around 5 minutes after adding the soy bits. Simmer for 5 minutes with 4 cups of water, tomatoes, celery, salt, Worcestershire sauce, bay leaf, and pepper. Cook for around 30 minutes with the potatoes, peas, and carrots.
- Thicken the stew to the appropriate consistency by dissolving the cornstarch with a few drops of water.

111. Smothered Cabbage

(Preparation time: 10 minutes | Cooking time: 30 minutes | Difficulty: Easy | Servings: 4)
Per serving: Calories 210, Total fat 6g, Protein 3g, Carbs 25g
Ingredients:

- 1/2 cup of water

- 1/2 teaspoon of salt
- 1/4 teaspoon of paprika
- 1/8 teaspoon of cayenne
- 2 tablespoons of extra-virgin olive oil
- 3 cloves of garlic crushed
- 1 red onion, diced - 1 cabbage, chopped

Instructions:

- When the oil is hot, add the onion, cabbage, & garlic, then cook for around 10 minutes, stirring frequently.
- Simmer for around 15 to 20 minutes, till the paprika, salt, cayenne, water, and pepper to taste are soft.

112. Rich Roasted Eggplant

(Preparation time: 10 minutes | Cooking time: 40 minutes | Difficulty: Easy | Servings: 4)
Per serving: Calories 190, Total fat 7g, Protein 5g, Carbs 15g
Ingredients:

- ¼ teaspoon of turmeric
- 1 garlic clove, crushed
- 1 tablespoon of fresh ginger, peeled and diced
- 2 tablespoons of extra-virgin olive oil
- 1 tablespoon of parsley, chopped
- 1 green chili
- 1 cup of red onion
- ½ cup of tomatoes, chopped
- 1 eggplant

Instructions:

- Preheat the oven at 450°F. Cut the eggplant in 1/2 and set the cut side down on a baking pan. Bake for around 30 to 40 minutes, or till the eggplant skin wrinkles and feels soft. Allow it cool for around 5 minutes before removing the skin, finely chopping the flesh, and rough chopping the flesh with a knife.
- Into a skillet over medium flame, heat the oil and cook the chilies for 1 minute. Add the onion and cook for 8 to 10

minutes, or till it is translucent. Toss in the tomatoes, ginger, green chili, garlic, turmeric, and salt. Cook for about 20 minutes, or till the tomatoes have formed a sauce.

- Add the eggplant & simmer for 10 minutes on low flame, covered, to blend flavors, stirring occasionally.
- Remove the pan from the flame. To mix the flavors, cover and set aside for 15 minutes. Add together the remaining ingredients & serve.

113. Red Cauliflower

(Preparation time: 10 minutes | Cooking time: 25 minutes | Difficulty: Easy | Servings: 4)
Per serving: Calories 190, Total fat 4g, Protein 8g, Carbs 20g
Ingredients:

- ¼ cup of water - 1 garlic clove crushed
- 2 tablespoons of extra-virgin olive oil
- 1 tablespoon of tomato paste
- 2 tablespoons of chopped parsley
- 1 cauliflower

Instructions:

- Divide the cauliflower into individual florets once it has been rinsed.
- In a saucepan, heat the extra-virgin olive oil & sauté the garlic for around 1 minute. Cook for 5 minutes with the cauliflower, occasionally stirring, before seasoning with salt and black pepper, water, & tomato paste.
- Cook, covered, over low flame till the vegetables are soft (around 15 to 20 minutes).

114. Raw Artichoke Salad

(Preparation time: 10 minutes | Cooking time: 0 minutes | Difficulty: Easy | Servings: 2)
Per serving: Calories 100, Total fat 11g, Protein 13g, Carbs 4g
Ingredients:

- Salt and black pepper - 1 lemon, juiced

- 1 teaspoon of extra-virgin olive oil
- 2 Roman artichokes

Instructions:

- Remove the outer leaves from the artichokes and wash them. Cut them in half and remove the hair from the inside. Cut them into extremely little pieces (using a mandolin if you have one)
- Put them in a bowl with water and lemon to keep them from browning.
- Drain the artichokes, mix them with olive oil, salt, a few drops of lemon & pepper, and place them on a serving plate when ready to serve.

115. Piquant Coleslaw

(Preparation time: 20 minutes | Cooking time: 0 minutes | Difficulty: Easy | Servings: 6)
Per serving: Calories 160, Total fat 7g, Protein 3g, Carbs 20g

Ingredients:

- 1 red onion - 1 green pepper
- 4 sticks of celery - 12 green olives
- 3 tablespoons of no-egg mayonnaise
- 5 drops of tabasco sauce
- 2 lbs. of white cabbage

Instructions:

- Prepare the cabbage by grating it. Cut the celery & green pepper into small pieces. Finely chop the onion and olives.
- In a mixing dish, combine all of the vegetables and whisk well. Toss in the mayonnaise, tabasco sauce, salt, & pepper to taste and serve.

116. Lemon Eggplant

(Preparation time: 10 minutes | Cooking time: 30 minutes | Difficulty: Easy | Servings: 2)
Per serving: Calories 265, Total fat 7g, Protein 2g, Carbs 18g

Ingredients:

- 2 cloves of garlic, crushed
- 3 tablespoons of lemon juice

- 1/2 cup of extra-virgin olive oil
- 6 tablespoons of parsley, finely chopped
- 1 green pepper, very finely chopped
- 1 eggplant, chopped

Instructions:

- Salt the eggplant slices and soak them in water for around 30 minutes before patting them dry with kitchen towels.
- Heat the oil in a frying pan and cook the eggplant till golden brown. Set them aside. Combine lemon juice, salt, & pepper to taste to make a sauce and sprinkle over the eggplant.
- Serve with a parsley garnish.

117. Ginger Zucchini

(Preparation time: 10 minutes | Cooking time: 15 minutes | Difficulty: Easy | Servings: 4)
Per serving: Calories 160, Total fat 4g, Protein 2g, Carbs 12g

Ingredients:

- 1 tablespoon of olive oil
- 2 teaspoons of light soy sauce
- 1 teaspoon of sesame oil
- 1/2 cup of vegetarian broth
- 1 lb. of zucchini chopped into 1/4-inch cuts - 1 tablespoon of red wine

Instructions:

- Heat the oil in a skillet and add the zucchini & ginger once it is heated. Stir for 1 minute before adding the red wine, soy sauce, & broth.
- Cook till the liquid has reduced & the zucchini is soft around 10 minutes. Serve with a drizzle of sesame oil.

118. Curry Chickpeas

(Preparation time: 10 minutes | Cooking time: 25 minutes | Difficulty: Easy | Servings: 4)
Per serving: Calories 173, Total fat 8g, Protein 7g, Carbs 15g

Ingredients:

- 1/4 tablespoon of salt

- 1/2 tablespoon of pepper
- 1/2 tablespoon of ground turmeric
- 1/4 tablespoon of ground cumin
- 2 tablespoons of olive oil
- 1/8 teaspoon of ground cinnamon
- 1 handful of parsley, chopped
- 2 tablespoons of curry powder
- 2 tablespoons of red wine vinegar
- 2 cups of chickpeas, cooked

Instructions:

- In a medium-sized bowl, gently crush chickpeas using your hands, removing any skins. Toss in the oil and vinegar to coat. Mix in the curry powder, turmeric, and cinnamon till well combined.
- Cook chickpeas into a single layer in the oven at 400°F for around 15 minutes, shaking halfway through. Place chickpeas in a mixing bowl. Toss with salt, pepper, & parsley till well coated.

119. Chinese-Style Chili Green Beans

(Preparation time: 10 minutes | Cooking time: 15 minutes | Difficulty: Easy | Servings: 4)

Per serving: Calories 145, Total fat 4g, Protein 3g, Carbs 18g

Ingredients:

- 2 cloves of garlic, crushed
- 1 tablespoon of olive oil
- 1 teaspoon of sesame oil
- 2 tablespoons of soy sauce
- 1 lb. of green beans, trimmed
- 1/2 teaspoon of dried red chili flakes

Instructions:

- Heat the oil in a skillet over a high flame. Stir in the chili flakes, garlic, green beans, and soy sauce till the beans are cooked, around 10 minutes.
- Serve with a dash of sesame oil on top.
- When eaten at room temperature, these beans are also delicious.

120. Butternut and Chestnut Holiday Sauté

(Preparation time: 10 minutes | Cooking time: 45 minutes | Difficulty: Easy | Servings: 4)

Per serving: Calories 206, Total fat 6g, Protein 2g, Carbs 20g

Ingredients:

- 1 garlic clove, diced
- 6 tablespoons of olive oil
- 1/2 teaspoon of thyme
- 1 handful of parsley, chopped
- 4 scallions, chopped
- 1 lb. of tomatoes, chopped and peeled
- 1 cup of dried lentils, soaked overnight
- 1 butternut squash, chopped into cubes
- 1 cup of chestnuts, shelled

Instructions:

- Drain and rinse the lentils. Fill a pan halfway with fresh water and place them in it. Bring to the boil, then reduce to a low flame and cook for 30 minutes, or till the lentils are cooked. Cook the garlic & scallions in a sauté pan with the oil till soft. Cook for a few minutes after adding the squash. Cook for around 10 minutes after adding the tomatoes and thyme. Cook for another 10 minutes, or till all of the vegetables are tender.
- Warm the chestnuts in the pan. Serve.

121. Beets with Parsley and Leeks

(Preparation time: 10 minutes | Cooking time: 30 minutes | Difficulty: Easy | Servings: 4)

Per serving: Calories 178, Total fat 5g, Protein 4g, Carbs 15g

Ingredients:

- 1 teaspoon of ground cumin
- 1 tablespoon of parsley, chopped
- 1 lb. of trimmed leeks, thickly chopped
- 2 lbs. of beets, chopped
- 1/2 cups of red wine

Instructions:

- In a skillet, combine the beets, leeks, and spices. Bring the wine to a boil, then reduce to a low flame and cook for 30 minutes, or till the beets are soft.
- Season using salt and pepper to taste and serve hot or cold.

122. Bean Salad

(Preparation time: 15 minutes | Cooking time: 0 minutes | Difficulty: Easy | Servings: 4)
Per serving: Calories 210, Total fat 3g, Protein 3g, Carbs 20g
Ingredients:

- 1 tablespoon of cumin
- 1/3 cup of lime juice
- 1/2 cup of parsley, chopped
- 3 tablespoons of extra-virgin olive oil
- 1/4 red onions, chopped
- 1/4 cup of green onions, chopped
- 1 can of black beans, drained
- 1 can of corn, drained

Instructions:

- Combine all ingredients in a mixing bowl and set aside for overnight.

123. Baked Eggplant with Garlic and Turmeric

(Preparation time: 10 minutes | Cooking time: 20 minutes | Difficulty: Easy | Servings: 2)
Per serving: Calories 160, Total fat 7g, Protein 3g, Carbs 22g
Ingredients:

- 1/4 cup of water
- 1/2 teaspoon of salt
- 1/4 teaspoon of turmeric
- 1 teaspoon of green chili
- 1 1/2 tablespoons of garlic, diced
- 2 tablespoons of extra-virgin olive oil
- 2 tablespoons of white poppy seeds made into a paste - 2 chilies
- 1 eggplant

Instructions:

- To make a paste, crush the poppy seeds with a splash of olive oil. Preheat the oven at 450°F. Cut the eggplant lengthwise & place it cut side down on a baking sheet.
- Bake for around 30–34 minutes, or till the eggplant wrinkles and is tender when pushed. Cut. Remove from the equation.
- Over medium flame, heat the oil in a skillet. Red chilies should be cooked till soft.
- Garlic and green chilies should be added at this point. Stir till the garlic has turned a light brown color. Add the water and turmeric and bring to the boil. Reduce the flame to low and add the eggplant slices. Mix in the poppy seed paste and salt thoroughly. Cook, covered, for 20 minutes, stirring periodically.
- Serve garnished with green onions.

124. Thyme Mushrooms

(Preparation time: 10 minutes | Cooking time: 30 minutes | Difficulty: Easy | Servings: 4)
Per serving: Calories 251, Total fat 9g, Protein 6g, Carbs 13g
Ingredients:

- 1 tablespoon of thyme, chopped
- 2 tablespoons of parsley, chopped
- 4 garlic cloves, minced
- 2 tablespoons of extra-virgin olive oil
- 2 lbs. of halved white mushrooms

Instructions:

- Combine the mushrooms, garlic with the remaining ingredients in a baking pan, stir well and bake at 400°F for around 30 minutes.
- Serve by dividing the mixture across plates.

125. Sage Carrots

(Preparation time: 10 minutes | Cooking time: 30 minutes | Difficulty: Easy | Servings: 4)

Per serving: Calories 200, Total fat 9g, Protein 4g, Carbs 8g

Ingredients:
- ¼ teaspoon of black pepper
- 2 tablespoons of Extra-virgin olive oil
- 2 teaspoons of sweet paprika
- 1 tablespoon of sage, chopped
- 1 red onion, chopped
- 1 lb. of carrots, chopped

Instructions:
- Combine the carrots, oil, & remaining ingredients in a baking pan, mix, & bake at 380°F for around 30 minutes. Serve by dividing the mixture across plates.

126. Rosemary Endives

(Preparation time: 10 minutes | Cooking time: 20 minutes | Difficulty: Easy | Servings: 2)

Per serving: Calories 66, Total fat 7g, Protein 1g, Carbs 1g

Ingredients:
- ¼ teaspoon of black pepper
- ½ teaspoon of turmeric powder
- 1 teaspoon of rosemary
- 2 tablespoons of extra-virgin olive oil
- 2 halved endives

Instructions:
- Combine the endives with oil and the remaining ingredients in a baking pan, mix lightly, & bake at 400°F for around 20 minutes. Serve by dividing the mixture across plates.

127. Roasted Beets

(Preparation time: 10 minutes | Cooking time: 30 minutes | Difficulty: Easy | Servings: 4)

Per serving: Calories 156, Total fat 12g, Protein 4g, Carbs 11g

Ingredients:
- ¼ teaspoon of black pepper
- 2 garlic cloves, minced
- 2 tablespoons of extra-virgin olive oil
- ¼ cup of parsley, chopped
- 4 beets, peeled and sliced
- ¼ cup of walnuts, chopped

Instructions:
- Mix the beets with the oil & the remaining ingredients in a baking dish, toss to coat, and bake for around 30 minutes at 420°F.
- Serve by dividing the mixture across plates.

128. Rice with Arugula and Lemon

(Preparation time: 10 minutes | Cooking time: 40 minutes | Difficulty: Easy | Servings: 4)

Per serving: Calories 290, Total fat 6g, Protein 13g, Carbs 30g

Ingredients:
- Salt and pepper to taste
- 1 tablespoon of extra-virgin olive oil
- ¼ teaspoon of dill weed
- 2 cloves garlic, minced
- 3 tablespoons of lemon juice
- 1 red onion, chopped
- 1 cup of fresh mushrooms, sliced
- 3 cups of brown rice, steamed
- 1 1/4 cups of fresh arugula
- 1/3 cup of feta cheese, crumbled

Instructions:
- Preheat the oven at 350°F. Sauté the mushrooms, onion, & garlic in oil in a skillet till soft. Toss in the rice, dill, arugula, lemon juice, and season to taste using salt and pepper.
- One tablespoon of cheese is set aside, and the remainder is stirred into the skillet till thoroughly combined. Place in an 8-inch square baking dish that has been sprayed using nonstick cooking spray.

- Sprinkle with the cheese that was set aside. Bake for around 25 minutes with the lid on.
- Uncover & bake for another 5 to 10 minutes, or till cheese is melted and cooked thoroughly.

129. Purple Potatoes with Mushrooms, Onions and Capers

(Preparation time: 10 minutes | Cooking time: 30 minutes | Difficulty: Easy | Servings: 4)
Per serving: Calories 215, Total fat 6g, Protein 3g, Carbs 20g
Ingredients:

- ¼ teaspoon of chili pepper flakes
- 3 tablespoons of extra-virgin olive oil
- 1 teaspoon of fresh tarragon, chopped
- 1 tablespoon of capers, drained and chopped
- 1 red onion, chopped
- 6 purple potatoes, scrubbed
- 1 cup of mushrooms, sliced

Instructions:

- By quartering the potatoes and then slicing each quarter in half, you can make wedges out of them. Cook the onion and mushrooms in a skillet with olive oil over medium flame till the mushrooms start to release their liquid & the onion becomes transparent (about 5 minutes). Set aside the onion & mushrooms in a mixing dish.
- Heat two tablespoons of additional oil in the same skillet over high flame & add the potato wedges to the hot oil. Season using salt and pepper, and cook, tossing periodically, for approximately 10 minutes, or till the wedges are browned on both sides.
- Reduce the flame to medium, season the potato wedges using red pepper flakes, & simmer for another 10 minutes, or till soft. Toss the vegetables together with the onion & mushroom mixture, then add the capers and fresh tarragon.

130. Kale Walnut Bake

(Preparation time: 10 minutes | Cooking time: 30 minutes | Difficulty: Easy | Servings: 4)
Per serving: Calories 355, Total fat 31g, Protein 26g, Carbs 35g
Ingredients:

- ½ teaspoon of ground nutmeg
- 2 tablespoons of extra-virgin olive oil
- 1 red onion, finely chopped
- 1/3 cup of buckwheat or whole-wheat breadcrumbs
- 2 cups of kale
- ½ cup of half-and-half cream
- ½ cup of walnuts, coarsely chopped

Instructions:

- Preheat the oven at 350°F. Into a skillet, sauté onion till soft in olive oil. Cook the onion, kale, cream, salt, walnuts, breadcrumbs, nutmeg, and pepper to taste in a mixing bowl.
- Place the mixture in a greased 1-1/2-quart baking dish. Toss together the topping ingredients & sprinkle over the greens. Bake for around 30 minutes, uncovered, or till lightly browned.

131. Kale Sauté

(Preparation time: 10 minutes | Cooking time: 20 minutes | Difficulty: Easy | Servings: 2)
Per serving: Calories 200, Total fat 7g, Protein 6g, Carbs 6g
Ingredients:

- 1 tablespoon of lime juice
- 2 minced garlic cloves
- 1 tablespoon of chopped parsley
- 2 tablespoons of olive oil
- 1 chopped red onion
- 3 tablespoons of soya sauce
- 1 lb. of kale

Instructions:

- Heat the olive oil in a pan over medium flame, add the garlic and onions and cook for around 5 minutes.
- Toss in the greens and remaining ingredients, cook for 10 minutes over medium flame, divide among plates and serve.

132. Avocado with Raspberry Vinegar Salad

(Preparation time: 10 minutes | Cooking time: 20 minutes | Difficulty: Easy | Servings: 2)
Per serving: Calories 163, Total fat 4g, Protein 14g, Carbs 15g

Ingredients:

- 1 teaspoon of extra-virgin olive oil
- 1/2 cup of raspberries
- 2 firm-ripe avocados
- 1 red endive
- 6 tablespoons of red wine

Instructions:

- Half of the raspberries should be placed in a bowl. In a saucepan, heat the vinegar till it begins to bubble, then put it over the raspberries & steep for 5 minutes.
- Strain the raspberries, carefully pressing the fruit to obtain all of the juices but leaving the pulp behind.
- Combine the strained raspberry vinegar, oils, & seasonings in a mixing bowl. Set them aside.
- Remove the stone from each avocado by carefully halving it and twisting it out.
- Remove the skin & cut the flesh into the dressing directly.
- Gently fold the avocados into the dressing till they are completely covered.
- Refrigerate for around 2 hours after carefully covering.

- Separate the radicchio leaves, rinse & drain them, and dry them on kitchen paper in the meantime. In a plastic bag, store in the refrigerator.
- Place a few radicchio leaves on each plate to serve.
- Spread the avocado over the top, toss it in, and garnish with the leftover raspberries.

133. Avocado and Potato Salad

(Preparation time: 10 minutes | Cooking time: 15 minutes | Difficulty: Easy | Servings: 2)
Per serving: Calories 213, Total fat 9g, Protein 3g, Carbs 25g

Ingredients:

- 1 handful of parsley, chopped
- 1/2 cup of red onion, chopped
- 2 ribs of celery, chopped
- 1 ripe avocado, mashed
- 6 Yukon gold or red potatoes
- 1/2 cup of sweet red bell pepper

Instructions:

- Cook the potatoes till they are cooked but not mushy. Combine all of the ingredients in a large-sized mixing bowl and thoroughly combine. Keep it refrigerated till you're ready to eat it.

134. Tomato and Avocado Salad

(Preparation time: 10 minutes | Cooking time: 0 minutes | Difficulty: Easy | Servings: 1)
Per serving: Calories 165, Total fat 14g, Protein 5g, Carbs 7g

Ingredients:

- 1 pinch of sea salt
- 1 teaspoon of fresh oregano
- 1 tablespoon of extra-virgin olive oil
- 1 tomato
- 1/2 cup of cherry tomatoes
- 1 / 2 red onion
- 1 ripe avocado
- 1 teaspoon of red wine

Instructions:

- Tomatoes should be cut into thick slices. Half of the cherry tomatoes should be cut into slices, and the other half should be cut in half. Cut the red onion into half-rings that are super-thin. (If you have one, use it for this.)
- Using a knife, cut the avocado into six pieces. Place the tomatoes on a platter and top with the avocado.
- Dress the salad with red onion and oregano, as well as olive oil, vinegar, & a touch of salt.

135. Salad with Apple and Cranberries

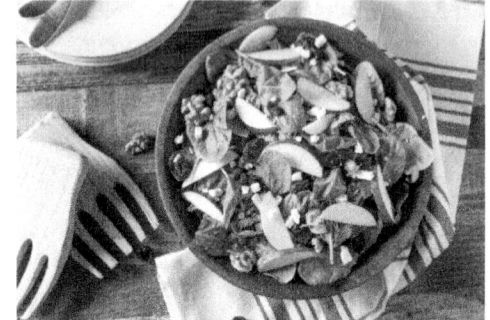

(Preparation time: 10 minutes | Cooking time: 0 minutes | Difficulty: Easy | Servings: 2)
Per serving: Calories 70, Total fat 3g, Protein 7g, Carbs 6g
Ingredients:

- 3 tablespoons of extra-virgin olive oil
- 1 teaspoon of mustard yellow
- 1 teaspoon of honey
- 1 / 2 red onion
- 1 / 2 apple
- 1 / 2 red bell pepper
- ½ cup of arugula
- 2 tablespoons of cranberries
- 10 Walnuts

Instructions:

- Half of the red onion should be cut into thin rings. The bell pepper should be cut into small bits. Remove the core from the apple and cut it into four pieces. After that, slice into thin wedges. To keep the apple wedges from becoming brown, drizzle them with lemon juice.
- Walnuts should be roughly chopped. In a mixing basin, combine the dressing ingredients. Salt & pepper to taste. Season the lettuce with red pepper, apple slices, red onions, and walnuts on a platter.
- Toss the salad with bacon and cranberries. Serve the salad with the dressing drizzled over it.

136. Roasted Butternut and Chickpeas Salad

(Preparation time: 10 minutes | Cooking time: 35 minutes | Difficulty: Easy | Servings: 4)
Per serving: Calories 353, Total fat 5g, Protein 28g, Carbs 22g
Ingredients:

- ½ lemon, juiced - 2 cloves of garlic
- ½ teaspoon of honey
- 2 teaspoons of oil - 1 green apple
- 1 cup of chickpeas, drained
- 1 lb. of butternut squash
- 2 cups of kale

Instructions:

- Preheat the oven at 400°F.
- Squash should be cut into medium pieces and placed in a baking dish with drained chickpeas, salt, garlic, 1 tablespoon oil, & pepper. The cooking time is 25 minutes.
- Mix the kale with dressing (salt, pepper, olive oil, lemon, and honey) so that the squash softens and becomes more enjoyable to eat while it cooks.
- Put the squash and chickpeas aside for 10 minutes while you chop the apple and combine it with the kale.
- Serve heated with the squash & chickpeas on top.

137. Rainbow Salad

(Preparation time: 10 minutes | Cooking time: 0 minutes | Difficulty: Easy | Servings: 1)
Per serving: Calories 40, Total fat 1g, Protein 2g, Carbs 5g
Ingredients:

- 2 tablespoons of olive oil
- 1 tablespoon of red wine vinegar
- 1 egg
- 1/4 green pepper
- 1/4 red bell pepper
- ½ carrot, grated
- ½ red onion
- 2 tomatoes
- 1 cup of lettuce
- 1/2 piece of avocado

Instructions:

- Cook the egg till it is fully cooked (around 6 minutes for soft boiled, 8 minutes for hard-boiled). Under running water, cool it, peel it, and cut it into slices. Cut the peppers into thin strips after removing the seeds. Tomatoes should be cut into small cubes. Thinly slice the red onion into half-rings.
- Using a knife, slice the avocado into thin slices. Arrange the salad on a platter and arrange the vegetables in brightly colored rows.
- Drizzle olive oil & red wine vinegar over the vegetables. Add salt & pepper to taste.

138. Moroccan Leeks Salad

(Preparation time: 10 minutes | Cooking time: 0 minutes | Difficulty: Easy | Servings: 4)
Per serving: Calories 135, Total fat 1g, Protein 9g, Carbs 15g
Ingredients:

- A pinch of turmeric powder
- 2 tablespoons of extra-virgin olive oil
- 1 bunch of radishes, sliced
- 1 cup of parsley, chopped
- 3 cups of leeks, chopped
- 1 ½ cups of olives, pitted and sliced

Instructions:

- Combine radishes, olives, leeks, and parsley in a mixing dish. Toss in the black pepper, oil, & turmeric, and serve.

139. French Onion Soup

(Preparation time: 10 minutes | Cooking time: 55 minutes | Difficulty: Easy | Servings: 4)
Per serving: Calories 210, Total fat 10g, Protein 13g, Carbs 15g
Ingredients:

- 1 tablespoon of olive oil
- 1 tablespoon of butter
- 2 teaspoons of buckwheat flour
- 2 slices of whole-wheat bread
- 3 cups of vegetable stock
- 2 lbs. of red onions, thinly sliced
- 4 tablespoons of cheddar cheese, grated

Instructions:

- In a pan, melt the oil and butter together.
- Cook, stirring periodically, for around 25 minutes on low flame with the onions. Mix in the flour thoroughly. Put in the stock & continue to whisk. Bring to the boil, then reduce to a low flame and cook for around 30 minutes.
- Cut the bread slices into triangles, top with cheese, and set under a hot grill till the cheese melts. To serve, ladle the soup into bowls and top with two triangles of cheesy toast.

140. Kale and Shiitake Soup

(Preparation time: 10 minutes | Cooking time: 40 minutes | Difficulty: Easy | Servings: 4)
Per serving: Calories 124, Total fat 2g, Protein 9g, Carbs 15g
Ingredients:

- 3 garlic cloves, minced

- 3 tablespoons of extra-virgin olive oil
- 4 cups of vegetable broth
- 1 cup of kale
- 2 cups of red onions, chopped
- 2 lbs. of dry shiitake mushrooms

Instructions:

- Put the oil, garlic, onion, & kale in a pan over medium flame and cook for a few minutes to soften.
- Sauté the mushrooms for around 2 minutes. Bring the stock to the boil, then reduce to a low flame and leave to simmer for around 30 minutes.
- Serve right away.

141. Lentil Soup

(Preparation time: 10 minutes | Cooking time: 25 minutes | Difficulty: Easy | Servings: 4)
Per serving: Calories 196, Total fat 4g, Protein 4g, Carbs 3g
Ingredients:

- 1 teaspoon of ground turmeric
- 1 teaspoon of ground cumin
- 2 tablespoons of extra-virgin olive oil
- 1 clove of garlic, chopped
- ½ Bird's Eye chili
- 1 red onion, chopped
- 2 sticks of celery, chopped
- 2 carrots, chopped
- 2 pints of vegetable stock
- 1 cup of red lentils

Instructions:

- In a saucepan, heat the oil and sauté the onion for around 5 minutes. Cook for 5 minutes after adding the carrots, turmeric, lentils, celery, chili, cumin, and garlic.
- Add in the stock, bring to the boil, then reduce to a low flame and continue to cook for 45 minutes.
- In a food processor, puree the soup till it is smooth.
- Serve with a pinch of salt and pepper.

142. Spicy Squash Soup

(Preparation time: 10 minutes | Cooking time: 35 minutes | Difficulty: Easy | Servings: 4)
Per serving: Calories 298, Total fat 9g, Protein 5g, Carbs 20g
Ingredients:

- 2 teaspoons of turmeric
- 3 cloves of garlic
- 1 teaspoon of ground ginger
- 3 chilies, chopped
- 2 tablespoons of olive oil
- 1 red onion, chopped - 1/2 cup of kale
- 1 butternut squash, chopped
- 2 cups of vegetable stock

Instructions:

- In a saucepan, heat the olive oil and sauté the chopped butternut squash with onion for around 6 minutes, or till softened.
- Cook for around 2 minutes, stirring regularly, after adding the kale, turmeric, garlic, chili, and ginger.
- Cook for 20 minutes after adding the vegetable stock and bringing it to a boil. Blitz the soup in a food processor till it's completely smooth. Serve right away.

143. Meatballs Tomato Soup

(Preparation time: 10 minutes | Cooking time: 40 minutes | Difficulty: Easy | Servings: 2)
Per serving: Calories 348, Total fat 8g, Protein 23g, Carbs 25g
Ingredients:

- 1 clove of garlic, crushed
- 1 Bird's Eye chili, finely sliced
- 2 teaspoons of extra-virgin olive oil
- 1 red onion finely chopped
- 1 yellow pepper, chopped
- 1 red pepper, chopped
- 1 tablespoon of parmesan
- 1 tablespoon of whole-wheat breadcrumbs
- 1 egg - 3 ripe tomatoes, chopped

- 2 cups of stock - 1/2 cup of buckwheat
- 1 cup of soy mince, ready to cook

Instructions:

- Mix together the mince, egg, salt, breadcrumbs, parmesan, and pepper in a mixing bowl, then form tiny meatballs. In a large skillet, heat the oil and slowly sauté the garlic and onions till they are translucent. Cook for another 5 minutes after adding the meatballs. Add the peppers and chili, stir to combine flavors, then add the tomatoes, broth, & cook for around 20-25 minutes.
- Cook the buckwheat for around 25 minutes as the soup simmer, then drain and add it to the soup just before serving.

144. Black Bean Stew

(Preparation time: 10 minutes | Cooking time: 35 minutes | Difficulty: Easy | Servings: 4)
Per serving: Calories 199, Total fat 5g, Protein 18g, Carbs 20g

Ingredients:

- 1 cup of boiling water
- 1/2 teaspoon of black pepper
- 1 bird's eye chili, finely chopped
- 1 pinch of cayenne pepper, chopped
- 1/4 teaspoon of oregano
- 1/4 teaspoon of ground cumin
- 2 tablespoons of extra-virgin olive oil
- 1 red onion diced - 1 carrot diced
- 1 celery stalk diced -1/2 cup of tomatoes
- 2 cups of black beans

Instructions:

- In a medium-sized pot, heat the oil. Sauté the carrot, onion, and celery for 2–3 minutes, or till the onion is translucent. Add the tomatoes to the pot after blending for 1 minute, till smooth. Bring the puree, beans, oregano, pepper, and cumin to a boil in

the pot, then lower to low flame. After 30 minutes of simmering, puree the stew in a blender till smooth.
- Serve immediately.

145. Black Eyed Peas Soup

(Preparation time: 10 minutes | Cooking time: 35 minutes | Difficulty: Easy | Servings: 4)
Per serving: Calories 240, Total fat 5g, Protein 18g, Carbs 25g

Ingredients:

- 2 cups of water
- 1 pinch of cayenne pepper
- 1 teaspoon of parsley
- 1/8 teaspoon of ground cumin
- 3 tablespoons of extra-virgin olive oil
- 2 red onions diced
- 2 carrots chopped into 1/4-inch cuts
- 2 cups of black-eyed peas, rinsed

Instructions:

- Melt two tablespoons of extra-virgin olive oil in a cast-iron skillet over medium flame. Add the onions & cook for 3 to 5 minutes, or till golden. Cayenne pepper should be added.
- In a saucepan, combine the black-eyed peas, salt, carrots, parsley, and black pepper. Bring them to a boil. Simmer for 30 to 40 minutes with the sautéed onions & cayenne pepper.
- Combine the remaining 1 tablespoon of extra-virgin olive oil & the cumin in a food processor and puree. Serve.

146. Celery Stew

(Preparation time: 10 minutes | Cooking time: 25 minutes | Difficulty: Easy | Servings: 2)
Per serving: Calories 142, Total fat 3g, Protein 8g, Carbs 10g

Ingredients:

- 1/2 tablespoon of extra-virgin olive oil
- 2 cloves of garlic, diced
- 1/4 teaspoon of dill - 1 cup of soy milk

- 1/2 cup of red onion, chopped
- 4 cups of celery, chopped
- 2 cups of vegetable stock or water

Instructions:

- When the oil is hot, add the celery, onion, and garlic to the pot. Add the stock & cook till the vegetables are tender.
- Blend till smooth and creamy. Return to the pot and season to taste using salt and pepper. Serve immediately with dill and soymilk.

147. Chipotle Split Pea Stew

(Preparation time: 10 minutes | Cooking time: 45 minutes | Difficulty: Easy | Servings: 4)
Per serving: Calories 206, Total fat 3g, Protein 9g, Carbs 20g
Ingredients:

- 3 cups of boiling water
- 2 cloves of garlic diced
- 1 tablespoon of soy sauce
- 1 red onion chopped
- 1/2 cup of chopped parsley
- 1/2 chipotle, finely chopped
- 2 carrots chopped diagonally
- 2 stalks of celery, chopped diagonally
- 2 cups of dried split peas

Instructions:

- Cook the split peas for 40 minutes in salted water till tender.
- Cook till the vegetables are soft, then add the onion, garlic, parsley, carrots, celery, chipotle, and soy sauce.
- Serve immediately.

148. Chickpea Soup

(Preparation time: 10 minutes | Cooking time: 1 hour 25 minutes | Difficulty: Easy | Servings: 4)
Per serving: Calories 205, Total fat 5g, Protein 11g, Carbs 22g
Ingredients:

- ½ teaspoon of turmeric

- 1/2 teaspoon of cayenne
- 1/4 teaspoon of mustard
- 2 tablespoons of extra-virgin olive oil
- 4 cloves of garlic, crushed
- 2 red onions, chopped
- 1/2 cup of parsley
- 3 cups of vegetable broth
- 1 cup of dried chickpeas, soaked overnight

Instructions:

- Drain chickpeas after boiling them in water for around 65-70 minutes.
- In a frying pan, heat the oil and stir fry the garlic and onions till they start to brown. Toss in the parsley, chickpeas, cayenne, mustard, and season with salt and black pepper to taste. Cook for another 5 minutes before adding 3 cups of vegetable broth.
- Cook for 15 minutes, covered, over medium flame. To thicken, quickly whiz with a hand blender for a few pulses & continue to cook for 5 minutes. Serve.

149. Coconut Kale Soup

(Preparation time: 10 minutes | Cooking time: 20 minutes | Difficulty: Easy | Servings: 2)
Per serving: Calories 234, Total fat 5g, Protein 8g, Carbs 9g
Ingredients:

- ½ teaspoon of turmeric
- 1/2-inch of fresh ginger, grated
- 1 teaspoon of curry paste
- 1 tablespoon of soy sauce
- 3 cups of kale
- 1 cup of coconut milk

Instructions:

- In a saucepan, combine the kale, coconut milk, ginger, curry, turmeric, and soy sauce and heat for around 15 minutes, or till the kale is cooked.

150. French Pea Stew

(Preparation time: 10 minutes | Cooking time: 35 minutes | Difficulty: Easy | Servings: 4)

Per serving: Calories 203, Total fat 4g, Protein 17g, Carbs 19g

Ingredients:

- 1 bay leaf - 2 cloves of garlic
- 1 teaspoon of cumin
- 2 tablespoons of olive oil
- 1 red onion chopped
- 1 cup of yellow split peas

Instructions:

- Sauté bay leaf, onions, and garlic in a soup pot till tender.
- Wash the peas, then combine them with the garlic, salt and pepper to taste. Add 2 cups of water & cumin in a large pot.
- Cook for around 35 minutes on medium-high, stirring frequently & adjusting the water to achieve the desired consistency.

151. Golden Chickpea Soup

(Preparation time: 10 minutes | Cooking time: 35 minutes | Difficulty: Easy | Servings: 6)

Per serving: Calories 224, Total fat 5g, Protein 8g, Carbs 25g

Ingredients:

- 1/4 teaspoon of ground black pepper
- 2 bay leaves
- 1 tablespoon of extra-virgin olive oil
- 2 tablespoons of parsley
- 6 cloves of garlic, crushed
- 1 red onion, chopped
- 2 carrots, peeled and diced
- 6 cups of vegetable broth
- 1 lb. of chickpeas, cooked
- 1/2 cup of buckwheat pasta

Instructions:

- Heat the olive oil in a pot, then add the garlic & cook for around 2 minutes. Bring the chickpeas, bay leaf, red onion,

carrots, and broth to a boil, then reduce to a low flame and cook for around 30 minutes. Remove the bay leaves out from the soup and discard them.
- Two cups of the soup should be blended till smooth, then returned to the stove.
- Simmer for around 8 minutes after adding the noodles. Serve immediately.

152. Green Soup

(Preparation time: 10 minutes | Cooking time: 25 minutes | Difficulty: Easy | Servings: 4)

Per serving: Calories 164, Total fat 3g, Protein 8g, Carbs 12g

Ingredients:

- 1 teaspoon of turmeric
- 1 teaspoon of marjoram
- 1 onion, chopped
- 2 zucchinis, chopped
- 2 bell peppers, chopped
- 4 cups of vegetable broth
- 4 cups of leafy greens, including kale, chopped

Instructions:

- Cook the leafy greens, onion, zucchini, bell peppers, & broth in a pot over medium flame for around 25 minutes, or till the vegetables are soft. To taste, season using salt and pepper.
- Turn off the flame, set aside to cool, and then puree till smooth.

153. Italian Bean Stew

(Preparation time: 10 minutes | Cooking time: 55 minutes | Difficulty: Easy | Servings: 4)

Per serving: Calories 226, Total fat 3g, Protein 18g, Carbs 24g

Ingredients:

- ½ turmeric
- 1/2 teaspoon of basil leaves
- 2 tablespoons of extra-virgin olive oil
- 1 red onion, chopped
- 2 celery stalks, chopped

- 2 carrots, chopped
- 1 zucchini, chopped
- 1/2 cup of kale
- 2 cups of tomatoes, diced
- 2 cups of vegetable broth
- 2 1/2 cups of white kidney beans, cooked

Instructions:

- In a bowl, mash half of the white kidney beans using a potato masher or fork.
- Cook the carrots, basil, onion, zucchini, and pepper in a saucepan over medium-high flame till the veggies are soft and beginning to brown, around 15 minutes.
- Add 2 cups of water, tomatoes, kale, vegetable broth, and mashed white beans. Bring to the boil, then reduce to a low flame, cover, and leave to simmer for 15 minutes to mix the flavors. Heat through the remaining beans.
- Serve.

154. Simple Kale Stew

(Preparation time: 10 minutes | Cooking time: 45 minutes | Difficulty: Easy | Servings: 4)
Per serving: Calories 41, Total fat 10g, Protein 3g, Carbs 7g
Ingredients:

- 2 teaspoons of thyme
- 2 teaspoons of sage
- 1 red onion, chopped
- 5 cups of vegetable broth
- 2 cups of squash, diced
- 3 cups of kale, stems removed and chopped

Instructions:

- In a pot, heat 1 tablespoon of stock and cook the onion for 5 minutes over high flame.
- Bring the remainder of the broth to a boil. Reduce flame to low, add squash,

and cook for around 25 minutes, or till squash is soft.
- Cook for another 5 minutes after adding the kale, thyme, & sage. Serve immediately.

155. Lima Bean Stew

(Preparation time: 10 minutes | Cooking time: 45 minutes | Difficulty: Easy | Servings: 6)
Per serving: Calories 179, Total fat 4g, Protein 8g, Carbs 18g
Ingredients:

- 8 cups of water
- 1 1/2 teaspoons of salt
- 1 garlic clove, diced
- 1/4 teaspoon of cayenne
- 2 teaspoons of extra-virgin olive oil
- 1 red onion, diced
- 1 bell pepper, diced
- 1/2 cup of fresh parsley, diced
- 4 stalks of celery, diced
- 1 lb. of lima beans, cooked

Instructions:

- In a large pot, heat the oil and sauté the onion, celery, garlic, and bell pepper for around 5 minutes.
- Bring the beans, water, cayenne pepper, salt, & pepper to taste to the boil, then reduce to a simmer for around 40 minutes.
- Serve with a garnish of parsley.

156. Tomato Bisque

(Preparation time: 10 minutes | Cooking time: 40 minutes | Difficulty: Easy | Servings: 2)
Per serving: Calories 190, Total fat 6g, Protein 11g, Carbs 20g
Ingredients:

- 1 cup of water
- ½ teaspoon of turmeric
- 2 tablespoons of tomato paste
- ½ red onion, chopped
- 1 cup of vegetable broth

- 2 cups of tomatoes, diced
- 1 1/2 cups of tofu

Instructions:

- To make the tofu smooth, combine it with the water in a blender. Simmer for 40 minutes with the tomatoes, turmeric, tomato paste, red onion, and broth.
- Serve warm.

157. Fuss-Free Veggies Bake

(Preparation time: 10 minutes | Cooking time: 20 minutes | Difficulty: Easy | Servings: 6)
Per serving: Calories 206, Total fat 15g, Protein 10g, Carbs 7g
Ingredients:

- Salt and freshly ground black pepper to taste
- 1 teaspoon of ground cumin
- ½ teaspoon of paprika
- 2 teaspoons of curry powder
- 1 large zucchini, chopped
- 2 tablespoons of olive oil
- 1 red onion, sliced thinly
- ¼ cup of vegetable broth
- 1 medium green bell pepper, seeded and cubed
- 1 medium red bell pepper, seeded and cubed - ¼ cup of parsley, chopped
- 1 large yellow squash, chopped

Instructions:

- Preheat the oven at 375°F. Grease a large-sized baking dish lightly.
- Combine all of the ingredients, except for the parsley, in a large-sized mixing dish and stir till well blended.
- Spread the vegetable mixture equally in the baking dish that has been prepared.
- Bake for around 15-20 minutes, or till the vegetables are done to your liking.
- Remove from oven and serve right away with parsley on top.

158. Green Veggie Curry

(Preparation time: 10 minutes | Cooking time: 25 minutes | Difficulty: Easy | Servings: 2)
Per serving: Calories 324, Total fat 24g, Protein 17g, Carbs 8g
Ingredients:

- 1 teaspoon of garlic, minced
- ¼ teaspoon of red pepper flakes, crushed
- 1 teaspoon of fresh ginger, minced
- 1 teaspoon of fresh parsley, chopped finely
- 3 tablespoons of olive oil, divided
- 2 teaspoons of low-sodium soy sauce
- 1 tablespoon of red curry paste
- 2 teaspoons of red boat fish sauce
- ¼ small yellow onion, chopped
- 1 cup of broccoli florets
- 2 cups of fresh kale, torn
- ½ cup of coconut cream

Instructions:

- Heat two tablespoons of olive oil in a large-sized skillet over medium-high flame, sauté the onion for around 3-4 minutes. Sauté for 1 minute after adding the garlic and ginger.
- Stir in the broccoli till everything is nicely combined. Reduce the flame to medium-low & cook, constantly stirring, for around 1-2 minutes.
- Cook, constantly stirring, for around 1 minute after adding the curry paste.
- Cook, stirring regularly, for around 2 minutes after adding the kale.
- Stir in the remaining coconut oil & coconut cream till smooth. Stir in the fish sauce, soy sauce, and red pepper flakes, and cook, stirring regularly, for around 5-10 minutes, or till the curry achieves the desired thickness.
- Remove from the flame and garnish with parsley before serving.

159. Stewed Vegetables

(Preparation time: 10 minutes | Cooking time: 25 minutes | Difficulty: Easy | Servings: 4)
Per serving: Calories 310, Total fat 26g, Protein 8g, Carbs 6g
Ingredients:

- Salt and black pepper to taste
- 1 garlic clove, minced
- 1 teaspoon of paprika
- 2 tablespoons of butter
- 2 tablespoons of parsley, chopped
- 1 red onion, chopped
- 1 carrot, chopped
- 2 tomatoes, chopped
- 2 bell peppers, sliced
- 1 head of cabbage, shredded
- 1 cup of vegetable broth
- 2 cups of green beans, chopped

Instructions:

- In a medium-sized saucepan, heat the oil and cook the garlic and onions till aromatic, around 2 minutes.
- Stir in the bell peppers, cabbage, carrots, and green beans, as well as the paprika, salt, & pepper. Add the vegetable broth & tomatoes and cook for around 25 minutes on low flame to soften. Serve with a parsley garnish.

160. Balsamic Veggies with Feta and Walnuts

(Preparation time: 10 minutes | Cooking time: 35 minutes | Difficulty: Easy | Servings: 4)
Per serving: Calories 276, Total fat 23g, Protein 8g, Carbs 8g
Ingredients:

- Sea salt and cayenne pepper to taste
- 2 garlic cloves, halved
- 1 teaspoon of dried sage, crushed
- 2 thyme sprigs, chopped
- 4 tablespoons of olive oil
- 2 tablespoons of balsamic vinegar
- 8 red onions, peeled
- 1 red bell pepper, sliced
- 1 orange bell pepper, sliced
- 1 green bell pepper, sliced
- ½ head of broccoli, cut into florets
- 2 zucchinis, sliced
- 1 cup of feta cheese, crumbled
- ½ cup of walnuts, toasted and chopped

Instructions:

- Preheat the oven at 375°F. Shake well to combine all veggies with olive oil, spices, & balsamic vinegar. In a baking dish, spread out the vegetables and roast for around 40 minutes, or till tender, flipping halfway through.
- Remove the dish from the oven and place it on a serving plate. Serve with feta cheese and walnuts scattered over the top.

161. Veggie Noodles with Avocado Sauce

(Preparation time: 10 minutes | Cooking time: 15 minutes | Difficulty: Easy | Servings: 4)
Per serving: Calories 373, Total fat 39g, Protein 23g, Carbs 10g
Ingredients:

- Salt and black pepper to taste
- 1 lemon, juiced and zested
- 1 bird's eye chili, deveined and minced
- 2 tablespoons of olive oil
- 2 tablespoons of sesame oil
- 2 tablespoons of cilantro, chopped
- 2 tablespoons of pumpkin seeds
- 1 red onion, chopped
- ½ pound of pumpkin, spiralized
- ½ pound of bell peppers, spiralized
- 2 avocados, chopped

Instructions:

- In a dry skillet, toast pumpkin seeds for 1 minute, turning regularly; set aside. Sauté bell peppers with pumpkin in oil for 8 minutes. Place on a serving dish and serve.

- In a food processor, pulse avocados, olive oil, lemon juice, onion, chili, and lemon zest to make a creamy consistency. Season to taste, then spoon over the vegetable noodles, sprinkle with pumpkin seeds, and serve.

162. Tamari Toasted Almonds

(Preparation time: 10 minutes | Cooking time: 10 minutes | Difficulty: Easy | Servings: 4)
Per serving: Calories 89, Total fat 8g, Protein 4g, Carbs 3g
Ingredients:
- 2 tablespoons of tamari or soy sauce
- 1 teaspoon of toasted sesame oil
- ½ cup of raw almonds or sunflower seeds

Instructions:
- Heat the walnuts in a dry skillet over medium-high flame, often turning to prevent them from browning. Pour the tamari with olive oil into the hot skillet & whisk to coat the walnuts, which should take around 7 to 8 minutes.
- Turn off the flame, and the tamari mixture will stick to & dry on the walnuts as they cool.

163. Garden Salad Wraps

(Preparation time: 10 minutes | Cooking time: 15 minutes | Difficulty: Easy | Servings: 4)
Per serving: Calories 152, Total fat 10g, Protein 5g, Carbs 8g
Ingredients:
- 1/2 teaspoon of salt
- 1/4 teaspoon of ground black pepper
- 6 tablespoons olive oil
- 1 tablespoon of soy sauce
- 1 teaspoon of yellow or spicy brown mustard
- 1/4 cup of apple cider vinegar
- 1/3 cup of minced red onion

- 1 medium English cucumber, peeled and chopped
- 1 large carrot, shredded
- 3 ripe Roma tomatoes, finely chopped
- 3 cups shredded romaine lettuce
- 1/4 cup of sliced pitted green olives
- 1-pound of extra-firm tofu, drained, patted dry, & cut into 1/2-inch strips
- 4 (10-inch) whole-grain flour tortillas

Instructions:
- Heat 2 tablespoons of oil in a large-sized frypan over medium flame. Toss in the tofu. Cook for around 10 minutes, or till golden brown. Set aside to cool after sprinkling with soy sauce. Stir together the remaining 4 tablespoons of oil, vinegar, salt, mustard, and pepper till well combined. Set them aside.
- Combine the lettuce, tomatoes, onion, carrots, cucumber, and olives. Pour the dressing on top and toss to coat.
- To make the wraps, spread one tortilla with roughly a fourth of the salad on a work surface. Place a few tofu strips on the tortilla & tightly fold it up. Cut in half.

164. Garden Patch Sandwiches

(Preparation time: 15 minutes | Cooking time: 0 minutes | Difficulty: Easy | Servings: 4)
Per serving: Calories 299, Total fat 25g, Protein 9g, Carbs 17g
Ingredients:
- 1/2 teaspoon of salt
- 1/4 teaspoon of ground black pepper
- 1 celery rib, finely chopped
- 3 red onions, minced
- 4 (1/4-inch) slices ripe tomato
- 1 medium red bell pepper, finely chopped
- 4 lettuce leaves
- 8 slices of whole-grain bread

- 1/4 cup of shelled sunflower seeds
- 1 pound of extra-firm tofu drained and patted dry
- 1/2 cup of vegan mayonnaise, homemade or store-bought

Instructions:

- Tofu should be ground and placed in a large-sized mixing dish. Combine the bell pepper, red onion, celery, and sunflower seeds. Mix the mayonnaise, salt, and pepper in a mixing bowl and stir well.
- If desired, toast the bread. Using four slices of bread, evenly spread the contents. Add a tomato slice, a lettuce leaf, & the remaining bread to each. Serve the sandwiches by cutting them in half diagonally.

165. Egg Avocado Salad

(Preparation time: 10 minutes | Cooking time: 0 minutes | Difficulty: Easy | Servings: 4)
Per serving: Calories 224, Total fat 18g, Protein 11g, Carbs 6g
Ingredients:

- Salt and pepper to taste
- 2 tablespoons of lemon juice
- 2 tablespoons of parsley, chopped
- ¼ cup of celery, chopped
- 1 tablespoon of mayonnaise
- 6 hard-boiled eggs, peeled and chopped
- 1 avocado

Instructions:

- In a large-sized mixing dish, mash the avocado.
- Using a fork, mash the avocado.
- Mash the eggs after adding the egg.
- Combine the mayonnaise, lemon juice, celery, parsley, salt, & pepper.
- Refrigerate for a few hours. Before serving, let it sit for at least 30 minutes.

166. Zucchini Pasta Salad

(Preparation time: 10 minutes | Cooking time: 0 minutes | Difficulty: Easy | Servings: 10)
Per serving: Calories 299, Total fat 25g, Protein 7g, Carbs 11g
Ingredients:

- 1 clove of garlic, grated
- ¼ teaspoon of red pepper flakes
- 5 tablespoons of olive oil
- 2 tablespoons of fresh oregano, chopped
- 2 teaspoons of Dijon mustard
- 1 red onion, chopped
- 3 cups of cherry tomatoes, sliced in half
- ¼ cup of Kalamata olives pitted
- 2 cups of zucchini noodles
- ¾ cup of Parmesan cheese shaved
- 3 tablespoons of red-wine vinegar

Instructions:

- In a bowl, whisk together the olive oil, Dijon mustard, oregano, red wine vinegar, garlic, red onion, and red pepper flakes.
- Add the zucchini noodles and mix well.
- Olives, tomatoes, & Parmesan cheese should be sprinkled on top.

167. Rice and Veggie Bowl

(Preparation time: 10 minutes | Cooking time: 15 minutes | Difficulty: Easy | Servings: 6)
Per serving: Calories 260, Total fat 9g, Protein 9g, Carbs 29g
Ingredients:

- 1 teaspoon of salt, to taste
- Ground black pepper
- 1 teaspoon of ground turmeric
- 1 teaspoon of chili powder
- 1 teaspoon of ground cumin
- 2 tablespoons of coconut oil
- 1 teaspoon of tomato paste
- 2 garlic cloves, minced
- 1 large red onion, sliced

- 1 red bell pepper, chopped
- 1 bunch of broccoli, cut into bite-sized florets with short stems
- 1 head of cauliflower, sliced into bite-sized florets
- 2 cups of cooked brown rice

Instructions:

- Into a large-sized pan, melt the olive oil on a medium-high flame.
- Stir in the turmeric, salt, cumin, chili powder, & tomato paste once the oil is hot.
- For 1 minute, cook the contents. Stir the spices in a circular motion till they are aromatic. Combine the onion and garlic. Sauté the onions for 3 minutes, or till they are softened. Combine the broccoli, cauliflower, & bell pepper. Cover the pot with a lid. Cook, stirring periodically, for around 3 to 4 minutes. Add the rice that has been cooked. Cook for around 2 to 3 minutes, frequently stirring to ensure that it is well combined with the veggies. Stir till the rice is thoroughly warmed.
- Make sure the seasoning is correct. And, if desired, make flavor changes.
- Reduce the flame to low and simmer for another 2 to 3 minutes to allow the flavors to mingle.
- Season using ground black pepper before serving.

168. High Protein Salad

(Preparation time: 10 minutes | Cooking time: 10 minutes | Difficulty: Easy | Servings: 6)
Per serving: Calories 205, Total fat 2g, Protein 13g, Carbs 21g
Ingredients:
For the salad:

- 4 tablespoons of capers
- 4 handfuls of arugula
- 2 cups of lentils

- 2 cups of green kidney beans

For the dressing:

- 1 tablespoon of balsamic vinegar
- 1 tablespoon of tahini
- 2 tablespoons of peanut butter
- 1 tablespoon of caper brine
- 1 tablespoon of tamari
- 2 tablespoons of hot sauce

Instructions:

- To make the dressing, combine the following ingredients.
- Stir all of the ingredients together in a mixing bowl until they form a creamy dressing. To make the salad:
- Combine the beans, capers, arugula, & lentils in a mixing bowl. Serve with the dressing on top.

169. Green Beans Stew

(Preparation time: 10 minutes | Cooking time: 25 minutes | Difficulty: Easy | Servings: 4)
Per serving: Calories 281, Total fat 5g, Protein 11g, Carbs 14g
Ingredients:

- A pinch of black pepper
- 2 garlic cloves, minced
- 1 tablespoon of parsley, chopped
- 2 tablespoons of olive oil
- 1 red onion, chopped
- 2 carrots, chopped
- 1 cup of tomatoes, chopped
- 2 1/2 cups of green beans
- 5 cups of low-sodium veggie stock

Instructions:

- Over medium flame, heat the oil in a pot, then add the onion, stir, & cook for around 5 minutes.
- Stir in the carrots, green beans, black pepper, garlic, tomatoes, and stock, then cover and cook for 20 minutes over medium flame.
- Serve for lunch by adding parsley and dividing it into bowls.

170. Carrot Stew

(Preparation time: 10 minutes | Cooking time: 35 minutes | Difficulty: Easy | Servings: 6)
Per serving: Calories 123, Total fat 4g, Protein 5g, Carbs 15g
Ingredients:

- 1 teaspoon of salt
- ½ teaspoon of ground black pepper
- 1 tablespoon of lemon juice
- 1 tablespoon of olive oil
- ½ teaspoon of ground cumin
- 1 bird's eye chili, chopped
- 1 teaspoon of dried thyme
- 1 tablespoon of tomato paste
- 1/3 cup of fresh parsley, chopped
- 1 tablespoon of sour cream
- 4 carrots, peeled
- 1 ½ cup of potatoes, chopped
- 5 cups of vegetable broth

Instructions:

- Baking paper should be used to line the baking tray.
- Sprinkle olive oil and salt over the sweet potatoes and carrots on the tray.
- Preheat the oven at 365°F and bake the vegetables for around 25 minutes.
- In the meantime, bring the beef stock to a boil in the pan.
- Add tomato paste, dried thyme, crushed cumin, and minced chili pepper. Add the vegetables to the pan once they've finished cooking.
- Bring the vegetables to a boil and cook till they are tender. Then, using the blender, blend the mixture till it is completely smooth. Cook for around 2 minutes before adding the lemon juice. Stir everything together thoroughly.
- Then stir in the sour cream and parsley. Stir everything together thoroughly.
- Continue to cook the soup for another 3 minutes.

171. Eggplant Stew

(Preparation time: 10 minutes | Cooking time: 20 minutes | Difficulty: Easy | Servings: 4)
Per serving: Calories 270, Total fat 4g, Protein 9g, Carbs 10g
Ingredients:

- 1 teaspoon of lime juice
- A pinch of cinnamon powder
- ½ teaspoon of turmeric powder
- ½ teaspoon of cumin seeds
- 1 tablespoon of coriander seeds
- 1 tablespoon of olive oil
- 2 garlic cloves, minced
- 1 tablespoon of ginger, grated
- ½ teaspoon of mustard seeds
- 1 bird's eye chili, chopped
- 1 tablespoon of parsley, chopped
- ½ teaspoon of cardamom, ground
- 1 cup of low-sodium veggie stock
- 4 baby eggplants, cubed

Instructions:

- Heat the oil in a pot over medium-high flame, then add the coriander, cumin, and mustard seeds, stirring constantly. Cook for 5 minutes.
- Stir in the ginger, garlic, cardamom, chili, cinnamon, and turmeric, then cook for another 5 minutes.
- Stir in the lime juice, eggplants, & stock, then cover and simmer for 15 minutes over medium flame. Stir in the parsley, divide into dishes, & serve for lunch.

172. Eggplant Soup

(Preparation time: 10 minutes | Cooking time: 30 minutes | Difficulty: Easy | Servings: 4)
Per serving: Calories 137, Total fat 6g, Protein 4g, Carbs 19g
Ingredients:

- 1 teaspoon of salt
- 1 garlic clove, peeled
- ½ teaspoon of ground cumin

- ½ teaspoon of cayenne pepper
- 1 tablespoon of olive oil
- ¼ cup of fresh parsley, chopped
- ¼ cup of fresh cilantro, chopped
- 1 celery stalk, chopped
- ½ cup of tomatoes, chopped
- 1 red onion, diced
- 2 eggplants, trimmed
- 1 teaspoon of butter
- 4 cups of vegetable stock

Instructions:

- Remove the skins off the eggplants and season them using salt and olive oil.
- Preheat the oven at 360°F.
- Place the eggplants in the baking tray and bake for around 20 minutes.
- Bake the veggies for around 25 minutes.
- Fill the pan halfway with stock.
- Add the tomatoes parsley, parsley, ground cumin, celery stalk, cayenne pepper, and garlic clove.
- Cook for around 5 minutes, stirring occasionaly.
- In a separate skillet, heat the butter.
- Roast the onion till it's transparent.
- Toss the onion into the stock that has been cooked.
- Transfer the cooked eggplants to a food processor and pulse till smooth.
- The pureed eggplants should then be added to the stock mixture.
- Hand-blender the soup till it reaches a creamy consistency.
- Cook for around 5 minutes on low flame.

173. Chard and Lentil Stew

(Preparation time: 10 minutes | Cooking time: 40 minutes | Difficulty: Easy | Servings: 4)
Per serving: Calories 286, Total fat 9g, Protein 14g, Carbs 22g
Ingredients:

- A pinch of salt and black pepper

- ½ teaspoon of ground turmeric
- ½ teaspoon of red chili flakes
- 2 garlic cloves, minced
- ½ teaspoon of ground ginger
- 1 teaspoon of ground cumin
- 2 tablespoons of olive oil
- 1 red onion, chopped
- 2 carrots, chopped
- 2 cups of tomatoes, chopped
- 1 cup of red lentils
- 2 quarts of veggie stock
- 1 bunch of chard, roughly chopped

Instructions:

- Heat the oil in a pot over medium flame.
- Cook for around 7 minutes after adding the onion and carrot.
- Stir in the chili flakes, garlic, cumin, salt, ginger, turmeric, and pepper and simmer for an additional minute.
- Cook for another 5 minutes after adding the tomatoes and stirring them in.
- Stir in the lentils & stock, bring to the boil, then reduce to medium-low flame and cook for 10 minutes.
- Toss in the chard, heat for 5 minutes, then ladle into serving bowls.

174. Spicy Pumpkin Soup

(Preparation time: 10 minutes | Cooking time: 45 minutes | Difficulty: Easy | Servings: 4)
Per serving: Calories 249, Total fat 9g, Protein 25g, Carbs 15g
Ingredients:

- 2 teaspoons of turmeric
- 1 teaspoon of ground ginger
- 3 cloves of garlic
- 2 tablespoons of olive oil
- 3 bird's-eye chilies, chopped
- 1 red onion, chopped
- 1/2 cup of kale
- 1 butternut squash, peeled, de-seeded, and chopped
- 1 pint of vegetable stock (broth)

Instructions:

- Prepare all of the ingredients & heat the olive oil in a skillet, then add the butternut squash & onion and simmer for 6 minutes, or till softened.
- Cook for around 2 minutes, stirring regularly, after adding the kale, garlic, chili, turmeric, & ginger.
- Bring the vegetable stock (broth) to a boil, then reduce to a low flame and cook for around 20 minutes.
- Process till smooth in a food processor.
- A hand blender can also be used.
- Serve with a swirl of cream or on its own. Enjoy.

175. Greens and Grains Soup

(Preparation time: 10 minutes | Cooking time: 45 minutes | Difficulty: Easy | Servings: 3)
Per serving: Calories 155, Total fat 2g, Protein 17g, Carbs 34g
Ingredients:
- Salt to taste
- Freshly ground pepper to taste
- ½ tablespoon of extra-virgin olive oil
- 1 clove of garlic, peeled, minced
- 3 cups of vegetable broth or chicken broth
- ½ cup of whole grains of your choice like wheat berries, brown rice, barley etc., rinsed well
- 1 cup of kale, chopped (leaves and stems, but keep them separate)

Instructions:
- In a saucepan, combine the grains. Pour just enough water to completely submerge the grains. Place the saucepan on the stovetop over medium flame.
- Reduce the flame to low and simmer, covered, till the grains are tender.
- Drain into a colander.

- Place a soup pot on the stovetop over medium-high flame. Allow the oil to heat up.
- Once the oil is hot, add the kale stems and cook till soft.
- Cook for a few seconds, till the garlic is aromatic.
- Pour the stock into the pot & scrape the bottom to deglaze it. Toss in some grains. When the soup has to a boil, add the kale leaves and simmer till the leaves have wilted. Season to taste using salt and pepper.
- Pour the soup into soup bowls. Serve with a drizzle of olive oil on top.

176. Kale and Feta Salad with Cranberry Dressing

(Preparation time: 10 minutes | Cooking time: 0 minutes | Difficulty: Easy | Servings: 2)
Per serving: Calories 300, Total fat 8g, Protein 14g, Carbs 1g
Ingredients:
- 4 Medjool dates, chopped
- 1 apple, peeled, cored, and sliced
- 1 cup of kale, finely chopped
- 1/4 cup of feta cheese, crumbled
- 4 tablespoons of walnuts, chopped

For the dressing
- 3 tablespoons of water
- Sea salt
- 2 teaspoons of honey
- 3 tablespoons of olive oil
- ½ red onion, chopped
- 1 tablespoon of red wine vinegar
- 1/4 cup of cranberries

Instructions:
- In a food processor, combine all of the dressing ingredients and process until smooth. In a large mixing bowl, combine all of the salad ingredients.
- Toss the salad with the dressing & toss it again.

177. Onion, Tomato, Chickpeas and Parsley Salad

(Preparation time: 10 minutes | Cooking time: 0 minutes | Difficulty: Easy | Servings: 2)
Per serving: Calories 238, Total fat 15g, Protein 6g, Carbs 18g
Ingredients:
- 1 tablespoon of chopped parsley
- 1/2 red onion, chopped
- 1/2 cup of chopped tomatoes
- 1 cup of cooked chickpeas

For the dressing:
- a pinch of sea salt
- 1 tablespoon of fresh lemon juice
- 1 tablespoon of olive oil
- 1 tablespoon of chia seeds
- 1 tablespoon of flax seeds

Instructions:
- Dressing, chickpeas, tomatoes, onions, & parsley should be placed in this order.

178. Strawberry, Arugula and Orange Bowls

(Preparation time: 15 minutes | Cooking time: 0 minutes | Difficulty: Easy | Servings: 4)
Per serving: Calories 107, Total fat 3g, Protein 2g, Carbs 19g
Ingredients:
- 2 oranges, peeled and segmented
- 1½ cups of fresh strawberries, hulled and sliced
- 6 cups of fresh baby arugula

For the dressing:
- Salt and ground black pepper, as required
- 2 tablespoons of fresh lemon juice
- 2 teaspoons of extra-virgin olive oil
- 1 tablespoon of raw honey
- 1 teaspoon of Dijon mustard

Instructions:
- Combine all ingredients in a salad bowl and toss to combine.

- To make the dressing, combine the following ingredients.
- In a separate bowl, whisk together all of the ingredients till smooth.
- Toss them with the dressing to coat it evenly.
- Serve right away.

179. Orange and Beet Bowls

(Preparation time: 10 minutes | Cooking time: 0 minutes | Difficulty: Easy | Servings: 4)
Per serving: Calories 233, Total fat 16g, Protein 5g, Carbs 20g
Ingredients:
- Pinch of salt
- 3 tablespoons of olive oil
- 3 large oranges, peeled
- 6 cups of fresh rocket
- 2 beets, trimmed, peeled, and sliced
- ¼ cup of walnuts, chopped

Instructions:
- Place all ingredients in a salad bowl and gently toss to coat.
- Serve right away.

180. Kale and Raspberry Salad

(Preparation time: 15 minutes | Cooking time: 0 minutes | Difficulty: Easy | Servings: 2)
Per serving: Calories 228, Total fat 16g, Protein 7g, Carbs 16g
Ingredients:
- ½ cup of fresh raspberries
- 3 cups of fresh baby kale
- ¼ cup of walnuts, chopped

For the dressing:
- Salt and ground black pepper, as required
- 1 tablespoon of extra-virgin olive oil
- 1 tablespoon of apple cider vinegar
- ½ teaspoon of pure maple syrup

Instructions:
- Combine all ingredients in a salad bowl and toss to combine.

- To make the dressing, whisk together all of the ingredients in a separate dish till smooth.
- Toss the salad with the dressing to coat it evenly. Serve right away.

181. Leek and Sun Roasted Tomatoes Frittata

(Preparation time: 10 minutes | Cooking time: 20 minutes | Difficulty: Easy | Servings: 4)
Per serving: Calories 211, Total fat 13g, Protein 15g, Carbs 12g
Ingredients:
- Salt and freshly ground black pepper
- 1 tablespoon of olive oil - 4 eggs
- 2 tablespoons of kale (frozen or fresh)
- 1 sliced leek
- 6 sliced sun roasted tomatoes

Instructions:
- Cook the leeks in olive oil in a medium-sized nonstick frying pan till soft.
- Heat till the kale has wilted, then add the kale & tomatoes (season using salt and black pepper).
- Separate the eggs and whisk them separately before pouring them into the pan, covering the majority of the other ingredients. While the eggs are cooking, carefully slide around the pan's sides to allow the uncooked egg on top to cook in the pan's bottom. After the frittata is finished, place it on the grill to crisp up the top without scorching the bottom.
- It's a lot of fun to eat it by slicing it into slices.

182. Vegetarian Kebabs

(Preparation time: 10 minutes | Cooking time: 10 minutes | Difficulty: Easy | Servings: 4)
Per serving: Calories 88, Total fat 4g, Protein 2g, Carbs 12g
Ingredients:
- 2 tablespoons of water

- 1 tablespoon of olive oil
- 1 tablespoon of dried parsley
- 2 tablespoons of balsamic vinegar
- 2 sweet peppers
- 2 peeled red onions
- 2 trimmed zucchinis

Instructions:
- Cut the sweet peppers and onions into medium-sized squares.
- After that, the zucchini should be sliced.
- Thread all of the vegetables together using skewers.
- After that, in a small dish, mix olive oil, water, dried parsley, & balsamic vinegar.
- Place the veggie skewers on a hot 390°F grill and drizzle with the olive oil mixture.
- Cook for 3 minutes per side, or till the vegetables are light brown.

183. Vegetarian Lasagna

(Preparation time: 10 minutes | Cooking time: 25 minutes | Difficulty: Easy | Servings: 4)
Per serving: Calories 77, Total fat 3g, Protein 5g, Carbs 9g
Ingredients:
- 1 tablespoon of olive oil
- 1 teaspoon of chili powder
- 1 eggplant, sliced
- 1/2 cup of diced bell pepper
- 1 cup of diced tomatoes
- 1 cup of diced carrot
- 1 cup of vegetable broth
- 1 cup of chopped spinach
- 1/2 cup of feta cheese

Instructions:
- Combine the carrot, bell pepper, & kale in a saucepan.
- Add the olive oil & chili powder and stir till the vegetables are completely covered. Cook for approximately 5 minutes.

- Create a layer of sliced eggplants in the casserole shape, then cover with the vegetable mixture.
- Combine the tomatoes & feta cheese.
- Preheat the oven at 400°F and bake for around 25 minutes.

184. Vegetarian Chili

(Preparation time: 10 minutes | Cooking time: 25 minutes | Difficulty: Easy | Servings: 4)
Per serving: Calories 234, Total fat 2g, Protein 14g, Carbs 34g
Ingredients:

- 1 teaspoon of tomato paste
- 1 chopped bird's eye chili, chopped
- 2 cups of vegetable broth
- 1/2 cup of chopped celery stalk
- 1 cup of chopped tomatoes
- 1 cup of cooked red kidney beans
- 1/2 cup of buckwheat

Instructions:

- Combine all of the ingredients in a large pot and well combine.
- Close the lid & cook the chili for around 25 minutes on medium-low flame.

185. Aromatic Spaghetti

(Preparation time: 10 minutes | Cooking time: 15 minutes | Difficulty: Easy | Servings: 4)
Per serving: Calories 128, Total fat 2g, Protein 5g, Carbs 20g
Ingredients:

- 2 cups of water
- 1 teaspoon of parsley
- 1 teaspoon of ground nutmeg
- 1/2 cup of buckwheat spaghetti
- 1/4 cup of soy milk

Instructions:

- Bring a saucepan of water to the boil, then add the spaghetti & cook for around 8 to 10 minutes, depending on how long you want it to cook.
- Meanwhile, bring the soy milk to a boil.

- Drain the spaghetti and mix it with the soy milk, powdered nutmeg, & parsley.
- Stir the meal thoroughly.

186. Chunky Tomatoes

(Preparation time: 10 minutes | Cooking time: 15 minutes | Difficulty: Easy | Servings: 3)
Per serving: Calories 250, Total fat 2g, Protein 3g, Carbs 8g
Ingredients:

- 1 teaspoon of olive oil
- 1/2 teaspoon of chopped garlic
- 1 teaspoon of Italian seasonings
- 1 chopped bird's eye chili
- ½ cup of diced red onion
- 2 cups of roughly chopped plum tomatoes

Instructions:

- Heat the olive oil in a saucepan.
- Combine the chili and onion. Cook the vegetables for around 5 minutes. They should be stirred once in a while.
- After that, add the tomatoes, garlic, & Italian spices.
- Close the lid and cook the meal for around 10 minutes.

187. Baked Falafel

(Preparation time: 10 minutes | Cooking time: 25 minutes | Difficulty: Easy | Servings: 4)
Per serving: Calories 216, Total fat 11g, Protein 13g, Carbs 28g
Ingredients:

- 1/2 teaspoon of coriander
- 1 teaspoon of ground cumin
- 2 diced garlic cloves
- 3 tablespoons of olive oil
- 1 diced yellow onion
- 1 cup of chopped fresh parsley
- 2 cups of cooked chickpeas

Instructions:

- Combine all of the ingredients in a food processor and pulse till smooth.

- Preheat the oven at 375°F.
- Then line the baking pan using baking paper.
- Make falafel shapes out of the chickpea mixture by rolling it into balls and gently flattening them.
- In a baking pan, place the falafel & bake for around 25 minutes.

188. Vegetarian Paella

(Preparation time: 10 minutes | Cooking time: 20 minutes | Difficulty: Easy | Servings: 4)
Per serving: Calories 170, Total fat 3g, Protein 4g, Carbs 22g
Ingredients:
- 2 cups of water
- 1 teaspoon of chili flakes
- 1 tablespoon of olive oil
- 1 sliced onion
- 1/2 cup of green peas
- 1 cup of diced bell pepper
- 1 cup of chopped artichoke hearts
- 1 cup of brown rice
- 1 teaspoon of saffron

Instructions:
- In a skillet, heat the olive oil.
- Combine the saffron, chili flakes, onion, & bell pepper.
- For around 5 minutes, roast the vegetables.
- Combine them with the cooked rice.
- Toss in the artichoke hearts & green peas after that. Cook the paella over low flame for about 10 minutes, stirring frequently.

189. Mushroom Cakes

(Preparation time: 10 minutes | Cooking time: 10 minutes | Difficulty: Easy | Servings: 4)
Per serving: Calories 103, Total fat 5g, Protein 4g, Carbs 12g
Ingredients:
- 1 teaspoon of chili powder

- 1 tablespoon of parsley
- 1 tablespoon of olive oil
- 3 chopped garlic cloves, chopped
- 1 beaten egg
- 1/4 cup of cooked brown rice
- 2 cups of chopped mushrooms

Instructions:
- Grind the mushrooms in a food processor.
- Combine the garlic, parsley, egg, rice, & chili powder.
- Blend the ingredients together for 10 seconds.
- After that, heat olive oil for around 1 minute.
- Make medium mushroom cakes & cook them in olive oil that has been heated.
- Cook the mushroom cakes for around 5 minutes on each side over medium flame.

190. Sweet Potato Balls

(Preparation time: 10 minutes | Cooking time: 10 minutes | Difficulty: Easy | Servings: 4)
Per serving: Calories 133, Total fat 8g, Protein 3g, Carbs 12g
Ingredients:
- 1/2 teaspoon of ground turmeric
- 1 teaspoon of ground paprika
- 2 tablespoons of olive oil
- 2 tablespoons of chopped fresh parsley
- 1 beaten egg
- 1 cup of sweet potato, mashed and cooked
- 3 tablespoons of ground buckwheat

Instructions:
- In a mixing bowl, combine the mashed sweet potato, paprika, fresh parsley, egg, ground buckwheat, and turmeric.
- To make the little balls, combine all of the ingredients in a mixing bowl and stir till smooth.
- Heat the olive oil in a saucepan.

- Place the sweet potato balls in the olive oil that has been heated.
- Cook till golden brown on both sides.

191. Quinoa Bowls

(Preparation time: 10 minutes | Cooking time: 15 minutes | Difficulty: Easy | Servings: 4)
Per serving: Calories 190, Total fat 6g, Protein 8g, Carbs 30g

Ingredients:

- 2 cups of water
- 1 tablespoon of lemon juice
- 1/2 teaspoon of grated lemon zest
- 1 tablespoon of olive oil
- 1 cup of diced tomatoes
- 1 cup of diced sweet pepper
- 1 cup of quinoa
- 1/2 cup of cooked rice

Instructions:

- After combining water with quinoa, cook for around 15 minutes. Remove it from the flame & set it aside to cool for 10 minutes. In a large-sized mixing bowl, place the cooked quinoa.
- Add in the tomatoes, lemon juice, sweet pepper, rice, lemon zest, & olive oil.
- Before transferring the mixture to the serving dishes, give it a good stir.

192. Vegetarian Meatloaf

(Preparation time: 10 minutes | Cooking time: 20 minutes | Difficulty: Easy | Servings: 4)
Per serving: Calories 162, Total fat 5g, Protein 7g, Carbs 15g

Ingredients:

- 1/2 teaspoon of chili flakes
- 1 tablespoon of ground flax seeds
- 1 tablespoon of tomato paste
- 1 tablespoon of olive oil
- 1 diced red onion
- 1/2 cup of diced carrot
- 1/2 cup of chopped celery stalk
- 1 cup of cooked chickpeas

Instructions:

- Heat the olive oil in a saucepan.
- In a large pot, combine the carrots, onion with a celery stalk. Cook for 8 minutes, or till the vegetables are soft.
- After that, add the chickpeas, chili flakes, & crushed flax seeds.
- Puree the ingredients in an immersion blender till smooth. Then line the loaf form with baking paper and pour the blended ingredients inside. Cover it with tomato paste & flatten it out. Preheat the oven at 365°F and bake the meatloaf for around 20 minutes.

193. Cauliflower Steaks

(Preparation time: 10 minutes | Cooking time: 20 minutes | Difficulty: Easy | Servings: 4)
Per serving: Calories 92, Total fat 7g, Protein 2g, Carbs 7g

Ingredients:

- A pinch of salt
- 1 teaspoon of ground turmeric
- 1/2 teaspoon of minced garlic
- 1/2 teaspoon of cayenne pepper
- 2 tablespoons of olive oil
- 1-pound of the cauliflower head

Instructions:

- The cauliflower head steaks are coated with cayenne pepper, ground turmeric, salt and garlic.The cauliflower steaks should next be lined on the oven pan with baking paper. Sprinkle with olive oil & bake at 375°F for about 25 minutes, or till the vegetable steaks are done.

194. Tofu Tikka Masala

(Preparation time: 10 minutes | Cooking time: 25 minutes | Difficulty: Easy | Servings: 4)
Per serving: Calories 155, Total fat 8g, Protein 12g, Carbs 18g

Ingredients:

- 1 teaspoon of garam masala
- 1 teaspoon of ground paprika

- 1 tablespoon of olive oil
- 1/2 cup of soy milk - 1/2 diced onion
- 1/2 cup of chopped tomatoes
- 1 cup of chopped plain tofu

Instructions:

- Heat the olive oil in a saucepan.
- Cook till the chopped onion is light brown. The tomatoes, paprika powder, and garam masala are then added. Bring the mixture to the boil in a pot.
- Well incorporate the soy milk. Cook on low flame for about 5 minutes.
- After adding the chopped tofu, cook for another 3 minutes. Allow 10 minutes for the dish to rest after it has been prepared.

195. Mushroom Stroganoff

(Preparation time: 10 minutes | Cooking time: 25 minutes | Difficulty: Easy | Servings: 4)
Per serving: Calories 70, Total fat 4g, Protein 3g, Carbs 7g

Ingredients:

- 1 diced garlic clove
- 1 teaspoon of ground black pepper
- 1 tablespoon of coconut oil
- 1 teaspoon of dried thyme
- 1 teaspoon of buckwheat flour
- 1 chopped onion - 1/2 cup of soy milk
- 2 cups of sliced mushrooms

Instructions:

- Heat the olive oil in a saucepan.
- With the mushrooms & onion, cook for almost 10 minutes. Stir the vegetables every now and then.
- Season using black pepper, salt, thyme, and garlic powder after that.
- With the soy milk, bring the mixture to the boil. The flour is then added and thoroughly mixed in till the mixture is perfectly smooth. Cook till the mushroom stroganoff thickens, around 10 minutes.

196. Chana Masala

(Preparation time: 10 minutes | Cooking time: 25 minutes | Difficulty: Easy | Servings: 4)
Per serving: Calories 235, Total fat 7g, Protein 10g, Carbs 25g

Ingredients:

- 2 cups of water
- 1 teaspoon of minced garlic
- 1 teaspoon of minced ginger
- 1 tablespoon of garam masala
- 1 chopped bird's eye chili
- 1 tablespoon of olive oil
- 3 tablespoons of chopped fresh parsley
- 1 diced red onion
- 1 cup of chopped tomatoes
- 1 cup of cooked chickpeas

Instructions:

- In a blender, combine the bird's eye chili, garlic, ginger, & fresh parsley.
- Then heat the olive oil in a saucepan. Roast the onion till it has turned a light brown color.
- Combine the chili mixture, garam masala, & chopped tomatoes.
- Bring the mixture to the boil in a pot.
- Add the chickpeas and water. On a low flame, cook the meal for around 10 minutes.

197. Vegetarian Korma

(Preparation time: 10 minutes | Cooking time: 20 minutes | Difficulty: Easy | Servings: 3)
Per serving: Calories 245, Total fat 29g, Protein 6g, Carbs 18g

Ingredients:

- 1/2 teaspoon of curry powder
- 1 teaspoon of garam masala
- 1 tablespoon of olive oil
- 1 diced red onion
- 1 cup of frozen mixed vegetables
- 1 cup of coconut milk
- 1/4 cup of chopped walnuts

Instructions:

- The walnuts & coconut milk should be combined in a blender.
- Heat the olive oil in a saucepan, then add the onion. Cook for about 3 minutes, stirring occasionally.
- After that, add the mixture & bring it to the boil.
- Combine the frozen vegetables, garam masala, & curry powder.
- Cook the korma on a medium flame for about 10 minutes with the lid closed.

198. Bake Walnut Eggplant

(Preparation time: 10 minutes | Cooking time: 25 minutes | Difficulty: Easy | Servings: 3)
Per serving: Calories 244, Total fat 23g, Protein 6g, Carbs 6g
Ingredients:

- 2 minced cloves of garlic
- 2 tablespoons of finely chopped fresh parsley
- 6 tablespoons of olive oil
- 2 eggplants
- 1/2 cup of raw walnuts

Instructions:

- Preheat the oven at 340°F.
- Place the eggplants cut side up onto a baking sheet after slicing them in half.
- Then sprinkle one tablespoon of olive oil over the top and bake till cooked. This should take you about 20 minutes to complete.
- Combine the walnuts, garlic, parsley, & 5 tablespoons of olive oil in a food processor and process till a thick paste forms. If necessary, thin the mixture with just a little water.
- Cook the eggplants for another 5 minutes underneath the grill, evenly distributing the walnut paste on top.
- Serve with your favorite salad or an onion, tomato, & parsley salad.

199. Seasoned Bitter Gourd

(Preparation time: 10 minutes | Cooking time: 25 minutes | Difficulty: Easy | Servings: 4)
Per serving: Calories 95, Total fat 9g, Protein 2g, Carbs 2g
Ingredients:

- 1/2 lemon juice
- 1 teaspoon of turmeric powder
- 1/2 teaspoon of garam masala
- 1 finely bird's eye chili
- 2 tablespoons of olive oil
- 2 teaspoons of finely chopped fresh coriander
- 2 mediums bitter gourd
- Salad, for serving

Instructions:

- Remove the tough skin of the bitter gourd and chop it into circular slices.
- Preheat the oven at 400°F.
- In a mixing bowl, combine the turmeric, parsley, chili, garam masala, lemon juice, & olive oil.
- For around 10 minutes, marinate the bitter gourd slices.
- Bake for around 10 to 15 minutes, then flip and continue baking for another 10 minutes, or till crisp.

200. Zesty Squash and Zucchini

(Preparation time: 10 minutes | Cooking time: 15 minutes | Difficulty: Easy | Servings: 4)
Per serving: Calories 43, Total fat 1g, Protein 2g, Carbs 9g
Ingredients:

- A pinch of salt
- 1 garlic minced to taste
- 1/2 chopped onion
- 1 cup of diced tomatoes with bird's eye chili
- 3 medium cubed small yellow squash
- 3 cubed small zucchinis

Instructions:

- Combine the squash, zucchini, salt, tomatoes, chilies, onion, & garlic in a large pot. On a medium-high burner, bring to a simmer.
- Reduce the flame to low and simmer till they are soft and crispy.

201. Stuffed Portobello

(Preparation time: 10 minutes | Cooking time: 10 minutes | Difficulty: Easy | Servings: 4)

Per serving: Calories 24, Total fat 1g, Protein 2g, Carbs 3g

Ingredients:

- A pinch of salt - 1 teaspoon of parsley
- 1 teaspoon of minced garlic
- 1 tablespoon of olive oil
- 1 diced tomato - 1/4 grated zucchini
- 4 Portobello mushroom caps

Instructions:

- In a mixing bowl, combine diced tomato, salt, grated zucchini, parsley, & minced garlic.
- Place the mushroom caps on a baking tray coated with baking paper and stuff them with the zucchini mixture.
- Bake for about 20 minutes, or till soft.

202. Quinoa Burger

(Preparation time: 10 minutes | Cooking time: 20 minutes | Difficulty: Easy | Servings: 4)

Per serving: Calories 158, Total fat 4g, Protein 7g, Carbs 24g

Ingredients:

- A pinch of salt
- 1 tablespoon of olive oil
- 1 teaspoon of Italian seasonings
- 1/2 minced red onion
- 1/3 cup of cooked chickpeas
- 1/2 cup of cooked quinoa

Instructions:

- Puree the chickpeas in a blender till smooth.

- Then, in a mixing bowl, blend them with quinoa, Italian spices, salt & onion. In a mixing bowl, mix all of the ingredients and stir till smooth.
- After that, shape the burgers from the mixture & place them on the prepared baking tray.
- Preheat the oven at 275°F and bake the quinoa patties for around 20 minutes.

203. Eggplant Croquettes

(Preparation time: 10 minutes | Cooking time: 10 minutes | Difficulty: Easy | Servings: 4)

Per serving: Calories 180, Total fat 9g, Protein 4g, Carbs 18g

Ingredients:

- 1 teaspoon of bird's eye chili
- 1 tablespoon of olive oil
- 1 tablespoon of coconut oil
- 1/4 teaspoon of ground cinnamon
- 2 tablespoons of almond meal
- 2 mashed potatoes
- 1 peeled and boiled eggplant

Instructions:

- Using a blender, puree the eggplant till it is smooth. Then toss in the mashed potatoes, coconut oil, chili, and powdered cinnamon.
- Make croquettes with the eggplant mixture.
- Heat the olive oil in a skillet.
- Cook the croquettes in the hot oil for 2 minutes on each side, or till browned.

204. Vegan Grilled Eggplant Tahini Satay Kebabs

(Preparation time: 10 minutes | Cooking time: 20 minutes | Difficulty: Easy | Servings: 4)

Per serving: Calories 97, Total fat 7g, Protein 2g, Carbs 7g

Ingredients:

- A pinch of salt
- 1/2 lime juice

- 2 teaspoons of grated garlic
- 2 teaspoons of olive oil
- 1 tablespoon of tomato paste
- 2 teaspoons of low-sodium soy sauce
- 2 teaspoons of shallot finely chopped
- 1/4 cup of parsley finely chopped
- 1 large eggplant
- 1/4 cup of tahini
- 1/3 cup of coconut milk

Instructions:

- Whisk together all of the ingredients except for the eggplant in a large-sized mixing bowl.
- Toss the eggplant with the marinade after slicing it into 2 1/2-centimeter (1-inch) pieces. Toss to combine and leave aside for 30 minutes to marinate. While you're waiting, soak eight skewers in water.
- Preheat the grill to medium-low or use a grill pan on the stovetop over medium-low flame. After threading the eggplant onto the skewers, tap to remove any excess marinade.
- Cook for 5 to 7 minutes on each side after brushing a little oil on the grill. To help the grilled eggplant complete cooking, close the lid on a grill with a lid. Top your pan with a heavy lid if you're cooking on the stove.
- Remove the kebabs from the grill and brush them with some of the remaining marinade before serving with a crisp salad & the rest of the marinade.

205. Vegan Mushroom Bourguignon

(Preparation time: 10 minutes | Cooking time: 40 minutes | Difficulty: Easy | Servings: 4)
Per serving: Calories 242, Total fat 10g, Protein 7g, Carbs 21g
Ingredients:

- Salt and black pepper to taste
- 4 tablespoons of olive oil
- 6 sprigs of thyme
- 3 bay leaves
- 4 peeled red onion
- 2 zucchini roughly chopped
- 2 stalks of celery
- 6 large carrots peeled and roughly chopped
- 4 to 5 large Portobello mushrooms (remove the stalks and cut into bite-size pieces)
- 1 1/2 cups of button mushrooms quartered
- 1 cup of vegetable stock
- 1/3 cup of almond flour
- 1/4 bottle of red wine

Instructions:

- In a very big skillet, heat 2 tablespoons of olive oil; add the onions and sauté till softly browned around 5 minutes. Increase the heat to medium-high and cook the garlic, carrots, & celery till the carrots are golden brown. Take the pan off the flame and set it aside.
- In a mixing bowl, season the flour using pepper and salt. Set aside the Portobello mushrooms after coating them with flour. Increase the flame to medium-high and brown the mushrooms in the pot with 2 tablespoons of olive oil. You may need to do this in two batches, depending on the size of your pan. Reduce the flame to medium, add the wine, bay leaves, vegetable stock, & thyme, and bring to a simmer till all the Portobello mushrooms have been browned. Reduce to a low flame and simmer, covered, for 15 minutes, stirring occasionally. After adding the vegetables, zucchini, and button mushrooms to the pan, cook for around 15 minutes.

206. Vegan Chili, Lime and Roasted Pumpkin Quinoa Salad

(Preparation time: 10 minutes | Cooking time: 30 minutes | Difficulty: Easy | Servings: 4)

Per serving: Calories 263, Total fat 6g, Protein 8g, Carbs 36g

Ingredients:

- 3/4 cup of water
- A pinch of salt and freshly ground pepper
- Zest and juice of 2 unwaxed limes
- 1 bird's eye chili deseeded and finely chopped - Olive oil as required
- 1 1/2 cups of mint and parsley leave roughly torn - 3/4 cup of white quinoa
- 1/4 cup of sunflower seeds
- 1 medium butternut pumpkin squash

Instructions:

- Rinse the quinoa thoroughly under cold running water. Drain and place them in a saucepan with just enough water to cover them. Using a pastry brush, brush any quinoa that has adhered to the pot's edges into the water. Bring the pot to a boil over high flame, then lower to low flame and cover. Cook for around 12 to 15 minutes, or till tender. Remove the pot from the flame and cover it while the pumpkin cooks. Preheat the oven at 200°F (400 Fahrenheit). After peeling and deseeding the butternut pumpkin, cut it into bite-sized pieces. You can leave the pumpkin bits larger if you prefer, but the cooking time will need to be modified. On a large dish, toss the pumpkin with just enough olive oil to moisten it and season using salt and black pepper. Roast for 15 minutes, or till soft and slightly browned on the edges. Remove the pan from the oven and allow it to cool. In a small-sized frying pan over low flame, toast

the sunflower seeds, turning occasionally. Allow time for chilling.
- Place the quinoa in a large serving dish, fluff it up using a fork, and season with salt and pepper to taste. Serve with parsley, mint leaves, or your favorite salad greens. On top of the pumpkin, sprinkle the chili and sunflower seeds. Finally, grate the lime over the top & drizzle with extra virgin olive oil and lime juice.

207. Vegan Museli

(Preparation time: 10 minutes | Cooking time: 30 minutes | Difficulty: Easy | Servings: 4)

Per serving: Calories 292, Total fat 24g, Protein 7g, Carbs 21g

Ingredients:

- 1/2 lemon, juiced - 3 tablespoons of chia seeds - 2 peeled and grated Granny Smith apples - 2 tablespoons of sugar-free maple syrup
- 2 cups of rolled oats
- 2 cups of strawberries sliced
- 1 cup of blueberries
- 2 cups of coconut milk

Instructions:

- Combine the coconut milk, oats, & chia seeds in a mixing bowl.
- Fold the apples into the oat mixture after tossing them with the lemon juice till they are equally coated. Combine blueberries, strawberries, & agave nectar in a mixing bowl. Refrigerate for at least 8 hours, if not all day.

208. Vegetarian Gravy

(Preparation time: 10 minutes | Cooking time: 20 minutes | Difficulty: Easy | Servings: 4)

Per serving: Calories 134, Total fat 11g, Protein 2g, Carbs 7g

Ingredients:

- A pinch of salt
- 1/4 teaspoon of ground black pepper

- 3 minced cloves of garlic
- 3 tablespoons of olive oil
- 1 cup of vegetable broth
- 1/3 cup of chopped red onion
- 1/2 teaspoon of dried sage
- 2 teaspoons of nutritional yeast
- 2 tablespoons of low-sodium soy sauce
- 4 tablespoons of almond flour

Instructions:

- In a medium-sized saucepan, heat the oil over medium flame. Cook till the garlic and onions are tender and transparent, about 5 minutes.
- To make a smooth paste, combine nutritional yeast, flour, & soy sauce. Pour the broth in slowly. Season with sage, salt and pepper to taste. Keep around 2–3 minutes at a boil. Reduce the flame to low and continue to stir for another 8 to 10 minutes, or till sauce thickens.

209. Garbanzo Stir Fry

(Preparation time: 10 minutes | Cooking time: 25 minutes | Difficulty: Easy | Servings: 4)

Per serving: Calories 231, Total fat 7g, Protein 11g, Carbs 31g

Ingredients:

- A pinch of salt - 1 diced zucchini
- 1 teaspoon of ground black pepper
- 1 tablespoon of lemon juice
- 1 tablespoon of olive oil
- 1 tablespoon of chopped fresh parsley
- 1 cup of cooked garbanzo beans
- 1/2 cup of chopped cremini mushrooms

Instructions:

- Heat the olive oil in a saucepan.
- After adding the mushrooms, cook for around 10 minutes.
- Then add the zucchini & garbanzo beans that have been cooked. After properly

tossing the ingredients, cook for another 10 minutes.

- Season the vegetables with a dash of salt and black pepper and a squeeze of lemon juice after that. Cook for approximately 5 minutes.
- Stir in the parsley well. Cook for an additional 5 minutes.

210. Zucchini and Peas Pasta

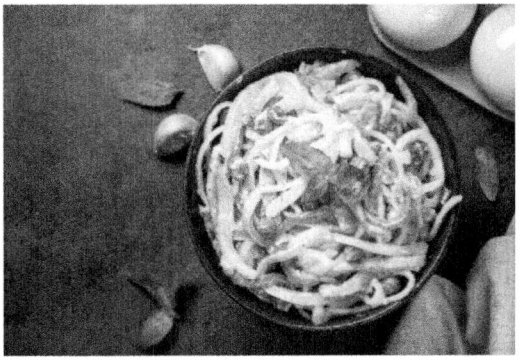

(Preparation time: 10 minutes | Cooking time: 15 minutes | Difficulty: Easy | Servings: 4)

Per serving: Calories 125, Total fat 21g, Protein 21g, Carbs 12g

Ingredients:

- 1/2 teaspoon of Italian seasoning
- 2 tablespoons of olive oil
- 2 tablespoons of homemade pesto
- 4 tablespoons of grated cheese
- 1 cup of frozen peas, thawed
- 2 chopped medium Zucchini
- 2 cups of cooked buckwheat pasta

Instructions:

- Heat the olive oil in a pan.
- Simmer for two minutes on medium flame with the frozen peas.
- Sauté the diced zucchini for another 2-3 minutes on low flame.
- After the zucchini is well sautéed, add the chili flakes (if using) and pesto.
- Cook for another minute after giving it a thorough stir. (Because the pan

contains cheese, the pesto may begin to stick as soon as it is poured.)

- Scrape the bottom of the pan with the spatula to ensure that the vegetables are evenly coated.
- Continue to sauté everything together, including the prepared buckwheat spaghetti.
- Add the cheese and Italian spice last.
- Cook for another minute on medium flame after combining all of the ingredients.
- Place the pasta in a serving dish after removing it from the flame.
- Serve warm or chilled.

211. Basil-Caper Roasted Red Peppers

(Preparation time: 10 minutes | Cooking time: 25 minutes | Difficulty: Easy | Servings: 4)
Per serving: Calories 84, Total fat 6g, Protein 2g, Carbs 6g
Ingredients:

- 2 garlic cloves crushed
- A handful of fresh basil leaves
- 3 leaves of fresh thyme sprigs
- 3 tablespoons of olive oil extra-virgin
- 2 tablespoons of balsamic vinegar
- 2 tablespoons of capers rinsed and drained
- 6 halved cherry tomatoes
- 3 red peppers large-sized

Instructions:

- Scrape the seeds out of the pepper by cutting it in half lengthwise. Place the garlic, thyme leaves, tomatoes, & capers cut side up on the nonstick baking pan between the red peppers. Place the tray in the oven with a drizzle of oil on it. Season using and salt black pepper to taste.
- Preheat the oven at 370°F and bake for about 10 minutes. Pour the balsamic

vinegar over the top of the dish after 10 minutes & bake for another 5 minutes, or till the sauce has caramelized. Serve with a fresh basil garnish.

212. Vegan Ginger Noodles Bowl

(Preparation time: 10 minutes | Cooking time: 15 minutes | Difficulty: Easy | Servings: 4)
Per serving: Calories 260, Total fat 10g, Protein 11g, Carbs 25g
Ingredients:

- 1 teaspoon of ground cumin
- 2 tablespoons of ginger and garlic grated
- 2 tablespoons of coconut oil
- 2 trimmed and thinly sliced red onions
- 3 cups of shredded carrots
- 3 cups of fresh bean sprouts
- 2 1/2 pounds of bok choy, bite-sized pieces
- 2 teaspoons of Chinese five-spice powder
- 2 cups of buckwheat noodles
- 12 cups of vegetable broth

Instructions:

- Heat the olive oil in a large-sized saucepan over medium-high flame. Cook, occasionally stirring, till the bok choy has wilted, about 3 to 5 minutes. Simmer for 1 minute, or till fragrant, after adding the ginger and garlic. Combine the carrots, cumin, & five-spice powder.
- Fill a pot halfway with vegetable broth. Bring the soup to a boil in a pot with enough water to cover it. Reduce the flame to low and simmer for 3 minutes, or till the noodles are softened. Mix in the bean sprouts & onions thoroughly. Remove the soup from the flame and leave it aside for 5 minutes to let the flavors mingle.

213. Stir-Fry Sesame Broccoli

(Preparation time: 10 minutes | Cooking time: 20 minutes | Difficulty: Easy | Servings: 4)

Per serving: Calories 99, Total fat 5g, Protein 5g, Carbs 12g

Ingredients:

- 1 teaspoon of fresh ginger finely chopped
- 3 cloves of minced garlic
- Toasted sesame seeds for garnish optional
- 1 tablespoon of olive oil
- 1 bunch of broccoli around 1 pound

For the sauce:

- 1 tablespoon of water
- 1/4 teaspoon of chili flakes
- 1 tablespoon of low-sodium soy sauce
- 1 teaspoon of toasted sesame oil
- 1 tablespoon of agave nectar

Instructions:

- Broccoli florets should be chopped into small pieces. After peeling off the rough outer coating, cut the broccoli stalk into 1" pieces.
- In a separate bowl, set aside the sauce ingredients. Heat the oil in a skillet over a medium-high flame before adding the broccoli. Cook for two minutes at most. Add 2 tablespoons of water or broth to the pan and cook for another 2 minutes, or till the water has evaporated.
- Cook, stirring regularly, for 1 minute, or till the garlic & ginger are fragrant. Cook for a further 2 minutes, or till the sauce mixture is well heated. Serve with a sprinkling of sesame seeds on top.

214. Roasted Lime-Parsley Cauliflower

(Preparation time: 10 minutes | Cooking time: 25 minutes | Difficulty: Easy | Servings: 4)

Per serving: Calories 91, Total fat 7g, Protein 2g, Carbs 4g

Ingredients:

- 1 fresh lime medium
- 1 teaspoon of cumin
- 3 cloves of garlic
- 2 tablespoons of chili powder
- 2 tablespoons of chopped cilantro
- 6 cups of cauliflower florets heaping
- 3 tablespoons of olive oil extra-virgin

Instructions:

- In a large-sized mixing dish, combine the olive oil & the cauliflower. Chili powder, cumin, salt & garlic should be sprinkled over the top. Crush the garlic clove with the side of a knife.
- Spread seasoned cauliflower & smashed garlic on a nonstick pan. Cook for 12 to 15 minutes over a medium flame. The cauliflower will be bubbly and golden around the edges. Place on a serving platter. Squeeze fresh lime juice over the cauliflower slices before serving. Serve with a garnish of parsley.

215. Mediterranean Herb Vegetables

(Preparation time: 10 minutes | Cooking time: 25 minutes | Difficulty: Easy | Servings: 2)

Per serving: Calories 142, Total fat 7g, Protein 3g, Carbs 15g

Ingredients:

- A pinch of salt
- Freshly ground black pepper
- 1 tablespoon of olive oil extra-virgin
- 1/2 chopped red onion
- 2 teaspoons of dried Italian herb mix
- 1 thinly sliced fennel bulb
- 1 cubed red bell pepper - 2 sliced carrots
- 1 cubed green bell pepper

Instructions:

- In a large-sized skillet, heat the olive oil & sauté the onion till soft and transparent, for around 5 minutes. Cook for 5 to 10 minutes, stirring periodically, or till bell peppers, carrots, & fennel are softened but still firm to the pinch. If preferred, season using salt and black pepper and Italian herbs.

216. Mediterranean-Style Vegetable Medley

(Preparation time: 10 minutes | Cooking time: 25 minutes | Difficulty: Easy | Servings: 4)
Per serving: Calories 107, Total fat 5g, Protein 2g, Carbs 9g
Ingredients:

- 1 teaspoon of lemon zest
- 1/2 teaspoon of dried oregano
- 2 minced cloves garlic
- 2 tablespoons of olive oil extra-virgin
- 1/2 small-sized eggplant, make 1/4-inch slices - 1 small-sized zucchini, make 1/4-inch slices
- 1 cup of shiitake mushrooms, sliced and stemmed - 1 cup of grape tomatoes
- 1 small-sized summer squash, make 1/4-inch slices

Instructions:

- Place the eggplant slices in a large-sized mixing dish, cut into wedges. Combine the zucchini, summer squash, mushrooms, olive oil, garlic, tomatoes, and oregano.
- Simmer the vegetables in a nonstick pan for around 10 to 15 minutes. Cook for another 5 minutes, frequently stirring, till the vegetables are tender and the edges are lightly browned.
- Before serving, grate some lemon zest over the vegetables.

217. Sautéed Zucchini

(Preparation time: 10 minutes | Cooking time: 25 minutes | Difficulty: Easy | Servings: 4)
Per serving: Calories 68, Total fat 3g, Protein 3g, Carbs 9g

Ingredients:

- Salt and black pepper to taste
- 1 minced clove of garlic
- 1/2 diced red onion
- 1 tablespoon of olive oil extra-virgin
- 1 teaspoon of Italian seasoning
- 1 diced tomato
- 4 halved and sliced zucchinis
- 1/2 pound of sliced fresh mushrooms

Instructions:

- In a large-sized skillet, heat the oil over medium flame. After adding the onion, cook for about 2 minutes using salt and black pepper. Combine the zucchini & mushrooms. Add the garlic, tomatoes, & Italian spice when the zucchini starts to soften. Cook till all the ingredients are ready.

218. Tomato Casserole

(Preparation time: 10 minutes | Cooking time: 25 minutes | Difficulty: Easy | Servings: 4)
Per serving: Calories 319, Total fat 30g, Protein 17g, Carbs 13g
Ingredients:

- 2 tablespoons of flat-leaf parsley, finely chopped - 2 eggs - 1/4 cup of olive oil
- 1/3 cup of chopped red onion
- 1 3/4 pounds of sliced tomatoes
- 1 1/4 cups of shredded vegan Parmesan cheese, divided
- 1 cup of vegan sour cream

Instructions:

- In a medium-low flame pan, heat oil and sauté onion and parsley till tender, about 5 minutes.
- Preheat the oven to 350°F.
- Brush a casserole dish using butter and set it aside. Arrange tomato slices in a single layer in the casserole dish. On top, sprinkle half of the onion mixture & half of the Parmesan cheese. Sprinkle the remaining 1/2 of the onions on top

of the tomato slices before adding another layer. Season using salt and black pepper before adding the last layer of tomatoes.

- In a mixing dish, whisk together the eggs and sour cream, then pour over the tomatoes. Over the top, sprinkle the remaining Parmesan cheese. Bake for around 25 minutes in a preheated oven or till firm and gently browned.

219. Tomato and Chickpea Salsa

(Preparation time: 10 minutes | Cooking time: 10 minutes | Difficulty: Easy | Servings: 2)
Per serving: Calories 293, Total fat 18g, Protein 14g, Carbs 20g
Ingredients:

- Salt and freshly ground black pepper
- Fresh parsley - 2 tablespoons of olive oil
- 4 tablespoons of buckwheat
- 1 cup of vine cherry tomatoes
- 1/2 cup of chickpeas cooked

Instructions:

- Pour half a cup of boiling water into a bowl & add just enough buckwheat to cover it. Cover the bowl with plastic wrap and set it aside for 30 minutes. Toss the cherry tomatoes & chickpeas together. Toss the chickpea & tomato mixture with the parsley, which has been carefully chopped.
- Now pour in half of the olive oil.
- To taste, season using salt and black pepper.
- With the remaining basil & olive oil, season the buckwheat to taste.

220. Broccoli Balls

(Preparation time: 10 minutes | Cooking time: 10 minutes | Difficulty: Easy | Servings: 2)
Per serving: Calories 82, Total fat 3g, Protein 5g, Carbs 9g
Ingredients:

- 1/2 teaspoon of ground coriander

- 2 tablespoons of olive oil
- 1 beaten egg
- 1 tablespoon of flax meal
- 1 teaspoon of nutritional yeast
- 1 cup of shredded broccoli
- 1/4 cup of cooked quinoa

Instructions:

- Broccoli, quinoa, nutritional yeast, ground coriander, flax flour, & egg must all be mixed together.
- Stir till the mixture is totally homogeneous.
- To make the medium-sized balls, combine all of the ingredients in a mixing bowl.
- For around 1 minute, heat olive oil.
- Cook the broccoli balls in the hot olive oil for about 2 minutes on each side or till light brown.

221. Vegetarian Sloppy Joes

(Preparation time: 10 minutes | Cooking time: 40 minutes | Difficulty: Easy | Servings: 2)
Per serving: Calories 316, Total fat 21g, Protein 15g, Carbs 23g
Ingredients:

- 2 cups of water
- 1 tablespoon of sesame oil
- 1 teaspoon of bird's eye chili
- 1 diced red onion
- 2 tablespoons of tomato paste
- 1 teaspoon of liquid honey
- 1/2 teaspoon of smoked paprika
- 1/2 cup of green lentils
- 1/2 cup of coconut milk

Instructions:

- Pour olive oil into a saucepan.
- With the red onion, bird's eye chili, and smoky paprika, cook for around 5 minutes.
- Then comes the green lentils, liquid honey, tomato paste, & water.

- Mix in the coconut milk till everything is well blended.
- Sloppy joes should be cooked for around 40 minutes over medium flame with the lid closed. Season using salt and black pepper.
- Remove the food from the heat and leave it aside for 10 minutes to cool down.

222. Tofu Stroganoff

(Preparation time: 10 minutes | Cooking time: 25 minutes | Difficulty: Easy | Servings: 2)
Per serving: Calories 270, Total fat 12g, Protein 13g, Carbs 25g
Ingredients:

- 1/2 cup of water
- 1 teaspoon of salt and ground black pepper
- 1/2 teaspoon of smoked paprika
- 1 tablespoon of olive oil
- 1 tablespoon of almond flour
- 1 sliced red onion
- 1 cup of chopped firm tofu
- 1/2 cup of buckwheat noodles
- 1/2 cup of soy milk

Instructions:

- Roast the chopped onion in olive oil till light brown in a pot.
- The buckwheat noodles, ground black pepper, salt, smoked paprika, and water are then added. Bring the mixture to the boil, then reduce to a low flame and allow it to simmer for 10 minutes.
- After that, in a mixing bowl, combine the flour-mixed soy milk, then add the liquid into the stroganoff mixture.
- Toss in the tofu and mix everything together completely.
- Close the cover and cook the tofu stroganoff for about 5 minutes. Allow 10 minutes for the meal to rest once it has been made.

223. Turmeric Cauliflower Florets

(Preparation time: 10 minutes | Cooking time: 25 minutes | Difficulty: Easy | Servings: 4)
Per serving: Calories 50, Total fat 4g, Protein 2g, Carbs 4g
Ingredients:

- A pinch of salt and ground black pepper
- 1 tablespoon of olive oil
- 1 tablespoon of ground turmeric
- 1 teaspoon of smoked paprika
- 2 cups of cauliflower florets

Instructions:

- The cauliflower florets are dusted with ground turmeric, smoky paprika, salt, black pepper, and olive oil.
- Then, using a baking paper, line the baking sheet with a single layer of cauliflower florets.
- Bake at 375°F for about 25 minutes or till the cauliflower florets are tender.

224. Italian-Style Vegetarian Patties

(Preparation time: 15 minutes | Cooking time: 15 minutes | Difficulty: Easy | Servings: 4)
Per serving: Calories 242, Total fat 8g, Protein 11g, Carbs 20g
Ingredients:

- 3 cups of water
- 1 1/2 teaspoons of minced garlic
- 2 teaspoons of dried basil
- 5 tablespoons of olive oil
- 1 egg
- 1 cup of red lentils
- 3/4 cup of uncooked brown rice
- 1 cup of vegan grated Parmesan cheese
- 1 cup of buckwheat breadcrumbs

Instructions:

- Heat two tablespoons of oil, heated in a big saucepan. Cook, constantly stirring, till the brown rice is golden brown. In a pot, bring the lentils & water to a boil. Reduce the flame to low, cover, and cook for 20 minutes, or till the rice is tender and the liquid has evaporated. Add more water if necessary; the mixture should be exceedingly thick. Take the pan from the heat and set it aside to cool.

- Combine the cooked rice mixture, eggs, breadcrumbs, basil, Parmesan cheese, & garlic in a food processor. Process till the mixture is well combined and resembles ground beef in texture. To form a 1/4 to 1/2-inch-thick patties, use about 3 tablespoons of the ingredients per patty.

- Heat three tablespoons of oil in a big skillet Patties should be fried in batches till golden brown, about 2 to 3 minutes per side. Place the paper towels to absorb the excess liquid & set them aside to cool. Fry the remaining patties in the same manner as the first. Keep the leftovers refrigerated or frozen in airtight containers.

225. Lentil Quiche

(Preparation time: 10 minutes | Cooking time: 35 minutes | Difficulty: Easy | Servings: 4)
Per serving: Calories 251, Total fat 12g, Protein 17g, Carbs 31g
Ingredients:

- 1 teaspoon of salt and ground black pepper
- 1 tablespoon of olive oil
- 1 diced red onion
- 1/2 cup of grated carrot
- 1 cup of boiled green lentils
- 1/4 cup of flax seeds meal
- 1/4 cup of soy milk

Instructions:

- In a pan with olive oil, sauté the onion till light brown.
- Then add the onions, lentils, and carrots that have been sautéed.

- Combine flaxseed meal, salt, ground black pepper, and soy milk. Stir the mixture thoroughly to ensure that it is totally homogenous.
- After that, level it out in the baking pan.
- Preheat the oven to 400°F and bake the quiche for around 35 minutes.

226. Corn Patties

(Preparation time: 10 minutes | Cooking time: 15 minutes | Difficulty: Easy | Servings: 4)
Per serving: Calories 168, Total fat 6g, Protein 7g, Carbs 20g
Ingredients:

- 1/2 teaspoon of ground coriander
- 1 teaspoon of chili powder
- 1 tablespoon of tomato paste
- 1 tablespoon of olive oil
- 1 tablespoon of chopped fresh parsley
- 1 tablespoon of almond meal
- 1 cup of cooked corn kernels
- 1/2 cup of cooked chickpeas

Instructions:

- In a large-sized mixing bowl, combine the cooked chickpeas, corn kernels, parsley, chili powder, powdered coriander, black pepper, tomato paste, salt, and almond meal.
- Stir till the mixture is totally homogeneous.
- Assemble all of the ingredients & form a shape to make the little patties.
- Then heat the olive oil in the skillet.
- Place the prepared patties in the hot oil and cook for 3 minutes per side, or till golden brown.
- Dry the cooked patties with a paper towel if required.

227. Vegan Meatballs

(Preparation time: 15 minutes | Cooking time: 15 minutes | Difficulty: Easy | Servings: 4)
Per serving: Calories 109, Total fat 3g, Protein 5g, Carbs 15g
Ingredients:

- 1 teaspoon of salt and ground black pepper
- 1/2 teaspoon of chili flakes
- 1 tablespoon of olive oil
- 2 tablespoons of chopped fresh parsley
- 1 tablespoon of tomato paste
- 1/2 cup of tomato puree
- 1/2 cup of cooked quinoa
- 1/2 cup of cooked white beans
- 4 tablespoons of grated vegan parmesan

Instructions:

- Combine white beans, buckwheat, and vegan parmesan in a blender.
- Combine the parsley, chili flakes, & tomato paste in a blender and blend till smooth.
- Form the meatballs from the mixture and roast them in warmed olive oil for about 3 minutes on each side, or till golden brown.
- Then, to taste, add the tomato puree, salt & black pepper. Close the lid & cook the meatballs for about 5 minutes on medium flame.

228. Vegan Shepherd Pie

(Preparation time: 15 minutes | Cooking time: 25 minutes | Difficulty: Easy | Servings: 4)
Per serving: Calories 136, Total fat 5g, Protein 4g, Carbs 18g
Ingredients:

- 1 teaspoon of chili powder
- 1 tablespoon of olive oil
- 1 chopped red onion
- 1/2 cup of diced carrot
- 1/2 cup of tomato puree
- 1/2 cup of cooked quinoa
- 1/2 cup of sliced mushrooms
- 1/2 cup of cooked and mashed potato

Instructions:

- Combine the onions, carrots, and mushrooms in a saucepan.
- With the olive oil, heat for around 10 minutes, or till the vegetables are cooked but not soft. Combine the chili powder, cooked vegetables, and tomato puree.
- Pour the mixture into the casserole dish and firmly pack it down.
- After that, cover the vegetables with mashed potatoes on top. Cover the shepherd pie with a baking sheet & bake at 450°F for around 20 minutes.

229. Vegan Lentil Salad

(Preparation time: 10 minutes | Cooking time: 15 minutes | Difficulty: Easy | Servings: 4)
Per serving: Calories 120, Total fat 2g, Protein 2g, Carbs 4g
Ingredients:

- A pinch of salt and black pepper
- 2 tablespoons of olive oil
- 2 tablespoons of chopped parsley
- 1 peeled and chopped red onion
- 1 chopped red bell pepper
- 1 1/4 cups of pre-cooked steamed lentils

Instructions:

- Cook the lentils according to the package instructions. In most circumstances, microwaving takes 3-5 minutes.
- Meanwhile, in a frying pan over medium-high flame, heat the olive oil.
- Cook, occasionally stirring, for 3-4 minutes, or till the red bell pepper & onion are softened. In a large-sized mixing bowl, combine the red bell pepper, cooked lentils, & onion.

- Drizzle a little more olive oil on top. Season using salt and black pepper to taste. Make a thorough mix.
- Before serving, garnish with parsley.

230. Vegan Baked Stuffed Tomatoes

(Preparation time: 10 minutes | Cooking time: 25 minutes | Difficulty: Easy | Servings: 3)
Per serving: Calories 50, Total fat 1g, Protein 2g, Carbs 10g
Ingredients:

- Salt and black pepper to taste
- Juice of 1/2 a lime
- 1/2 peeled and chopped red onion
- 1 chopped large tomato
- 1/2 cup of chopped parsley
- 3 large-sized tomatoes for the stuffing
- 1 cup of Riced Cauliflower frozen, prepared as per as package directions

Instructions:

- Preheat the oven at 375°F.
- The tops of the tomatoes should be removed and sliced off. Using a spoon, scrape out the seeds and pulp.
- Combine the chopped tomatoes, parsley, onion, & lime juice in a bowl to make the Pico de Gallo Cauliflower Rice. Season using salt and black pepper to taste.
- Tomatoes should be packed with the cauliflower rice mixture. It's great if they're a little too full.
- Arrange tomatoes in an oven-safe baking dish.
- Bake for around 25 minutes.

231. Vegan Mexican-Style Bean Stew

(Preparation time: 10 minutes | Cooking time: 25 minutes | Difficulty: Easy | Servings: 4)
Per serving: Calories 326, Total fat 6g, Protein 23g, Carbs 36g

Ingredients:

- A pinch of salt
- A pinch of cayenne pepper
- A pinch of black pepper to taste
- 1 teaspoon of ground cumin
- 1/2 teaspoon of ground cinnamon
- 4 cloves of crushed garlic
- 1 tablespoon of olive oil
- 1 diced red onion
- 2 cups of crushed tomatoes
- 1 cup of cooked pinto beans, black beans. and garbanzo beans each
- 2 cups of fresh corn kernels

Instructions:

- Heat the oil in a small saucepan over medium-high flame. Cook till the onion and garlic are transparent and aromatic. At this point, cumin should be added. Toss the cooked beans with the onions, garlic, & smashed tomatoes. Cook on low flame for 20 minutes. After adding the corn & cinnamon, cook for another 15 minutes. Season using pepper, salt and cayenne to taste before serving.

232. Vegan Cauliflower and Potatoes in Coconut Milk

(Preparation time: 10 minutes | Cooking time: 25 minutes | Difficulty: Easy | Servings: 4)
Per serving: Calories 244, Total fat 17g, Protein 5g, Carbs 18g
Ingredients:

- 1/2 cup of water
- A pinch of salt and freshly ground black pepper
- 1 teaspoon of ground turmeric
- 2 tablespoons of chopped fresh cilantro
- 2 tablespoons of olive oil
- 1 chopped onion
- 1 cup of new potatoes
- 1 head of cauliflower, florets
- 1 1/2 cups of coconut milk

Instructions:

- Heat the olive oil in a medium-sized saucepan & sauté the onion till soft and transparent, around 5 minutes. Toss the potatoes with the water & bring to a boil. Cook, covered, for about 10 minutes, or till potatoes are nearly tender.
- Combine the coconut milk, cauliflower, & turmeric; cover and cook on low heat for around 10 minutes, or till the cauliflower is soft. Before adding the parsley, remove the top and season using salt and black pepper.

233. Vegan Baked Chocolate Blended Oats

(Preparation time: 10 minutes | Cooking time: 25 minutes | Difficulty: Easy | Servings: 2)
Per serving: Calories 279, Total fat 11g, Protein 8g, Carbs 31g
Ingredients:

- A pinch of cinnamon powder
- 1/2 teaspoon of vanilla extract
- 1 teaspoon of baking powder
- 2 tablespoons of cocoa powder
- 2 tablespoons of maple syrup
- 1 mashed large ripe banana
- 1 cup of rolled oats
- 2/3 cup of almond milk
- 2 tablespoons of vegan chocolate chips

Instructions:

- Preheat the oven at 350°F.
- Cooking spray the bottom and sides of two 8-ounce ramekins.
- Blend the oats, cocoa powder, almond milk, banana, maple syrup, vanilla extract, cinnamon powder and baking powder together in a blender. Blend for 30 to 60 seconds, or till all ingredients are well combined. Half-fill the ramekins

with the mixture and 1 tablespoon of dark chocolate chips on top.
- In a preheated oven, bake for around 25 minutes or till firm.

234. Vegan Coconut Curry with Tofu

(Preparation time: 10 minutes | Cooking time: 25 minutes | Difficulty: Easy | Servings: 4)
Per serving: Calories 277, Total fat 25g, Protein 10g, Carbs 32g
Ingredients:

- 1 teaspoon of minced ginger and garlic each
- 2 finely chopped green onions
- 3 tablespoons of vegetable oil
- 1 teaspoon of vegetable oil
- 3 tablespoons of cornstarch
- 1 tablespoon of green curry paste
- 2 cups of low-sodium vegetable broth
- 2 cups of buckwheat noodles
- 2 cups of firm tofu, sliced into small cubes
- 1 1/2 cups of light coconut milk

Instructions:

- Add the noodles to a large-sized mixing bowl halfway filled with boiling water. Allow for a 15-minute rest period or till the noodles have softened. Drain and rinse completely.
- Set aside tofu that has been tossed in cornstarch. Heat three tablespoons of oil in a medium-sized pan Tofu should be fried for around 5 minutes or till crisp. Heat 1 teaspoon of oil, curry paste, garlic, & ginger in a separate pan over medium flame. Cook for 2 minutes, stirring occasionally, or till fragrant. Pour in the vegetable broth & coconut milk in a slow, steady stream. Cook, frequently stirring, for about 10 minutes, or till sauce is well heated.
- Combine the noodles, curry sauce, tofu, & green onion in each serving dish.

235. Vegan Tomato and Peanut Stew

(Preparation time: 10 minutes | Cooking time: 25 minutes | Difficulty: Easy | Servings: 4)

Per serving: Calories 134, Total fat 8g, Protein 5g, Carbs 14g

Ingredients:

- 1 1/2 cups of water
- Onion powder to taste
- Garlic powder to taste
- Ground cayenne pepper to taste
- 2 tablespoons of olive oil
- 6 chopped cloves of garlic
- 1 1/2 chopped red onion
- 4 coarsely chopped large tomatoes
- 2 diced green bell peppers
- 1/3 cup of crushed peanuts

Instructions:

- Heat the oil in a medium-sized saucepan over medium flame. With onion, bell pepper, garlic, & peanuts, cook for 2 to 3 minutes. With the tomatoes, water, onion powder, salt, garlic powder, & cayenne pepper, bring to the boil. Reduce the flame to low & cook for at least 30 minutes, ideally 1 1/2 hours.

236. Vegan Sweet Potato and Chickpea Curry

(Preparation time: 10 minutes | Cooking time: 25 minutes | Difficulty: Easy | Servings: 4)

Per serving: Calories 293, Total fat 22g, Protein 5g, Carbs 20g

Ingredients:

- A pinch of salt
- 1 teaspoon of turmeric
- 1 teaspoon of ground cumin
- 1 teaspoon of red chili flakes
- 1 teaspoon of garam masala
- 3 tablespoons of olive oil
- 2 cloves of minced garlic
- 2 teaspoons of minced fresh ginger root
- 1 chopped red onion

- 1 cubed sweet potato
- 1 cup of diced tomatoes
- 1 cup of cooked chickpeas
- 1 cup of kale
- 1 cup of coconut milk

Instructions:

- In a pan over medium flame, cook the onion, garlic, & ginger till softened, around 5 minutes. Combine the chickpeas, coconut milk, tomatoes, & sweet potato. Bring to a boil, then reduce to a low flame and cook for 15 minutes, or till the veggies are tender.
- Season the meal with garam masala, cumin, turmeric, salt and chili flakes. Toss in the spinach right before serving.

237. Vegan Curried Cauliflower, Lentils and Sweet Potato Soup

(Preparation time: 10 minutes | Cooking time: 25 minutes | Difficulty: Easy | Servings: 4)

Per serving: Calories 213, Total fat 5g, Protein 16g, Carbs 30g

Ingredients:

- A pinch of salt
- 2 teaspoons of ground cumin
- 2 teaspoons of ground coriander
- 2 tbsp. of minced ginger and garlic
- 2 tablespoons of olive oil
- 1 tablespoon of curry powder
- 1 chopped red onion
- 1 head of cauliflower, florets
- 8 cups of vegetable broth
- 1 cup of dry red lentils, rinsed and drained
- 2 cups of sweet potato cubed
- 3 cups of kale

Instructions:

- Heat the olive oil in a large-sized saucepan over medium flame. Cook for around 5–6 minutes, or till the garlic & onions are translucent. Cook for another 2 minutes, or till fragrant, after adding the ginger, 1 tablespoon coriander, curry powder, and cumin. Mix the broth and lentils till everything is well incorporated. Bring the mixture to a low boil, then reduce to a low flame and continue to cook for 5 minutes.

- Combine the cauliflower and sweet potato. Cook for 20 to 25 minutes, or until cauliflower and sweet potato are tender, covered, on medium-low heat. Season using salt and black pepper and more curry powder if desired. Cook, stirring periodically, for 3 to 5 minutes, or till the kale has wilted.
- Serve and enjoy!

238. Vegan Seitan Curry

(Preparation time: 10 minutes | Cooking time: 25 minutes | Difficulty: Easy | Servings: 2)
Per serving: Calories 347, Total fat 11g, Protein 36g, Carbs 31g
Ingredients:

- A pinch of salt
- A pinch of ground black pepper
- 2 garlic cloves minced
- 1/2 teaspoon of ground turmeric
- 1 tablespoon of cumin
- 1 tablespoon of ground coriander
- 1 tablespoon of olive oil
- 1 teaspoon of curry powder
- 1/2 od cubed red onion
- 1 small cubed zucchini
- 1/2 cup of sliced seitan

Instructions:

- Combine the zucchini & onion in a saucepan of water, bring to a boil, and simmer for around 20 minutes. Drain. In a blender, combine all of the ingredients and blend till smooth.
- Pour the pureed zucchini mixture into a medium-sized pot. Seitan is seasoned using cumin, coriander, pepper, curry powder, turmeric, salt and garlic powder. Cook for 30 minutes, or till the sauce is thick, adding a tablespoon of water as needed to avoid burning.

239. Vegan Zoodles with Chickpeas

(Preparation time: 10 minutes | Cooking time: 15 minutes | Difficulty: Easy | Servings: 2)
Per serving: Calories 248, Total fat 28g, Protein 6g, Carbs 19g
Ingredients:

- A pinch of salt and black pepper
- 2 cloves of minced garlic
- 4 tablespoons of olive oil
- A handful of parsley, chopped
- 2 medium zucchinis, make noodles with a spiralizer - 12 zucchini blossoms, remove the pistils, sliced into strips
- 1/2 cup of drained and rinsed chickpeas

Instructions:

- Heat olive oil in a large-sized skillet over low flame and cook garlic till softened, about 10 minutes. Toss zucchini & zucchini blossoms in olive oil until well coated. Stir in the chickpeas till thoroughly incorporated. Toss in the parsley and season using salt and pepper. Serve immediately.

240. Vegan African-Style Stew

(Preparation time: 10 minutes | Cooking time: 35 minutes | Difficulty: Easy | Servings: 4)
Per serving: Calories 279, Total fat 20g, Protein 10g, Carbs 24g
Ingredients:

- A pinch of salt
- 1/4 teaspoon of cayenne pepper
- 1 tablespoon of minced ginger and garlic
- 2 tablespoons of olive oil
- 2 chopped red onions
- 6 tablespoons of flaked coconut
- 1 large chopped green bell pepper

- 3 cups of tomato juice plus 2 tomatoes chopped
- 2 cups of chopped cabbage
- 3 cups of chopped yams
- 1 cup of apple juice
- 1/2 cup of peanut butter

Instructions:

- Heat the olive oil in a saucepan or pot over medium-high flame. In the hot oil, cook & stir the yams, onions, coconut, cabbage, tomatoes, & garlic for 4 to 5 minutes, or till the vegetables are lightly browned.
- Season with ginger, salt and cayenne pepper and combine the tomato liquid and apple juice. Reduce the flame to a medium-low setting.
- Combine the bell pepper and the peanut butter. Close the lid and cook for about 30 minutes, or till the peanut butter has completely melted into the soup, stirring regularly.

241. Vegan Oats with Chia Seeds and Fruits

(Preparation time: 10 minutes | Cooking time: 10 minutes | Difficulty: Easy | Servings: 2)
Per serving: Calories 171, Total fat 12g, Protein 13g, Carbs 28g

Ingredients:

- 3/4 cup of water
- 1/2 teaspoon of ground cinnamon
- 4 tablespoons of chia seeds
- 2 mashed ripe bananas
- 1/4 cup of fresh blackberries
- ¼ cup of fresh blueberries
- 1 peeled and diced nectarine
- 1 ¼ cups of rolled oats
- 1 1/3 cups of almond milk

Instructions:

- Combine almond milk, bananas, chia seeds, oats, water, & cinnamon in a jar

or airtight container; stir well. Cover and refrigerate for 8 hours to overnight.

- Slowly boil the oat mixture in a saucepan on low flame for about 5 minutes. Divide between two bowls after garnishing with blueberries, blackberries, & nectarine.

242. Vegan Golden Cauli Rice with Garden Veggies

(Preparation time: 10 minutes | Cooking time: 15 minutes | Difficulty: Easy | Servings: 4)
Per serving: Calories 90, Total fat 6g, Protein 3g, Carbs 8g

Ingredients:

- A pinch of salt
- 1 teaspoon of ground turmeric
- 1 tablespoon of minced fresh garlic
- A handful of chopped fresh parsley
- 2 tablespoons of extra-virgin olive oil
- 1/4 teaspoon of sweet paprika
- 1/8 teaspoon of curry powder, or to taste - 2 tablespoons of blanched slivered almonds
- 1 pound of frozen riced cauliflower
- 1/4 cup of red bell pepper thinly sliced
- 1/2 cup of each julienned carrot, chopped onion, diced mushrooms, French cut green beans

Instructions:

- Heat the oil in a 12-inch nonstick skillet over medium flame. For about 1 minute, sauté the onion in the hot oil. The carrots, mushrooms, green beans, & bell pepper are then added. Cook, stirring periodically, for 3 to 4 minutes.
- Combine the cauliflower rice, curry powder, garlic, turmeric, salt, paprika, & pepper. Cook, stirring regularly, on medium flame till the vegetables have reached the desired texture, about 5 minutes. Serve warm, garnished with almonds & parsley.

243. Vegan Banana Chocolate Oatmeal

(Preparation time: 10 minutes | Cooking time: 15 minutes | Difficulty: Easy | Servings: 2)
Per serving: Calories 268, Total fat 28g, Protein 5g, Carbs 32g
Ingredients:

- A pinch of ground cinnamon
- 1/2 sliced banana
- 1 teaspoon of unsweetened cocoa powder - 2 teaspoons of maple syrup
- 1 tablespoon of vegan dark chocolate chips - 1/4 cup of quick-cooking oats
- 3/4 cup of cashew milk

Instructions:

- Bring cashew milk to the boil in a saucepan over medium-high flame. Reduce the flame to a low setting and stir in the oats. Combine cocoa powder & cinnamon. To sweeten the dish, maple syrup might be utilized.
- Cook on low flame for about 5 minutes. Stir in the chocolate chunks & continue to cook for an additional 1 to 2 minutes, or till the oatmeal has reached the desired consistency.
- In a bowl, place the banana on top of the oats.

244. Vegetable Ratatouille

(Preparation time: 10 minutes | Cooking time: 30 minutes | Difficulty: Easy | Servings: 4)
Per serving: Calories 153, Total fat 8g, Protein 4g, Carbs 19g
Ingredients:

- A pinch of salt
- A pinch of black pepper to taste
- 1 tablespoon of garlic
- 1 tablespoon of vinegar
- 2 tablespoons of olive oil extra-virgin
- 1 red onion
- 1 tablespoon of herbs de Provence

- 2 yellow peppers medium-sized
- 3 tomatoes medium-sized
- 1 eggplant medium-sized
- 1 zucchini medium-sized

Instructions:

- Using a sharp knife, cut the peppers, tomatoes, onions, zucchini, & eggplant into 2-inch pieces. Garlic needs to be minced.
- In a nonstick pan, toss the vegetables with the garlic, vegetables, & herbs de Provence. To taste, season with salt and black pepper.
- Drizzle extra virgin olive oil & balsamic vinegar over the top. Combine all ingredients.
- Cook for around 20 minutes on medium-low flame. Stir once during the cooking process.

245. Garden Stuffed Squash

(Preparation time: 10 minutes | Cooking time: 20 minutes | Difficulty: Easy | Servings: 2)
Per serving: Calories 289, Total fat 13g, Protein 5g, Carbs 29g
Ingredients:

- 1 tablespoon of olive oil
- A handful of parsley
- 1 chopped bell pepper
- 1/2 cup of chopped leek
- 1 1/2 cup of halved butternut squash
- 4 tablespoons of shredded vegan Mozzarella

Instructions:

- Heat the olive oil in a skillet.
- In the same pan, add the bell pepper & leek. It only takes 3 minutes. After that, thoroughly combine the parsley.
- Fill the butternut squash using the veggie mixture and top with vegan Mozzarella.
- Preheat the oven at 400°F and roast the squash halves for around 25 minutes.

246. Vegetarian Borscht

(Preparation time: 10 minutes | Cooking time: 20 minutes | Difficulty: Easy | Servings: 4)
Per serving: Calories 264, Total fat 6g, Protein 10g, Carbs 33g

Ingredients:

- A pinch of salt and black pepper
- 2 tablespoons of olive oil, or as needed
- 3 tablespoons of vinegar
- 2 tablespoons of chopped fresh dill
- 2 tablespoons of tomato paste
- 1 chopped red onion
- 2 tablespoons of sour cream, or more to taste
- 1/4 medium shredded head cabbage
- 3/4 cup dry yellow lentils
- 3 medium sweet potatoes, peeled and diced
- 2 peeled and coarsely grated each small beets and carrots

Instructions:

- Combine the beets & vinegar in a small-sized frying pan over low flame. Cook, stirring periodically, for about 15 minutes, or till the veggies are soft.
- Heat the oil in a big frying pan over a low flame while the beets are cooking. For 2 minutes, stir in the onion. Cook, turning periodically, till carrots are soft, about 10 minutes. Set them aside.
- Meanwhile, bring water to a simmer in a large saucepan. In a large-sized mixing dish, combine the cabbage and lentils. Cook for about 10 minutes. After adding the potatoes, cook for another 10 minutes. Combine the cooked beets with the onion-carrot mixture. Toss in a pinch of salt and black pepper to taste. Cook for another 10 minutes, or till all of the vegetables are tender, before adding the tomato paste. Serve with a sour cream dollop and a dill sprig.

247. Vegetarian Pasta

(Preparation time: 10 minutes | Cooking time: 20 minutes | Difficulty: Easy | Servings: 3)
Per serving: Calories 241, Total fat 27g, Protein 15g, Carbs 30g

Ingredients:

- A pinch of salt and black pepper
- 1 minced clove of garlic
- 2 tablespoons of olive oil
- 1/2 thinly sliced red onion
- 1 chopped red bell pepper
- 1/2 cup of frozen peas
- 3 1/2 cups of broccoli florets
- 1 cup of buckwheat pasta
- 3 tablespoons of vegan half and half cream - 1/2 cup of vegan cheese

Instructions:

- Bring a large-sized pot of salted water to a rolling boil. Boil pasta for about 8 minutes, occasionally stirring, until cooked but still firm to the bite. Drain.
- Meanwhile, bring the second pot of water to a boil. Broccoli should be cooked for about 8 minutes or till tender but firm to the biting. Drain.
- Heat the olive oil in a large-sized skillet or wok over medium flame and sauté the garlic & onions till soft and translucent, about 5 minutes. After adding the bell pepper, cook for about 2 minutes. Toss in a pinch of salt and black pepper to taste. Toss in the peas and pour in the cream. Stir in the vegan cheese till it is melted and cooked through.
- Combine the cooked noodles and broccoli. Toss in a pinch of black pepper to taste.

248. Briam

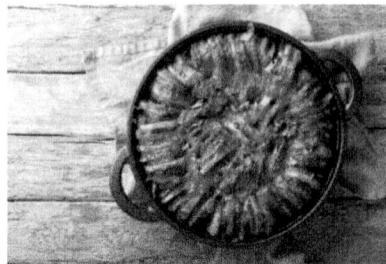

(Preparation time: 10 minutes | Cooking time: 30 minutes | Difficulty: Easy | Servings: 4)
Per serving: Calories 187, Total fat 4g, Protein 6g, Carbs 3g
Ingredients:
- A pinch of salt and black pepper
- 1 tablespoon of olive oil
- 1/2 teaspoon of dried rosemary
- 1 teaspoon of dried oregano
- 1/2 cup of chopped fresh parsley
- 1 sliced red onion - 2 sliced potatoes
- 2 sliced zucchinis
- 1 cup of marinara sauce

Instructions:
- Combine the zucchinis, potatoes, & onion in a large-sized mixing bowl.
- The vegetables are seasoned with oregano, rosemary, salt, black pepper and parsley.
- Give the vegetables a brisk shake after adding the olive oil.
- After that, place them in the baking sheet one by one and cover them with marinara sauce.
- Cover the vegetables with foil & bake at 450°F for around 30 minutes.

249. Oatmeal with Peas and Beans

(Preparation time: 10 minutes | Cooking time: 30 minutes | Difficulty: Easy | Servings: 4)
Per serving: Calories 293, Total fat 11g, Protein 20g, Carbs 32g
Ingredients:
- 2 cups of water
- A pinch of salt
- 1 tablespoon of olive oil
- 2 tablespoons of paprika
- 1 tablespoon of cornstarch
- 1 egg
- 1/2 cup of ground oats
- 1 cup of cooked peas
- 1 cup of cooked beans of your choice

Instructions:
- Combine water, egg, buckwheat, paprika, salt, and cornstarch in a medium-sized saucepan over medium flame; mix in beans and peas.
- Cook, stirring regularly, for around 20 to 30 minutes, or till the mixture thickens. Remove the pan from the flame and stir in the olive oil. The mixture should be poured into the plates.

250. Buckwheat Cereal with Mushrooms and Onion

(Preparation time: 10 minutes | Cooking time: 25 minutes | Difficulty: Easy | Servings: 4)
Per serving: Calories 243, Total fat 8g, Protein 8g, Carbs 23g
Ingredients:
- 2 cups of water
- A pinch of sea salt
- A pinch of ground black pepper to taste
- 1 tablespoon of olive oil to taste
- 1 tablespoon of butter to taste
- 1 diced red onion
- 1 diced carrot
- 1 cup of buckwheat groats
- 1/2 pound of diced mushrooms

Instructions:
- After rinsing with cold water in a sieve, drain the buckwheat.
- Buckwheat should be toasted and aromatic after 5 to 10 minutes of cooking and stirring in a pan over medium flame. In a mixing bowl, combine all of the ingredients.

- Heat the olive oil in a pan over medium flame; sauté and stir the onion and carrot till brown, about 5 to 10 minutes. After adding the mushrooms, cook & stir for another 5 minutes.

- Melt the butter in a medium saucepan; add the buckwheat and stir to coat. Bring the onion mixture, water, & pepper to a boil. Reduce to a low flame, cover, and simmer for 15 minutes, or till the liquid has been absorbed.

CHAPTER 8:

Healthy, Easy, and Tasty Recipes

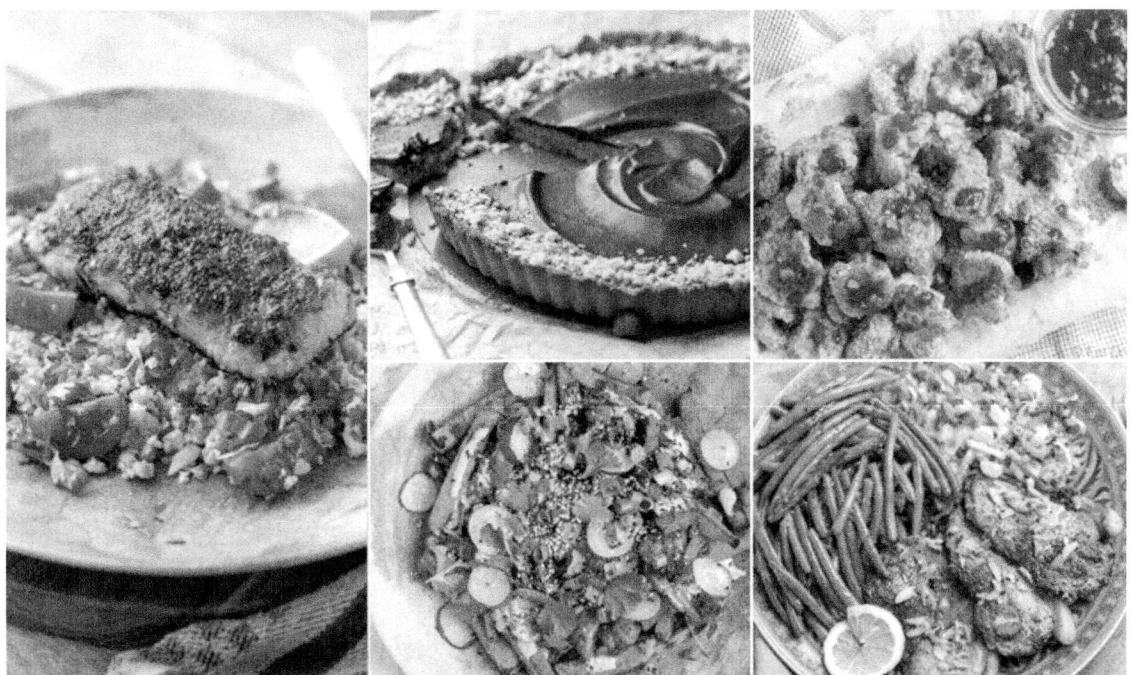

Adopting a diet high in 'sirtfoods' is part of the Sirtfood diet. These foods operate by activating special proteins in the body called sirtuins, according to the diet's creators. These are thought to assist prevent cells in the body from dying when they are stressed and regulate inflammation, metabolism, and the aging process.

In this chapter, we have compiled sirtfood breakfast, lunch, dinner, snack, dessert, and non-alcoholic and alcoholic cocktails recipes for you to continue including these recipes in your daily life.

CHAPTER 9:

Breakfast Recipes

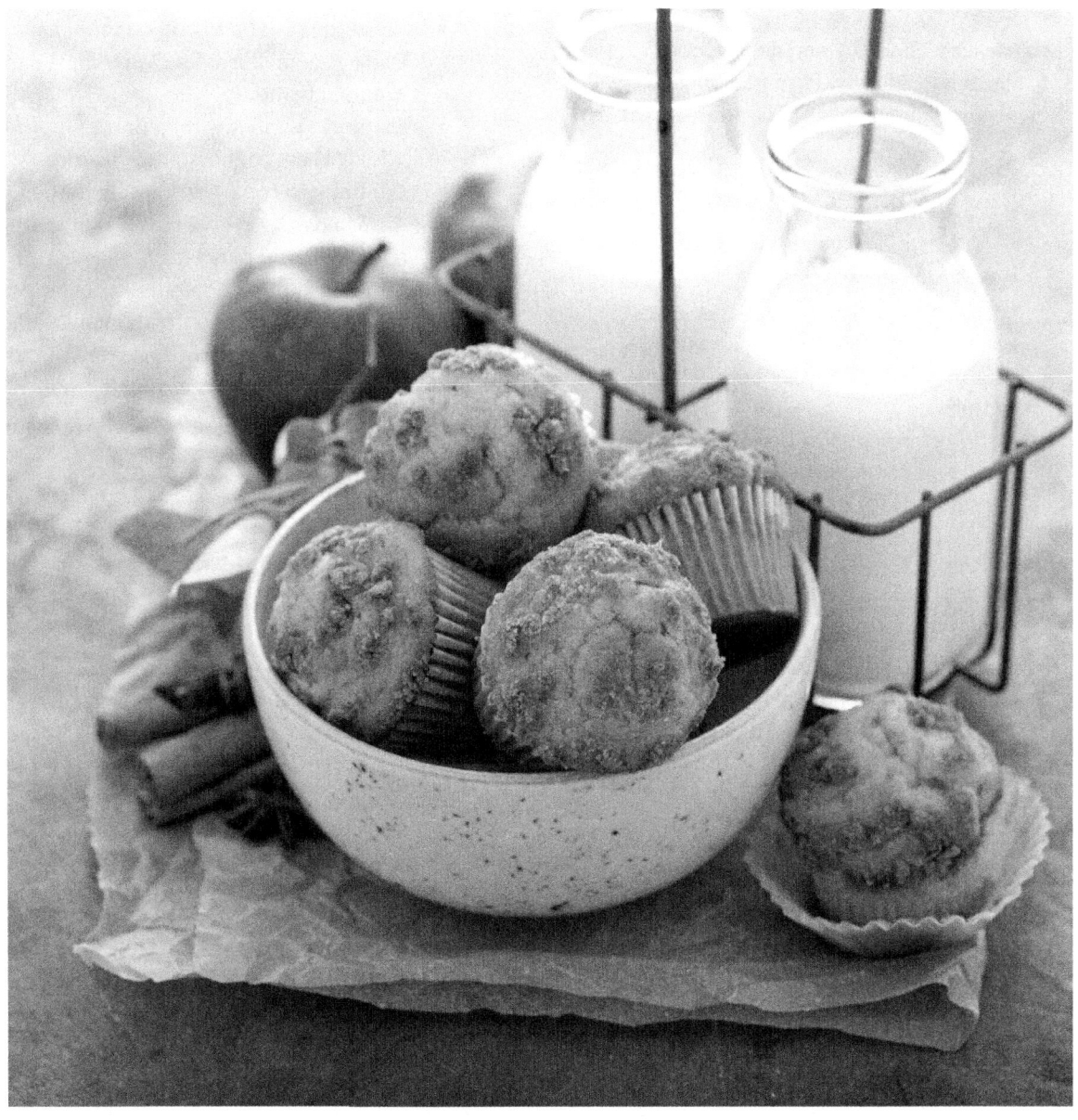

Smoked Salmon Omelet

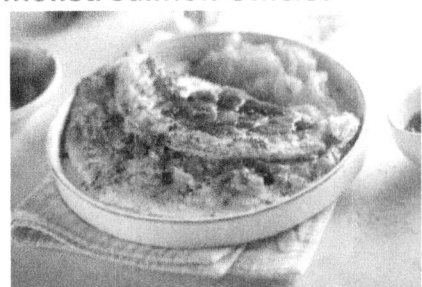

(Preparation time: 10 minutes | Cooking time: 15 minutes | Difficulty: Easy | Servings: 2)

Per serving: Calories 148, Total fat 9g, Protein 16g, Carbs 1g

Ingredients:

- 1 teaspoon extra virgin olive oil
- 1 teaspoon Parsley, shredded
- 2 medium eggs
- 1/2 teaspoon of Capers
- 1 tablespoon of rocket, shredded
- 100g of Smoked salmon, cut

Instructions:

- In a mixing dish, crack the eggs and whisk them thoroughly. Combine the salmon, tricks, rocket, & parsley in a mixing bowl.
- In a nonstick skillet, heat the olive oil till it is hot but not smoking. Using a spatula, move the egg mixture around the dish till it is evenly distributed.
- Reduce the flame and allow the omelet to finish cooking. To serve, run the spatula over the sides of the omelet and fold it in half.

2. Breakfast Quinoa Bowls

(Preparation time: 10 minutes | Cooking time: 15 minutes | Difficulty: Easy | Servings: 6)

Per serving: Calories 348, Total fat 14g, Protein 10g, Carbs 28g

Ingredients:

- 2 cups of water
- 2 cups of quinoa
- 1 cup of blueberries
- 1 cup of coconut milk, unsweetened
- 2 tablespoons of walnuts
- 1 teaspoon of pistachio
- 2 tablespoons of honey

Instructions:

- In a saucepan, combine the coconut milk and water and whisk thoroughly to combine.
- Close the cover and add the quinoa.
- Cook the mixture for 5 minutes over medium flame.
- Carefully wash the blueberries before adding them to the quinoa mixture.
- Continue to cook, stirring constantly.
- Pistachios and walnuts should be combined and crushed.
- Cook for another 3 minutes after adding the smashed nuts to the quinoa.
- Add the honey and whisk the mixture till it has completely dissolved.
- Enjoy by transferring to serving bowls.
- Enjoy!

3. Spiced Morning Omelet

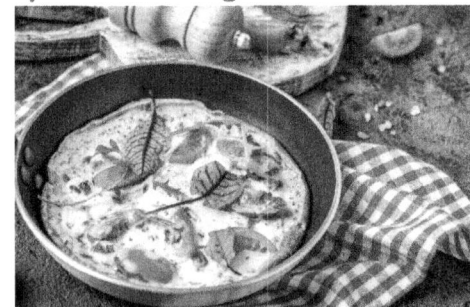

(Preparation time: 10 minutes | Cooking time: 15 minutes | Difficulty: Easy | Servings: 3)

Per serving: Calories 179, Total fat 12g, Protein 14g, Carbs 4g

Ingredients:

- 1 teaspoon of turmeric
- 3 garlic cloves
- ¼ teaspoon of ground ginger
- 1 teaspoon of olive oil

- 1 teaspoon of cilantro
- ¼ teaspoon of nutmeg
- 1 tablespoon of chives
- 7 eggs
- 1/3 cup of skim milk

Instructions:

- In a mixing dish, whisk together the eggs.
- Whisk in the skim milk once more.
- Sprinkle the nutmeg, ground ginger, cilantro, & turmeric over the egg mixture.
- Peel and mince the garlic cloves.
- Chop the chives & mix them in with the garlic.
- Stir the herb mixture into the eggs once more.
- Preheat a skillet over a high flame and add the olive oil.
- Preheat the olive oil over a medium flame before pouring in the egg mixture.
- Cook the omelet for around 15 minutes with the cover closed.
- Allow the dish to cool slightly before cutting into serving portions.

4. Rice Pudding

(Preparation time: 10 minutes | Cooking time: 15 minutes | Difficulty: Easy | Servings: 5)
Per serving: Calories 323, Total fat 27g, Protein 6.5g, Carbs 23g
Ingredients:

- 1 teaspoon of lemon zest
- 1 teaspoon of cinnamon
- 1 teaspoon of ginger
- 1/3 teaspoon of thyme
- 2 tablespoons of honey
- 1 cup of brown rice
- 1/3 cup of walnuts
- 2 cups of coconut milk, unsweetened

Instructions:

- Heat the coconut milk in a saucepan over medium flame.

- Stir in the brown rice till it is thoroughly combined.
- Cook the brown rice for around 10 minutes with the cover closed over medium flame.
- Meanwhile, combine the walnuts, lemon zest, thyme, ginger, & cinnamon in a mixing bowl.
- Sprinkle the almond mixture over the brown rice and gently toss it in.
- Cook the dish for around 5 minutes with the lid closed.
- Remove the pudding from the saucepan & place it in a large mixing bowl once it has finished cooking.
- Stir in the honey into the pudding.
- Serve it right away.

5. Creamy Millet

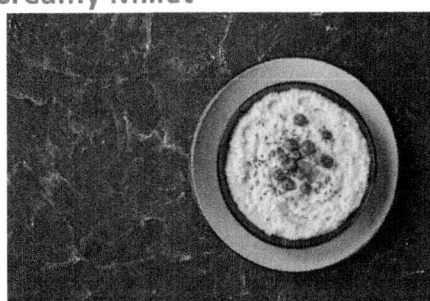

(Preparation time: 10 minutes | Cooking time: 15 minutes | Difficulty: Easy | Servings: 8)
Per serving: Calories 384, Total fat 20g, Protein 12g, Carbs 32g
Ingredients:

- 1 cup of water
- ¼ teaspoon of salt
- ½ teaspoon of ground ginger
- 1 teaspoon of cinnamon
- 1 tablespoon of chia seeds
- 1/2 cup of Parmesan cheese, grated
- 1 tablespoon of cashew butter
- 2 cups of millet
- 1 cup of almond milk, unsweetened
- 1 cup of coconut milk, unsweetened

Instructions:

- In a saucepan, add the coconut milk, almond milk, plus water.
- Add millet to the liquid and gently stir it in.
- Close the lid after properly mixing.
- Cook the millet for around 5 minutes over medium flame.
- Cinnamon, ground ginger, salt, & chia seeds should be sprinkled over the meal.
- Stir the mixture well with a spoon and simmer for another 5 minutes on medium flame.
- Cook the millet for around 5 minutes with the cashew butter.
- Remove the millet from the flame & transfer it to serving bowls.
- Grate the cheese over the top of the dish and serve.

6. Apple Muffins

(Preparation time: 10 minutes | Cooking time: 20 minutes | Difficulty: Easy | Servings: 5)
Per serving: Calories 200, Total fat 6g, Protein 12g, Carbs 22g
Ingredients:

- ½ teaspoon of salt
- 1 tablespoon of olive oil
- ½ teaspoon of baking soda
- 1 teaspoon of apple cider vinegar
- 3 apples, washed and peeled
- 2 eggs
- ½ cup of skim milk
- 1 cup of buckwheat flour
- 2 tablespoon of stevia

Instructions:

- In a mixing dish, whisk together the eggs thoroughly.
- Combine the skim milk, salt, baking soda, stevia, & apple cider vinegar.
- Carefully stir the mixture.

- Grate the apples & combine them with the egg mixture.
- Add the buckwheat flour and stir well.
- Blend in the olive oil till the batter is smooth.
- Preheat the oven at 350°F.
- Place the muffins in the oven halfway filled with batter.
- Allow 15 minutes for the meal to cook.
- Take the baked muffins out of the oven.
- Allow the baked muffins to cool completely before serving.

7. Breakfast Mushroom Frittata

(Preparation time: 10 minutes | Cooking time: 20 minutes | Difficulty: Easy | Servings: 5)
Per serving: Calories 250, Total fat 15g, Protein 19g, Carbs 11g
Ingredients:

- 1 teaspoon of salt
- 5 garlic cloves
- 1 tablespoon of olive oil
- 1 teaspoon of oregano
- 1 teaspoon of basil
- 1 teaspoon of cilantro
- ½ teaspoon of ground ginger
- 7 eggs
- 1 cup broccoli
- 1 cup of shiitake mushrooms
- 1/2 cup of Parmesan cheese
- ½ cup of low-fat milk

Instructions:

- Wash and slice the shiitake mushrooms well.
- In a mixing bowl, chop the broccoli & mix it with the mushrooms.
- Beat the eggs in a separate dish.
- Add the parsley, basil, oregano, & ground ginger to the egg mixture. It should be thoroughly mixed.
- Combine the low-fat milk & broccoli. The egg mixture should be thoroughly mixed. Peel and mince the garlic cloves.

- In the egg mixture, gradually whisk in the minced garlic. Preheat the oven to 350°F. Using olive oil, coat a deep pan.
- Fill the pan with the egg mixture and bake it into the preheated oven.
- Cook for 20 minutes on the frittata.
- Remove the dish from the oven once it is done cooking and allow it to cool slightly.
- Serve the frittata as soon as possible.

8. Simple Breakfast Porridge

(Preparation time: 10 minutes | Cooking time: 15 minutes | Difficulty: Easy | Servings: 1)
Per serving: Calories 142, Total fat 1g, Protein 4g, Carbs 20g
Ingredients:
- 1 cup of water
- 1/2 cup of buckwheat groats

Instructions:
- In a small pot over medium-high flame, combine water and buckwheat groats.
- Bring to a boil, then lower to a low flame.
- Cover the saucepan with the lid and set the flame to low.
- Cook for around 10 minutes, taking care not to overcook.
- Allow it to steam for another 5 minutes without opening the cover. Using a fork, fluff the mixture.
- Serve with almond milk, cherries, a dash of cinnamon, a splash of vanilla, a drizzle of honey or maple syrup, and a drizzle of honey or maple syrup on top. Enjoy.

9. Kale with Scrambled Egg

(Preparation time: 10 minutes | Cooking time: 10 minutes | Difficulty: Easy | Servings: 1)
Per serving: Calories 48, Total fat 1g, Protein 7g, Carbs 2g
Ingredients:
- 1/6 teaspoon of garlic salt

- 1/4 cup of chopped red onion
- 1 tablespoon of parmesan cheese
- 1/2 cup of beaten eggs
- Fresh baby kale

Instructions:
- Spray a large chopped yellow skillet using cooking spray.
- Cook for around 2 minutes over medium heat, or until crisp-tender.
- Add the garlic, salt, and greens to the pan. Cook for another minute, constantly stirring, till the kale wilts.
- Add the egg beaters and cook, shredded, till the bottom and edges of the parmesan cheese begin to solidify.
- Scramble the eggs gently. Cook till the sauce has thickened.
- Place a slice of cheese on top. Serve right away and enjoy.

10. Sirtfood-Friendly Breakfast Omelet

(Preparation time: 10 minutes | Cooking time: 10 minutes | Difficulty: Easy | Servings: 1)
Per serving: Calories 321, Total fat 24g, Protein 43g, Carbs 2g
Ingredients:
- 1 teaspoon turmeric
- 1 teaspoon extra virgin olive oil
- 1 tablespoon parsley – finely chopped
- 3 eggs – medium
- 50g of chicken breasts – no skin
- 1/3 red endive – sliced

Instructions:
- To begin, dice the chicken breasts & heat the skillet or frying pan.
- Toss the diced chicken breasts in the skillet with a teaspoon of extra virgin olive oil. Stir the chicken chunks occasionally as they cook. Remove the chicken from the skillet once it has been browned and set it aside. Combine the

eggs, endive, parsley, & chicken in a mixing bowl, then add the turmeric.

- To combine the ingredients, whisk them together. Return the skillet to the stovetop and reheat it. Fill the skillet with the egg mixture. Make a beautiful omelet by moving the ingredients around the pan with a spatula to ensure that it cooks evenly.
- Reduce the flame to low and allow the omelet to settle before folding the edges with the spatula to roll up the omelet. Take pleasure in your breakfast.

11. Date and Walnut Strawberry Porridge

(Preparation time: 10 minutes | Cooking time: 20 minutes | Difficulty: Easy | Servings: 4)
Per serving: Calories 137, Total fat 3g, Protein 3g, Carbs 25g
Ingredients:

- 2 Medjool dates – chopped
- 1/3 cup of buckwheat flakes
- 1/2 cup of strawberries – hulled
- 1 cup of skim milk
- Walnut – 4 chopped halves

Instructions:

- Add the chopped dates to the milk in a boiling pot. Allow the milk to heat up over medium flame, stirring constantly.
- Stir in the buckwheat flakes till everything is well combined.
- Cook the flakes till they reach your desired consistency, stirring occasionally. Toss in the walnuts and whisk to mix. When serving, top with cherries & enjoy your Sirtfood morning.

12. Mushroom Scramble

(Preparation time: 10 minutes | Cooking time: 10 minutes | Difficulty: Easy | Servings: 3)
Per serving: Calories 223, Total fat 20g, Protein 16g, Carbs 5g

Ingredients:

- 1 teaspoon of ground turmeric
- 1 teaspoon of extra virgin olive oil
- 2 eggs – medium
- ½ thinly sliced bird's eye chili
- 1 teaspoon of parsley
- 1 teaspoon of mild curry powder
- 1/4 cup of chopped kale
- 1 cup of button mushrooms – thinly sliced

Instructions:

- Leave the kale to steam for a few minutes till it softens, then set it aside.
- Meanwhile, make a paste with the turmeric & curry powder and some water; set it away while you mix the eggs.
- Toss the paste into the mixing bowl with the eggs. Incorporate the greens into the egg mixture as well.
- Add the oil to the frying pan after it has heated up.
- In a hot skillet, add the bird's eye chili and thinly sliced mushrooms.
- Cook for 3 minutes, or till golden brown.
- Combine the mushrooms & the bird's eye chili.
- Return the pan to the flame and pour the egg mixture into it.
- Stir in the parsley & continue to simmer. Serve and have fun.

13. Chia and Almonds Blueberry Bowl

(Preparation time: 10 minutes | Cooking time: 20 minutes | Difficulty: Easy | Servings: 10)
Per serving: Calories 243, Total fat 16g, Protein 12g, Carbs 20g
Ingredients:

- Pinch of salt
- 2 Medjool dates
- ½ tablespoon of almonds
- ½ tablespoon of almond butter

- 1/4 teaspoon of cardamom - powdered
- 1/8 cup of chia seeds
- 1/8 cup of blueberries
- 1/8 cup of buckwheat groats - raw
- 3/8 cup of coconut milk
- ½ tablespoon of cocoa nibs

Instructions:

- Place the coconut milk, dates, cardamom, salt, & almond butter in a
- lender and blend till smooth.
- Blend the mixture till it is completely smooth.
- In a mixing bowl, combine the chia seeds & buckwheat groats, then add the mixed mixture and toss to integrate.
- Refrigerate the bowl for at least 15 minutes after covering it.
- Add almonds, cocoa nibs, & blueberries to the bowl delight.

14. Mushroom and Buckwheat Breakfast Bowl

(Preparation time: 10 minutes | Cooking time: 10 minutes | Difficulty: Easy | Servings: 2)
Per serving: Calories 204, Total fat 3g, Protein 8g, Carbs 34g
Ingredients:

- Pinch of salt - 2 tablespoons of butter
- 3 sprigs of flat-leaf parsley
- 1 teaspoon of oregano
- 1 boiled egg per serving
- 1 red onion – medium, chopped
- 2 cups of buckwheat groats – toasted
- 8 chestnut mushrooms

Instructions:

- In a cooking pot, combine the buckwheat, water, & salt.
- Cook till the buckwheat is tender, and the water has evaporated.
- Remove the saucepan from the flame and cover it. Allow the buckwheat to rest for another 15 minutes.

- Meanwhile, melt the butter in a pan over medium flame.
- Once the butter has melted, add the sliced mushrooms & chopped onions and cook, occasionally turning, till the mushrooms and onions have caramelized. Once the mushrooms have browned, add the chopped parsley and cook for another 5 minutes. Stir in the buckwheat till it is well combined with the other ingredients.
- Finally, add the oregano and simmer for another two minutes.
- Serve immediately with a boiled egg on top.

15. Sirtfood Diet Chicken Breakfast Salad

(Preparation time: 10 minutes | Cooking time: 15 minutes | Difficulty: Easy | Servings: 1)
Per serving: Calories 294, Total fat 17g, Protein 3g, Carbs 7g
Ingredients:

- 1 teaspoon of turmeric
- ¼ lemon – freshly juiced
- 1 teaspoon of coriander – chopped
- ½ teaspoon of curry powder – mild
- 1 Medjool date – chopped
- 1 sliced bird's eye chili
- 1/4 cup of red onion – chopped
- 1/2 cup of rocket lettuce
- 1/3 cup of yogurt
- 100g of chicken – cooked and cut into bite-sized strips
- 6 chopped walnut halves

Instructions:

- Toss together the yogurt, spices, lemon juice, & coriander in a mixing bowl.
- Stir in the remaining ingredients (except for the rocket salad) till everything is well combined. On a serving plate, make a bed of rocket salad and pour the chicken & yogurt mixture over it. Enjoy!

16. Breakfast Shakshuka

(Preparation time: 10 minutes | Cooking time: 20 minutes | Difficulty: Easy | Servings: 1)
Per serving: Calories 309, Total fat 34g, Protein 23g, Carbs 22g
Ingredients:

- 1 teaspoon of turmeric
- 1 tablespoon of extra-virgin olive oil
- 1 chopped garlic clove
- 1 tablespoon of chopped parsley
- 1 sliced bird's eye chili
- 1 teaspoon of cumin – ground
- 1 teaspoon of paprika - ground
- 1/4 cup of red onion – chopped
- 2 eggs
- 1/4 cup of celery – chopped
- 2 cups of tomatoes – tinned, chopped
- 1/4 cup of kale – chopped

Instructions:

- On low-medium flame, heat a small deep pan. Add the garlic, onions, chili, celery, & spices once the olive oil has been added.
- Cook for two minutes, or till softened somewhat.
- Toss in the tomatoes and toss well to integrate all of the ingredients.
- To prevent the sauce from burning, keep it on a low flame setting and mix it occasionally.
- Cook for another 5 minutes after adding the kale. If the sauce appears to be excessively thick, thin it out with a little water. When the sauce has reached the desired consistency, whisk in the parsley thoroughly. Reduce to a low flame setting and poke two holes in the sauce. Cover the pan with the lid & cook for 10 to 12 minutes, cracking one egg into each sauce hole.

- Cook for a few minutes longer if you prefer your egg yolks hard.
- Serve immediately, ideally straight from the pan.

17. Moroccan Eggs

(Preparation time: 10 minutes | Cooking time: 20 minutes | Difficulty: Easy | Servings: 1)
Per serving: Calories 394, Total fat 1g, Protein 16g, Carbs 37g
Ingredients:

- ½ teaspoon salt
- 1 garlic clove – chopped
- ½ teaspoon chili powder
- ½ teaspoon cumin - ground
- 1 tablespoon olive oil
- ½ teaspoon cinnamon – ground
- 1 teaspoon of chopped parsley
- 1 tablespoon of tomato puree
- 1 red bell pepper – chopped
- ½ half small zucchini
- 1 cup of chopped tomatoes
- 1 cup of chickpeas
- 2 eggs

Instructions:

- Add the oil to the pot and heat it up.
- Cook for 5 minutes after adding the peppers.
- Cook for another minute after adding the garlic and zucchini.
- Stir in the tomato puree, spices, & salt to mix.
- With a little water, add the diced tomatoes and chickpeas.
- Reduce the flame to medium-low and cook the sauce for around 30 minutes, or till it has reduced by a third. While you're waiting for the sauce to reduce, preheat the oven at 350°F.
- Place the sauce in a baking dish, and then break the eggs over it.
- Place in the oven, covered in foil. Serve after baking for 10 to 15 minutes.

18. Buckwheat Granola

(Preparation time: 10 minutes | Cooking time: 30 minutes | Difficulty: Easy | Servings: 5)
Per serving: Calories 252, Total fat 14g, Protein 8g, Carbs 25g
Ingredients:

- 1 teaspoon of ground cinnamon
- 2 tablespoons of olive oil
- 1 teaspoon of ground ginger
- 2 tablespoons of maple syrup
- 1 ripe banana, peeled
- 1 cup of raw buckwheat groats
- 1/4 cup pumpkin seeds
- 1/4 cup almonds, chopped
- 1/2 cup of unsweetened coconut flakes

Instructions:

- Preheat the oven at 350ºF.
- Mix the buckwheat groats, coconut flakes, pumpkin seeds, almonds, & spices together in a bowl.
- Add the banana to a separate bowl and mash well with a fork.
- Mix the maple syrup and oil into the buckwheat mixture till everything is thoroughly incorporated.
- Spread the mixture evenly on the baking sheet that has been prepared.
- Bake for around 25–30 minutes, stirring halfway through.
- Take the baking sheet out of the oven and place it on a cooling rack.

19. Matcha Pancakes

(Preparation time: 10 minutes | Cooking time: 25 minutes | Difficulty: Easy | Servings: 6)
Per serving: Calories 232, Total fat 5g, Protein 6g, Carbs 36g
Ingredients:

- 5 tablespoons of warm water
- Pinch of salt
- 1 tablespoon of olive oil
- 1 tablespoon of baking powder

- 1 teaspoon of vanilla extract
- 1 tablespoon of matcha powder
- 2 tablespoons of flax meal
- 1 cup of spelt flour
- 1 cup of buckwheat flour
- ¾ cup of unsweetened almond milk
- 1/3 cup of raw honey

Instructions:

- Combine the flax meal and warm water in a mixing dish and stir well. Allow for a 5-minute rest period.
- Mix the flours, matcha powder, baking powder, and salt together in a separate dish.
- Add the almond milk, oil, and vanilla extract to the flax meal mixture in the mixing dish and mix well.
- Place the flour mixture in a mixing bowl and stir until a smooth textured mixture forms.
- Over medium-high heat, gently butter a nonstick wok.
- Pour in the necessary amount of mixture and spread it out evenly with a spoon.
- Cook for 2–3 minutes at a low temperature.
- Flip the side carefully and cook for about 1 minute.
- Rep with the rest of the mixture.
- Serve warm with honey drizzled over the top.

20. Eggs with Kale

(Preparation time: 10 minutes | Cooking time: 25 minutes | Difficulty: Easy | Servings: 4)
Per serving: Calories 175, Total fat 12g, Protein 8g, Carbs 11g
Ingredients:

- Salt and ground black pepper, to taste
- 2 garlic cloves, minced
- ¼ teaspoon of red pepper flakes, crushed

- 1 teaspoon of ground cumin
- 2 tablespoons of olive oil
- 2 tablespoons of fresh parsley, chopped
- 4 eggs
- 1 red onion, chopped
- 1 cup of tomatoes, chopped
- ½ pound of fresh kale, tough ribs removed and chopped

Instructions:

- In a large-sized wok, heat the oil over medium flame & sauté the onion for around 4–5 minutes.
- Add the garlic and cook for 1 minute.
- Cook for 2–3 minutes, constantly stirring, after adding the tomatoes, spices, salt, & black pepper.
- Cook for around 4–5 minutes after adding the kale. Crack eggs carefully on top of the kale mixture. Cover the pan with the lid & cook for around 10 minutes, or till the eggs are done to your liking. Serve immediately with a parsley garnish.

21. Soy and Zucchini Omelet

(Preparation time: 10 minutes | Cooking time: 10 minutes | Difficulty: Easy | Servings: 2)
Per serving: Calories 115, Total fat 1g, Protein 6g, Carbs 20g
Ingredients:

- 2 pinches of salt
- 2 teaspoons of olive oil
- 2 small zucchini
- 3 teaspoons of buckwheat flour
- ⅓ cup of glass soy milk

Instructions:

- Using a vegetable slicer, cut the zucchini into very thin strips (with a grater or with a potato peeler, not using a knife).
- In a soup plate, combine the flour & salt, add the soy milk a little at a time, and 2 fingers of water, stirring quickly with a fork to avoid lumps. You need a batter that isn't too dense and is rather watery.
- Stir in the zucchini slices thoroughly.
- Heat 2 teaspoons of oil in a nonstick frying pan (just enough to cover the bottom) over high heat. Pour the batter into the hot oil and smooth it out with a wooden spatula. Cover the fire and leave it on high for about half a minute, then reduce the flame a little.
- The omelet should cook for around 10 minutes, during which time it should be turned over several times to brown both sides (you can cut it into 4 slices & turn them one at a time).

22. Kale Mushroom Scramble

(Preparation time: 10 minutes | Cooking time: 10 minutes | Difficulty: Easy | Servings: 1)
Per serving: Calories 116, Total fat 5g, Protein 6g, Carbs 13g
Ingredients:

- 1 teaspoon of ground turmeric
- 1 teaspoon of extra virgin olive oil
- ½ thinly sliced bird's eye chili
- 1 teaspoon of mild curry powder
- 2 tablespoons of kale, roughly chopped
- Handful thinly sliced button mushrooms

Instructions:

- To make a light paste, combine the curry powder, turmeric with a splash of water.
- Place the kale in a steamer basket & steam for around 2-3 minutes in boiling water. In a frying pan, heat the oil over medium flame and cook the mushrooms and chilies for around 2 to 3 minutes, till softened, then continue till they turn brown.

23. Chia Breakfast Bowl

(Preparation time: 10 minutes | Cooking time: 0 minutes | Difficulty: Easy | Servings: 1)
Per serving: Calories 220, Total fat 11g, Protein 8g, Carbs 25g
Ingredients:

- A pinch of salt
- 1-3 teaspoons of chia seeds
- ⅔ cup of nut milk (almond or coconut)
- Coconut flakes or seasonal fruit like blueberries as a topper
- Maple syrup, honey or nectar to taste

Instructions:

- Begin by stirring the chia seeds into the almond milk till they are thoroughly combined.
- Allow the seeds to sit for around 12 minutes or till they are totally swelled.
- Finally, add the honey, desired fruit, and a pinch of salt. Now it's time to enjoy and serve.

24. Blueberries Pancake

(Preparation time: 10 minutes | Cooking time: 10 minutes | Difficulty: Easy | Servings: 2)
Per serving: Calories 308, Total fat 14g, Protein 10g, Carbs 33g
Ingredients:

- A pinch of ground cinnamon
- Olive oil cooking spray
- 1 banana, peeled
- 1 tablespoon of agave syrup
- 4 tablespoons of peanut butter
- 4 tablespoons of blueberries
- ¼ cup of buckwheat flour
- ½ cup of almond milk, unsweetened

Instructions:

- In a blender, combine all of the ingredients and pulse for 2 minutes, or till smooth. Coat a skillet pan in cooking spray and heat over medium flame till hot.

- Pour a small amount of batter into the pan, shape it into a pancake, & cook for around 2 to 3 minutes per side, or till golden brown.
- Repeat with the remaining batter and transfer cooked pancakes to a platter. Serve immediately.
- Pancakes can be kept in the fridge for up to three days if stored in an airtight container with a lid. Once ready to eat, warm for around 1 to 2 minutes in the microwave till hot, then serve.

25. Chocolate Waffles

(Preparation time: 10 minutes | Cooking time: 25 minutes | Difficulty: Easy | Servings: 8)
Per serving: Calories 297, Total fat 10g, Protein 11g, Carbs 25g
Ingredients:

- ¼ teaspoon of kosher salt
- 1 tablespoon of fresh lemon juice
- 1 teaspoon of baking soda
- 1 teaspoon of baking powder
- 2 teaspoons of vanilla extract
- 2 cups of unsweetened almond milk
- ½ cup of coconut oil, melted
- 2 large eggs
- ¼ cup of stevia
- 4 tablespoons of unsweetened dark chocolate, chopped roughly
- 1 cup of buckwheat flour
- ½ cup of cacao powder
- ¼ cup of flaxseed meal

Instructions:

- Combine the almond milk & lemon juice in a mixing dish and stir well.
- Allow for a 10-minute rest period.
- In a mixing dish, combine buckwheat flour, cacao powder, baking powder, flaxseed meal, baking soda, & salt.
- Place the eggs, stevia, coconut oil, & vanilla extract in the bowl with the

almond milk mixture and whisk till smooth.

- Put the flour mixture in a mixing bowl & beat till smooth.
- Fold the chocolate bits in gently.
- Grease the waffle iron after it has been preheated.
- Place the necessary amount of the mixture in the waffle iron & cook for around 3 minutes, or till golden brown.
- Rep with the rest of the mixture.
- Warm the dish before serving.

26. Buckwheat Pancakes

(Preparation time: 10 minutes | Cooking time: 15 minutes | Difficulty: Easy | Servings: 5)
Per serving: Calories 143, Total fat 3g, Protein 4g, Carbs 19g
Ingredients:

- ¼ teaspoon of sea salt
- 1 tablespoon of baking powder
- 1 teaspoon of vanilla extract
- 1 tablespoon of coconut oil
- 2 teaspoons of apple cider vinegar
- 2 tablespoons of ground flax seed
- ¼ cup of maple syrup
- 1 cup of coconut milk
- 1 cup of buckwheat flour

Instructions:

- Combine the coconut milk & vinegar in a medium-sized mixing dish. Set them aside.
- Combine the flour, flaxseed, baking powder, & salt in a large-sized mixing dish.
- Blend in the coconut milk mixture, maple syrup, & vanilla extract till smooth.
- Melt coconut oil in a nonstick skillet over medium flame.
- Spread approximately a third of a cup of the mixture in an even circle.
- Cook for 1-2 minutes at a time.

- Cook for a further minute on the other side before removing it from the pan.
- Rep with the rest of the mixture.
- Warm the dish before serving.

27. Apple Cinnamon Wraps

(Preparation time: 15 minutes | Cooking time: 15 minutes | Difficulty: Easy | Servings: 4)
Per serving: Calories 278, Total fat 24g, Protein 19g, Carbs 37g
Ingredients:

- A dash of salt
- 1 teaspoon of baking powder
- 2 teaspoons of extra virgin olive oil
- 2 egg whites
- 2 tablespoons of raw honey
- 2 Apples, cut into small chunks
- 2 cups of quick-cooking oats
- 1 cup of buckwheat flour
- 1 ¼ cups of milk (or soy/almond/coconut)

For the berry topping:

- 3 tablespoons of water
- 1 cup of blackcurrants, washed and stalks removed
- 2 tablespoons of stevia

Instructions:

- In a mixing bowl, whisk the eggs with the almond milk, olive oil, & salt.
- Whisk together the tapioca & coconut flour till a smooth batter forms.
- 1/6 of the batter should go into a greased pan.
- Wraps with a diameter of about 15 cm should be used.
- Cook till the wraps are golden brown on both sides.
- Using a pan, heat the oil.
- Cook over medium flame till the apple is mushy, then add the chopped apple, cinnamon, cranberries, & lemon juice.
- Fold the wrap in half and place the apple on top.

28. Breakfast Chicken Wraps

(Preparation time: 15 minutes | Cooking time: 15 minutes | Difficulty: Easy | Servings: 2)
Per serving: Calories 256, Total fat 42g, Protein 52g, Carbs 35g
Ingredients:

- 1/4 teaspoon of sea salt
- 1 teaspoon of olive oil
- 3 tablespoons of coconut flour
- 2 pieces Egg
- 10 slices of chicken breast
- 1/3 cup of buckwheat flour
- 1 cup of Almond milk

Instructions:

- In a container, whisk the eggs, then add the almond milk, olive oil, & salt.
- Stir in the buckwheat flour & coconut flour with a whisk till you have a smooth mixture. 1/6 of the batter should be poured into a greased pan.
- Fry the wraps till golden brown on both sides. Carry on with the rest of the dough in the same manner.
- As desired, top the wraps with chicken & more salad or raw vegetables.

29. Kale, Red onion and Cheese Frittata

(Preparation time: 10 minutes | Cooking time: 25 minutes | Difficulty: Easy | Servings: 1)
Per serving: Calories 260, Total fat 15g, Protein 13g, Carbs 20g
Ingredients:

- 1 small clove of garlic
- 1 teaspoon chopped parsley
- 1 teaspoon extra virgin olive oil
- ½ teaspoon herbs of Provence
- 1/3 cup of red onion, cut
- 3 medium-sized eggs
- 4 tablespoons of cheese (feta, cheddar)
- 1/3 cup of cut kale (weight with stems removed)

Instructions:

- Preheat the oven at 360°F.
- Crack the eggs into a mixing dish and whisk them thoroughly.
- In an ovenproof pan over low to medium flame, heat the olive oil and sauté the onion, kale, & garlic for 3-4 minutes, or till soft.
- Combine the cooked veggies with the egg mixture. Stir in the herbs and parsley well. You can either rub or crumble the cheese into the egg.
- Return the pan to a high flame setting and pour in the egg mixture. Allow sitting for 30 seconds or till the egg peels away from the pan's side. Shift the pan and bake for around 15 minutes, or till the egg is completely set.
- If the middle is still a bit runny, remove it from the oven and let it aside for 5 minutes before serving, as the residual heat will finish cooking the frittata.
- Serve with a sprinkle of arugula and a drizzle of olive oil on top.

30. Scrambled Eggs with Kale, Red onion and Tomatoes

(Preparation time: 10 minutes | Cooking time: 10 minutes | Difficulty: Easy | Servings: 1)
Per serving: Calories 110, Total fat 9g, Protein 13g, Carbs 5g
Ingredients:

- 1 teaspoon of ground turmeric
- 1 teaspoon of extra virgin olive oil
- 1 tablespoon of chopped parsley
- ½ cut bird's eye chili
- 2 tablespoons of cut red onion
- 5 halved cherry tomatoes
- 2 tablespoons of cut celery
- 3 tablespoons of chopped kale (weight with stems removed)
- 1/2 cup of extra firm tofu

Instructions:

- To remove any extra water, cover the tofu in kitchen paper & set something heavy on top. Cook the greens for 2-3 minutes in a steamer. To make a light paste, combine the turmeric and a little water. Heat the olive oil in a pan over medium flame, then add the onion, celery, and chilies and cook for 2-3 minutes.
- Toss the tofu with the cherry tomatoes in the pan, then pour in the turmeric paste and stir well. Toss in the kale and continue to stir and sauté till the tofu is browned. Serve with parsley.

31. Turmeric Couscous with Edamame Beans

(Preparation time: 10 minutes | Cooking time: 15 minutes | Difficulty: Easy | Servings: 2)
Per serving: Calories 342, Total fat 5g, Protein 32g, Carbs 15g
Ingredients:

- 1 tablespoon of turmeric
- 2 teaspoons of extra virgin olive oil
- 2 tablespoons of parsley, finely chopped
- ½ cup of red onion, finely sliced
- ¼ cup of cherry tomatoes, chopped
- ½ eggplant - ½ yellow pepper, cubed
- ½ red pepper, cubed
- 1 ½ edamame beans
- 1/2 cup of couscous

Instructions:

- Set aside edamame after steaming for 5 minutes. Toss the couscous with 1 cup of salted boiling water and set aside to absorb the liquid.
- Meanwhile, preheat a pan over medium-high flame.
- Oil, eggplant, peppers, onion, and tomatoes, as well as turmeric, salt, and pepper, are added to the pan. Cook on high flame for around 5 minutes.

- Combine the couscous & edamame in a mixing bowl.
- Serve with fresh parsley as a garnish.

32. Red Onion Frittata with Chili Grilled Zucchini

(Preparation time: 10 minutes | Cooking time: 30 minutes | Difficulty: Easy | Servings: 2)
Per serving: Calories 359, Total fat 8g, Protein 21g, Carbs 18g
Ingredients:

- Salt and pepper to taste
- 1 clove of garlic, crushed
- 2 tablespoons of oil
- ½ bird's eye chili, finely sliced
- 1 teaspoon of white vinegar
- 1 ½ cups of red onion, finely sliced
- 3 eggs
- 2 tablespoons of skim milk
- 2 zucchinis
- 6 tablespoons of cheddar cheese

Instructions:

- Preheat the oven at 350°F. Slice the zucchini into thin pieces and broil them before serving.
- Whisk together 3 eggs, salt, shredded cheddar cheese, milk, and pepper, then pour into a silicone baking tray and bake for around 25-30 minutes.
- Combine the garlic, oil, salt, pepper, and vinegar in a bowl and pour over the zucchini. Serve the zucchini frittata beside it.

33. Matcha Overnight Oats

(Preparation time: 10 minutes | Cooking time: 0 minutes | Difficulty: Easy | Servings: 2)
Per serving: Calories 324, Total fat 14g, Protein 22g, Carbs 30g
Ingredients:

- 2 pinches of ground cinnamon
- 2 teaspoons of Chia seeds
- 1 teaspoon of Honey

- 1/2 cup of Rolled oats
- 1 Apple, peeled, cored and chopped
- 1 teaspoon of Matcha powder
- 4 walnuts
- 1 ½ cups of Almond milk

Instructions:

- In a jar or bowl, combine the chia seeds with oats.
- In a separate jug or dish, whisk together the matcha powder & one tablespoon of almond milk with a hand-held mixer till a smooth paste forms, then add the remaining milk and thoroughly combine.
- Pour the milk mixture over the oats, then toss in the honey and cinnamon. Refrigerate the bowl overnight after covering it with a lid.
- Transfer the oats to two serving bowls when ready to eat, then top with the walnuts & diced apple.

34. Scrambled Eggs with Parsley and Red Onion

(Preparation time: 5 minutes | Cooking time: 10 minutes | Difficulty: Easy | Servings: 1)

Per serving: Calories 278, Total fat 6g, Protein 19g, Carbs 13g

Ingredients:

- Salt and pepper
- 1 tablespoon of parsley, finely chopped
- 2 eggs
- ½ cup of red onion
- 1 tablespoon of Parmesan

Instructions:

- In a mixing dish, combine eggs, cheese, a touch of salt and pepper, parsley and finely sliced onion. Quickly whisk the ingredients together.
- In a skillet, scramble the eggs for 2 minutes, stirring constantly till done.

35. Pancakes with Caramelized Strawberries

(Preparation time: 10 minutes | Cooking time: 15 minutes | Difficulty: Easy | Servings: 2)

Per serving: Calories 272, Total fat 4g, Protein 24g, Carbs 22g

Ingredients:

- 1 egg - 2 tsp honey
- 4 tablespoons of almond flour
- 1/3 cup of skimmed milk
- 4 tablespoons of buckwheat flour
- 1 cup of strawberries

Instructions:

- In a mixing dish, combine the flours, the yolk, and a small amount of the mixture to make a thick batter. To avoid lumps, add the milk in little increments.
- In a separate dish, whisk the egg white till stiff, then delicately fold it into the batter.
- Make a 5-inch circular pancake with enough batter to cook for around 2 minutes per side till done. Continue till all the pancakes are cooked.
- Place half of the strawberries on top of each serving after caramelizing them in a hot skillet with honey.

36. Chicken Breast Skillet

(Preparation time: 10 minutes | Cooking time: 30 minutes | Difficulty: Easy | Servings: 2)

Per serving: Calories 341, Total fat 19g, Protein 36g, Carbs 1g

Ingredients:

- ½ teaspoon ground black pepper
- 1 teaspoon of minced garlic
- 1 tablespoon of olive oil
- 2 eggs
- 1 chicken breast
- 3 ounces ground sausage
- 3 slices bacon

Instructions:

- Chop the bacon and the chicken breast into one-inch chunks. Cook in the oil for around 2 minutes, constantly turning, in a pan over medium flame with bacon. Stir in diced chicken & ground or crumbled sausage once the bacon fat has started to gather in the pan.
- Season the meat in the skillet using garlic and pepper. Brown the meat for around 6 to 8 minutes over medium-high flame.
- Reduce to a medium flame setting. Clear two pockets of room for the eggs on opposite sides of the pan. Break the yolks apart and crack the eggs into the skillet. Cover the skillet & cook for 10 minutes, or till the egg whites are hard. To serve, remove the cover & scoop onto a plate.

37. Buckwheat and Brown Rice Crepes

(Preparation time: 10 minutes | Cooking time: 10 minutes | Difficulty: Easy | Servings: 4)
Per serving: Calories 121, Total fat 6g, Protein 5g, Carbs 13g
Ingredients:

- 1 teaspoon of butter, or as needed
- 1 tablespoon of olive oil - 2 eggs
- 1 cup of skim milk
- 1/2 cup of brown rice flour
- 3 tablespoons of buckwheat flour

Instructions:

- Combine the eggs, milk, & olive oil in a mixing bowl. Sift in the brown rice & buckwheat flours one at a time, constantly stirring until the batter is extremely runny.
- Melt butter in an 8-inch skillet or crepe pan over medium flame. In the skillet, 1/4 cup of batter should be poured. Rotate the skillet till the bottom is

covered in a thin coating of batter. Cook for 1–2 minutes, or till the crepe's top is no longer moist & the bottom is light brown. Run a spatula along the edge of the pan to release the crepe; flip the crepe and cook till the second side is gently brown, around 1 minute more. Allow to cool on a cooling rack. Continue with the rest of the batter, stirring it in a small amount before using.

38. Blueberry Banana Buckwheat Pancakes

(Preparation time: 10 minutes | Cooking time: 10 minutes | Difficulty: Easy | Servings: 4)
Per serving: Calories 239, Total fat 14g, Protein 6g, Carbs 35g
Ingredients:

- 1/2 teaspoon of baking soda
- 1/2 teaspoon of ground cinnamon
- 1 tablespoon of raw honey
- 2 tablespoons of olive oil, divided
- 2 eggs - 1 mashed banana
- 1 cup of fresh blueberries
- 1 cup of buckwheat flour
- 1 cup of coconut milk

Instructions:

- Combine buckwheat flour & cinnamon in a large-sized mixing bowl. Make a well in the center and add the coconut milk, honey, eggs, 1 tablespoon of oil, and baking soda. Blend till the batter is entirely smooth.
- To integrate the blueberries & banana into the batter, stir gently.
- Melt the remaining 1 tablespoon of oil on a skillet over medium-low flame. Cook for around 3 to 4 minutes, or till bubbles form & the sides are dry, by dropping 1/4 cup of batter onto the griddle. On the other side, cook for 2 to 3 minutes, or till golden brown. Repeat with the remaining batter.

39. Quinoa Buckwheat Pancakes

(Preparation time: 10 minutes | Cooking time: 10 minutes | Difficulty: Easy | Servings: 4)
Per serving: Calories 104, Total fat 5g, Protein 3g, Carbs 12g
Ingredients:
- 1/2 teaspoon of baking soda
- 1 teaspoon of baking powder
- 1 tablespoon of honey
- 1 lightly beaten egg
- 2 tablespoons of olive oil
- 1/2 cup of quinoa flour
- 1/2 cup of buckwheat flour
- 1 cup of buttermilk

Instructions:
- Combine the olive oil, buttermilk, egg, & honey in a large-sized mixing bowl. Mix together the buckwheat flour, baking powder, quinoa flour, & baking soda. Stir the flour and buttermilk mixture together till it is evenly spread.
- Heat a lightly oiled griddle over medium flame. Pour 1/4 cup of batter onto the griddle for each pancake and cook for 3 to 4 minutes, or till bubbles form & the edges are dry. Cook for 2 to 3 minutes on the other side, or till browned. Carry on with the rest of the batter.

40. Buckwheat and Avocado Breakfast Salad

(Preparation time: 10 minutes | Cooking time: 10 minutes | Difficulty: Easy | Servings: 2)
Per serving: Calories 264, Total fat 30g, Protein 12g, Carbs 26g
Ingredients:
- 1 cup of water
- 1 lime, juiced
- 1 1/2 tablespoons of extra-virgin olive oil
- 1 tablespoon of chopped fresh flat-leaf parsley

- 1/2 teaspoon of each fennel seed
- 1/2 teaspoon of ground mixed peppercorns
- 1/2 teaspoon of cayenne pepper
- 2 tablespoons of thinly sliced red onion
- 5 diced cherry tomatoes
- 1 small peeled, pitted, and diced avocado
- 1/4 cup of low-fat crumbled soft goat cheese
- 1/2 cup of buckwheat groats

Instructions:
- Bring the water, buckwheat, and salt to a boil in a saucepan. Reduce the flame to medium-low, cover the saucepan, and cook for around 8 minutes, or till the buckwheat is firm to the bite but still soft. After rinsing buckwheat in cold water, drain it.
- Combine the avocado, red onion, cherry tomatoes, lime juice, olive oil, cayenne pepper, parsley, fennel seed, & mixed pepper in a large-sized mixing bowl. Carefully fold in the buckwheat groats, then top with goat cheese.

41. Nut and Date Millet Porridge

(Preparation time: 10 minutes | Cooking time: 25 minutes | Difficulty: Easy | Servings: 2)
Per serving: Calories 312, Total fat 18g, Protein 12g, Carbs 28g
Ingredients:
- 1/2 teaspoon of ground cinnamon
- 1/4 teaspoon of ground nutmeg
- 3 pitted and diced Medjool dates
- 2 tablespoons of pumpkin seeds
- 2 tablespoons of slivered almonds
- 1 tablespoon of flax seeds
- 1/2 cup of hulled millet
- 2 tablespoons of shredded and unsweetened coconut
- 2 cups of unsweetened almond milk, divided

Instructions:

- Pulse millet in a blender or food processor till it resembles finely ground coffee. Set them aside.
- Heat a nonstick saucepan over medium-high flame. Toast the walnuts for around 2 minutes, stirring halfway through, till golden brown. Continue to stir & toast the pepitas till golden brown, around 3 minutes. Toss in the flax seeds and coconut, & toast for another 5 minutes, or till golden. Place the ingredients in a mixing bowl and set aside.
- Add the millet that has been ground to the same pan. Toast for around 3 minutes, or till fragrant. Add 1 1/2 cups almond milk, properly combine to ensure no lumps. Bring the bring to the boil, then add the dates. Reduce the flame to low and simmer for another 10 minutes, stirring occasionally.
- Add 2 teaspoons of toasted seed mixture, mix well into the porridge Mix in the cinnamon & nutmeg. Toss everything together thoroughly. Cook for around 6–10 minutes more, or until the sauce has thickened.
- Porridge should be divided into two bowls. In separate bowls, serve the remaining seed mixture & 1/2 cup of almond milk.

42. Whole Grain Carrot Peach Breakfast Muffins

(Preparation time: 10 minutes | Cooking time: 20 minutes | Difficulty: Easy | Servings: 4)
Per serving: Calories 214, Total fat 13g, Protein 3g, Carbs 22g
Ingredients:

- 1 teaspoon of ground cinnamon
- 1/2 teaspoon of baking soda
- 1 1/2 teaspoon of baking powder
- 1 teaspoon of vanilla extract
- 1/2 cup of olive oil
- 2 large eggs
- 1 cup of grated carrots
- 1 1/2 cups of diced peaches
- 1/2 cup of stevia
- 1/2 cup of almond flour
- 1/2 cup of oat flour
- 1/2 cup of buckwheat flour

Instructions:

- Preheat the oven at 350°F. A muffin tray should be lined using paper liners.
- 1/2 cup of almond flour, 1 teaspoon of cinnamon, whole-wheat flour, buckwheat flour, baking powder, and baking soda should all be combined.
- Combine the oil, eggs, sweetener, & vanilla essence in a separate bowl. Fold the batter into the flour mixture till barely combined. Fold in the peaches & carrots gently.
- Fill muffin tins two-thirds of the way with batter.
- In a preheated oven, bake for around 15 minutes till a toothpick inserted in the center comes out clean. Cool in the pan for 5 to 10 minutes before transferring to a wire rack to cool completely.

43. Buckwheat Cinnamon and Raisin Bagels

(Preparation time: 10 minutes | Cooking time: 20 minutes | Difficulty: Easy | Servings: 4)
Per serving: Calories 182, Total fat 1g, Protein 5g, Carbs 28g
Ingredients:

- 2 cups of warm water
- 1 teaspoon of cinnamon
- 1/2 cup of honey
- 1/2 cup of raisins
- 2 tablespoons of molasses
- 3 cups of buckwheat flour

Instructions:

- Combine warm water and yeast in a large-sized mixing bowl and set aside for around 5 minutes to dissolve.
- Gently combine the molasses, honey, & cinnamon.
- Combine the flour and raisins in the same bowl as the yeast-honey mixture. Mix thoroughly; the final product will be crumbly. Knead the dough for about 10 minutes till it is smooth. Cover the dough with a towel and set aside for 20 minutes.
- Bring a large saucepan of water to a low simmer.
- Pinch off a 2-inch ball of dough & roll it into a snake form to make a snake. Wrap it around four fingers & gently pinch the ends together to form a bagel shape. Repeat with the remaining dough to make more bagels.
- Preheat the oven at 400°F. Two baking sheets should be greased.
- In boiling water, cook bagels for around 2 minutes on each side. Remove them from the water and place them on the prepared baking sheets.
- In a preheated oven, bake for around 10 to 15 minutes, or till golden brown. Allow the wire racks to cool.

44. Breakfast Buckwheat Scones with Oatmeal and Blueberries

(Preparation time: 10 minutes | Cooking time: 20 minutes | Difficulty: Easy | Servings: 6)
Per serving: Calories 223, Total fat 11g, Protein 5g, Carbs 18g
Ingredients:

- 1 teaspoon of ground cinnamon
- 3 teaspoons of baking powder
- 1 beaten egg
- 1 cup of half-and-half
- 1/2 cup of rolled oats

- 1/2 cup of stevia
- 2 tablespoons of granulated sweetener
- 3 cups of buckwheat flour
- 1 cup of blueberries

Instructions:

- Preheat the oven at 400°F. A baking sheet should be lightly oiled.
- Combine flour, baking powder, sweetener, & cinnamon in a mixing bowl. Cut in butter cubes with a pastry cutter or two knives.
- Combine half-and-half and egg in a mixing bowl. In a mixing dish, combine the flour and butter. Combine the blueberries & oats.
- On a lightly floured board, divide the dough in half & roll it out. Make a circle out of each side and cut it into eight wedges. Place the scones on a parchment-lined baking sheet and top with granulated sweetener.
- In a preheated oven, bake for around 12 to 15 minutes, or till golden brown.

45. Buckwheat Breakfast Muffins

(Preparation time: 10 minutes | Cooking time: 20 minutes | Difficulty: Easy | Servings: 4)
Per serving: Calories 183, Total fat 7g, Protein 3g, Carbs 21g
Ingredients:

- 2 teaspoons of baking powder
- 1 egg
- 1/3 cup of olive oil
- 1 pint of fresh blueberries
- 1/3 cup of skim milk
- 3/4 cup of stevia
- 1 cup of buckwheat flour
- 1/2 cup of unsweetened applesauce

Instructions:

- Preheat the oven at 400°F. The muffin cups should be greased or coated with paper liners. Combine the flour, sweetener, & baking powder in a large-sized mixing bowl.

- Whisk the olive oil, egg, milk, & applesauce together in a separate bowl till smooth, then pour the liquid components into the flour mixture till moistened. Gently fold in the blueberries. Fill the muffin tins two-thirds of the way with batter.
- In a preheated oven, bake muffins for around 20 minutes, or till they rise & the tops are golden brown, and in the middle of a muffin, a toothpick must come out clean.

46. Oatmeal Cake

(Preparation time: 10 minutes | Cooking time: 15 minutes | Difficulty: Easy | Servings: 4)
Per serving: Calories 264, Total fat 13g, Protein 3g, Carbs 25g
Ingredients:

- 1 teaspoon of ground cinnamon
- 1 teaspoon of baking soda
- 2 eggs
- 4 tablespoons of evaporated milk
- 1/2 cup of unsalted butter
- 2 cups of stevia
- 1 cup of flaked coconut
- 1 cup of quick-cooking oats
- 1 1/3 cups of whole-wheat flour
- 1 cup of chopped walnuts

Instructions:

- Preheat the oven at 350°F. The cake pan should be greased and floured.
- Bring the bring to the boil and then pour it over the oats. Set them aside.
- In a sifter, combine the flour, baking soda, & cinnamon. Set them aside.
- Cream Combine 1/2 cup of butter, 1 cup of stevia, and eggs in a mixer and beat till frothy. Incorporate the flour mixture. Toss in the oats that have softened. Half-fill a baking pan with batter.

- Bake for around 20–25 minutes. Remove the cake from the oven.
- Preheat the broiler in the oven.
- In a saucepan, combine milk, 1/2 cup butter, & 1 cup of stevia.
- Stir in the coconut & sliced almonds after the butter has melted. Apply to a cake that has been heated.
- Under the broiler, cook the cake for around 2 to 3 minutes.

47. Baked Cranberry Oatmeal

(Preparation time: 10 minutes | Cooking time: 25 minutes | Difficulty: Easy | Servings: 4)
Per serving: Calories 252, Total fat 10g, Protein 7g, Carbs 25g
Ingredients:

- 1 teaspoon of ground cinnamon
- 1/4 teaspoon of ground nutmeg
- 1/4 teaspoon of ground cloves
- 3/4 cup of chopped apples
- 1 1/2 cups of skim milk
- 3 tablespoons of stevia
- 3/4 cup of rolled oats
- 1/3 cup of chopped walnuts
- 1/3 cup of dried cranberries

Instructions:

- Preheat the oven at 350°F.
- Using cooking spray, coat an 8x8-inch baking dish.
- Bring the milk, nutmeg, stevia, cinnamon, and cloves to a boil in a saucepan; remove from the flame. In a baking dish, combine the oats, dried cranberries, apples, & walnuts. Over the oats, pour the milk mixture.
- In a preheated oven, bake for around 20 to 25 minutes, or till lightly browned.

48. Greek Breakfast Pasta Salad

(Preparation time: 10 minutes | Cooking time: 15 minutes | Difficulty: Easy | Servings: 4)

Per serving: Calories 337, Total fat 12g, Protein 11g, Carbs 24g

Ingredients:

- Salt and ground black pepper to taste
- 1 tablespoon of lemon juice
- 2 cloves of diced garlic
- 1 tablespoon of fresh parsley
- 2 tablespoons of olive oil
- 1 tablespoon of balsamic vinegar
- 1/4 finely diced red onion
- 1 peeled and diced cucumber
- 1/4 cup of grape tomatoes
- 1/4 cup of sliced black olives
- 1/2 cup of garbanzo beans
- 1 1/2 cups of buckwheat pasta
- 1/2 cup of low-fat crumbled feta cheese

Instructions:

- Toss the garbanzo beans, red onion, grape tomatoes, cucumber, black olives, olive oil, garlic, basil, salt, balsamic vinegar, lemon juice, & black pepper in a large-sized salad dish.
- Bring a large pot of water to the boil, then add the pasta and cook for about 10 minutes, or till soft but firm to the biting. Toss the pasta gently into the salad and chill for 15 to 20 minutes to let the flavors mingle. Toss the salad with feta cheese before serving.

49. Brown Rice Pudding with Strawberries

(Preparation time: 10 minutes | Cooking time: 15 minutes | Difficulty: Easy | Servings: 4)

Per serving: Calories 302, Total fat 4g, Protein 2g, Carbs 25g

Ingredients:

- 1/2 cup of water
- A pinch of ground cinnamon
- A pinch of ground nutmeg
- 1/2 teaspoon of vanilla extract
- 1 tablespoon of unsalted butter
- 1 1/2 tablespoons of stevia
- 1 cup of brown rice cooked
- 2 cups of strawberry juice

Instructions:

- Combine strawberries, stevia, 1/4 cup of water, rice, & vanilla essence in a saucepan over low flame. Simmer for around 3 to 5 minutes, or till the strawberries wilt. After plating, add the butter and stir thoroughly; sprinkle with cinnamon and nutmeg.

50. Buckwheat with Pineapple, Pecans and Parsley

(Preparation time: 10 minutes | Cooking time: 25 minutes | Difficulty: Easy | Servings: 4)

Per serving: Calories 300, Total fat 12g, Protein 6g, Carbs 36g

Ingredients:

- 2 cups of water
- 1 1/2 teaspoons of olive oil
- 2 tablespoons of chopped Italian parsley
- 2 tablespoons of chopped fresh basil
- 1/2 cup of pineapple chunks
- 1 cup of buckwheat
- 1/2 cup of chopped pecans

Instructions:

- Cook buckwheat according to package directions. Then add pineapple chunks, parsley, pecans, basil, & oil to the buckwheat. Allow cooling completely before serving.

51. Avocado Meyer Lemon Toast

(Preparation time: 10 minutes | Cooking time: 5 minutes | Difficulty: Easy | Servings: 2)

Per serving: Calories 72, Total fat 1g, Protein 4g, Carbs 12g

Ingredients:

- A pinch of salt

- A pinch of cayenne pepper
- 1 teaspoon of Meyer lemon juice
- 1/4 teaspoon of Meyer lemon zest
- 1/4 teaspoon of chia seeds
- 2 tablespoons of fresh parsley chopped
- 2 slices of buckwheat or whole-grain bread
- 1/2 avocado

Instructions:

- For 3 to 4 minutes, toast the bread slices.
- In a medium-sized mixing bowl, mash the avocado with the parsley, Meyer lemon juice, cayenne pepper, salt & Meyer lemon zest. On top of the avocado mixture on the toast, sprinkle the chia seeds.

52. Breakfast Mushroom Surprise

(Preparation time: 10 minutes | Cooking time: 15 minutes | Difficulty: Easy | Servings: 2)
Per serving: Calories 184, Total fat 16g, Protein 8g, Carbs 7g
Ingredients:

- A pinch of black pepper and salt
- 1 teaspoon of finely chopped garlic
- 4 teaspoons of olive oil
- 1 teaspoon of dried thyme or rosemary
- 1 tablespoon of finely grated cheddar cheese
- 2 large-sized eggs
- 2 Portobello mushrooms

Instructions:

- Preheat the oven at 390°F.
- Arrange the mushrooms in a foil-lined roasting pan. Combine the mushrooms, garlic, salt & pepper.
- Bake for around 10 minutes, or until it is soft. Meanwhile, in a mixing bowl, whisk the eggs & season using salt and black pepper to taste.
- Scramble the egg with the olive oil in a frying pan over a low to medium

temperature. Cook, stirring regularly until the egg is set and fully cooked.

- Pour a quarter of the egg mixture over each mushroom once they've been cooked.
- Sprinkle cheese and parsley/thyme/rosemary on top. Serve right away.

53. Creamy Breakfast Vegetable Frittata

(Preparation time: 10 minutes | Cooking time: 20 minutes | Difficulty: Easy | Servings: 4)
Per serving: Calories 168, Total fat 12g, Protein 10g, Carbs 7g
Ingredients:

- A pinch of salt and black pepper
- 6 large size eggs
- 1/2 cup of grape tomatoes
- 1/2 cup of kale chopped
- 1/2 cup of broccoli chopped
- 1/4 cup of green bell pepper chopped
- 1/4 cup of yellow onion chopped
- 1/4 cup of half and half

Instructions:

- Preheat the oven at 350°F.
- In a large-sized mixing bowl, whisk together the whipping cream and eggs. Toss together the kale, onion, bell pepper, tomatoes, & broccoli. Season using black pepper and salt.
- Bake the mixture for around 30 minutes in a greased 6-inch round oven-safe baking dish.
- Bake for around 12 to 15 minutes.

54. Zucchini Waffles

(Preparation time: 10 minutes | Cooking time: 10 minutes | Difficulty: Easy | Servings: 4)
Per serving: Calories 69, Total fat 4g, Protein 4g, Carbs 5g
Ingredients:

- A pinch of cinnamon

- 2 whisked eggs
- 1/4 teaspoon of baking powder
- 1 tablespoon of olive oil
- 2 tablespoons of buckwheat flour
- 1/2 cup of grated zucchini
- 1 cup of skim milk

Instructions:

- In a mixing dish, mix together the zucchini, milk, and the other ingredients (excluding the oil).
- Grease the waffle iron using olive oil and fill each mold with 1/3 of the batter.
- Waffles should be cooked for around 3-4 minutes.

55. Roasted Kale and Sweet Potato Hash

(Preparation time: 10 minutes | Cooking time: 20 minutes | Difficulty: Easy | Servings: 4)
Per serving: Calories 217, Total fat 12g, Protein 9g, Carbs 19g

Ingredients:

- Salt and ground black pepper to taste
- 1 teaspoon of minced garlic
- 2 tablespoons of olive oil
- 1 medium sliced red onion
- 4 large eggs
- 1 pound of sweet potatoes peeled and cubed
- 4 cups of kale

Instructions:

- Set the oven temperature at 425 °F.
- Arrange a big baking sheet in the oven & heat it evenly.
- Combine the onion and sweet potatoes in a medium-sized mixing dish with 1/2 tablespoon of oil and 1/4 teaspoon of minced garlic. Toss the vegetables with the seasonings till they are uniformly covered. Shift to the oven with the coated vegetables onto the baking sheet. For approximately 20 minutes, roast the vegetables. Meanwhile, combine the kale, 1/2 tablespoon of oil, and 1/4 teaspoon of garlic powder in the same bowl. Toss the kale till it is uniformly covered. Take the baking pan out of the oven & toss the vegetables around. Cook for another 10 minutes with the spice-coated kale on top of the sweet potatoes. Remove the baking sheet out from the oven and place the roasted vegetables in a mixing dish.
- Meanwhile, fill a stockpot halfway with water & place it over a high flame. Reduce the flame to medium-low after the water begins to boil. Create a whirlpool in the water using a spoon.
- In a bowl, crack an egg open and place it in the whirlpool's center. For approximately 4 minutes, poach the egg. Transfer the egg to a plate using a slotted spoon. Carry on with the rest of the eggs in the same manner. Place 1/4 of the roasted vegetables on a dish and cover using one of the poached eggs to serve. Season the egg with salt and fresh cracked pepper to finish. Serve!

56. Oat, Walnut, and Raspberry Breakfast Cookies

(Preparation time: 10 minutes | Cooking time: 15 minutes | Difficulty: Easy | Servings: 4)
Per serving: Calories 86, Total fat 3g, Protein 2g, Carbs 13g

Ingredients:

- 1/2 teaspoon of cinnamon
- 1 mashed ripe banana
- 1/4 cup of porridge oats
- 2 tablespoons of walnuts
- 1/4 cup of frozen fresh raspberries

Instructions:

- Preheat the oven at 400 °F and prepare 2 baking sheets using parchment paper. In a mixing bowl, incorporate the banana, cinnamon, oats, & walnuts to make a sticky dough. Stir in the raspberries gently; take care not to break them. Scoop tablespoons of the mixture and create them into balls, then place them on a baking sheet and flatten using your fingers.

- Bake the cookies for around 15 minutes, or till golden brown & firm around the edges. Allow time for chilling. In an airtight container, it may last up to three days.

57. Breakfast Berries Mix

(Preparation time: 10 minutes | Cooking time: 15 minutes | Difficulty: Easy | Servings: 4)
Per serving: Calories 243, Total fat 34g, Protein 8g, Carbs 20g
Ingredients:
- 4 tablespoons of chia seeds
- 1 cup of strawberries and raspberries
- 1 cup of oats - 2 cups of coconut milk

Instructions:
- Mix all ingredients into a mixing dish and pour into serving glasses.
- Refrigerate the meal for at least 8 hours prior to serving.

58. Breakfast Apple Muffins

(Preparation time: 10 minutes | Cooking time: 20 minutes | Difficulty: Easy | Servings: 4)
Per serving: Calories 98, Total fat 3g, Protein 3g, Carbs 15g
Ingredients:
- 1/2 teaspoon of ground cinnamon
- 2 teaspoons of baking powder
- 1/4 teaspoon of nutmeg
- 3 tablespoons of olive oil
- 1 lightly beaten egg
- 1 tablespoon of stevia sugar substitute
- 1/2 cup of apple minced
- 1/4 cup of skim milk
- 1/2 cup of buckwheat flour

Instructions:
- Preheat the oven at 400°F. Using the nonstick cooking spray, coat muffin pans evenly.
- Combine buckwheat flour, baking powder, stevia, cinnamon, and nutmeg in a large-sized mixing dish. Whisk the skim milk, egg, and olive oil together in a separate bowl; pour into the flour mixture & stir them till the dry ingredients are moistened. Mix the apple mince into the batter softly. Half-fill muffin cups using the prepared batter. In a preheated oven, bake for approximately 20 minutes or till the tops are lightly browned. Serve and enjoy.

59. Breakfast Walnut and Almond Cookies

(Preparation time: 10 minutes | Cooking time: 15 minutes | Difficulty: Easy | Servings: 4)
Per serving: Calories 83, Total fat 5g, Protein 3g, Carbs 10g
Ingredients:
- 1 teaspoon of vanilla extract
- 1 mashed banana
- 2 tablespoons of honey
- 1/4 cup of almond butter
- 1/2 cup of flax meal, grinded
- 1/4 cup of chopped walnuts

Instructions:
- Mix all of the ingredients in a mixing dish. Spoon the mixture into medium balls and arrange them onto a baking sheet lined using parchment paper.
- Preheat the oven at 350°F & bake the cookies for around 15 minutes.

60. Coconut Banana and Berry Porridge

(Preparation time: 10 minutes | Cooking time: 25 minutes | Difficulty: Easy | Servings: 4)
Per serving: Calories 227, Total fat 6g, Protein 6g, Carbs 20g
Ingredients:

- 1/2 cup of water - 1/2 cup of quinoa
- 1 teaspoon of ground cinnamon
- 1 medium sliced banana
- 1/2 cup of blackberries and blueberries
- 1 tablespoon of coconut shavings
- 3 tablespoons of walnuts
- 1 1/2 cups of almond milk unsweetened
- 2 tablespoons of dried cranberries

Instructions:

- Bring the quinoa, milk, and water to the boil in a saucepan. Reduce to medium flame and simmer for another 15 minutes.
- Toss in the blueberries, blackberries and cranberries. Combine the ground cinnamon with the rest of the ingredients till everything is thoroughly mixed. In four breakfast dishes, sprinkle walnuts, coconut shavings, and banana slices over the mixture.

61. Chia Oatmeal

(Preparation time: 10 minutes | Cooking time: 0 minutes | Difficulty: Easy | Servings: 2)
Per serving: Calories 234, Total fat 12g, Protein 12g, Carbs 20g
Ingredients:

- A pinch of cinnamon
- 1 teaspoon of olive oil
- 1 tablespoon of chia seeds
- 1 teaspoon of liquid honey
- 1/2 cup of oatmeal
- 1/2 cup of hot skim milk

Instructions:

- Mix all the contents in a glass jar & seal their top.
- Put the meal in the refrigerator for around 6 hours to cool.

62. Avocado on Pita with Fried Egg

(Preparation time: 10 minutes | Cooking time: 15 minutes | Difficulty: Easy | Servings: 2)
Per serving: Calories 225, Total fat 18g, Protein 7g, Carbs 14g
Ingredients:

- Dash of salt and black pepper
- Dash of parsley
- 1 teaspoon of minced garlic
- 2 eggs
- 2 whole-wheat mini pitas
- 1 mashed avocado

Instructions:

- Preheat a sauté pan over medium flame. Lightly fry the eggs, sunny side up.
- Cook the tiny pitas in a toaster oven till light golden.
- In a mixing dish, combine the avocado & minced garlic. Evenly distribute the filling among the pitas.
- Place one egg on each pita. Serve with parsley and a dash of salt and black pepper.

63. Low-Fat Feta Hash

(Preparation time: 10 minutes | Cooking time: 20 minutes | Difficulty: Easy | Servings: 4)
Per serving: Calories 302, Total fat 17g, Protein 8g, Carbs 25g
Ingredients:

- 1 tablespoon of olive oil
- 1 chopped of red onion
- A dash of soy - 4 beaten eggs
- 1/2 cup of crumbled low-fat feta
- 2 cups of hash browns
- 1/3 cup of soy milk

Instructions:

- In a skillet over medium flame, heat the oil, then add the hash browns & cook for around 5 minutes.
- Add the remaining ingredients, except for the cheese, and cook for another 5 minutes.
- Bake for around 15 minutes at 390°F after layering the cheese on top and splash of soy on top.

64. Almond Breakfast Porridge

(Preparation time: 10 minutes | Cooking time: 10 minutes | Difficulty: Easy | Servings: 4)
Per serving: Calories 292, Total fat 27g, Protein 30g, Carbs 22g
Ingredients:

- A pinch of cinnamon
- 2 teaspoons of vanilla extract
- 1 tablespoon of margarine
- 1 mashed banana
- 1 chopped apple
- 2 cups of skim milk
- 1/2 cup of chopped walnuts
- 1/2 cup of raw and chopped almonds
- 1/2 cup of raw cashews

Instructions:

- All of the nuts, including almonds, cashews, walnuts, & bananas, should be mashed together.
- In a saucepan over medium flame, heat the oil, then add the apple, vanilla, milk, & nut mixture, stirring well to combine. Bring to the boil, then reduce to a low flame and simmer for 5 minutes. Serve with a pinch of cinnamon.

65. Crunchy Chocolate Breakfast Granola

(Preparation time: 10 minutes | Cooking time: 10 minutes | Difficulty: Easy | Servings: 2)
Per serving: Calories 137, Total fat 13g, Protein 4g, Carbs 1g

Ingredients:

- 1 teaspoon of ground cinnamon
- 1 extra-large egg white
- 5 tablespoons of stevia
- 3 tablespoons of dark chocolate grated (85 % cocoa solids)
- 1/3 cup of blanched almonds
- 1/3 cup of sunflower seeds
- 1/3 cup of walnuts
- 1/3 cup of pecan nuts

Instructions:

- Preheat the oven at 350°F. Using parchment paper, line a baking sheet.
- In a food processor, combine the mixed nuts, sweetener, & cinnamon. In a food processor, combine the ingredients and process them till they resemble a coarse meal. Combine the ingredients in a separate bowl. Stir the egg whites together till they are thoroughly combined.
- Bake the mixture for around 25 minutes on a parchment-lined baking sheet. Using a spoon, evenly distribute the ingredients. It should be as small as possible, with some open areas.
- Bake for around 8–12 minutes, or till golden brown on top. Keep an eye on the nuts & seeds because they can burn and become brown quickly.
- Set the baking sheet aside after removing it from the oven. Sprinkle the crushed chocolate on top as soon as possible. Serve and have fun.

66. Sesame, Parsley and Chives Omelet

(Preparation time: 10 minutes | Cooking time: 15 minutes | Difficulty: Easy | Servings: 4)
Per serving: Calories 79, Total fat 5g, Protein 6g, Carbs 2g
Ingredients:

- A pinch of salt and black pepper

- 1 tablespoon of olive oil
- 1 tablespoon of chopped chives
- 1 tablespoon of parsley
- 1 teaspoon of sesame seeds
- 4 whisked eggs -
- 1/2 cup of skim milk

Instructions:
- Heat the olive oil in a pan.
- In a bowl, whisk together the milk, salt, black pepper and eggs, then pour into the skillet. Add the chives, parsley and sesame seeds. Cook the omelet for around 8 minutes.
- Cook for another 6 minutes on low flame after flipping the omelet.

67. Fruity Millet Raisin Breakfast

(Preparation time: 10 minutes | Cooking time: 25 minutes | Difficulty: Easy | Servings: 4)
Per serving: Calories 368, Total fat 24g, Protein 9g, Carbs 20g
Ingredients:
- 2 cups of water
- 1 teaspoon of cinnamon
- 1 teaspoon of vanilla extract
- 2 tablespoons of sunflower seeds
- 1 tablespoon of agave nectar
- 1/2 cup of strawberries and raspberries
- 1/4 cup of raisins
- 1 cup of millet
- 1 1/2 cups of almond milk unsweetened
- 1/2 cup of roughly chopped walnuts
- A few sprigs of fresh mint for garnishing

Instructions:
- In a medium-sized saucepan, combine the millet & water and bring to the boil.
- Reduce the flame to low and add the raisins carefully, being careful not to spill the hot water. Cook for around 10 minutes, or till all the liquid has been absorbed, covered. Allow the millet to

cool for 10 minutes after turning off the flame.
- Mix together almond milk, cinnamon, vanilla essence, & agave nectar.
- Reheat for a minute or two more, or till the almond milk has been absorbed & the mixture has thickened to a creamy consistency.
- Top with walnuts, raspberries, strawberries, sunflower seeds, & mint springs and divide the mixture among four plates.
- Enjoy with a splash of almond milk on top!

68. Walnut Breakfast Pudding

(Preparation time: 10 minutes | Cooking time: 25 minutes | Difficulty: Easy | Servings: 4)
Per serving: Calories 369, Total fat 6g, Protein 9g, Carbs 28g
Ingredients:
- A pinch of cinnamon
- 1 teaspoon of vanilla extract
- 1 cup of brown rice
- 1 1/2 cups of skim milk
- 1/4 cup of soy milk
- 2 tablespoons of chopped walnuts

Instructions:
- Add all of the ingredients to the pan and close the lid.
- On low flame, cook the dish for around 25 minutes.

69. Chia Nut and Berry Porridge

(Preparation time: 10 minutes | Cooking time: 0 minutes | Difficulty: Easy | Servings: 2)
Per serving: Calories 210, Total fat 15g, Protein 6g, Carbs 10g
Ingredients:
- A pinch of cinnamon
- 1/4 tsp. of vanilla extract
- Seeds of cardamom pods
- 3 drops of liquid Stevia (optional)

- 1/2 tablespoon of chia seeds
- 1 tablespoon of chopped walnuts
- 1/2 tablespoon of dried cranberries
- Chopped raspberries, strawberries, and blueberries (for the topping)
- 1 1/2 cups of cold almond milk unsweetened

Instructions:

- Place the chia seeds on top of the almond milk in a bowl (it doesn't have to be very big).
- To break up any clumps, stir vigorously.
- Combine the cranberries, Stevia, cinnamon, cardamom, & vanilla essence in a large-sized mixing bowl and stir well.
- Allow 20-30 minutes for the mixture to thicken. Add the berries & chopped walnuts last but not least.

70. Breakfast Chia Wonder

(Preparation time: 10 minutes | Cooking time: 20 minutes | Difficulty: Easy | Servings: 2)
Per serving: Calories 159, Total fat 6g, Protein 6g, Carbs 15g
Ingredients:

- 1/2 cup of water
- Stevia, to sweeten
- 1/2 cup of quinoa
- 3 1/2 tablespoons of chia seeds
- 1 tablespoon of raw dark cocoa powder
- 1 cup of almond milk unsweetened
- Chopped walnuts as required

Instructions:

- Bring the quinoa, milk, & water to the boil in a saucepan.
- Allow 15 minutes for the mixture to boil.
- Combine the cooked quinoa, chocolate powder, chia seeds, & Stevia in a large-sized mixing dish.
- Serve the mixture with fruit & walnuts.

71. Sausage Breakfast Casserole

(Preparation time: 10 minutes | Cooking time: 30 minutes | Difficulty: Easy | Servings: 4)
Per serving: Calories 73, Total fat 6g, Protein 3g, Carbs 3g
Ingredients:

- A pinch of salt and black pepper
- 1 tablespoon of olive oil
- 1 chopped bird's eye chili
- 1 chopped onion - 2 beaten eggs
- 1 cup of ground sausages
- 1 teaspoon of chili flakes

Instructions:

- Combine the olive oil, onion, & ground sausages in a pan. Combine all of the remaining ingredients in a large-sized mixing bowl. Season using black pepper and salt.
- Roast the mixture for around 5 minutes.
- Then bake it for around 20 minutes at 370°F.

72. Breakfast Berry Salad

(Preparation time: 10 minutes | Cooking time: 0 minutes | Difficulty: Easy | Servings: 4)
Per serving: Calories 296, Total fat 34g, Protein 4g, Carbs 25g
Ingredients:

- 4 cups of chopped salad greens (Rocket, romaine lettuce etc.)
- 3 cups of chopped orange
- 4 cups of blackberries

For the vinaigrette:

- A pinch of sea salt - 1 cup of olive oil
- 2 teaspoons of minced red onion
- 1/2 teaspoon of ground paprika

Instructions:

- Whisk together all of the ingredients for the vinaigrette.
- After that, add all of the remaining ingredients to a salad plate.
- To incorporate the vinaigrette, give it a good shake.

73. Breakfast Veggie and Chicken Omelet

(Preparation time: 10 minutes | Cooking time: 25 minutes | Difficulty: Easy | Servings: 4)

Per serving: Calories 200, Total fat 10g, Protein 19g, Carbs 7g

Ingredients:

- 3 tablespoons of olive oil
- 1 cup of carrots grated
- 1 cup of sliced red onions
- 8 eggs - 1 teaspoon of Dijon mustard
- 4 cups of baby spinach
- 1/4 cup of plain fat-free Greek yogurt
- 1/2 pound of chicken breasts skinless and boneless - 3 tablespoons of grated asiago cheese

Instructions:

- Chicken breasts should be cut into 1/2-inch pieces.
- In a medium-sized skillet, heat 1 teaspoon of olive oil and cook chicken breasts with onions till golden brown, about 10 minutes. Return to the pan with the leftover olive oil after transferring to a dish.
- Whisk together the eggs & Dijon mustard in a mixing dish till fully combined. Fill the nonstick pan halfway with batter. Over the egg mixture, cooked chicken, & onion, evenly distribute the spinach and shredded carrot. Push the spinach down on top of it. Cook for 15 minutes each side on each side, turning halfway through. Cut into six pieces and top with Asiago cheese. To complete the meal, serve with a green salad.

74. Crustless Caprese Quiche

(Preparation time: 10 minutes | Cooking time: 25 minutes | Difficulty: Easy | Servings: 4)

Per serving: Calories 218, Total fat 15g, Protein 17g, Carbs 4g

Ingredients:

- 1/4 teaspoon of black pepper and salt
- 4 garlic cloves minced
- 1 tablespoon of olive oil
- 1 1/2 cup of halved grape tomatoes
- 10 eggs
- 1/2 cup of chopped fresh parsley
- 1 cup of grated fresh mozzarella cheese
- 1/2 cup of the almond milk unsweetened

Instructions:

- Preheat the oven at 380°F.
- In a medium-sized mixing dish, combine the garlic, olive oil, tomatoes, parsley, & 2/3 of the mozzarella bites. In a 9-inch glass or ceramic pan, combine the ingredients halfway (round or square).
- Whisk together the eggs, salt, black pepper, & milk in a mixing bowl. Spread the egg mixture over the tomatoes and parsley in the pan.
- Bake for around 20 minutes. After 20 minutes, top the quiche with the remaining mozzarella slices and bake for another 20 minutes. Bake till the timer on the oven goes off.
- Drain any liquid around the dish's edges before serving (from the tomatoes). As a finishing touch, scatter more parsley leaves on top.

75. Mixed Veggie and Egg Breakfast Cups

(Preparation time: 10 minutes | Cooking time: 25 minutes | Difficulty: Easy | Servings: 4)

Per serving: Calories 195, Total fat 12g, Protein 13g, Carbs 7g

Ingredients:

- A pinch of black pepper and salt to taste
- 1 tablespoon of olive oil
- Olive oil cooking spray
- 1 tablespoon of chopped parsley
- 4 free-range eggs

- 4 tablespoons of half and half
- 1 cup of diced mixed vegetables of your choice
- 1 cup of shredded cheese of your choice

Instructions:

- Preheat the oven to 380°F.
- Coat four ramekins using nonstick cooking spray.
- In a mixing dish, combine half-and-half vegetables, olive oil, eggs, half-cheese, parsley, & pepper.
- Distribute the batter evenly between the ramekins.
- Bake the ramekins for around 12–15 minutes.
- In the ramekins, bake for another 2 to 3 minutes, or just till the cheese has melted.

76. Onion Risotto

(Preparation time: 10 minutes | Cooking time: 25 minutes | Difficulty: Easy | Servings: 4)
Per serving: Calories 241, Total fat 6g, Protein 7g, Carbs 20g

Ingredients:

- A pinch of salt
- 1/2 teaspoon of white pepper
- 1 tablespoon of olive oil
- 2 tablespoons of chopped red onion
- 2 tablespoons of grated low-fat mozzarella
- 1 cup of cooked brown rice
- 4 slices of bacon, low-sodium and chopped

Instructions:

- Heat the oil in a skillet over medium-high flame, then add the bacon & cook for about 5 minutes.
- With the other ingredients, cook for 15 minutes on medium flame.

77. Veggies with Hash Browns

(Preparation time: 10 minutes | Cooking time: 20 minutes | Difficulty: Easy | Servings: 4)
Per serving: Calories 290, Total fat 19g, Protein 12g, Carbs 18g

Ingredients:

- 1 tablespoon of olive oil
- 1/2 teaspoon of chili flakes
- 1 tablespoon of chopped parsley
- 1 diced red onion
- 1 chopped green bell pepper
- 1 shredded carrot - 4 beaten eggs
- 1 cup of hash browns
- 1/2 cup of low-fat cheese

Instructions:

- Heat the oil in a large-sized skillet, then add the hash browns & onion. Cook the mixture for around 5 minutes.
- Simmer for another 5 minutes after adding the bell peppers & carrots.
- Then add the eggs, black pepper, salt and cheese, and continue to cook, stirring periodically, for another 10 minutes.
- Cook for another 10 seconds after adding the parsley.

78. Breakfast Banana Cookies

(Preparation time: 10 minutes | Cooking time: 15 minutes | Difficulty: Easy | Servings: 4)
Per serving: Calories 280, Total fat 16g, Protein 8g, Carbs 10g

Ingredients:

- 1 teaspoon of cinnamon powder
- 1 teaspoon of vanilla extract
- 1 peeled and mashed banana
- 1/4 cup of stevia
- 1/4 cup of raisins
- 1 cup of gluten-free oats
- 1/2 cup of almond butter
- 1/2 cup of chopped walnuts

Instructions:

- In a mixing bowl, beat together the butter, stevia, & other ingredients with a hand mixer till smooth.
- Fill medium molds halfway with the ingredients & flatten them on a parchment-lined baking sheet.
- Serve for breakfast after baking for around 15 minutes at 325°F.

79. Quinoa Cakes

(Preparation time: 10 minutes | Cooking time: 20 minutes | Difficulty: Easy | Servings: 4)
Per serving: Calories 280, Total fat 8g, Protein 15g, Carbs 20g
Ingredients:

- 1 cup of water
- 1/2 teaspoon of ground black pepper and salt - 1 tablespoon of olive oil
- 1 beaten egg
- 1 cup of shredded cauliflower
- 1 cup of quinoa
- 1/2 cup of grated parmesan

Instructions:

- In a medium-sized saucepan, add the quinoa, broccoli, salt, water, and ground black pepper, stir to incorporate, and cook for around 15 minutes over medium flame.
- Allow the mixture to cool completely before tossing in the parmesan and eggs. Make medium cakes with the batter. In a skillet over medium-high flame, heat the oil, then add the quinoa cakes. Cook each side for around 4-5 minutes.

80. White Beans with Eggs, Fennel, and Pancetta

(Preparation time: 10 minutes | Cooking time: 20 minutes | Difficulty: Easy | Servings: 4)
Per serving: Calories 288, Total fat 15g, Protein 16g, Carbs 21g

Ingredients:

- 1/4 teaspoon of salt and ground Pepper
- 2 teaspoons of olive oil
- 2 teaspoons of dried oregano
- 3 large cloves of minced garlic
- 1 diced red onion
- Parsley leaves
- 4 large eggs
- 1 thinly sliced fennel bulb
- 1 cup of cherry tomatoes (halved)
- 2 cups of cannellini beans, low-sodium and rinsed
- 1/2 cup of diced Bacon

Instructions:

- Begin by heating a large-sized skillet over medium flame. In the same pan, cook for around 5 minutes or till the bacon is crispy.
- Remove the bacon to a plate and add the fennel, sliced onion, garlic, and oregano to the bacon grease, simmering for about 8 minutes. The fennel should be wilted, and the onion should be translucent.
- After adding the tomatoes and beans, cook for another 5 minutes, tossing occasionally.
- On a medium temperature, pour the oil into a third nonstick pan.
- Once the oil begins to sizzle, crack the eggs open & cover the pan with a lid. Reduce the flame to medium-low and cook the eggs for an additional 4-5 minutes. The yolks should be runny, while the whites should be firm.
- To serve, top a quarter of the vegetable & bean mixture on a dish with a fried egg.
- Season using salt and black pepper, and parsley before serving.
- Serve right away.

81. Artichoke Eggs

(Preparation time: 10 minutes | Cooking time: 20 minutes | Difficulty: Easy | Servings: 4)

Per serving: Calories 177, Total fat 12g, Protein 11g, Carbs 7g

Ingredients:

- 1 tablespoon of olive oil
- 1 tablespoon of chopped parsley
- 1 chopped red onion
- 1 cup of artichoke hearts
- 5 beaten eggs
- 4 tablespoons of low-fat feta

Instructions:

- Grease four ramekins using the oil.
- In a mixing bowl, combine the remaining ingredients & divide the mixture among the ramekins.
- Preheat the oven to 380°F and bake the food for 20 minutes.

82. Breakfast Black Bean Pasta

(Preparation time: 10 minutes | Cooking time: 20 minutes | Difficulty: Easy | Servings: 4)

Per serving: Calories 348, Total fat 7g, Protein 7g, Carbs 10g

Ingredients:

- 3/4 teaspoon of salt and freshly ground pepper - 2 minced garlic cloves
- 1 tablespoon of olive oil
- 2 large chopped tomatoes
- 1 medium sliced zucchini
- 4 tablespoons of sliced ripe olives
- 2 1/2 cups of uncooked buckwheat pasta- 2 cups of rinsed and drained cannellini beans
- 1/2 cup of crumbled feta cheese

Instructions:

- For instructions on how to cook your pasta, see on the package. Half a cup of the cooking water should be saved, with the rest being drained.
- Heat the oil in a pan over medium-high flame. When the pan is hot, add the zucchini and cook till crisp, about 4 minutes. After adding the garlic, cook for around 30 seconds. Tomatoes, peppers, beans, & olives are added at this point. Reduce the flame to low and simmer, occasionally stirring, for around 5 minutes.
- Toss the pasta with just enough of the reserved water to keep it wet. Gently fold in the cheese till it is evenly distributed.

83. Fruity Breakfast Granola

(Preparation time: 10 minutes | Cooking time: 15 minutes | Difficulty: Easy | Servings: 4)

Per serving: Calories 340, Total fat 27g, Protein 7g, Carbs 8g

Ingredients:

- 2 tablespoons of honey - 4 small bananas, peeled and halved lengthwise
- 2 cups of fat-free vanilla Greek yogurt
- 2 tablespoons of toasted chopped walnuts
- 2 tablespoons of sunflower kernels
- 2 small peaches sliced
- 1 cup of fresh strawberries
- 1/2 cup of granola without raisins

Instructions:

- It's best if the walnuts are lightly roasted. After spreading them out on a pan, bake them for 5 minutes at 350°F. Continue to bake for 5 minutes more, or till the nuts are lightly browned.
- Fill four shallow dishes with an equal amount of bananas in each. On top of that, layer the remaining ingredients.

84. Fruity Muffins

(Preparation time: 10 minutes | Cooking time: 30 minutes | Difficulty: Easy | Servings: 4)

Per serving: Calories 380, Total fat 8g, Protein 11g, Carbs 20g

Ingredients:

- 1 cup of water

- 1 teaspoon of ground cinnamon
- 1 teaspoon vanilla extract
- 1 tablespoon of olive oil
- 1 tablespoon of liquid honey
- 1 cup of grated apple
- 2 cups of oatmeal
- 1 cup of quinoa
- 1/2 cup of coconut milk

Instructions:

- Fluff using a fork and transfer to a bowl after 15 minutes of mixing water and quinoa.
- Combine the remaining ingredients in a large-sized mixing bowl.
- Place the batter in muffin tins & bake at 375°F for around 20 minutes.

85. Strawberry Sandwich

(Preparation time: 10 minutes | Cooking time: 0 minutes | Difficulty: Easy | Servings: 2)
Per serving: Calories 84, Total fat 1g, Protein 5g, Carbs 12g
Ingredients:

- 4 buckwheat bread slices
- 4 tablespoons of low-fat yogurt
- 4 sliced strawberries

Instructions:

- Top the bread with a dollop of yogurt and sliced strawberries.

86. Banana Tahini Date Shake

(Preparation time: 10 minutes | Cooking time: 0 minutes | Difficulty: Easy | Servings: 2)
Per serving: Calories 299, Total fat 12g, Protein 6g, Carbs 15g
Ingredients:

- 1/4 cup of crushed ice
- A pinch of ground cinnamon
- 2 frozen bananas chunks
- 4 medium Medjool dates pitted
- 1/4 cup of tahini
- 1 1/2 cups of almond milk unsweetened

Instructions:

- In a blender, combine the frozen banana chunks and the remaining ingredients. Blend till a thick, creamy smoothie forms.
- Serve the smoothie in glasses with a pinch of cinnamon powder sprinkled on top.

87. Cheese Omelet

(Preparation time: 10 minutes | Cooking time: 10 minutes | Difficulty: Easy | Servings: 4)
Per serving: Calories 117, Total fat 10g, Protein 6g, Carbs 2g
Ingredients:

- 1/2 teaspoon of salt and ground black pepper - 1 tablespoon of olive oil
- 1 tablespoon of chopped parsley
- 3 beaten eggs
- 4 tablespoons of low-fat feta cheese
- 1 cup of chopped baby spinach

Instructions:

- In a skillet over medium-high flame, heat the oil, then add the spinach & cook for around 3 minutes.
- After that, carefully incorporate the other ingredients. Cover the omelet and cook it on low flame for around 7 minutes, or till it is firm.

88. Fruit Scones

(Preparation time: 10 minutes | Cooking time: 15 minutes | Difficulty: Easy | Servings: 4)
Per serving: Calories 156, Total fat 4g, Protein 6g, Carbs 25g
Ingredients:

- A pinch of cinnamon
- 1/2 teaspoon of baking powder
- 1 tablespoon of liquid honey
- 1/2 whisked egg
- 1/4 cup of chia seeds
- 1/4 cup of chopped walnuts
- 1/4 cup of chopped apricots

- 1/4 cup of dried cranberries
- 1 cup of whole-grain wheat flour

Instructions:

- In a mixing bowl, combine all of the ingredients and knead the dough.
- Cut into 16 pieces using a knife (scones)
- Bake for about 12 minutes at 350°F on a prepared baking paper sheet.
- Before serving, let the scones cool fully.

89. Breakfast Salsa Eggs

(Preparation time: 10 minutes | Cooking time: 10 minutes | Difficulty: Easy | Servings: 4)
Per serving: Calories 140, Total fat 8g, Protein 7g, Carbs 11g
Ingredients:

- 1 cup of water
- 1 tablespoon of lemon juice
- 1 tablespoon of olive oil
- 2 tablespoons of chopped parsley
- 1 chopped bird's eye chili
- 4 eggs - 1 chopped red onion
- 2 chopped tomatoes
- 2 chopped cucumbers

Instructions:

- In a kettle of water, boil the eggs for around 7 minutes. After letting the cooked eggs to cool in cold water, peel them. To make the salsa salad, in a large mixing bowl, add tomatoes, chili, cucumbers, olive oil, red onion, parsley, & lemon juice.
- Half the eggs & top with a generous helping of prepared salsa salad.

90. Yogurt with Raspberry and Strawberry

(Preparation time: 10 minutes | Cooking time: 10 minutes | Difficulty: Easy | Servings: 4)
Per serving: Calories 77, Total fat 3g, Protein 4g, Carbs 8g
Ingredients:

- 1/2 cup of low-fat yogurt

- 1/2 cup of raspberries and strawberries
- 1 tablespoon of chopped walnuts
- Chia seeds as required
- Flaxseeds as required

Instructions:

- In the serving cups, combine the yogurt, strawberries and raspberries.
- Top the yogurt with chopped walnuts, flaxseeds and chia seeds.

91. Classic Vegetable Frittata

(Preparation time: 10 minutes | Cooking time: 15 minutes | Difficulty: Easy | Servings: 2)
Per serving: Calories 232, Total fat 15g, Protein 18g, Carbs 7g
Ingredients:

- Salt and ground black pepper
- 1 tablespoon of olive oil
- 3 eggs
- 2 tablespoons of minced red onion
- 1 small zucchini, make 1/4-inch slices
- 1/2 cup of thinly sliced mushrooms
- 1/2 cup of part-skim ricotta cheese
- Nonstick cooking spray

Instructions:

- In a medium-sized mixing bowl, mix together the eggs. Whisk the eggs till they become frothy, then fold in the ricotta. Season with a sprinkle of salt and black pepper.
- Using cooking spray, coat an 8- to 10-inch oven-safe (i.e., cast-iron) pan. Add the oil and cook it for around 1 to 2 minutes over medium flame.
- Cook for around 3 to 4 minutes, till the zucchini, mushrooms, and red onion are soft. Turn on the broiler & set it at 450°F while the vegetables are cooking.
- Pour the egg mixture over the veggies and shake the skillet to evenly distribute the eggs. Reduce the flame to low & cook the eggs for around 2 minutes, uncovered.

- Broil the skillet in the oven for 1 to 2 minutes on high, till gently browned.
- Take the skillet out of the oven. Remove the frittata from the pan with a metal spatula, place a big plate on top of the skillet, gently flip the frittata onto the platter.
- Serve & enjoy.

92. Breakfast Egg Toasts

(Preparation time: 10 minutes | Cooking time: 10 minutes | Difficulty: Easy | Servings: 3)
Per serving: Calories 157, Total fat 7g, Protein 9g, Carbs 13g
Ingredients:

- 1/4 teaspoon of salt and ground black pepper
- 1/4 teaspoon of minced garlic
- 1 tablespoon of olive oil
- 3 medium eggs
- 3 buckwheat bread slices

Instructions:

- Into a skillet, heat the olive oil.
- Cook the eggs for around 4 minutes after breaking them within.
- Meanwhile, massage the garlic cloves into the bread pieces.
- Cooked eggs, salt and ground black pepper, are sprinkled on top of the toast.

93. Veggie Scramble Soft Taco

(Preparation time: 10 minutes | Cooking time: 15 minutes | Difficulty: Easy | Servings: 2)
Per serving: Calories 297, Total fat 30g, Protein 16g, Carbs 21g
Ingredients:

- Salt and freshly ground black pepper
- 1/2 teaspoon of paprika
- 1 tablespoon of olive oil
- 1 finely chopped red onion
- 3 large eggs
- 1 medium finely chopped bell pepper

- 2 cups of finely chopped fresh baby spinach
- 2 whole-grain tortillas
- 1/4 cup of skim milk
- 1 small sliced avocado

Instructions:

- In a medium-sized skillet, heat the oil on medium flame.
- Sauté the peppers and onion for around 3 minutes, or till the onion is transparent. Reduce the flame to low, cover, & simmer for approximately 2 minutes, just till the spinach has wilted.
- While the spinach is boiling, mix together the eggs, milk, paprika, and a sprinkle of salt and pepper in a small-sized bowl.
- Layout the egg mixture on top of the veggies in the pan and stir for around 2 minutes, or till the eggs are done.
- Top with sliced avocado & divide the eggs among two dishes.
- If desired, serve in a tortilla or with a piece of whole-wheat bread.

94. Breakfast Granola

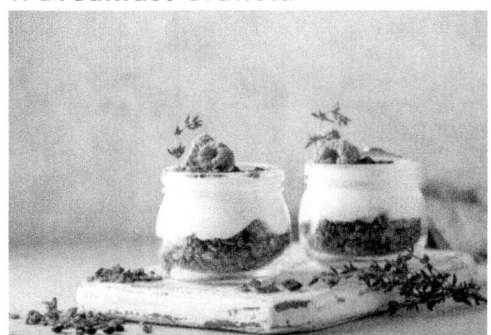

(Preparation time: 10 minutes | Cooking time: 20 minutes | Difficulty: Easy | Servings: 2)
Per serving: Calories 203, Total fat 11g, Protein 6g, Carbs 20g
Ingredients:

- Cooking spray
- 1/4 teaspoon of ground cinnamon
- 2 tablespoons of olive oil

- 1 tablespoon of liquid honey
- 1 teaspoon of sesame seeds
- 1 tablespoon of chia seeds
- 2 tablespoons of cut oats
- 1/4 cup of chopped walnuts

Instructions:

- Heat the olive oil with liquid honey till a smooth consistency is achieved.
- Then toss in the sesame seeds, ground cinnamon, chia seeds, walnuts, and oats.
- Stir them till the mixture is completely smooth.
- Place the almond mixture on the baking pan after spraying it using cooking spray. Make a square out of it by flattening it. Preheat the oven at 345°F and bake the granola for around 20 minutes. Before serving, it should be cut into portions.

95. Banana Split in a Bowl

(Preparation time: 10 minutes | Cooking time: 0 minutes | Difficulty: Easy | Servings: 4)
Per serving: Calories 340, Total fat 6g, Protein 17g, Carbs 35g
Ingredients:

- A pinch of cinnamon
- 2 tablespoons of honey
- 4 peeled and sliced in half bananas
- 2 sliced peaches
- 1 cup of fresh strawberries and raspberries
- 2 tablespoons of sunflower seeds
- 2 cups of non-fat vanilla Greek yogurt
- 1/2 cup of granola
- 2 tablespoons of toasted walnuts

Instructions:

- In a bowl, arrange the banana slices.
- On top, spread the yogurt.
- Add the strawberries, raspberries and peaches on top.

- Sunflower seeds, walnuts, and granola are sprinkled over the top.
- Drizzle the honey over the top.

96. Omelet with Asparagus

(Preparation time: 10 minutes | Cooking time: 10 minutes | Difficulty: Easy | Servings: 2)
Per serving: Calories 115, Total fat 7g, Protein 10g, Carbs 4g
Ingredients:

- A pinch of salt
- 1/2 teaspoon of ground cumin
- 1/4 teaspoon of ground paprika
- 1 tablespoon of avocado oil
- 2 tablespoons of chopped parsley
- 3 beaten eggs
- 2 tablespoons of skim milk
- 1/2 cup of chopped and boiled asparagus

Instructions:

- Into a skillet, heat the olive oil.
- Meanwhile, combine the salt, paprika and cumin powders. Whisk milk with eggs. Cook for around 2 minutes into a heated skillet with the liquid.
- After that, add the chopped asparagus and parsley, then cover the pot.
- Cook the omelet on low flame for around 5 minutes.

97. Apple Oats

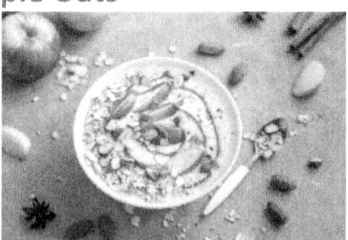

(Preparation time: 10 minutes | Cooking time: 10 minutes | Difficulty: Easy | Servings: 2)
Per serving: Calories 159, Total fat 5g, Protein 29g, Carbs 4g
Ingredients:

- 1 cup of water

- A pinch of cinnamon
- 1/2 teaspoon of vanilla extract
- 1 teaspoon of olive oil
- 1 chopped apple
- 1/2 cup of oats

Instructions:

- Toss the oats with the olive oil in a saucepan. Cook for 2 minutes, stirring constantly.
- Mix in the water after that.
- Cook the oats on low flame for 5 minutes with the lid closed.
- After that, add the diced apples, cinnamon and vanilla extract. Mix the ingredients together.

98. Apple Sandwich

(Preparation time: 10 minutes | Cooking time: 0 minutes | Difficulty: Easy | Servings: 2)

Per serving: Calories 100, Total fat 6g, Protein 3g, Carbs 10g

Ingredients:

- A pinch of cinnamon - 1 apple
- 2 teaspoons of peanuts, optional
- 1 1/2 tablespoon of peanut butter
- 1 teaspoon of golden raisins
- Dark chocolate chips as required

Instructions:

- Remove the core from the apple and slice it into 4-5 pieces.
- Take a number of equal-sized pieces and apply peanut butter liberally on each. Distribute the butter evenly.
- One slice should be covered with chocolate chips and raisins. Place the second slice on top and push it down lightly with the palm of your hand.
- Sprinkle with cinnamon. As soon as possible, eat!

99. Deluxe Berries Oatmeal

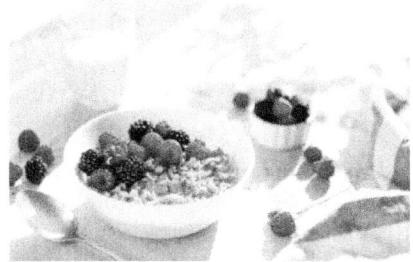

(Preparation time: 10 minutes | Cooking time: 0 minutes | Difficulty: Easy | Servings: 2)

Per serving: Calories 261, Total fat 10g, Protein 7g, Carbs 6g

Ingredients:

- A pinch of cinnamon
- 1/8 teaspoon vanilla extract
- 2 tablespoons of toasted pecans
- 3/4 cup of coarsely chopped blueberries, blackberries, and strawberries
- 1 cup of old-fashioned oats
- 1 1/2 cups of unsweetened almond milk

Instructions:

- Warm the almond milk and vanilla essence in a small-sized saucepan over medium flame. Add the oats when the mixture begins to boil, and stir for 4 minutes, or till the liquid is mostly absorbed. Mix in the berries thoroughly. Divide the mixture between two bowls & top with roasted pecans and a pinch of cinnamon.

100. Scramble Eggs with Spinach and Raspberries

(Preparation time: 10 minutes | Cooking time: 15 minutes | Difficulty: Easy | Servings: 2)

Per serving: Calories 296, Total fat 16g, Protein 18g, Carbs 20g

Ingredients:

- A pinch of cinnamon
- 1 tablespoon of olive oil

- 1 1/2 cups of baby spinach
- A pinch of salt and ground black pepper
- 2 large, lightly beaten eggs
- 1/2 cup of fresh raspberries
- 2 slices of whole-grain bread

Instructions:

- To begin, toast the entire piece of whole-grain bread till golden brown.
- In the meantime, heat a skillet over medium-high flame. Heat the oil fully before adding it.
- Cook for just a few minutes till the spinach has wilted. Place the spinach on a plate to serve.
- After wiping the skillet clean using a kitchen towel, return it to a medium flame. Pour in the eggs & cook, occasionally stirring, for around 12 minutes.
- At this time, add the wilted spinach and season using salt and pepper. Mix together the eggs and spinach until thoroughly incorporated.
- Arrange the bread on a plate with the scrambled eggs & spinach on top.
- Toss raspberries on top of the eggs to finish.
- Serve right away!

CHAPTER 10:

Lunch Recipes

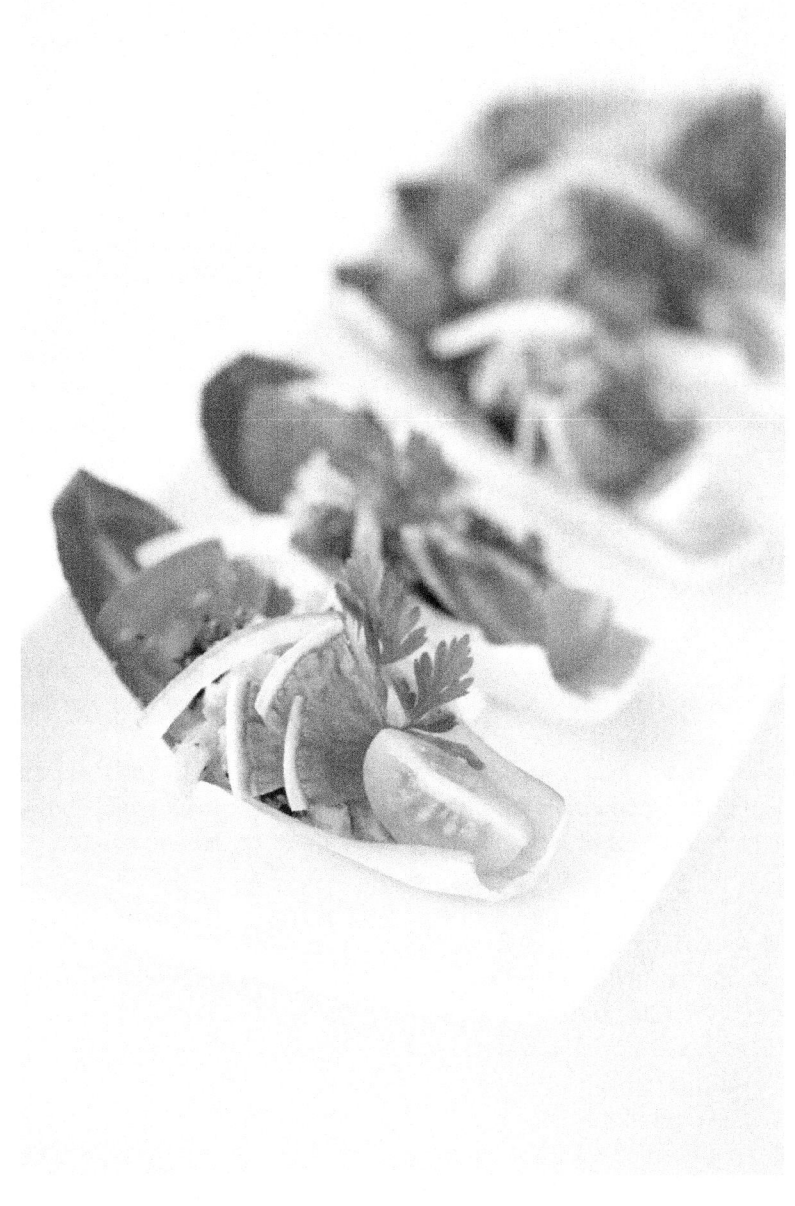

101. Asian King Prawn Stir-Fry with Buckwheat Noodles

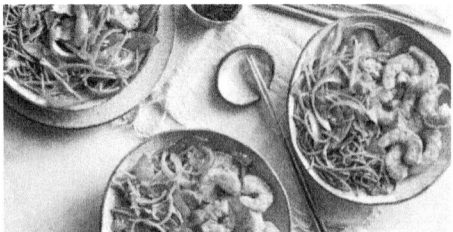

(Preparation time: 15 minutes | Cooking time: 20 minutes | Difficulty: Easy | Servings: 2)
Per serving: Calories 251, Total fat 23g, Protein 23g, Carbs 24g
Ingredients:

- 1 clove of garlic, finely chopped
- 1 teaspoon of finely chopped fresh ginger - 2 teaspoons of extra virgin olive oil
- 1 finely chopped bird's eye chili
- 1/4 cup of red onion, cut into slices
- 2 teaspoons of tamari
- 1/4 cup of celery, trimmed and cut into slices - 1 tablespoon of lovage or celery leaves 1/4 cup of kale, coarsely chopped
- 75g chopped green beans
- 2 tablespoons of chicken stock
- 1/2 cup of raw royal shrimps in shelled skins
- 1/4 cup of soba (buckwheat noodles)

Instructions:

- Cook the prawns in 1 teaspoon of tamari and 1 teaspoon oil in a frying pan over high heat for 2–3 minutes. Place the prawns on a serving plate. Because you'll be using the pan again, wipe it out with oven paper.
- Cook the noodles in boiling water for 5–8 minutes, or according to the package directions. Drain and store the water.
- Meanwhile, in the remaining oil, sauté the garlic, chili, and ginger, beans, red onion, celery, and kale for 2–3 minutes

over medium-high flame. Remove the stock from the flame and return to a boil, then cook for one or two minutes, or till the veggies are tender but still crisp. Return the pan to a boil with the prawns, noodles, & lovage/celery leaves, then remove from the flame and serve.

102. Easy Shrimp Salad

(Preparation time: 10 minutes | Cooking time: 0 minutes | Difficulty: Easy | Servings: 2)
Per serving: Calories 353, Total fat 5g, Protein 28g, Carbs 21g
Ingredients:

- ½ lemon, juiced
- 1 teaspoon of extra virgin olive oil
- 1 tablespoon of parsley, chopped
- 4 tablespoons of red onion-sliced
- 1 cup of yellow pepper, cubed
- 1 cup of cherry tomatoes, halved
- 2 cups of red endive, finely sliced
- 1/2 cup of celery, sliced
- 6 walnuts, chopped
- 1/2 cup of steamed shrimps

Instructions:

- On a large-sized platter, arrange the red endive. Distribute finely sliced onion, celery, yellow pepper, cherry tomatoes, walnuts, and parsley evenly over the top.
- Spread the dressing on top by combining oil, lemon juice, and a pinch of salt and pepper.

103. Turmeric Turkey Breast with Cauli Rice

(Preparation time: 10 minutes | Cooking time: 25 minutes | Difficulty: Easy | Servings: 2)
Per serving: Calories 107, Total fat 3g, Protein 2g, Carbs 20g
Ingredients:

- 2 teaspoons ground turmeric

- 1 clove of garlic, crushed
- 2 teaspoons extra virgin olive oil
- 2 tablespoons of parsley, finely chopped
- 1/2 red onion, sliced
- 1/2 pepper, chopped - 1 large tomato
- 2 cups of cauliflower, grated
- 2 teaspoons of buckwheat flour
- 1 cup of milk, skimmed
- 8 oz. turkey breast, cut into slices

Instructions:

- Using flour, coat the turkey slices.
- Heat 1/2 of the oil in a skillet on medium flame, and add the turkey once it is hot. Allow the meat to brown on all sides before adding milk, salt, pepper, & 1 teaspoon turmeric. Cook for 10 minutes, or till the turkey is cooked through, and the sauce has thickened.
- Heat the remaining oil in a separate pan over medium flame. Add the pepper, onion, and tomato, as well as 1 teaspoon turmeric, and cook for 3 minutes. Cook for another 2 minutes after adding the cauliflower. Season using salt and pepper and set aside for 2 minutes.
- Serve the turkey alongside cauliflower rice.

104. Garlic Chicken Burgers

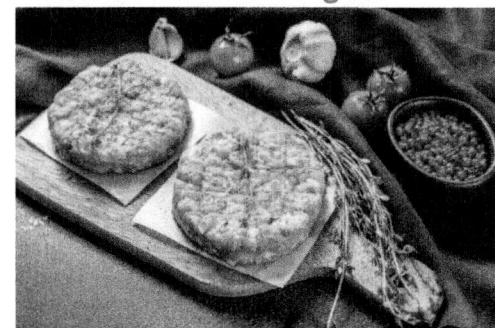

(Preparation time: 10 minutes | Cooking time: 25 minutes | Difficulty: Easy | Servings: 2)
Per serving: Calories 353, Total fat 5g, Protein 28g, Carbs 25g

Ingredients:

- 1 clove of garlic, crushed
- 3 teaspoons of extra virgin olive oil
- ¼ red onion, finely chopped
- 1 cup of cherry tomatoes
- 1 handful of parsley, finely chopped
- 1 cup of arugula - ½ orange, chopped
- 8 oz. of chicken mince

Instructions:

- In a mixing bowl, combine the chicken mince, parsley, onion, garlic, and salt & pepper. Form 2 patties & set aside for 5 minutes to rest. Cook 3 minutes per section in a pan with olive oil when it is extremely hot.
- If you want to grill them, brush them with a little oil immediately before cooking. Place the arugula on two dishes, top with the cherry tomatoes and orange, then drizzle with the remaining olive oil and salt. Serve with the patties on top.

105. Mustard Salmon with Baby Carrots

(Preparation time: 10 minutes | Cooking time: 40 minutes | Difficulty: Easy | Servings: 2)
Per serving: Calories 314, Total fat 9g, Protein 41g, Carbs 15g

Ingredients:

- Salt and pepper to taste
- 2 teaspoons of extra virgin olive oil
- 1 tablespoon white vinegar
- 1 teaspoon of parsley, finely chopped
- 2 tablespoons of mustard
- 2 cups of baby carrots
- 1/2 cup of buckwheat
- 8 oz. salmon fillet

Instructions:

- Preheat the oven at 400°F.
- Boil the buckwheat for around 25 minutes in salted water, then drain. 1 teaspoon of olive oil is used to dress the

salad. Set them aside. Place the fish on a sheet of aluminum foil. In a small-sized bowl, combine the mustard and vinegar; spread the mixture over the salmon and seal the foil packet. Cook for around 35 minutes in the oven. While the salmon is cooking, steam the young carrots for 6 minutes, then brown them in a pan with 1 tablespoon of olive oil, salt, and pepper over medium flame.

- Serve the salmon with a side of tiny carrots and buckwheat.

106. Smoked Trout with Curd Cheese and Caper Crackers

(Preparation time: 10 minutes | Cooking time: 10 minutes | Difficulty: Easy | Servings: 1)
Per serving: Calories 80, Total fat 3g, Protein 4g, Carbs 12g
Ingredients:
- Lemon juice
- 1 teaspoon of chopped parsley
- 1 1/2 tablespoons of rocket
- 2 1/2 tablespoons of diced red onion
- 1 teaspoon of capers
- 1/4 cup of cottage cheese
- 75g of sliced smoked trout
- 2–3 buckwheat crackers (store-bought or homemade)

Instructions:
- In a mixing bowl, combine the cottage cheese, capers, parsley, & red onion. Over the crackers, spread the mixture & top with the rocket & smoked trout.
- To serve, squeeze the lemon juice over the top.

107. Chicken, Arugula, Avocado and Buckwheat Crackers

(Preparation time: 10 minutes | Cooking time: 15 minutes | Difficulty: Easy | Servings: 1)
Per serving: Calories 200, Total fat 11g, Protein 27g, Carbs 6g

Ingredients:
- juice from ¼ lemon
- 1 teaspoon of extra virgin olive oil
- 1 1/2 tablespoons of rocket
- 1/2 red onion, diced
- 1/4 cup of celery, diced
- ½ avocado
- 100g of cooked chicken breast, cut into bite-sized pieces
- 2–3 buckwheat crackers (store-bought or homemade)

Instructions:
- Mash the avocado with the back of a fork after peeling it.
- Mix in the lemon juice, olive oil, celery, & red onion. Add the chicken and mix well. Cover the crackers with the mixture and then the rocket.

108. Sirt Chicken Salad

(Preparation time: 10 minutes | Cooking time: 0 minutes | Difficulty: Easy | Servings: 1)
Per serving: Calories 310, Total fat 14g, Protein 22g, Carbs 24g
Ingredients:
- juice from ¼ lemon
- 1 teaspoon of ground turmeric
- 1 teaspoon of chopped coriander
- 1/2 diced red onion - 1 bird's eye chili
- ½ teaspoon of mild curry powder
- 1 Medjool date, finely chopped
- 1/4 cup of natural yogurt
- 100g of cooked chicken breast, cut into bite-sized pieces
- 1/4 cup of arugula to serve
- 6 chopped walnut halves

Instructions:
- In a mixing bowl, combine the yogurt, lemon juice, coriander, & spices. Serve on a bed of arugula with the remaining ingredients.

109. Tuna and Chicory Boats

(Preparation time: 10 minutes | Cooking time: 0 minutes | Difficulty: Easy | Servings: 1)

Per serving: Calories 430, Total fat 25g, Protein 26g, Carbs 18g

Ingredients:

- ¼ lemon juice
- 1 teaspoon of extra virgin olive oil
- 1 teaspoon of capers
- 1 teaspoon of chopped parsley
- 1/4 diced red onion
- 2 tablespoons of diced celery
- 1 head of chicory
- 5–6 chopped walnut halves
- 1 × 150 g can of drained tuna (in oil or brine)

Instructions:

- Toss the tuna with the onion, celery, parsley, capers, lemon juice, & olive oil in a mixing bowl. Mix thoroughly.
- Cut the chicory head off at the end & separate the leaves. Place the tuna in as many leaves as you can and top with chopped walnuts.

110. Lemon Herb Sardines with Avocado, Rocket and Caper Salad

(Preparation time: 15 minutes | Cooking time: 0 minutes | Difficulty: Easy | Servings: 1)

Per serving: Calories 170, Total fat 23g, Protein 8g, Carbs 16g

Ingredients:

- Juice of ½ lemon
- 1 teaspoon of extra virgin olive oil
- 1 tablespoon of chopped parsley
- 1 teaspoon of capers
- 1 cut red onion
- 1/4 cup of rocket
- 1/4 cup of sliced celery
- ½ avocado
- 2 chopped walnut halves
- 120g of drained canned sardines (boneless, best in olive oil or brine)

Instructions:

- Combine the red onion & celery with half of the lemon juice. Slice the avocado and combine it with the arugula, capers, walnuts, and olive oil in a bowl.
- Serve the sardines on top of the avocado and arugula mixture, along with the parsley & the rest of the lemon juice.

111. Chicken Skewers with Buckwheat and Satay Sauce

(Preparation time: 15 minutes | Cooking time: 1 hour 30 minutes | Difficulty: Easy | Servings: 1)

Per serving: Calories 310, Total fat 13g, Protein 26g, Carbs 11g

Ingredients:

- 1 teaspoon of ground turmeric
- ½ teaspoon of extra virgin olive oil
- 1/4 cup of celery cut into slices
- 1/4 cup of kale (weight without stems removed)
- 150g of chicken breast, cut into pieces
- 1/4 cup of buckwheat
- 4 walnut halves sliced, chopped, to refine

For the sauce:

- 1 teaspoon of ground turmeric
- 1 clove of garlic diced
- 1 teaspoon of extra virgin olive oil chopped
- 1 tablespoon of chopped coriander
- 1 teaspoon of curry powder
- 1/2 red onion
- 2 tablespoons of chicken broth
- 1/4 cup of coconut milk
- 1 tablespoon of walnut butter or peanut butter

Instructions:

- Set aside for 30 minutes to 1 hour to marinate the chicken with turmeric & olive oil, but if you're short on time, leave it for as long as possible.
- Cook the buckwheat as per the package guidelines, then add the kale & celery for the last 5–7 minutes of cooking.
- Drain. Preheat the grill to high heat.
- To make the sauce
- In a small amount of olive oil, fry the red onion & garlic till soft, about 2-3 minutes. Cook for another minute after adding the spices. Bring the stock & coconut milk to a boil, then mix in the walnut butter. Reduce the flame to low and cook for 8-10 minutes, or till the sauce is creamy and rich.
- While the sauce is cooking, insert the chicken onto the skewers and cook for 10 minutes on a hot grill.
- Flip it over.

112. Baked Cod with Chicory, Kale and White Beans

(Preparation time: 15 minutes | Cooking time: 20 minutes | Difficulty: Easy | Servings: 1)
Per serving: Calories 430, Total fat 26g, Protein 31g, Carbs 16g
Ingredients:

- ½ teaspoon of extra virgin olive oil
- 1 teaspoon of chopped parsley
- 150g of cod fillet

For the beans:

- 1 clove of garlic sliced
- 1 teaspoon of extra virgin olive oil
- 1/2 red onion - 1/4 cup of kale, sliced, the stems removed
- 5 tablespoons of vegetable stock
- 1 head of chicory, halved lengthways and sliced
- 1/2 cup of white beans such as cannellini or haricot

Instructions:

- Preheat the oven at 400°F. Use parchment paper to line a small-sized baking sheet.
- Set aside the kale after steaming or cooking it for around 5–7 minutes till soft. Rub the fish with the olive oil & parsley, then bake for around 10 minutes on the preheated tray.
- Meanwhile, in a small-sized saucepan over low to medium flame, heat the olive oil and cook the red garlic and onions till soft, about 2-3 minutes.
- Bring the stock & beans to a boil together. Cook for a couple more minutes on low to medium flame with the chicory.
- Make sure you don't overcook it. Serve the greens with the fish after stirring it into the mixture.

113. Tuna Noodles

(Preparation time: 10 minutes | Cooking time: 15 minutes | Difficulty: Easy | Servings: 1)
Per serving: Calories 260, Total fat 12g, Protein 21g, Carbs 8g
Ingredients:

- 1 clove of garlic, chopped
- 1 tablespoon of chopped parsley
- 1 teaspoon of extra virgin olive oil
- 1 teaspoon of capers
- 1 teaspoon of herbs of Provence
- 1 red onion
- 1/4 cup of celery cut into slices
- 1/4 cup of sliced kale (weight without stems), finely chopped
- 1/3 cup of buckwheat noodles
- 1/2 cup of vegetable broth
- 1 × 150 g can of tuna (in oil or salt solution), drained

Instructions:

- Cook the pasta as per the package instructions. Meanwhile, sauté the onion, celery, kale, garlic, & dry herbs in olive oil till soft, about 3 to 4 minutes over low to medium flame.

- Cook for a few minutes longer over the same heat with the broth. Stir in the parsley, capers, and tuna once all of the vegetables are cooked to your liking. Toss in the cooked noodles, heat through, and serve.

114. Fried Thai Prawns

(Preparation time: 10 minutes | Cooking time: 15 minutes | Difficulty: Easy | Servings: 1)

Per serving: Calories 230, Total fat 10g, Protein 25g, Carbs 8g

Ingredients:

- 1 teaspoon of ground turmeric
- 4–5 basil leaves
- 1/4 cup of kale (weight with stems removed), cut
- 1/4 cup of celery, cut diagonally into 1 cm slices
- 1/2 cup of chicken broth or vegetable broth
- 125g of chicken breast, sliced or cut into bite-sized pieces or raw king prawns, peeled and deveined
- 1/4 cup of buckwheat

For the stir-fry dishes:

- 1 teaspoon of ground turmeric
- 1 clove of garlic chopped
- 1 cm of fresh ginger chopped, chopped
- 1 teaspoon of ground cumin
- 1 tablespoon of chopped parsley
- 1 teaspoon of extra virgin olive oil
- 1 bird's eye chili, chopped
- 1 red onion
- 1 teaspoon of fish sauce, soy sauce or tamari - 1 lemongrass stalk chopped

Instructions:

- Cook the buckwheat as per the package directions, adding the turmeric into the water halfway through.

- Meanwhile, combine all of the ingredients inside a food processor and process till smooth. If you don't have a food processor, finely chop everything and mix thoroughly. In a medium-sized saucepan, cook the pasta. Add the chicken or shrimp, celery, and kale to the pan & cook for around 4 to 5 minutes, or till chicken or shrimp is well cooked. Cook for another 1-2 minutes after adding the broth. Cut the basil leaves in half and toss them into the pan. Serve with buckwheat on the side.

115. Grilled Turkey Schnitzel with Walnut, Herb and Cheddar Crust

(Preparation time: 10 minutes | Cooking time: 15 minutes | Difficulty: Easy | Servings: 1)

Per serving: Calories 330, Total fat 17g, Protein 27g, Carbs 9g

Ingredients:

- Juice of ¼ lemon
- ½ teaspoon of extra virgin olive oil
- 1 tablespoon of chopped parsley
- 1/4 red onion, diced
- 150g of turkey schnitzel or turkey breast steak
- 2 tablespoons of cheddar cheese, grated
- 1 tablespoon of walnuts, chopped

For the salad:

- 1 teaspoon of extra virgin olive oil
- 1 teaspoon of balsamic vinegar
- 1/2 red onions, cut
- 1/2 cup of tomato slices
- 1/4 cup of rocket - 1 teaspoon of capers
- 1/4 cup of celery, cut

Instructions:

- Preheat the grill to high heat. Grill the turkey for around 4 minutes on each side after brushing it with olive oil and placing it on a baking sheet. Combine the cheese, parsley, red onions, and

walnuts in a small-sized bowl. In a separate bowl, combine all of the salad ingredients. Cover one side of the turkey with the cheese mixture and return it to the grill for around 2-3 minutes, or till the cheese & walnuts start to brown.
- Serve with the salad and lemon juice squeezed over the schnitzel.

116. Lamb Date Kofta with Tzatziki, Chili and Rocket Buckwheat

(Preparation time: 10 minutes | Cooking time: 45 minutes | Difficulty: Easy | Servings: 1)
Per serving: Calories 420, Total fat 23g, Protein 25g, Carbs 19g
Ingredients:
- 1 small clove of garlic
- 1 Medjool dates, chopped
- 1 teaspoon of ground turmeric
- 1 teaspoon of ground cumin
- 1 teaspoon of chopped parsley
- 1/2 red onion - 1 medium egg yolk
- 150g of minced lamb

For the buckwheat:
- 1 bird's eye chili, chopped
- 1 teaspoon of chopped parsley
- 30 g buckwheat

For the tzatziki:
- ¼ lemon
- ½ teaspoon of dried or fresh mint juice (optional)
- 5 tablespoons of natural yogurt
- 3 tablespoons of cucumber, grated

For the salad:
- ¼ lemon
- 1 teaspoon of extra virgin olive oil juice
- 1/4 cup of tomato, diced
- 1/4 cup of rocket

Instructions:
- To create the kofta, combine all of the ingredients in a food processor, except the meat, and process till smooth.
- Remove the paste and mix it with the lamb and knead it in. Refrigerate the meat for 30 minutes before frying it into two sausages. Cook the buckwheat as per the package directions.
- Simply combine all of the ingredients for the tzatziki and set them aside. Preheat the grill to high heat.
- Place your kofta underneath the grill for around 8-10 minutes, occasionally flipping, till well browned & cooked through.
- Meanwhile, toss in the chopped chilies & parsley to the buckwheat.
- Simply combine all of the ingredients in a bowl for the salad. Serve the entire meal at the same time.

117. Beef Burger with Sweet Potato Fries

(Preparation time: 10 minutes | Cooking time: 35 minutes | Difficulty: Easy | Servings: 1)
Per serving: Calories 410, Total fat 31g, Protein 28g, Carbs 21g
Ingredients:
- 1 teaspoon of extra virgin olive oil
- 1 teaspoon of finely chopped parsley
- 1/2 red onion, finely chopped
- 125g of lean ground beef (5 percent fat)
- For the fries:
- 1 clove of garlic, unpeeled
- 1 teaspoon of extra virgin olive oil
- 1 teaspoon of dried rosemary
- 1 cup of sweet potatoes
- For serving:
- 2 tablespoons of rocket
- 1/4 cup of tomato, cut
- 2 red onions, cut into rings
- 2 tablespoons of cheddar cheese, sliced or grated
- 1 pickle (optional)

Instructions:

- Preheat the oven at 400°F. Start with the fries.
- Cut the sweet potato into 1 cm thick French fries after peeling it. Combine them with olive oil, rosemary, & a garlic clove.
- Cook for 30 minutes, till crispy, on a baking sheet.
- Combine the onion & parsley with the ground beef to make the burger. If you have cookie cutters, use the largest cookie cutter in the set to shape your burger.
- Otherwise, make a lovely, even pie with your hands. Lay the burger on one side of the pan, and the onion rings on the other. Heat a pan over medium flame, add the olive oil, and place the burger on one side of the pan & the onion rings on the other.
- Check the burger for doneness after 6 minutes on each side. To taste, fry the onion rings.
- When the burger is done, top it with the cheese and red onion, and bake for a minute to melt the cheese.
- Remove the tomatoes, rocket, and pickles from the can & set them on top. Serve alongside the fries.

118. Salmon Tartare with Rocket Salad

(Preparation time: 10 minutes | Cooking time: 35 minutes | Difficulty: Easy | Servings: 1)
Per serving: Calories 390, Total fat 25g, Protein 23g, Carbs 15g
Ingredients:

- Salt and pepper
- ¼ lemon juice
- 1 teaspoon extra virgin olive oil
- 1/2 red onion
- 1 tablespoon of chopped parsley

- 1 teaspoon of capers
- 125g skinless salmon fillet without bones

For the salad:

- 1 teaspoon of extra virgin olive oil
- 1 teaspoon of balsamic vinegar
- 1/4 cup of rocket
- 1/4 celery, cut
- Walnut halves, chopped

Instructions:

- Cut the salmon fillet in half. After that, chop each half into little cubes by cutting it into thin strips.
- Mix the red onions & capers with the fish in as small a dice as feasible.
- You can chop it up in a small food processor if you have one.
- Combine olive oil, parsley, and a pinch of salt and pepper in a mixing bowl. To make the salad, combine all of the ingredients and top with the salmon.
- Simply squeeze the lemon juice over the salmon & serve (do not add the lemon juice before serving since it will react with the raw fish and cause it to cook).

119. Spiced Burger

(Preparation time: 10 minutes | Cooking time: 35 minutes | Difficulty: Easy | Servings: 2 to 4)
Per serving: Calories 122, Total fat 2g, Protein 7g, Carbs 25g
Ingredients:

- 1 clove of garlic
- 1 teaspoon of Paprika powder
- 1 teaspoon of dried oregano
- 250g of ground beef

Toppings:

- ½ pieces red onion
- 1 piece of little gem
- 1 tomato
- ¼ pieces of zucchini
- 4 pieces of mushrooms

Instructions:

- Squeeze the garlic clove.
- In a mixing bowl, combine all of the burger ingredients. Divide the mixture in 1/2 and form each half into a hamburger.
- Place the burgers onto a plate and chill for a few minutes.
- Cut the zucchini into 1 cm slices on the diagonal.
- The red onion should be cut into half-rings. Cut the tomato into thin slices & the salad leaves into small pieces.
- Grill the hamburgers till they are done on the grill.
- Grill the mushrooms alongside the burgers till cooked but firm on all sides.
- Grill the zucchini slices with it for a few minutes.
- It's time to assemble the burger!
- Put two mushrooms onto a plate, then layer lettuce, zucchini slices, and tomatoes on top. The burger should then be placed on top, followed by the red onion.

120. Chicken Skewers with Cashew Sauce

(Preparation time: 15 minutes | Cooking time: 30 minutes | Difficulty: Easy | Servings: 3)
Per serving: Calories 219, Total fat 45g, Protein 15g, Carbs 21g
Ingredients:

- 1 clove of garlic
- 1 tablespoon of olive oil
- 1 tablespoon of sesame seeds
- ½ spring onions
- 1 1/2 tablespoons of coconut amino
- 2 pieces of chicken legs
- 4 toothpicks

For the Cashew Sauce:

- 1 clove of garlic
- 1 1/2 tablespoons of coconut amino

- 1/4 cup of unsalted cashew nuts
- 1/4 cup of Coconut milk

Instructions:

- Place the chicken legs in a dish and cut them into pieces.
- Mix in the coconut amino & olive oil, as well as the garlic clove.
- Allow 30 minutes to marinate after stirring with a spoon.
- Meanwhile, soak several long wooden skewers in water.
- Using the skewers, thread the chicken cubes.
- In a food processor, combine all of the ingredients for the cashew sauce and pulse till smooth.
- In a saucepan, steadily cook the sauce till it is hot. (Slow cooking is essential; else, the sauce will separate.)
- Spring onions should be cut into rings.
- Grill the chicken skewers and serve with spring onions & sesame seeds on the side. Serve with warm cashew sauce on the side.

121. Pork Chops with Orange and Mustard Glaze

(Preparation time: 15 minutes | Cooking time: 45 minutes | Difficulty: Easy | Servings: 4)
Per serving: Calories 230, Total fat 36g, Protein 42g, Carbs 2g
Ingredients:

- 2 sprigs of fresh rosemary
- 1 tablespoon of olive oil
- 1 piece of orange
- 1 tablespoon of mustard yellow
- 2 pieces of Rib cutlet

Instructions:

- In a bowl, place the pork chops.
- Squeeze the orange & combine it with the mustard & olive oil in a mixing bowl.
- Add the rosemary leaves to the orange juice mixture.

- After a minute of vigorous beating, pour the mixture over the pork chops.
- Allow at least 45 minutes for the treatment to take effect.
- On the grill, cook the pork chops.

122. Bacon with Sweet Potato Salad

(Preparation time: 15 minutes | Cooking time: 30 minutes | Difficulty: Easy | Servings: 4)
Per serving: Calories 405, Total fat 11g, Protein 12g, Carbs 18g
Ingredients:

- 1 tablespoon of lemon juice
- Garlic clove (squeezed)
- 1 tablespoon of olive oil
- Balsamic vinegar
- Sweet potato (peeled and diced)
- 5 slices of bacon

Instructions:

- Preheat the oven at 380°F and line the baking sheet using parchment paper.
- Cook the bacon on a baking pan till it is crispy (around 20 minutes).
- Remove the bacon out from the skillet and crisp it before chopping it up.
- In the same pot, combine the sweet potato cubes with the garlic, season with some olive oil, and bake for around 30 minutes.
- In a bowl, combine the olive oil, vinegar, and lime juice. Take the French fries out of the oven, combine them with the bacon French fries, & season with seasonings. Add rockets & pine nuts at the end if desired.

123. Veggie and Nut Loaf

(Preparation time: 15 minutes | Cooking time: 60 minutes | Difficulty: Medium | Servings: 3)
Per serving: Calories 297, Total fat 18g, Protein 10g, Carbs 15g
Ingredients:

- 1/2 cup of water

- 2 teaspoons of turmeric powder
- 2 tablespoons of olive oil
- 2 cloves of garlic, chopped
- 1 bird's-eye chili, finely chopped
- 1 red onion, finely chopped
- 4 tablespoons of fresh parsley, chopped
- 1 egg, beaten
- 2 tablespoons of soy sauce
- 1 carrot, finely chopped
- 3 sticks of celery, finely chopped
- 1 cup of mushrooms, finely chopped
- 1/2 cup of haricot beans
- 1/2 cup of peanuts, finely chopped
- 1/2 cup of walnuts, finely chopped
- 1/3 cup of red wine

Instructions:

- Add the garlic, chili, carrot, celery, onion, mushrooms, & turmeric to a pan of hot oil. Cook them for around 5 minutes.
- Combine the haricot beans, nuts, red wine, veggies, soy sauce, egg, parsley, & water.
- Grease a large loaf pan and line it with greaseproof paper. Pour the mixture into the loaf tin, cover with foil, and bake for around 60-90 minutes at 380°F. Allow it to cool for 10 minutes before turning it out onto a serving platter.

124. Turmeric Chicken and Kale with Food, Lemon and Honey

(Preparation time: 15 minutes | Cooking time: 20 minutes | Difficulty: Easy | Servings: 4)
Per serving: Calories 232, Total fat 11g, Protein 14g, Carbs 8g
Ingredients:
For the chicken:

- ½ teaspoon of salt + pepper
- 1 teaspoon of lime zest
- ½ lime juice
- 1 teaspoon of turmeric powder
- 1 large garlic clove, diced

- 1 tablespoon of olive oil
- ½ red onion, diced
- 250-300g of minced chicken meat or diced chicken legs

For the salad:

- A handful of fresh coriander leaves, chopped
- A handful of fresh parsley leaves, chopped
- 6 stalks of broccoli
- 2 tablespoons of pumpkin seeds (seeds)
- 3 large cabbage leaves, stems removed and chopped
- ½ sliced avocado

For the dressing:

- ½ teaspoon of sea salt with pepper
- 1 small garlic clove, diced or grated
- 3 tablespoons of lime juice
- 3 tablespoons of virgin olive oil
- 1 teaspoon of raw honey
- ½ teaspoon of whole or Dijon mustard

Instructions:

- In a pan, melt the olive oil. Add the onion and cook for 4-5 minutes over medium flame, till golden brown. Separate the minced chicken & garlic by stirring for 2-3 minutes over medium-high flame.
- Cook, constantly stirring, for another 3-4 minutes after adding the turmeric, lime zest, salt, lime juice, and pepper.
- Bring a small saucepan of water to a boil while the chicken is cooking. Cook for 2 minutes after adding the broccoli. After rinsing with cold water, cut each piece into 3-4 pieces.
- Toast the pumpkin seeds in the chicken pan for 2 minutes over medium flame, stirring regularly to avoid scorching. Season with a pinch of salt and pepper. Set them aside. You can also use raw pumpkin seeds.

- In a salad dish, combine the chopped cabbage and the dressing. Mix and rub the cabbage with the dressing with your hands. This softens the cabbage in the same way that citrus juice softens fish or beef Carpaccio by "cooking" it a little.
- Finally, combine the cooked chicken, broccoli, fresh herbs, pumpkin seeds, & slices of avocado in a mixing bowl.

125. Asian King Jumped Jamp

(Preparation time: 15 minutes | Cooking time: 15 minutes | Difficulty: Easy | Servings: 4)
Per serving: Calories 223, Total fat 2g, Protein 34g, Carbs 6g

Ingredients:

- 1 garlic clove, finely chopped
- 1 teaspoon of finely chopped fresh ginger.
- 1 bird's eye chili, finely chopped
- 2 teaspoons of extra virgin olive oil
- 1 sliced red onion
- 1 tablespoon of celery or celery leaves
- 1/4 cup of celery, cut and sliced
- 2 teaspoons of tamari or soy sauce
- ½ cup of chicken broth
- 1/4 cup of chopped cabbage
- 1/2 cup of chopped green beans
- 1/2 cup of soba (buckwheat pasta)
- 1/2 cup of raw shelled prawns, not chopped

Instructions:

- Cook the prawns in 1 teaspoon of tamari & 1 teaspoon of oil in a pan over high flame for around 2-3 minutes. Place the prawns on a platter and set them aside. Because the pan will be reused, clean it using kitchen paper. Cook your noodles for around 5-8 minutes in boiling water or as directed on the package. Drain the water and set it aside.
- Meanwhile, in the remaining oil, sauté the garlic, chili, ginger, beans, red

onion, celery, and cabbage for around 2-3 minutes over medium-high flame. Allow the broth to come to a boil, then reduce to a low flame and cook for a minute or two, till the veggies are tender but still crisp.

- Return the pan to a boil with the shrimp, noodles, & celery/celery leaves, then remove from the flame and serve.

126. Sesame Chicken Salad

(Preparation time: 20 minutes | Cooking time: 0 minutes | Difficulty: Easy | Servings: 4)
Per serving: Calories 345, Total fat 5g, Protein 4g, Carbs 10g
Ingredients:

- ½ red onion, thinly sliced
- 1 tablespoon of sesame seeds
- 2 tablespoons of chopped large parsley
- 1/2 cup of cabbage, chopped
- 1 cucumber, peeled, halved lengthwise, without a teaspoon, and sliced.
- 1/4 cup of bok choi, finely chopped
- 150g of cooked chicken, minced

For the dressing:

- 1 lime juice
- 1 tablespoon of extra virgin olive oil
- 1 teaspoon of sesame oil
- 1 teaspoon of light honey
- 2 teaspoons of soy sauce

Instructions:

- In a dry pan, toast sesame seeds for around 2 minutes, or till they are slightly brown and aromatic.
- Allow to cool on a platter.
- To make the dressing, whisk together olive oil, sesame oil, lime juice, honey, & soy sauce in a small-sized dish.
- In a large-sized mixing dish, carefully combine the cucumber, red onion, black cabbage, bok choi, & parsley.

- Pour in the dressing and toss to combine.
- Serve the salad between two plates with the shredded chicken on top. Just before serving, sprinkle with sesame seeds.

127. Beef and Kale Salad

(Preparation time: 15 minutes | Cooking time: 10 minutes | Difficulty: Easy | Servings: 2)
Per serving: Calories 262, Total fat 12g, Protein 25g, Carbs 15g
Ingredients:
For the Steak:

- Salt and ground black pepper, to taste
- 2 teaspoons of olive oil
- 2 (4-ounce) strips of steaks

For the Salad:

- ¼ cup of cherry tomatoes halved
- ¼ cup of carrot, peeled and shredded
- ¼ cup of radish, sliced
- ¼ cup of cucumber, peeled, seeded, and sliced
- 3 cups of fresh kale, tough ribs removed and chopped

For the Dressing:

- Salt and ground black pepper, to taste
- 1 tablespoon of fresh lemon juice
- 1 tablespoon of extra-virgin olive oil

Instructions:

- For the steak, heat the oil in a big heavy-bottomed wok over a high flame and fry the steaks for around 3-4 minutes per side using salt & black pepper.
- Before slicing, place the steaks on a cutting board for around 5 minutes.
- To make the salad, combine all of the ingredients into a salad bowl and toss well. To make the dressing, put all of the ingredients in a separate bowl and whisk till smooth.
- Cut the steaks against the grain into appropriately sized slices.

- Arrange the salad on each of the serving plates. The steak slices should be placed on top of each plate.
- Serve with the dressing drizzled on top.

128. Sweet Potato and Salmon Patties

(Preparation time: 15 minutes | Cooking time: 30 minutes | Difficulty: Easy | Servings: 4)
Per serving: Calories 116, Total fat 2g, Protein 9g, Carbs 13g
Ingredients:
- Herb salt and pepper to taste
- Rice flour or buckwheat flour
- 1 1/2 cups of sweet potato cooked and mashed
- 225g of wild salmon, cooked or tinned

Instructions:
- Preheat the oven at 360°F.
- Combine the sweet potato, salmon, & herbal salt and pepper in a mixing bowl. Shape a tiny quantity of the mixture into a ball with your hands. Flatten into a burger shape, then dip each side into the flour. Place it on a parchment-lined baking sheet. Repeat till all the blend has been consumed.
- Cook for around 20 minutes, rotating only once. Serve alongside a large green salad.

129. Sirtfood Miso Marinated Cod with Greens and Sesame

(Preparation time: 10 minutes | Cooking time: 20 minutes | Difficulty: Easy | Servings: 6)
Per serving: Calories 244, Total fat 16g, Protein 16g, Carbs 11g
Ingredients:
- 1 teaspoon of ground turmeric
- 1 tablespoon of extra-virgin olive oil
- 1 garlic clove, finely chopped
- 1 teaspoon of finely chopped fresh ginger - 1 bird's eye chili, finely chopped

- 1 teaspoon of sesame seeds
- 1 tablespoon of parsley, roughly chopped
- 1 tablespoon of tamari or soya sauce
- 1/2 red onion, sliced - 1/4 cup of buckwheat - 1/4 cup of celery, sliced
- 1/4 kale, roughly chopped
- 1/4 cup of green beans
- 20g miso - 1 tablespoon of mirin
- 200g of skinless cod fillet

Instructions:
- Combine the miso, mirin, and 1 teaspoon of oil in a mixing bowl. Rub it all over the fish and set it aside for around 30 minutes to marinate. Preheat the oven at 220ºF.
- Cook the cod for around 10 minutes in the oven. Meanwhile, heat the remaining oil in a large-sized frying pan or wok. Stir-fry for a few minutes with the onion before adding the celery, garlic, chili, ginger, green beans, & kale. Toss and sauté till the kale is cooked through and tender. To aid the cooking process, you may have to add a little water to the pan.
- Cook the buckwheat for around 3 minutes with the turmeric, as directed on the box.
- Serve with the greens & fish after adding the sesame seeds, parsley, & tamari to the stir-fry.

130. Chicken and Kale with Spicy Salsa

(Preparation time: 10 minutes | Cooking time: 50 minutes | Difficulty: Easy | Servings: 1)
Per serving: Calories 169, Total fat 7g, Protein 5g, Carbs 15g
Ingredients:
- ¼ lemon, juiced
- 2 teaspoons of ground turmeric
- 1 teaspoon of fresh ginger, chopped

- 1 tablespoon of extra virgin olive oil
- ½ red onion, sliced - 1 cup of kale, chopped - 1 skinless, boneless chicken filet or breast - ¼ cup of buckwheat

For the Salsa:
- ¼ lemon, juiced
- 3 sprigs of parsley, chopped
- 1 bird's eye chili, deseeded and minced use less if desired - 1 tomato
- 1 tablespoon of chopped capers

Instructions:
- Set aside into a bowl all of the ingredients listed above, except for the salsa. Preheat the oven at 425°F.
- Cover the chicken with a teaspoon of turmeric, a squeeze of lemon juice, and a drizzle of oil, and lay aside for around 10 minutes. Slide the chicken & marinade onto a heated pan and sear for around 2-3 minutes on each side on high flame. Then, transfer everything to an oven-safe dish & bake for around 20 minutes, or till everything is cooked and pink. Steam the kale for around 5 minutes in a steamer or on the stovetop with a lid and some water. The goal is to wilt the kale rather than boil or burn it.
- After 4-5 minutes of sautéing the red onions & ginger, add the cooked kale, then toss for 1 minute. Cook the buckwheat as directed on the package, then add the turmeric. Serve the chicken with buckwheat, kale, & spicy salsa on the side.

131. Chicken Skewers with Satay Sauce

(Preparation time: 15 minutes | Cooking time: 30 minutes | Difficulty: Easy | Servings: 1)
Per serving: Calories 398, Total fat 21g, Protein 24g, Carbs 19g
Ingredients:
- 1 teaspoon of ground turmeric

- ½ teaspoon of extra virgin olive oil
- 1/4 cup of celery, sliced
- 1/4 cup of kale, stalks removed and sliced
- 150g of chicken breast, cut into chunks
- 50g of buckwheat
- 4 walnut halves, chopped, to garnish

For the sauce:
- 1 teaspoon of ground turmeric
- 1 garlic clove, chopped
- 1 teaspoon of extra virgin olive oil
- 1 tablespoon of coriander, chopped
- 1 teaspoon of curry powder
- 1 red onion, diced - 1/4 chicken stock
- 1/2 cup of coconut milk
- 1 tablespoon of walnut butter

Instructions:
- Set aside for 30 minutes to 1 hour to marinate the chicken with the turmeric and olive oil, but if you're short on time, just leave it for as long as you can.
- Cook the buckwheat according to package directions, adding the kale & celery for the last 5-7 minutes. Drain.
- Preheat the grill to high flame.
- To make the sauce, gently sauté the red garlic and onions in the olive oil till tender, around 2-3 minutes. Cook for another minute after adding the spices. Bring the stock and coconut milk to a boil, then add the walnut butter & whisk till it's combined. Reduce the flame to low and cook for around 8-10 minutes, or till the sauce is creamy and rich.
- While the sauce is simmering, insert the chicken onto the skewers & cook for around 10 minutes on a hot grill, rotating after 5 minutes.
- Stir the coriander into the sauce before pouring it over the skewers and scattering the chopped walnuts on top.

132. Strawberry Buckwheat Tabbouleh

(Preparation time: 15 minutes | Cooking time: 20 minutes | Difficulty: Easy | Servings: 3)
Per serving: Calories 246, Total fat 18g, Protein 2g, Carbs 19g
Ingredients:

- ½ lemon - 1 tablespoon of turmeric
- 1 tablespoon of extra virgin olive oil
- 2 tablespoons of parsley
- 1 tablespoon of caper
- 1 red onion - 2 tablespoons of rocket
- 1/4 cup of tomato
- 1/4 cup of buckwheat
- 3 Medjool dates pitted
- 1/2 cup of strawberries, billed
- 1/2 cup of avocado

Instructions:

- Cook the buckwheat according to the package directions, then add the turmeric. Drain the water and set it aside to cool.
- Tomato, red onion, avocado, dates, parsley, & caper should all be finely chopped. Combine the warm buckwheat with the chilly buckwheat.
- Slice the strawberries & toss them with the lemon juice & oil in the salad. Serve and have fun.

133. Chicken Curry

(Preparation time: 15 minutes | Cooking time: 30 minutes | Difficulty: Easy | Servings: 3)
Per serving: Calories 398, Total fat 21g, Protein 24g, Carbs 15g
Ingredients:

- 2 teaspoons of ground turmeric
- 1 tablespoon of olive oil
- 3 garlic cloves, roughly chopped
- 2 teaspoons of garam masala
- 2 teaspoons of ground cumin
- 1 red onion, roughly chopped
- 2cm fresh ginger, peeled and roughly chopped - 1 cinnamon stick (optional)
- 6 cardamom pods (optional)
- 2 tablespoons of fresh coriander, chopped (plus extra for garnish)
- 8 boneless, skinless chicken thighs (or 4 chicken breasts), cut into bite-size chunks - 1 x 400ml tin coconut milk
- 1 cup of buckwheat, brown rice or basmati rice to serve

Instructions:

- Into a food processor, combine the onion, garlic, and ginger till a paste forms. You can also use a hand blender, or if you don't have one, finely chop all three ingredients and proceed as directed below. Stir together the garam masala, cumin, and turmeric in the paste. Remove from the equation.
- In a large deep pan, pour 1 tablespoon of olive oil (ideally non-stick). Heat the pan for one minute over high heat before adding the chopped chicken thighs. Stir-fry the chicken for 2 minutes on high heat, then reduce the heat & add the curry paste. Allow the chicken to cook for 3 minutes in the paste before adding half of the coconut milk (200ml), as well as the cinnamon & cardamom (if using). Bring to a boil, then reduce to a low heat and continue to cook for 30 minutes, or till the curry sauce is thick & wonderful. Add more coconut milk if the curry becomes too dry. You might not need all, but if you want a saucier curry, go ahead and use a lot. Prepare your accompaniment (buckwheat/rice) & any side dishes while the curry is simmering. Add the chopped coriander when the curry is done & serve immediately with buckwheat or rice & a glass of chilled white wine or water.

134. Trout with Roasted Vegetables

(Preparation time: 15 minutes | Cooking time: 25 minutes | Difficulty: Easy | Servings: 2)
Per serving: Calories 154, Total fat 3g, Protein 10g, Carbs 11g
Ingredients:

- 1 lemon, juiced
- Olive oil
- Dried dill
- Tamari
- 2 turnips, peeled and cut into segments
- 2 carrots cut into batons
- 2 parsnips, peeled and cut into wedges
- 1 trout fillet per person

Instructions:

- Fill a baking tray halfway with cut vegetables. Add a splash of tamari & olive oil to finish. Preheat the oven at 400°F. Bake for around 25 minutes; after 25 minutes, remove the veggies from the oven and toss thoroughly.
- Place the fish on top of it. Drizzle with lemon juice & dill. Return to the oven, covered with foil.
- Reduce the oven temperature at 300°F and cook for around 20 minutes, or till the fish is cooked through.

135. Baked Salmon with Stir-Fried Vegetables

(Preparation time: 15 minutes | Cooking time: 30 minutes | Difficulty: Easy | Servings: 2)
Per serving: Calories 160, Total fat 4g, Protein 12g, Carbs 9g
Ingredients:

- Grated zest and juice of 1 lemon
- 2 teaspoon of root ginger, grated
- 2 teaspoons of olive oil
- 1 teaspoon of toasted sesame oil
- Bunch of kale, chopped
- 2 carrots cut into matchsticks
- 2 wild salmon fillets

- 1 tin of water chestnuts, drained, rinsed & chopped

Instructions:

- Combine the lemon juice, ginger, and zest in a mixing bowl. Pour the lemon-ginger mixture over the salmon in a shallow ovenproof dish. Wrap in foil and set aside to marinate for 30-60 minutes.
- While the salmon is baking at 380°F, heat a wok or frying pan and add the toasted sesame oil & olive oil. Cook, stirring regularly for a few minutes after adding the vegetables.
- When the salmon is done, ladle some of the salmon marinade over the vegetables and continue to simmer for a few minutes more.
- Serve the veggies on a platter with the salmon on top.

136. Chicken Breast with Kale and Red Onions

(Preparation time: 10 minutes | Cooking time: 1 hour 5 minutes | Difficulty: Easy | Servings: 4)
Per serving: Calories 107, Total fat 3g, Protein 2g, Carbs 20g
Ingredients:

- 1 lemon, juiced
- 1 teaspoon of chopped fresh ginger
- 2 ½ teaspoons of ground turmeric
- 1 bird's eye chili, finely chopped
- 1 ½ tablespoon of olive oil
- 2 tablespoons of parsley, finely chopped
- 1 red onion, sliced
- 2 tablespoons of celery
- 1/4 cup of kale, chopped
- 1/2 cup pf tomato
- 1/4 cup of buckwheat
- 140g of chicken breast

Instructions:

- Marinate the chicken breast in 1 teaspoon of turmeric, lemon juice, celery, & ginger for around 30 minutes.

- Cook the marinated chicken for around 10 to 12 minutes in the oven. Remove the dish from the oven, cover it with foil, and set it aside for around 5 minutes before serving.
- Meanwhile, steam the kale for around 5 minutes, then sauté the red onions and ginger in a little oil till tender, then add the cooked kale & fry for an additional minute.
- Cook the buckwheat per the instructions on the package. Serve with the chicken, vegetables, & salsa on the side.

137. Salmon with Chili and Turmeric

(Preparation time: 10 minutes | Cooking time: 30 minutes | Difficulty: Easy | Servings: 4)
Per serving: Calories 177, Total fat 15g, Protein 12g, Carbs 4g
Ingredients:

- ¼ lemon, juiced
- 1 garlic clove, finely chopped
- 1 teaspoon of ground turmeric
- 1 teaspoon of extra virgin olive oil
- 1 bird's eye chili, finely chopped
- 1 tablespoon of chopped parsley
- 1 teaspoon of mild curry powder
- 2 red onions, finely chopped
- 2 tomatoes, cut into 8 wedges
- 1 cup of celery cut into 2cm lengths
- 1/4 cup of tinned green lentils
- 1/2 cup of chicken or vegetable stock
- Skinned salmon

Instructions:

- Preheat the oven at 400°F.
- Begin with the spicy celery. Heat the olive oil in a frying pan over medium-low flame, then add the onion, garlic, ginger, chili, & celery. Cook, occasionally stirring, for 2-3 minutes, or till softened but not colored, then add the curry powder & cook for another minute.

- Simmer for 10 minutes after adding the tomatoes, stock, & lentils. Depending on how crunchy you prefer your celery, you may choose to increase or decrease the cooking time.
- Meanwhile, massage the salmon with a mixture of turmeric, oil, & lemon juice. Bake for around 8 to 10 minutes on a baking tray. Finish by stirring the parsley into the celery and serving the salmon with it.

138. Steak with Veggies

(Preparation time: 10 minutes | Cooking time: 15 minutes | Difficulty: Easy | Servings: 4)
Per serving: Calories 311, Total fat 14g, Protein 37g, Carbs 8g
Ingredients:

- Ground black pepper, as required
- 4 garlic cloves, minced
- 2 tablespoons of olive oil
- 3 tablespoons of tamari
- 1½ cups of carrots, peeled and cut into matchsticks
- 1½ cups of fresh kale, tough ribs removed and chopped
- 1 pound of beef sirloin steak, cut into bite-sized pieces

Instructions:

- In a pan over medium flame, melt the olive oil & sauté the garlic for around 1 minute.
- Stir in the meat and black pepper to mix.
- Raise the heat to medium-high & cook for around 3-4 minutes, or till both sides are browned.
- Cook for 4-5 minutes after adding the carrot, kale, & tamari.
- Remove the pan from the flame & serve immediately.

139. Shrimp with Vegetables

(Preparation time: 10 minutes | Cooking time: 15 minutes | Difficulty: Easy | Servings: 5)
Per serving: Calories 298, Total fat 11g, Protein 45g, Carbs 7g
Ingredients:
For the Sauce:
- 2 garlic cloves, minced
- 1 tablespoon of fresh ginger, grated
- ¼ teaspoon of red pepper flakes, crushed
- 1 teaspoon of brown sugar
- 3 tablespoons of low-sodium soy sauce
- 1 tablespoon of red wine vinegar

For Shrimp Mixture:
- 3 tablespoons of olive oil
- 1 1/4 cups of broccoli florets
- 1 cup of carrot, peeled and sliced
- 1½ pounds of medium shrimp, peeled and deveined

Instructions:
- To make the sauce, combine all of the ingredients in a mixing bowl and whisk till smooth. Set them aside.
- Cook the shrimp in a large-sized wok over medium-high flame for around 2 minutes, stirring occasionally.
- Cook, often stirring, for 3-4 minutes after adding the broccoli and carrot.
- Cook for around 1-2 minutes after adding the sauce mixture.
- Serve right away.

140. Chickpeas with Swiss Chard

(Preparation time: 10 minutes | Cooking time: 15 minutes | Difficulty: Easy | Servings: 4)
Per serving: Calories 217, Total fat 8g, Protein 9g, Carbs 25g
Ingredients:
- ¼ cup of water
- Salt and ground black pepper, as required
- 1 tablespoon of fresh lemon juice
- 2 tablespoons of olive oil
- 2 garlic cloves, sliced thinly
- 2 tablespoons of fresh parsley, chopped
- 1 large tomato, chopped finely
- 2 1/4 cups of chickpeas, drained and rinsed
- 2 bunches of fresh Swiss chard, trimmed

Instructions:
- In a large-sized nonstick wok, heat the oil over medium flame & sauté the garlic for around 1 minute.
- Cook for around 2-3 minutes, mashing the tomato with the back of a spoon.
- Cook for around 5-7 minutes, stirring in the remaining ingredients except for the lemon juice and parsley.
- Remove from the flame and drizzle with lemon juice.
- Serve immediately with a parsley garnish.

141. Buckwheat Noodles with Chicken

(Preparation time: 10 minutes | Cooking time: 25 minutes | Difficulty: Easy | Servings: 2)
Per serving: Calories 363, Total fat 12g, Protein 23g, Carbs 38g
Ingredients:
- 2 garlic cloves, chopped finely
- 1 tablespoon of olive oil
- 1 red onion, chopped finely
- 3 tablespoons of low-sodium soy sauce
- ½ cup of broccoli florets
- ½ cup of fresh green beans, trimmed and sliced
- 1 cup of fresh kale, tough ribs removed and chopped
- 1/2 cup of buckwheat noodles
- 1 (6-ounce) boneless, skinless chicken breast, cubed

Instructions:
- Cook the broccoli & green beans in a medium-sized pan of boiling water for around 4-5 minutes.
- Cook for 1-2 minutes after adding the kale.
- Drain the vegetables & place them in a big mixing dish. Set them aside.
- Cook the soba noodles for 5 minutes in a separate pan of lightly salted boiling water.
- Drain the noodles thoroughly before rinsing them underneath cold running water. Remove from the equation.
- Meanwhile, heat the olive oil in a big wok over medium flame & sauté the onion for around 2-3 minutes.
- Cook for 5-6 minutes after adding the chicken cubes.
- Cook for around 2-3 minutes, stirring regularly, after adding the garlic, soy sauce, and a splash of water.
- Cook for 1-2 minutes, constantly tossing, after adding the cooked veggies and noodles.
- Serve immediately with sesame seeds as a garnish.

142. One-Pot Pasta with Veggie Sausage and Sun-Dried Tomato

(Preparation time: 10 minutes | Cooking time: 25 minutes | Difficulty: Easy | Servings: 4)
Per serving: Calories 285, Total fat 3g, Protein 10g, Carbs 3g
Ingredients:
- 1-liter of water
- 2 tablespoons of olive or rapeseed oil
- 1 red onion, peeled and sliced
- 6-8 sun-dried tomatoes, roughly chopped
- 1 cup of cherry tomatoes, halved
- 2 teaspoons of vegetable stock powder
- 3 veggie sausages

- 2 cups of buckwheat pasta
- 1/2 cup of soya cream
- 1/2 cup of fresh baby spinach

Instructions:
- In a big, shallow dish, heat the oil and cook the sausage & onion till the sausages are golden. Remove them from the pan with care and cut each slice into four pieces, then return them to the saucepan for another 2 minutes.
- In a large pot, combine the pasta, tomatoes, sun-dried tomatoes, water, and powder. Bring to the boil, then lower to a low flame, cover, and simmer for 12-14 minutes, occasionally stirring, till the pasta is tender.
- Toss in the cream and spinach, then stir well and simmer for another minute, or till the spinach is completely gone.

143. Fennel, Broad Bean and Baby Carrot Pilaf

(Preparation time: 10 minutes | Cooking time: 15 minutes | Difficulty: Easy | Servings: 2)
Per serving: Calories 285, Total fat 9g, Protein 13g, Carbs 33g
Ingredients:
- 1 lemon
- Handful fresh parsley
- 2 cloves of garlic, peeled and chopped
- 2 tablespoons of olive oil
- 1 red onion
- 1 fennel bulb
- 1 cup of fresh or frozen broad beans
- 2 cups of vegetable stock
- 1/2 cup of baby carrots
- 1 cup of brown rice (rinsed well under cold water)
- 2 tablespoons of walnuts

Instructions:
- The onions should be peeled and chopped, the fennel should be chopped finely, and the garlic cloves should be

chopped. In a large pot or with a pot, heat the oil and soften the onion, fennel, & garlic for around 2 minutes.

- Cut the baby carrots in half and boil them. After that, store the vegetables in the pot with the beans and brown rice. Bring to a boil, then reduce to a low flame and simmer for 12 minutes, or till the rice is tender. Check the rice after a few minutes of cooking and, if it appears to be too dry, add a little more water. In the meantime, cut the nuts & parsley leaves and drizzle with lemon juice. Pour the lemon juice over the rice and crush the nuts & parsley. If required, serve right away.

144. Chicken and Berries Salad

(Preparation time: 20 minutes | Cooking time: 15 minutes | Difficulty: Easy | Servings: 8)
Per serving: Calories 377, Total fat 21g, Protein 34g, Carbs 12g
Ingredients:

- Salt and ground black pepper, as required
- ¼ cup of fresh lemon juice
- 1 garlic clove, minced
- ½ cup of olive oil
- 2 tablespoons of maple syrup
- 2 cups of fresh blueberries
- 2 cups of fresh strawberries, hulled and sliced
- 2 pounds of boneless, skinless chicken breasts
- 10 cups of fresh baby arugula

Instructions:

- In a large-sized mixing bowl, whisk together the oil, salt, lemon juice, Erythritol, garlic, and black pepper.
- Place the chicken and 3/4 cup of marinade in a large-sized resealable plastic bag.

- Seal the bag & shake it vigorously to coat everything evenly.
- Refrigerate for at least one night.
- Refrigerate the remaining marinade in the bowl before serving.
- Preheat the grill to medium-high temperature. Grease the grill grate with cooking spray.
- Take the chicken out of the package and throw away the marinade.
- Place the chicken onto the grill grate and cook for 5 to 8 minutes per side, covered. Cut the chicken into bite-sized pieces after removing it from the grill.
- Combine the chicken, strawberries, and spinach in a large-sized mixing dish.
- Toss with the leftover marinade to coat.
- Serve right away.

145. Beef and Kale Salad

(Preparation time: 10 minutes | Cooking time: 10 minutes | Difficulty: Easy | Servings: 2)
Per serving: Calories 262, Total fat 12g, Protein 25g, Carbs 15g
Ingredients:
For the steak:

- Salt and ground black pepper, as required
- 2 teaspoons of olive oil
- 2 (4-ounce) strips of steaks

For the salad:

- ¼ cup of cherry tomatoes halved
- ¼ cup of carrot, peeled and shredded
- ¼ cup of cucumber, peeled, seeded, and sliced
- 3 cups of fresh kale, tough ribs removed and chopped
- ¼ cup radish, sliced

For the dressing:

- 1 tablespoon of fresh lemon juice
- Salt and ground black pepper, as required
- 1 tablespoon of extra-virgin olive oil

Instructions:

- For the steak, prepare as follows:
- Heat the oil in a big heavy-bottomed wok over high flame, then season the steaks using salt and black pepper and cook for around 3 to 4 minutes per side.
- Before slicing, place the steaks on a cutting board for around 5 minutes.
- To make the salad:
- Mix all of the ingredients in a salad dish.
- To make the dressing, in a separate bowl, whisk together all of the ingredients till smooth.
- Cut the steaks against the grain into appropriately sized slices.
- Arrange the salad on each of the serving plates.
- Steak slices should be placed on top of each plate.
- Serve with a drizzle of dressing.

146. Chicken with Mole Salad

(Preparation time: 10 minutes | Cooking time: 40 minutes | Difficulty: Easy | Servings: 2)
Per serving: Calories 360, Total fat 10g, Protein 31g, Carbs 23g
Ingredients:

- 2 tablespoons of water
- Dash of salt
- 1 tablespoon of extra virgin olive oil
- 5 sprigs of parsley, chopped
- ½ red onion, diced
- 2 Medjool pitted dates, chopped
- 1 tablespoon of dark chocolate powder
- 1 skinned chicken breast
- ½ cup of arugula
- 2 cups of spinach, washed, dried, and torn in halves
- 2 celery stalks, chopped or sliced thinly

Instructions:

- Blend the dates, chocolate powder, water and oil, and salt in a food processor. Add the chili and continue to

process. Place the chicken breast in the refrigerator after applying the paste.
- Toss the other salad ingredients, veggies, & herbs in a bowl.
- Cook the chicken in a pan with a little oil till it's done, about 10 to 15 minutes over medium flame.
- Allow cooling before laying over the salad bed and serving.

147. Smoked Salmon Sirt Salad

(Preparation time: 10 minutes | Cooking time: 40 minutes | Difficulty: Easy | Servings: 4)
Per serving: Calories 368, Total fat 18g, Protein 14g, Carbs 30g
Ingredients:

- 1/4 of a lemon, juiced
- 1 tablespoon of extra virgin olive oil
- 5 sprigs of parsley, chopped
- 1 Medjool pitted date, chopped
- ½ small red onion, sliced thinly
- 1 tablespoon of capers
- 1 cup, or ¼ package if large of smoked salmon slices no cooking needed!
- 2 celery stalks, chopped or sliced thinly
- 1 avocado, pitted, sliced, and scooped out
- 10 walnuts, chopped
- 5 lovage or celery leaves, chopped

Instructions:

- Salad ingredients and vegetables should be washed and dried before being topped with salmon.

148. Chicken Leek Stew

(Preparation time: 10 minutes | Cooking time: 35 minutes | Difficulty: Easy | Servings: 4)
Per serving: Calories 222, Total fat 9g, Protein 25g, Carbs 9g
Ingredients:

- 4 cups of water
- 1 teaspoon salt
- 1 tablespoon of olive oil

- 1 tablespoon of butter
- ½ teaspoon of dried oregano
- ½ teaspoon of dried thyme
- ½ red onion, diced
- 1 cup of cabbage, shredded
- 1 cup of leek, chopped
- 1-pound of chicken breast, skinless, boneless

Instructions:

- Place the chicken breast in the pan after chopping it into cubes.
- Combine the butter & olive oil.
- Preheat the oven to 350°F and cook the chicken for around 5 minutes. From time to time, give it a stir.
- After that, add the chopped leek and yellow onion.
- Season using salt, oregano, and thyme. Combine all of the ingredients in a large-sized mixing bowl and cook for 5 minutes.
- Then add the cabbage and water.
- Cook the soup for around 25 minutes with the cover closed over medium flame.

149. Shrimp. Dates and Tomato Bowls

(Preparation time: 10 minutes | Cooking time: 0 minutes | Difficulty: Easy | Servings: 4)

Per serving: Calories 243, Total fat 5g, Protein 28g, Carbs 21g

Ingredients:

- 1 tablespoon of lemon juice
- 2 tablespoons of olive oil
- 1 cup of cherry tomatoes, halved
- ½ cup of Medjool dates, chopped
- 2 cups of baby spinach
- 2 tablespoons of walnuts, chopped
- 1-pound of shrimp, cooked, peeled, and deveined

Instructions:

- Toss the shrimp with spinach, walnuts, & other ingredients in a salad bowl and serve.

150. Tuna, Caper and Egg Salad

(Preparation time: 10 minutes | Cooking time: 0 minutes | Difficulty: Easy | Servings: 2)

Per serving: Calories 310, Total fat 15g, Protein 1g, Carbs 14g

Ingredients:

- 1 red onion, chopped
- 2 tomatoes, chopped
- 1/2 cup of cucumber
- 2 tablespoons of fresh parsley, chopped
- 1 tablespoon of capers
- 6 pitted black olives
- 1 stalk of celery
- 2 tablespoons of rocket arugula
- 2 tablespoons of garlic vinaigrette
- 2 hard-boiled eggs, peeled and quartered
- 1/2 cup of red chicory or yellow
- 150g of tinned tuna flakes in brine, drained

Instructions:

- In a mixing dish, combine the tuna, cucumber, olives, tomatoes, parsley, onion, chicory, celery, and rocket arugula.
- Serve on plates with the eggs & capers scattered on top.

151. Citrus Salmon

(Preparation time: 10 minutes | Cooking time: 45 minutes | Difficulty: Easy | Servings: 2)

Per serving: Calories 294, Total fat 3g, Protein 21g, Carbs 39g

Ingredients:

- Salt and pepper to taste
- 1 lemon, sliced thinly
- 2 teaspoons of lemon rind, grated
- 2 tablespoons of extra virgin olive oil

- 2 tablespoons of parsley, chopped
- 1 medium red onion, chopped
- 1 orange, sliced thinly
- 2 teaspoons of orange rind, grated
- 1 cup of vegetable broth
- 1 ½ lb. salmon fillet with skin on

Instructions:

- Cover the bottom of your crockpot using parchment paper and lemon wedges.
- Place the salmon on the lemon and season it with salt and pepper.
- Oil the fish and top it with the onion, parsley, and grated citrus rinds. Orange slices are sprinkled on top, with a few set aside for garnish.
- Pour the broth around the salmon, but not directly on top of it.
- Cook on low for around 2 hours, covered. Preheat the oven at 400°F.
- When the salmon is opaque & flaky, carefully take it from the crockpot using the parchment paper & place it on a baking sheet. Allow for 5–8 minutes in the oven for the salmon to brown on top.
- Serve with lemon and orange slices as garnish.

152. Scallops and Sweet Potatoes

(Preparation time: 10 minutes | Cooking time: 22 minutes | Difficulty: Easy | Servings: 4)
Per serving: Calories 211, Total fat 2g, Protein 21g, Carbs 25g
Ingredients:

- 2 tablespoons of olive oil
- ½ teaspoon of rosemary, dried
- ½ teaspoon of oregano, dried
- 1 red onion, chopped
- 1 tablespoon of parsley, chopped
- ½ cup of chicken stock
- 2 sweet potatoes, peeled and cubed
- 1 pound of scallops

Instructions:

- Heat the oil in a pan over medium flame, then add the onion & cook for 2 minutes.
- Toss in the sweet potatoes & stock, and simmer for another 10 minutes.
- Toss in the scallops and the rest of the ingredients, simmer for another 10 minutes, then divide into dishes and serve.

153. Minty Tomatoes and Corn

(Preparation time: 10 minutes | Cooking time: 0 minutes | Difficulty: Easy | Servings: 4)
Per serving: Calories 230, Total fat 7g, Protein 4g, Carbs 11g
Ingredients:

- ¼ teaspoon of black pepper
- 2 tablespoons of olive oil
- 1 tablespoon of rosemary vinegar
- 2 tablespoons of chopped mint
- 1 lb. of sliced tomatoes
- 2 cups of corn

Instructions:

- Combine the tomatoes, corn, and other ingredients in a salad dish, stir and serve.
- Enjoy!

154. Scallops with Walnuts and Mushrooms

(Preparation time: 10 minutes | Cooking time: 10 minutes | Difficulty: Easy | Servings: 4)
Per serving: Calories 322, Total fat 24g, Protein 22g, Carbs 8g
Ingredients:

- 2 tablespoons of olive oil
- 2 red onions, chopped
- ½ cup of mushrooms, sliced
- 2 tablespoons of walnuts, chopped
- 1 pound of scallops
- 1 cup of coconut cream

Instructions:

- Heat the oil in a skillet over medium flame, then add the red onions & mushrooms and cook for around 2 minutes.
- Cook for another 8 minutes over medium flame after adding other ingredients, then divide into bowls & serve.

155. Ginger and Lemongrass Mackerel

(Preparation time: 10 minutes | Cooking time: 25 minutes | Difficulty: Easy | Servings: 4)

Per serving: Calories 251, Total fat 3g, Protein 8g, Carbs 14g

Ingredients:

- Juice of 1 lime
- 2 tablespoons of olive oil
- 1 tablespoon of ginger, grated
- A handful of parsley, chopped
- 2 bird's eye chilies, chopped
- 2 lemongrass sticks, chopped
- 4 mackerel fillets, skinless and boneless

Instructions:

- Toss the mackerel with the oil, ginger, and other ingredients in a roasting pan and bake for around 25 minutes at 390°F.
- Serve by dividing everything amongst plates.

156. Tuna and Kale

(Preparation time: 10 minutes | Cooking time: 20 minutes | Difficulty: Easy | Servings: 4)

Per serving: Calories 251, Total fat 4g, Protein 7g, Carbs 14g

Ingredients:

- 2 tablespoons of olive oil
- 1 red onion, chopped
- ½ cup of cherry tomatoes, cubed
- 1 cup of kale, torn

- 1 pound of tuna fillets, boneless, skinless and cubed

Instructions:

- Heat the oil in a pan over medium flame, then add the onion & cook for around 5 minutes.
- Toss in the tuna and remaining ingredients, simmer for another 15 minutes, then divide amongst plates and serve.

157. Coronation Chicken Salad

(Preparation time: 10 minutes | Cooking time: 0 minutes | Difficulty: Easy | Servings: 2)

Per serving: Calories 20, Total fat 13g, Protein 7g, Carbs 14g

Ingredients:

- Juice of 1/4 of a lemon
- 1 teaspoon of ground turmeric
- 1 Medjool date, finely hacked
- 1 Bird's eye stew
- 1 teaspoon of parsley, chopped
- 1 Red onion, diced
- 1/2 teaspoon of mild curry powder
- 1/4 cup of Rocket, to serve
- 1/2 cup of natural yogurt
- 100g of Cooked chicken bosom, cut into scaled-down pieces
- 6 Walnut, finely chopped

Instructions:

- In a mixing bowl, combine the yogurt, lemon juice, parsley, & seasonings.
- Serve on a bed of rockets with all of the remaining fixings.

158. Serrano Ham and Rocket Arugula

(Preparation time: 10 minutes | Cooking time: 0 minutes | Difficulty: Easy | Servings: 2)

Per serving: Calories 165, Total fat 11g, Protein 7g, Carbs 9g

Ingredients:

- 1 tablespoon of orange juice

- 2 tablespoons of olive oil
- 1/2 cup of rocket arugula leaves
- 1 cup of Serrano ham

Instructions:

- Toss the rocket arugula with the oil and lemon juice in a mixing dish.
- Serve the rocket on plates with the ham on the side.

---

159. Country Chicken Breasts

(Preparation time: 10 minutes | Cooking time: 4 hours 10 minutes | Difficulty: Medium | Servings: 2)

Per serving: Calories 155, Total fat 4g, Protein 18g, Carbs 14g

Ingredients:

- Salt and pepper to taste
- Chopped parsley
- 1 teaspoon of turmeric
- 1 teaspoon of ground ginger
- 3 cloves of garlic, minced
- ¼ teaspoon of chili pepper flakes
- 1 tablespoon of curry powder
- 1 small red onion, finely diced
- ½ cup of chicken broth
- 2 cups of diced tomatoes
- 2 medium green apples, diced
- 1 small green bell pepper, chopped
- 2 tablespoons of dried currants
- 1 cup of brown rice
- 6 skinless, boneless chicken breasts, halved
- 1 pound of large raw shrimp, shelled and deveined
- 1/3 cup of walnuts

Instructions:

- Rinse the chicken and pat it dry before putting it aside.
- Combine apples, onion, bell pepper, garlic, currants, curry powder, turmeric, & chili pepper flakes in a large crockpot. Toss in the tomatoes.

- Arrange chicken on top of the tomato mixture, slightly overlapping pieces.
- Pour in the broth without mixing or stirring.
- Cook on high for around 3–4 hours, covered.
- Preheat the oven at 200 °F.
- Transfer the chicken to an oven-safe plate, wrap lightly, and place in the oven to keep warm.
- In a separate bowl, combine the rice and the remaining liquid. Increase the flame setting to high; cover and cook, stirring once or twice, for around 30 to 35 minutes, or till rice is almost soft to bite. Stir in the shrimp, cover, and cook for another 10 minutes, or till the shrimp are opaque in the center.
- Meanwhile, toast walnuts in a small-sized pan over medium flame for around 5 to 8 minutes, occasionally stirring, until golden brown. Set them aside.
- Season the rice mixture with salt and black pepper to taste before serving. Arrange chicken on top of the mound in a warm serving dish. Parsley and walnuts should be sprinkled on top.

---

160. Chicken Merlot with Mushrooms

(Preparation time: 10 minutes | Cooking time: 4 hours 10 minutes | Difficulty: Medium | Servings: 2)

Per serving: Calories 213, Total fat 4g, Protein 7g, Carbs 32g

Ingredients:

- Salt and pepper to taste
- 2 cloves of garlic, minced
- 1 large red onion, chopped
- ¾ cup of chicken broth
- 2 tablespoons of basil, chopped finely
- 2 tablespoons of Parmesan, shaved

- 2 teaspoons of sweetener
- 1 cup of tomato paste
- 3 tablespoons of chia seeds
- 3 cups of mushrooms, sliced
- 6 boneless, skinless chicken breasts, cubed
- 1 1/4 cups of package buckwheat ramen noodles, cooked
- ¼ cup of Merlot

Instructions:

- Rinse the chicken and leave it aside.
- Mix in the mushrooms, onion, & garlic in the crockpot.
- Do not mix the chicken cubes in with the veggies.
- Combine broth, basil, tomato paste, wine, chia seeds, sweetener, salt, & pepper in a large-sized mixing bowl. Pour the sauce over the chicken.
- Cook on low for around 7 to 8 hours or high for 3 12 to 4 hours, covered.
- Spoon the chicken, mushroom combination, and sauce over hot buckwheat ramen noodles to serve. Serve with shaved Parmesan cheese on top.

161. Chicken with Artichoke and Capers

(Preparation time: 10 minutes | Cooking time: 4 hours 5 minutes | Difficulty: Medium | Servings: 2)

Per serving: Calories 473, Total fat 22g, Protein 13g, Carbs 43g

Ingredients:

- Salt and pepper to taste
- 1 teaspoon of turmeric
- 1 medium red onion, diced
- 1 cup of chicken broth
- 3 tablespoons of chia seeds
- 3 teaspoons of curry powder
- 2 cups of diced tomatoes
- ½ cup of Kalamata olives, sliced

- 2 cups of mushrooms, sliced
- 1 (8 or 9 ounces) package frozen artichokes
- ¼ cup of capers, drained
- 6 boneless, skinless chicken breasts
- 3/4 teaspoon of dried lovage
- 3 cups of hot cooked buckwheat
- ¼ cup of dry white wine

Instructions:

- Set aside the chicken after rinsing it.
- Combine mushrooms, tomatoes (with juice), frozen artichoke hearts, olives, chicken broth, white wine, onion, and capers in a large-sized mixing bowl.
- Add the chia seeds, curry powder, salt, turmeric, lovage, and pepper and stir to combine.
- Pour half of the mixture into your crockpot, then top with the chicken and the remaining sauce.
- Cook on high for around 3 1/2 to 4 hours, covered.
- Serve with the cooked buckwheat.

162. Cheesy Crockpot Chicken and Veggies

(Preparation time: 10 minutes | Cooking time: 45 minutes | Difficulty: Easy | Servings: 2)

Per serving: Calories 417, Total fat 15g, Protein 16g, Carbs 35g

Ingredients:

- ¼ cup water
- 2 tablespoons of olive oil
- 1 tablespoon of parsley, chopped
- 1 small red onion, diced
- 3 stalks celery, chopped
- 3 carrots, chopped
- 1 cup of green beans, chopped
- 2 cups of mushrooms, sliced
- 1 cup of skim milk
- 1 tablespoon of buckwheat flour
- ¾ teaspoon of poultry seasoning

- 4 boneless, skinless chicken breasts, cubed
- 1/3 cup of ham, diced
- 1 cup of cheddar cheese, shredded
- ¼ cup of Parmesan, shredded

Instructions:

- Combine the ham, carrots, olive oil, mushrooms, celery, onion, and green beans in a large-sized mixing dish. Combine all ingredients in an instant pot.
- Without mixing, layer the chicken on top.
- Whisk broth, poultry seasoning, milk, parsley, and flour together in the now-empty dish till it's blended.
- Combine the cheddar & Parmesan cheeses.
- Over the chicken, pour the mixture. Do not mix them.
- Cook on high for around 30 minutes, covered.

163. Buckwheat Tuna Casserole

(Preparation time: 10 minutes | Cooking time: 35 minutes | Difficulty: Easy | Servings: 2)
Per serving: Calories 411, Total fat 17g, Protein 14g, Carbs 31g
Ingredients:

- 2 cups of boiling water
- 2 teaspoons of turmeric
- 2 tablespoons of olive oil
- 2 tablespoons of dried parsley
- ½ teaspoon of curry powder
- 2 tablespoons of buckwheat flour
- 1 cup of frozen peas
- 2 cups of celery, chopped
- 3 cups of skim milk
- 1 1/4 cups of buckwheat ramen noodles
- 1/3 cup of dry red wine
- 2 cans of tuna, drained

Instructions:

- Fill a large-sized bowl halfway with boiling water and add the buckwheat ramen noodles. Allow to settle for 5–8 minutes, or till fork-prodded noodles separate.
- Whisk together the red wine, turmeric, milk, parsley, and flour in a separate dish.
- Combine celery, peas, & tuna.
- Drain the ramen & add it to the olive oil greased baking dish, along with the tuna mixture. To combine, mix everything together. Bake for around 30 to 35 minutes at 380°F.

164. Chicken with Chili Salsa and Kale

(Preparation time: 10 minutes | Cooking time: 45 minutes | Difficulty: Easy | Servings: 1)
Per serving: Calories 135, Total fat 6g, Protein 7g, Carbs 13g
Ingredients:

- Juice of ½ lemon, divided
- 1 tablespoon of extra-virgin olive oil
- 2 teaspoons of ground turmeric
- 1 handful of parsley
- 1 teaspoon of chopped fresh ginger
- 1 bird's eye chili, chopped
- 1 red onion, sliced
- 1 tomato
- 1/4 cup of kale, chopped
- 1/4 cup of buckwheat
- 120g of skinless, boneless chicken breast

Instructions:

- To make the salsa, coarsely slice the tomatoes, discarding the seeds and retaining as much liquid as possible. Combine the chilies, parsley, & lemon juice in a mixing bowl. To get diverse effects, you may put everything in a blender.

- Preheat the oven at 320°F. With just a little oil, 1 teaspoon of turmeric, and lemon juice, marinate the chicken. Allow for 5-10 minutes of resting time.
- Heat a pan over medium flame till heated, then add the marinated chicken and cook for a minute on both sides till pale gold). If the pan isn't ovenproof, place the chicken in a baking tray & bake for around 8 to 10 minutes, or till it's cooked through. Remove the chicken from the oven, tent it with foil, and set it aside to rest for five minutes before serving. Meanwhile, cook the kale for around 5 minutes in a steamer.
- Sauté the ginger & red onions in a little oil till soft but not browned, then add the cooked kale & fry for a minute.
- With the remaining turmeric, cook the buckwheat according to the package guidelines. Serve with the vegetables, salsa, and chicken on the side.

165. Tofu with Cauliflower

(Preparation time: 10 minutes | Cooking time: 45 minutes | Difficulty: Easy | Servings: 2)
Per serving: Calories 298, Total fat 5g, Protein 7g, Carbs 31g
Ingredients:
- Juice of a 1/4 lemon
- 2 cloves of garlic
- 1 teaspoon of finely chopped ginger
- 2 teaspoons of turmeric
- 1 teaspoon of olive oil
- 1 pinch of cumin
- 1 pinch of coriander
- 2 red onions, finely chopped
- 2 tablespoons of parsley, chopped
- 1/4 cup of red pepper, seeded
- 1 Thai chili, cut in two halves, seeded
- 1/4 cup of dried tomatoes, finely chopped

- 1 cup of tofu
- 1 cup of cauliflower, roughly chopped

Instructions:
- Preheat the oven at 400°F. Slice the peppers & combine them with the chili and garlic in an ovenproof dish. Pour some olive oil on top, sprinkle with the dried herbs, and bake till the peppers are tender (approximately 20 minutes). Allow cooling before combining the peppers with the lemon juice in a blender & blending until smooth.
- To make the triangles, cut the tofu in half & then in half again. In a small-sized casserole dish, add the tofu, cover with the paprika mixture, and bake for around 20 minutes.
- Chop the cauliflower into small pieces, about the size of a grain of rice.
- Then, in a small-sized saucepan, cook the garlic, onions, chili, and ginger with the olive oil till the garlic, onions, chili, and ginger are translucent. Add the turmeric and cauliflower, stir to combine, and reheat. Remove from the flame and stir in the parsley and tomatoes. Toss the tofu in the sauce before serving.

166. Turmeric Baked Salmon

(Preparation time: 10 minutes | Cooking time: 50 minutes | Difficulty: Easy | Servings: 2)
Per serving: Calories 25, Total fat 1g, Protein 2g, Carbs 5g
Ingredients:
- 1/4 Juice of a lemon
- 1 teaspoon of ground turmeric
- 1 teaspoon of extra virgin olive oil
- 125-150g of skinned salmon

For the fiery celery
- 1 teaspoon of extra virgin olive oil
- 1 cm of fresh ginger, finely shredded
- 1 garlic clove, finely shredded

- 1 tablespoon of chopped parsley
- 1 red onion, finely shredded
- 2 to 3 tomatoes, cut into eight wedges
- 1 Bier's eye bean stew, finely shredded
- 1/4 cup of tinned green lentils
- 150g of celery, cut into 2cm lengths
- 1 teaspoon of mild curry powder
- 1/2 cup of chicken or vegetable stock

Instructions:

- Preheat the grill at 400°F.
- Begin with the smoky celery. Warm the olive oil in a skillet over medium-low flame, then add the ginger, onion, garlic, bean stew, & celery. Fry delicately for 2–3 minutes, or till softened but not colored, then add the curry powder & cook for a few more minutes. Cook for 10 minutes on low flame with the red tomato, stock, and lentils. Depending on how crispy you prefer your celery, you may need to increase or decrease the cooking time.
- In the meantime, combine the turmeric, oil, & lemon juice and spread it all over the salmon. Cook, covered, for 8–10 minutes on a hot plate. To finish, toss the parsley with the celery & serve with the salmon.

167. Prawn Arrabbiata

(Preparation time: 10 minutes | Cooking time: 55 minutes | Difficulty: Easy | Servings: 2)
Per serving: Calories 115, Total fat 30g, Protein 18g, Carbs 15g
Ingredients:

- 1 tablespoon of Extra virgin olive oil
- 1/4 cup of Buckwheat pasta
- 125-150g of raw or cooked prawns (Ideally ruler prawns)

For arrabbiata sauce

- 1 teaspoon of extra virgin olive oil
- 1 garlic clove, finely shredded
- 1 Bird's eye bean stew, finely hacked

- 1 tablespoon of chopped parsley
- 1 teaspoon of dried, blended herbs
- 1 red onion, finely shredded
- 1/4 cup of celery, finely shredded
- 2 cups of shredded tomatoes
- 2 tablespoons of white wine (discretionary)

Instructions:

- In a medium-low flame, fry the onion, bean stew, garlic, celery, and dry herbs in the oil for 1–2 minutes. Increase the flame to medium-high, then add the wine & cook for one minute. Add the tomatoes & simmer for 20–30 minutes over medium-low flame, till the sauce has a nice creamy consistency. If the sauce becomes too thick, a little water can be added to thin it up.
- Bring a pot of water to the boil as the sauce cooks, & cook the pasta according to the package directions. When everything is to your liking, channel, toss with the olive oil, and keep in the jar till needed.
- If using raw prawns, combine them with the sauce & bake for another 3–4 minutes, or till the sauce has turned pink & black. Garnish with parsley and serve. If using cooked prawns, combine them with the parsley and continue with the sauce.
- Add the pasta to the sauce, mix well but softly, and serve.

168. Lamb, Date and Butternut Squash Tagine

(Preparation time: 10 minutes | Cooking time: 25 minutes | Difficulty: Easy | Servings: 2)
Per serving: Calories 134, Total fat 2g, Protein 18g, Carbs 15g
Ingredients:

- ½ teaspoon of salt
- 2 tablespoons of olive oil

- 2 teaspoons of ground turmeric
- 1 cinnamon stick
- 3 garlic cloves, ground or squashed
- 2cm ginger, ground
- 1 red onion, cut
- 2 teaspoons of cumin seeds
- 2 tablespoons of coriander
- 1 teaspoon of stew pieces (or to taste)
- 1/4 cup of Medjool dates, hollowed and hacked
- 2 cups of chickpeas, depleted
- 2 cups of butternut squash, chopped
- 2 cups of tin chopped tomatoes
- 800g of sheep neck filet, cut into 2cm pieces
- Buckwheat, couscous, flatbreads or rice to serve

Instructions:

- Preheat your oven at 320°F.
- In a large-sized ovenproof pot or cast iron meal dish, drizzle around two teaspoons of olive oil. Add the sliced onion and cook for around 5 minutes on a low flame, covered, till the onions have mellowed but are not dark-colored.
- Add the garlic and ginger powders, as well as the bean stew, cumin, cinnamon, and turmeric. Cook, constantly stirring, for one minute at a time, with the cover off. If it becomes too dry, add a splash of water.
- Add the sheep pieces next. Mix thoroughly to coat the meat in the onions and spices, then add the salt, sliced dates, and tomatoes, as well as about a third of a jar of water (100-200ml).
- Bring the tagine to a boil, then cover it and place it in your preheated oven for 1 hour & 15 minutes.
- Add the sliced butternut squash & depleted chickpeas 30 minutes before

the end of the cooking time. Return to the stove for about the last 30 minutes of cooking after mixing everything together.
- When the tagine is finished, remove it from the flame and stir in the chopped coriander. Serve with buckwheat, couscous, flatbreads, or brown rice as an accompaniment.

169. Green Quinoa Tabbouleh

(Preparation time: 10 minutes | Cooking time: 20 minutes | Difficulty: Easy | Servings: 4)
Per serving: Calories 302, Total fat 23g, Protein 10g, Carbs 33g
Ingredients:

- 6 cups water
- 2 lemons, halved
- A pinch of freshly ground black pepper
- A pinch of cayenne pepper
- 2 cloves of garlic
- 1/2 cup of extra-virgin olive oil
- 1 large bunch of stemmed fresh mint
- 1 bunch of stemmed fresh tarragon
- 2 large bunches of stemmed curly parsley
- 2 cups of white quinoa

Instructions:

- Bring a pot of water to the boil, and have an ice water dish on hand. Combine half of the mint, half of the parsley, & half of the tarragon. Before scooping herbs into cold water, they must be blanched for 5 seconds. Allow 2 minutes for complete cooling. Drain and squeeze out as much water as possible.
- Rinse the quinoa thoroughly. Cook for around 12 minutes over medium flame, stirring occasionally, or till the quinoa is just barely cooked.
- In the meantime, chop the leftover herbs into tiny pieces.

- In a blender, combine the garlic and the blanched herbs. Drizzle with the olive oil and squeeze in the lemon juice. Blend on low speed till smooth & green dressing is achieved, then increase to high speed and blend till smooth & green dressing is achieved.
- Remove the quinoa from the flame and drain in a colander over a bowl for around 5 minutes, stirring occasionally. In a bowl, place the quinoa. To taste, season using black pepper and cayenne pepper. Allow it to cool for 5 to 10 minutes till it reaches a temperature that is between warm and room temperature.
- Combine the quinoa and the dressing in a mixing bowl. Continue cooling the salad for another 5 to 10 minutes if it is not at room temperature. Add the chopped herbs and stir until everything is nicely mixed. Wrap the dish in plastic wrap & chill for 2 hours, or until the flavors have blended.
- Season the salad to taste & make any necessary adjustments. A serving plate should be used to serve the salad.

170. Shredded Chicken Bowls

(Preparation time: 10 minutes | Cooking time: 35 minutes | Difficulty: Easy | Servings: 2)
Per serving: Calories 320, Total fat 6g, Protein 21g, Carbs 12g
Ingredients:

- ½ Lime
- 1 teaspoon of garlic powder
- 2 teaspoons of extra virgin olive oil
- 1 teaspoon of onion powder
- 2 cups of broth
- 1 cup of cherry tomatoes
- 2 cups of kale
- 8 oz. of chicken breast
- 2 ripe avocados

Instructions:

- In a saucepan, combine the chicken breasts, salt, pepper, onion, and garlic powder. Bring the stock to a boil, then cover and simmer for around 30 to 40 minutes, or till the meat begins to shred.
- Remove the chicken from the soup, shred it with a fork, and set aside.
- In a serving bowl, start with the kale.
- In a mixing dish, combine the shredded chicken, sliced avocado, and cherry tomatoes.
- Just before serving, make the dressing with lime, oil, salt, & pepper and spread it over the salad.

171. Creamy Turkey and Asparagus

(Preparation time: 10 minutes | Cooking time: 30 minutes | Difficulty: Easy | Servings: 2)
Per serving: Calories 353, Total fat 5g, Protein 28g, Carbs 20g
Ingredients:

- Salt and pepper
- 2 cloves garlic
- 2 teaspoons of extra virgin olive oil
- ½ bird's eye chili
- ½ red onion
- 2 cups of asparagus
- 8 oz. turkey breast
- ½ cup of full-fat coconut milk

Instructions:

- Heat the oil, onion, garlic, and chili in a pan over medium-high flame for around 5 minutes.
- Cook for another 5 minutes, or till the turkey is brown on all sides.
- Add the asparagus, chopped into 2-inch pieces, and the coconut milk after 2 minutes.
- Allow for a 25-minute simmer or till the sauce is creamy.

172. Asian Beef Salad

(Preparation time: 10 minutes | Cooking time: 10 minutes | Difficulty: Easy | Servings: 2)
Per serving: Calories 262, Total fat 12g, Protein 25g, Carbs 15g
Ingredients:

- ½ bird's eye chili
- 3 tablespoons of lemon juice
- 3 teaspoons of extra virgin olive oil
- 1 handful of parsley
- 1 tablespoon of soy sauce
- ½ red onion, finely sliced
- ½ cucumber, sliced
- ½ cup of cherry tomatoes halved
- 2 cups of lettuce
- 8 oz. sirloin steaks

Instructions:

- Crush the garlic and combine it with finely chopped chili and parsley, 2 tablespoons olive oil, and soy sauce in a mixing bowl. This is going to be the dressing.
- Place lettuce on the bottom of a salad bowl, followed by onion, cherry tomatoes, and cucumber.
- Heat a skillet over a high flame. Brush the remaining oil over the steaks, season using salt and pepper, and cook to your liking. Before slicing, place the steaks on a cutting board for 5 minutes.
- Drizzle the dressing over the salad and toss to combine. Serve with steak slices on top.

173. Creamy Chicken and Broccoli Casserole

(Preparation time: 10 minutes | Cooking time: 30 minutes | Difficulty: Easy | Servings: 2)
Per serving: Calories 353, Total fat 5g, Protein 28g, Carbs 20g
Ingredients:

- 1/2 red onion
- ½ cup of broth
- 1 tablespoon of almond flour
- 3 cups of broccoli
- 1 cup of mushrooms
- 2 tablespoons of Parmesan
- 8 oz. of chicken breast, cubed
- 2 tablespoons of red wine

Instructions:

- Preheat the oven at 350°F. To keep the vibrant green color, steam the broccoli for around 5 minutes, then drain and cool in water and ice.
- Chicken breasts should be cut into medium-sized cubes. Combine the chicken and broccoli in a baking dish.
- Make the creamy sauce by combining all of the ingredients. On a low flame, sauté the onion in olive oil, then increase to high flame, add the mushrooms, a pinch of salt & pepper, and the flour, and mix well.
- Mix in the wine till it has completely evaporated. Cook for around 5 minutes after adding the broth, then puree by hand till smooth.
- Cook in the oven for around 30-35 minutes after pouring the sauce over the chicken & broccoli and topping with 2 tablespoons of Parmesan. For the last 5 minutes, turn on the broiler.

174. Spicy Turmeric Salmon with Lentils

(Preparation time: 10 minutes | Cooking time: 30 minutes | Difficulty: Easy | Servings: 4)
Per serving: Calories 177, Total fat 20g, Protein 12g, Carbs 4g
Ingredients:

- 1/4 juice of a lemon
- 1 teaspoon of turmeric
- 1 garlic clove, finely chopped
- 1 teaspoon of extra virgin olive oil
- 1 tablespoon of parsley, chopped

- 1 bird's eye chili, finely chopped
- ½ red onion, finely chopped
- 1 large tomato, cut into 8 wedges
- 1 teaspoon of mild curry powder
- 1 cup of chicken or vegetable stock
- 1/2 cup of celery cut into 2cm sticks
- 1/2 cup of lentils, canned
- 8 oz. of Skinned salmon

Instructions:

- Preheat the oven at 400°F. Heat the olive oil in a frying pan over medium-low flame, then add the onion, garlic, ginger, chili, & celery.
- Cook for 2–3 minutes, or till softened, then add the curry powder & cook for another minute.
- Simmer for 10 minutes after adding the tomatoes, stock, and lentils. Depending on how crunchy you prefer your celery, you may choose to increase or decrease the cooking time.
- Meanwhile, massage the salmon with a mixture of turmeric, oil, & lemon juice. Cook for around 8–10 minutes on a baking tray.
- Finish by sprinkling parsley over the celery & serving with the fish.

175. Lemon Chicken Skewers with Peppers

(Preparation time: 10 minutes | Cooking time: 20 minutes | Difficulty: Easy | Servings: 8)
Per serving: Calories 315, Total fat 21g, Protein 16g, Carbs 5g
Ingredients:

- Salt and pepper
- ½ lemon, juiced
- ½ teaspoon of turmeric
- 1 garlic clove
- 3 teaspoons of extra virgin olive oil
- ½ teaspoon of paprika
- 1 handful of parsley, chopped
- 1 cup of tomatoes, chopped

- 2 cups of peppers, chopped
- 8 oz. of chicken breast

Instructions:

- Cut the breast into tiny cubes and marinate for 30 minutes in oil and spices.
- Set the skewers aside after preparing them.
- Oil should be heated in a pan. When the pan is hot, add the garlic and simmer for 5 minutes before removing the clove.
- Cook for around 5-10 minutes on high flame with peppers, tomatoes, salt, and pepper.
- Heat a second pan to high flame, then add the skewers and cook for 10-12 minutes, till brown on all sides. Along with the peppers, serve the skewers.

176. Ginger and Lemon Shrimp Salad

(Preparation time: 10 minutes | Cooking time: 10 minutes | Difficulty: Easy | Servings: 2)
Per serving: Calories 353, Total fat 5g, Protein 28g, Carbs 20g
Ingredients:

- Juice of ½ lemon
- 1 pinch of chili
- 2 teaspoons of extra virgin olive oil
- 1 cup of chicory leaves
- ½ cup of arugula
- ½ cup of baby spinach
- 1 avocado-peeled, stoned, and sliced
- 6 walnuts, chopped
- 8 oz. of shrimps

Instructions:

- On a big platter, combine chicory, baby spinach, and arugula. Heat a pan on medium flame with 1 tablespoon of oil and cook the shrimps with chili, salt, pepper and garlic till they are not transparent anymore. Combine the avocado, oil, lemon juice, and a bit of salt and pepper in a blender, then pour the dressing over the salad.

- Chop the walnuts and serve as the last element on the plate.

177. Creamy Chicken and Mushroom Soup

(Preparation time: 10 minutes | Cooking time: 40 minutes | Difficulty: Easy | Servings: 3)
Per serving: Calories 302, Total fat 4g, Protein 15g, Carbs 16g
Ingredients:

- 1 tablespoon of extra virgin olive oil
- 1 red onion, finely diced
- 3 leaves of sage
- 2 cups of vegetable stock
- 1 carrot, finely diced
- 1 stick of celery, finely diced
- 1 cup of mixed mushrooms, sliced
- 4 oz. chicken breast, cubed

Instructions:

- In a skillet, heat 1 tablespoon of oil & sauté the chicken till it is gently browned. Set them aside.
- Cook for around 3 to 5 minutes in a heated pan with 1 tablespoon of oil, celery, carrot, onion, & sage.
- Add the stock and cook for another 5 minutes, then puree the soup with a hand blender till smooth.
- Cook for another 8 to 10 minutes, or till the chicken is creamy.

178. Turkey and Arugula with Italian Dressing

(Preparation time: 10 minutes | Cooking time: 30 minutes | Difficulty: Easy | Servings: 2)
Per serving: Calories 165, Total fat 3g, Protein 26g, Carbs 14g
Ingredients:

- Salt and pepper to taste
- 2 teaspoons of extra virgin olive oil
- 1 tablespoon of cumin

- 2 teaspoons of oregano
- 2 teaspoons of Dijon mustard
- 1 cup of arugula - 1 cup of lettuce
- 1/4 cup of scallions, sliced
- 1/2 cup of celery, finely diced
- 8 oz. of turkey breast

Instructions:

- Shred the turkey once it has been grilled. Set them aside.
- On a plate, combine lettuce and arugula. Distribute the shredded turkey, celery, and scallions evenly.
- Combine all dressing ingredients in a small-sized bowl, including mustard, oil, salt, lemon juice, oregano, and pepper, and pour over the salad immediately before serving.

179. Mince Stuffed Peppers

(Preparation time: 10 minutes | Cooking time: 50 minutes | Difficulty: Easy | Servings: 4)
Per serving: Calories 375, Total fat 8g, Protein 15g, Carbs 24g
Ingredients:

- Salt and pepper, to taste
- Few drops of lemon juice
- 2 teaspoons of extra virgin olive oil
- 2 tablespoons of breadcrumbs
- Cooking spray - 1 egg
- 2 large yellow peppers
- 2 red bell peppers - 2 cups of arugula
- ¼ cup of brown rice, cooked
- 1 tablespoon of parmesan
- 1/4 cup of mozzarella
- ¼ cup of walnuts, chopped
- 4 oz. of lean mince

Instructions:

- Preheat the oven at 350°F.
- Combine the mince, egg, parmesan, brown rice, and mozzarella in a mixing bowl. Set aside after thoroughly mixing. Remove the seeds from the peppers, fill them with mince mixture, and place

them on a baking pan. To get a crispy top without adding calories, sprinkle breadcrumbs on top, then lightly spray using cooking spray.

- Cook till the peppers are tender, around 50-60 minutes. Allow cooling for a few minutes before serving. Serve the stuffed peppers alongside an arugula salad with olive oil, salt, and a squeeze of lemon.

180. Trout with Roasted Veggies

(Preparation time: 15 minutes | Cooking time: 20 minutes | Difficulty: Easy | Servings: 2)
Per serving: Calories 154, Total fat 2g, Protein 24g, Carbs 14g
Ingredients:

- 1 lemon, juiced
- Extra virgin olive oil - Dried dill
- 2 carrots cut into sticks
- 2 parsnips, peeled and cut into wedges
- 2 turnips, peeled and chopped
- 2 tablespoons of tamari
- 2 trout fillets

Instructions:

- Fill a baking tray halfway with cut vegetables. Add a splash of tamari & olive oil to finish. Preheat the oven at 400°F. After 25 minutes, remove the veggies from the oven and toss thoroughly. Place the fish on top of it. Drizzle with lemon juice & dill. Return to the oven, cover with foil.
- Reduce the oven temperature at 375°F & cook for around 20 minutes, or till the fish is cooked through.

181. Chicken Curry with Kale and Potatoes

(Preparation time: 15 minutes | Cooking time: 45 minutes | Difficulty: Easy | Servings: 4)
Per serving: Calories 394, Total fat 22g, Protein 25g, Carbs 32g

Ingredients:

- 3 tablespoons of turmeric
- 3 cloves of garlic, finely chopped
- 4 tablespoons of extra virgin olive oil
- 1 tablespoon of curry powder
- 1 tablespoon of coriander, chopped
- 2 tablespoons of parsley, chopped
- 2 pieces of cardamom
- 1 cinnamon stick
- 1 tablespoon of freshly chopped ginger
- 2 red onions, sliced
- 2 bird's eye chilies, finely chopped
- 3 cups of potatoes
- 2 cups of small tomatoes
- 1 cup of kale, chopped
- 2 cups of chicken broth
- 600g of chicken breast, cut into pieces
- 1 cup of coconut milk

Instructions:

- For around 30 minutes, marinate the chicken in a teaspoon of olive oil & a tablespoon of turmeric. Then cook for around 4 minutes in a hot frying pan over a high flame. Remove the pan from the flame and set it aside.
- In a pan with chili, garlic, onion, & ginger, heat a tablespoon of oil. Cook for another two minutes over medium flame, stirring regularly, after adding the curry powder & a tablespoon of turmeric. Cook for another two minutes with the tomatoes before adding the chicken stock, coconut milk, cardamom, & cinnamon stick. Cook for around 45 to 60 minutes, adding more broth as needed.
- Preheat the oven at 425°F. Potatoes should be peeled and chopped. Bring the water to a boil, then add the turmeric-infused veggies & cook for around 5 minutes. Then pour out the water and wait 10 minutes for it to evaporate. On a baking tray, toss the

potatoes with olive oil and bake for around 30 minutes.

- When the potatoes & curry are almost done, add the coriander, kale, & chicken and cook for another five minutes, or till the chicken is thoroughly heated.
- Serve the potatoes with the chicken curry and parsley.

182. Fried Chicken with Broccolini

(Preparation time: 15 minutes | Cooking time: 45 minutes | Difficulty: Easy | Servings: 4)
Per serving: Calories 198, Total fat 24g, Protein 48g, Carbs 9g
Ingredients:

- 2 tablespoons of olive oil
- 1 1/4 cups of broccolini
- 150g of bacon cubes
- 400g of chicken breast

Instructions:

- Chicken should be cut into cubes.
- In a pan over medium flame, heat the olive oil & brown the chicken with bacon cubes till done.
- Add chili flakes, salt, and pepper to taste.
- Toss in the broccolini and cook for a few minutes.
- Arrange on a plate & eat!

183. Chicken Rolls with Pesto

(Preparation time: 15 minutes | Cooking time: 20 minutes | Difficulty: Easy | Servings: 4)
Per serving: Calories 105, Total fat 36g, Protein 87g, Carbs 7g
Ingredients:

- 1 clove of garlic (chopped)
- 2 tablespoons of fresh basil
- 3 tablespoons of olive oil
- 2 tablespoons of pine nuts
- 2 tablespoons of yeast flakes
- 2 pieces of chicken breast

Instructions:

- Preheat the oven at 280°F.
- In a dry pan over medium flame, toast the pine nuts for around 3 minutes, or till golden brown. Place the chicken on a platter and set it aside.
- In a food processor, finely crush the pine nuts, yeast flakes, and garlic.
- Combine the basil & oil and stir briskly till a pesto forms.
- Add salt & pepper to taste.
- Each chicken breast should be sandwiched between two pieces of cling film.
- Using a saucepan or rolling pin, pound the chicken breasts till they are about 0.6 cm thick.
- Remove the cling film from the chicken and put the pesto on top.
- To keep the chicken breasts together, roll them up and secure them with cocktail skewers.
- Add salt & pepper to taste.
- In a saucepan, heat the olive oil and cook the chicken rolls on all sides over high flame.
- Set the chicken rolls into a baking tray, place in the oven, and bake till done around 15-20 minutes.
- Cut the rolls in half diagonally & serve with the remaining pesto.

184. Avocado and Salmon Salad Buffet

(Preparation time: 15 minutes | Cooking time: 0 minutes | Difficulty: Easy | Servings: 4)
Per serving: Calories 209, Total fat 21g, Protein 9g, Carbs 23g
Ingredients:

- ½ red onion
- ½ cucumber
- 1 piece of avocado

- 250g of mixed salad
- 4 slices of smoked salmon

Instructions:

- Cucumber and avocado should be cut into cubes, and the onion should be chopped.
- Place the lettuce leaves on deep plates & top them with the cucumber, avocado, and onion.
- Add salt and pepper to taste (you can also add a little olive oil to the salad).
- Serve with smoked salmon slices on top.

185. Tilapia Veracruz

(Preparation time: 10 minutes | Cooking time: 20 minutes | Difficulty: Easy | Servings: 4)
Per serving: Calories 148, Total fat 5g, Protein 22g, Carbs 6g
Ingredients:

- 1/4 cup of water
- 1 diced onion
- 1 tablespoon of olive oil
- 1 teaspoon of dried oregano
- 1 cup of chopped tomatoes
- 1/2 cup of chopped bell pepper
- 4 tilapia fillets

Instructions:

- Heat the olive oil in a pan & add the tilapia fillets.
- Cook the fish for about 4 minutes on each side. Remove the fish from the skillet.
- Cook for around 2 minutes in the skillet with the onion.
- Toss in the bell peppers, oregano, & tomatoes after that. Combine the ingredients in a saucepan and cook for 5 minutes.
- Add the fish and the water after that.
- Close the lid and cook for another 5 minutes.

186. Salmon with Capers

(Preparation time: 10 minutes | Cooking time: 15 minutes | Difficulty: Easy | Servings: 4)
Per serving: Calories 173, Total fat 8g, Protein 23g, Carbs 2g
Ingredients:

- Salt and black pepper to taste
- 2 tablespoons of olive oil
- 1 tablespoon of capers
- 1/2 cup of skim milk
- 1-pound of salmon fillet

Instructions:

- In a medium-high-heat pan, heat the oil, then add the salmon & roast for around 5 minutes.
- With capers, milk, salt and black pepper sauté the meal for 10 minutes over medium flame.

187. Curry Snapper

(Preparation time: 10 minutes | Cooking time: 15 minutes | Difficulty: Easy | Servings: 4)
Per serving: Calories 195, Total fat 6g, Protein 29g, Carbs 3g
Ingredients:

- 1/4 cup of water
- Salt and black pepper to taste
- 1 tablespoon of olive oil
- 1 teaspoon of curry powder
- 1/2 cup of low-fat yogurt
- 1 cup of chopped celery stalk
- 1-pound of snapper fillet, chopped

Instructions:

- Roast the snapper fillets in olive oil for around 2 minutes on each side.
- After that, add the celery stalk, low-fat yogurt, curry powder, salt, pepper and water.
- Stir the fish till it's all the same texture.
- Cook the fish for approximately 10 minutes on medium flame with the lid closed.

188. Shrimp Putanesca

(Preparation time: 10 minutes | Cooking time: 20 minutes | Difficulty: Easy | Servings: 3)
Per serving: Calories 128, Total fat 7g, Protein 12g, Carbs 6g
Ingredients:

- 1/4 cup of water
- Salt and black pepper to taste
- 1 teaspoon of garlic, diced
- 1 teaspoon of chili flakes
- 1 tablespoon of olive oil
- 1/2 diced red onion
- 1 cup of chopped tomatoes
- 1/4 cup of sliced olives
- 5 oz. of peeled shrimps

Instructions:

- Heat the olive oil in a saucepan.
- Combine the shrimp, pepper, salt and chili flakes in a mixing bowl. The cooking time for the shrimp is 4 minutes.
- Stir in the chopped onion, garlic, olives, tomatoes, & water till everything is well combined.
- Close the lid and cook the meal for around 15 minutes.

189. Parsley Trout

(Preparation time: 10 minutes | Cooking time: 15 minutes | Difficulty: Easy | Servings: 4)
Per serving: Calories 152, Total fat 9g, Protein 17g, Carbs 2g
Ingredients:

- Salt and black pepper to taste
- 2 tablespoons of olive oil
- 1 tablespoon of dried parsley
- 4 trout fillets

Instructions:

- The fish fillets should be massaged with salt, pepper and parsley.
- Then heat the olive oil in the same skillet. Cook for around 5 minutes on each side of the salmon fillets.

190. Salmon with Green Onions

(Preparation time: 10 minutes | Cooking time: 20 minutes | Difficulty: Easy | Servings: 4)
Per serving: Calories 272, Total fat 13g, Protein 35g, Carbs 3g
Ingredients:

- A pinch of salt - 1/2 tsp. of chili flakes
- 1/4 tsp. of ground black pepper
- 3 tablespoons of olive oil
- 2 tablespoons of chopped parsley
- 4 tablespoons of blended green onions
- 4 pitted and sliced green olives
- 4 salmon fillets, skinless and boneless

Instructions:

- In a blender, combine the green onions, ground black pepper, salt, chili flakes, avocado oil, & parsley.
- After that, the salmon fillets are coated with the green onion mixture before being placed in the heated skillet.
- Cook for around 5 minutes on each side.
- The grilled fish should be topped with sliced olives.

191. Cod Mash with Broccoli

(Preparation time: 10 minutes | Cooking time: 20 minutes | Difficulty: Easy | Servings: 4)
Per serving: Calories 186, Total fat 9g, Protein 22g, Carbs 6g
Ingredients:

- 1 cup of water
- A pinch of salt
- 1/2 teaspoon of ground black pepper
- 2 tablespoons of olive oil
- 1 chopped red onion
- 1 tablespoon of low-fat cream cheese
- 2 cups of chopped broccoli
- 4 cod fillets, boneless and chopped

Instructions:

- In a skillet with olive oil, roast the fish for around 2 minutes per side.

- Then, except for the cream cheese, combine all of the remaining ingredients & cook for around 18 minutes.
- After that, drain the water & completely combine the meal with the cream cheese.

192. Lemon Zested Seabass

(Preparation time: 10 minutes | Cooking time: 15 minutes | Difficulty: Easy | Servings: 4)
Per serving: Calories 215, Total fat 11g, Protein 27g, Carbs 2g
Ingredients:

- 1 cup of water
- A pinch of salt
- 1 diced garlic clove
- 2 tablespoons of olive oil
- 1 teaspoon of margarine
- 1/4 cup of lemon juice
- 1 tablespoon of grated lemon zest
- 1-pound of skinless and boneless sea bass fillets

Instructions:

- Melt the margarine in a skillet.
- Combine the garlic & olive oil. Do a one-minute roasting session.
- Before adding the seabass fillets to the skillet with the garlic, season them with salt, pepper, lemon zest and juice.
- Roast the fish for about 5 minutes per side on medium flame.

193. Stir-Fry Turkey

(Preparation time: 10 minutes | Cooking time: 25 minutes | Difficulty: Easy | Servings: 4)
Per serving: Calories 89, Total fat 1g, Protein 15g, Carbs 5g
Ingredients:

- A pinch of salt
- 1 teaspoon of olive oil
- 1 teaspoon of chili powder
- 1 teaspoon of potato starch

- 1 sliced red onion
- 1 julienned carrot
- ½ cup of low-sodium chicken broth
- 12 oz. of turkey fillet, sliced

Instructions:

- In a pot with olive oil, place the turkey fillet.
- Cook the chicken for 4 minutes on each side.
- Toss in the carrots, salt, onion, & chili powder after that. After stirring the ingredients, cook for about 10 minutes.
- In a mixing cup, add the chicken broth & potato starch.
- Pour the sauce over the turkey, then toss to combine.
- Cook for an additional 10 minutes.

194. Chicken Chop Suey

(Preparation time: 10 minutes | Cooking time: 30 minutes | Difficulty: Easy | Servings: 4)
Per serving: Calories 169, Total fat 6g, Protein 24g, Carbs 3g
Ingredients:

- A pinch of salt
- 1/2 teaspoon of chili flakes
- 2 tablespoons of avocado oil
- 1/2 chopped onion
- 1/4 cup of low-sodium soy sauce
- 1/2 cup of chopped mushrooms
- 1 cup of bean sprouts
- 1-pound of chicken fillet, chopped

Instructions:

- Heat the olive oil in a large-sized skillet.
- After adding the mushrooms, cook for around 2 minutes.
- After that, add the chopped onion and cook for around 5 minutes, stirring occasionally. Stir them occasionally to prevent them from burning.
- Place the cooked vegetables in the serving bowls.

- Then add the chicken to the same skillet & season it with salt and chili flakes. The cooking time is around 15 minutes. It should be stirred once in a while.
- Then add the bean sprouts and continue to cook for another 10 minutes.
- On top of the onion-mushroom combination, layer the chicken mixture.

195. Chicken and Veggie Wraps

(Preparation time: 10 minutes | Cooking time: 15 minutes | Difficulty: Easy | Servings: 3)
Per serving: Calories 217, Total fat 11g, Protein 25g, Carbs 3g
Ingredients:
- 1 tablespoon of olive oil
- 3 teaspoons of low-fat yogurt
- 3 lettuce leaves
- 3 celery stalks
- 1 teaspoon of rotisserie chicken seasonings - 1 carrot, cut into sticks
- 9 oz. of chicken fillet

Instructions:
- Once the chicken has been sliced, place it in the skillet.
- Roast the chicken slices for around 5 minutes on each side, or till light brown, after adding the olive oil.
- After that, allow the chicken to cool somewhat before placing it on the lettuce leaves.
- Put the carrots & celery stalks. Serve the ingredients wrapped in yogurt.

196. Piccata Chicken

(Preparation time: 10 minutes | Cooking time: 15 minutes | Difficulty: Easy | Servings: 3)
Per serving: Calories 188, Total fat 8g, Protein 25g, Carbs 3g
Ingredients:
- A pinch of salt
- 1 teaspoon of ground black pepper
- 3 tablespoons of lemon juice

- 1 tablespoon of olive oil
- 1 tablespoon of whole-grain wheat flour - 1 tablespoon of capers
- 1/3 cup of low-sodium chicken stock
- 9 oz. of chicken fillet

Instructions:
- Dust the chicken fillet with flour after cutting it into small pieces.
- Then, heat the olive oil in the skillet, add the chicken, then roast it for 2 minutes on each side.
- After that, add the ground black pepper, salt, chicken stock, lemon juice, and capers. After properly stirring the chicken, close the lid.
- Cook for another 5 to 7 minutes, then serve the chicken piccata.

197. Turkey Casserole

(Preparation time: 10 minutes | Cooking time: 25 minutes | Difficulty: Easy | Servings: 4)
Per serving: Calories 211, Total fat 9g, Protein 24g, Carbs 8g
Ingredients:
- A pinch of salt
- 1 teaspoon of chili flakes
- 1 tablespoon of olive oil
- 1 chopped bird's eye chili
- 1 cup of chopped broccoli
- 1 cup of low-fat sour cream
- 1/4 cup of low-fat cheese, shredded
- 1 cup of ground turkey

Instructions:
- Brush the casserole dish using olive oil all over. Preheat the oven at 450°F.
- Then, in a prepared casserole shape, combine the ground turkey, salt & chili flakes. Make sure the mixture is well flattened.
- After that, top with broccoli, bird's eye chili, and fat-free sour cream.
- Cover with foil and sprinkle with shredded cheese.

198. Tasty Onion Chicken

(Preparation time: 10 minutes | Cooking time: 35 minutes | Difficulty: Easy | Servings: 4)

Per serving: Calories 232, Total fat 13g, Protein 24g, Carbs 3g

Ingredients:

- 1 cup of water
- A pinch of salt
- 3 tablespoons of olive oil
- 1/2 teaspoon of dried oregano
- 1 tablespoon of chopped parsley
- 1 cup of chopped red onion
- 1-pound of chicken breast, skinless and boneless

Instructions:

- In a medium-low-heat pan, heat 2 tablespoons of oil, then add the onion & cook for 5 minutes.
- Continue to cook for another 10 minutes, except the water, with the remaining ingredients.
- After that, add the water and cook the chicken for around 25 minutes while continually stirring.

199. Turkey and Mushrooms

(Preparation time: 10 minutes | Cooking time: 25 minutes | Difficulty: Easy | Servings: 4)

Per serving: Calories 188, Total fat 8g, Protein 26g, Carbs 4g

Ingredients:

- 1/3 cup of water
- A pinch of salt
- 2 tablespoons of olive oil
- 1 teaspoon of minced garlic
- 1 tablespoon of chopped rosemary
- 1/2 diced red onion
- 1/2 pound of white mushrooms halved
- 1-pound of sliced turkey fillet

Instructions:

- In a medium-sized pan, heat the oil, then add the onions and garlic and sauté for around 5 minutes.

- Thoroughly combine the remaining ingredients.
- Afterward, bake the entrée for 20 minutes at 425°F in a preheated oven.

200. Spring Chicken Mix

(Preparation time: 10 minutes | Cooking time: 30 minutes | Difficulty: Easy | Servings: 4)

Per serving: Calories 169, Total fat 6g, Protein 25g, Carbs 2g

Ingredients:

- 2 cups of water - A pinch of salt
- 1 tablespoon of olive oil
- 2 minced garlic cloves
- 1/2 teaspoon of white pepper
- 1 chopped red onion
- 1 cup of chopped kale
- 1 cup of chopped radish
- 1-pound of chicken breast, skinless, and boneless, chopped

Instructions:

- Heat the olive oil in a saucepan.
- After adding the chicken, cook for around 10 minutes.
- After that, add the remaining ingredients, cover, & cook for another 20 minutes.

201. Chicken and Collard Greens

(Preparation time: 10 minutes | Cooking time: 25 minutes | Difficulty: Easy | Servings: 4)

Per serving: Calories 150, Total fat 3g, Protein 25g, Carbs 4g

Ingredients:

- 4 cups of water
- A pinch of salt
- 1 teaspoon of ground black pepper
- 1/2 teaspoon of turmeric
- 1/2 teaspoon of smoked paprika
- 1 chopped red onion
- 2 cups of chopped collard greens
- 1-pound of chicken breast, skinless and boneless, chopped

Instructions:

- Close the saucepan's lid & add all of the ingredients.
- On medium heat, cook the meal for around 25 minutes.

202. Beef Sirloin with a Green Salad

(Preparation time: 10 minutes | Cooking time: 30 minutes | Difficulty: Easy | Servings: 4)
Per serving: Calories 326, Total fat 43g, Protein 79g, Carbs 7g
Ingredients:

- A pinch of salt
- Freshly ground pepper
- 2 tablespoons of olive oil
- Small rocket bag
- 1 1/2 pounds of sirloin of beef

For the green salad:

- Juice of a lemon
- 5 tablespoons of extra-virgin olive oil
- 1 tablespoon of finely chopped parsley
- 4 finely chopped spring onions
- 1 1/2 tablespoons of finely chopped capers - 3 tablespoons of finely chopped gherkins

Instructions:

- Preheat the oven at 450°F.
- Massage the meat with the oil.
- Season using salt and black pepper to taste after that.
- Cook for 10 minutes in the oven with the meat onto a baking pan.
- Reduce the oven temperature to 400°F and roast for around 20 minutes.
- Take the baking sheet out of the oven and place it on a cooling rack.
- Combine the capers, gherkins, freshly chopped parsley, spring onions, lemon juice, and extra virgin olive oil in a mixing bowl to prepare the green salad.
- Serve the meat on a platter, sliced into thin slithers. Finish with a dollop of salsa Verde and a sprinkling of rocket leaves.

203. Spicy Beef Stew

(Preparation time: 10 minutes | Cooking time: 30 minutes | Difficulty: Easy | Servings: 4)
Per serving: Calories 338, Total fat 14g, Protein 33g, Carbs 25g
Ingredients:

- A pinch of salt
- 2 tablespoons of olive oil
- 3 finely chopped garlic cloves
- 1 finely chopped bird's eye chili
- 1 tablespoon of fresh coriander
- 1 finely chopped red onion
- 1 sliced celery stick
- 2 cups of tinned tomatoes
- 2 medium sliced red bell peppers
- 2 cups of cannellini beans
- 1/2 pound of lean beef mince

Instructions:

- In a large-sized saucepan, heat the vegetable oil over medium flame & sauté the onions for around 2 minutes.
- Cook for another 2 minutes after adding the garlic & chilies.
- Cook for another 4 minutes after adding the red bell peppers & celery.
- In a large-sized skillet, brown the lean beef mince on all sides. This task will take you about 4-5 minutes to complete.
- After that, toss in the tomatoes & beans. Reduce the flame to low and cook for an additional 20 minutes.
- Serve with brown rice & salsa on the side.

204. Beef Stuffed Eggplants

(Preparation time: 10 minutes | Cooking time: 30 minutes | Difficulty: Easy | Servings: 4)
Per serving: Calories 195, Total fat 5g, Protein 25g, Carbs 16g
Ingredients:

- 1/4 cup of water
- A pinch of salt

- 1 teaspoon of black pepper
- Chopped fresh parsley
- 1 1/2 teaspoons of chopped garlic
- A pinch of paprika
- 2 cups of sliced green and red bell peppers
- 2 halved lengthwise eggplants
- 2 cups of sliced mushrooms
- 1-pound of boneless beef sirloin steak, visible fat trimmed & cut into 1/4-inch strips

Instructions:

- Preheat the oven at 450°F. Coat a baking dish using nonstick cooking spray.
- In a large-sized baking dish, place the eggplant halves facing-up. Poke the sliced sides with a fork in about 8 places. Bake for around 10 minutes after covering with foil.
- Meanwhile, spray a big nonstick skillet using nonstick cooking spray. With the garlic, salt & black pepper, cook for about 2 minutes over medium flame, stirring frequently. Cook & stir for 5 minutes after adding the beef.
- Cook for 5 minutes after adding the bell peppers. Cook for another 5 minutes after adding the mushrooms. Cover and add the water while stirring. Take the skillet off the heat.
- Take the eggplant out of the oven and lay it aside for 5 minutes to cool. The cooked centers of eggplant, but not the shells, should be mashed with a fork.
- Add a quarter of the meat mixture & mashed eggplant on each side. Bake for about 5 minutes after covering with foil. Remove the casserole from the oven. Paprika & parsley are optional garnishes.

205. Coconut Flavored Kale Chicken

(Preparation time: 10 minutes | Cooking time: 30 minutes | Difficulty: Easy | Servings: 4)
Per serving: Calories 237, Total fat 13g, Protein 26g, Carbs 5g

Ingredients:

- A pinch of salt and black pepper
- 2 minced garlic cloves
- 1 tablespoon of olive oil
- 1/2 teaspoon of basil, dried
- 1/2 teaspoon of sweet paprika
- 2 tablespoons of chopped parsley
- 2 chopped red onions
- 2 cups of kale
- 1/4 cup of low-sodium veggie stock
- 2/3 cup of coconut cream
- 1 pound of chicken breast, skinless, boneless and cubed

Instructions:

- In a medium-high flame, heat the oil & brown the meat, basil, & black pepper for about 5 minutes.
- After adding the onions & garlic, cook for another 5 minutes.
- Add the other ingredients, reduce to a low flame, and cook for another 15 minutes over medium flame.
- After splitting across plates, serve immediately.

206. Lemony Chicken with Leek

(Preparation time: 10 minutes | Cooking time: 30 minutes | Difficulty: Easy | Servings: 4)
Per serving: Calories 199, Total fat 13g, Protein 17g, Carbs 7g

Ingredients:

- A pinch of salt and black pepper
- 1/2 cup of lemon juice
- 2 tablespoons of olive oil
- 1 tablespoon of tomato sauce, no-salt-added
- 4 roughly chopped leek

- 1 cup of low-sodium veggie stock
- 1-pound of chicken breast, skinless, boneless and cubed

Instructions:
- In a skillet over medium flame, heat the oil, then add the leeks, mix well, and cook for around 15 minutes.
- Cook for another 15 minutes on medium flame with the chicken and the accompanying ingredients, then divide among plates and serve.

207. Chicken with Parsley-Lemon Gravy

(Preparation time: 10 minutes | Cooking time: 25 minutes | Difficulty: Easy | Servings: 4)
Per serving: Calories 193, Total fat 8g, Protein 24g, Carbs 5g

Ingredients:
- A pinch of salt
- 1 tablespoon of lemon zest
- 3 tablespoons of fresh lemon juice
- 2 tablespoons of butter
- 3 tablespoons of chopped fresh basil
- 2 tablespoons of almond flour
- 1 cup of low-sodium chicken stock
- 4 chicken breast halves boned and skinned

Instructions:
- Arrange the chicken breasts on a cutting board. Flatten lightly with the smooth side of a meat mallet. Make a fine flour coating on all sides of the chicken. Heat the oil in a large-sized skillet over medium-high flame. Cook chicken breasts in a skillet till lightly browned on both sides, around 6 minutes per side. Set the fillets aside after removing them from the pan.
- Meanwhile, in the same pan, combine the chicken stock, parsley, fresh lemon juice, salt, pepper & lemon zest. Cook for around 5 minutes with the lid on.

Cook for another 5 minutes after adding the cooked chicken.
- Place the chicken on a serving tray and continue to cook for another 5 minutes, or till the sauce has thickened. Toss the chicken with the sauce to coat it.

208. Curry Pork Chops

(Preparation time: 10 minutes | Cooking time: 25 minutes | Difficulty: Easy | Servings: 2)
Per serving: Calories 358, Total fat 28g, Protein 20g, Carbs 8g

Ingredients:
- A pinch of salt
- 1 tablespoon of olive oil
- 1 teaspoon of curry powder
- 1 red onion, diced
- 1/4 cup of soy milk
- 2 pork loin chops

Instructions:
- Heat the olive oil in a skillet.
- Roast the pork chops for around 5 minutes on each side.
- Remove the meat from the skillet & add the diced onion. Cook for about 4 minutes, or till the onion is tender.
- Stir in the curry powder, salt & soy milk after that.
- Bring everything to a boil in the pot.
- Cook the pork chops & coat them completely in curry sauce.
- Cook for 10 minutes on low flame with the lid closed.

209. Pork Roast in Orange Sauce

(Preparation time: 10 minutes | Cooking time: 40 minutes | Difficulty: Easy | Servings: 4)
Per serving: Calories 292, Total fat 11g, Protein 33g, Carbs 12g

Ingredients:
- A pinch of salt
- 1 teaspoon of Italian seasonings
- 1/2 cup of red onion, diced

- 1 tablespoon of potato starch
- 1/2 cup of celery stalk, chopped
- 1/2 cup of carrot, diced
- 1 cup of orange juice
- 1-pound of pork of loin roast

Instructions:

- Pork loin roast should be seasoned with Italian spices.
- Then add the carrot, celery stalk, & diced onion to the tray.
- Arrange the meat and vegetables on top of each other. In a separate bowl, combine the orange juice and the water.
- Preheat the oven to 450°F and roast the meat for around 30 minutes.
- In a saucepan, combine all of the vegetables & liquid and bring to a boil.
- Blend the components with the aid of the blender. Stir in the potato starch well.
- On low flame, cook the sauce for around 2 minutes.
- Slice the cooked meat, then top it with the orange sauce.

210. Beef Stew with Celery

(Preparation time: 10 minutes | Cooking time: 30 minutes | Difficulty: Easy | Servings: 4)
Per serving: Calories 150, Total fat 8g, Protein 15g, Carbs 5g
Ingredients:

- 2 cups of water
- A pinch of salt
- 1 diced garlic clove
- 1 tablespoon of olive oil
- 1 teaspoon of chili powder
- 1 teaspoon of dried dill
- 1 tablespoon of tomato paste
- 1 red onion, diced
- 2 cups of chopped celery stalk
- 1-pound of beef loin, chopped

Instructions:

- Roast the beef loin in an instant pot with olive oil for around 5 minutes.
- After that, add the remaining ingredients & close the lid.
- Cook the stew for around 25 minutes on high.

211. Turmeric Flavored Meatloaf

(Preparation time: 10 minutes | Cooking time: 30 minutes | Difficulty: Easy | Servings: 4)
Per serving: Calories 136, Total fat 5g, Protein 16g, Carbs 4g
Ingredients:

- A pinch of salt
- 1 teaspoon of ground turmeric
- 1 teaspoon of chili flakes
- 4 tablespoons of minced onion
- 1 teaspoon of olive oil
- 1 tablespoon of ketchup
- 1 egg, beaten
- 2 tablespoons of semolina
- 2 cups of lean ground beef

Instructions:

- The meatloaf mold should be coated using olive oil.
- Then, in a mixing dish, combine all of the above-mentioned ingredients.
- Place the meat mixture in the meatloaf and firmly push it down.
- Preheat the oven at 425°F & bake the meatloaf for around 30 minutes.
- Then, before slicing into servings, let it cool fully.

212. Turkey Parsnip

(Preparation time: 10 minutes | Cooking time: 30 minutes | Difficulty: Easy | Servings: 4)
Per serving: Calories 177, Total fat 7g, Protein 18g, Carbs 9g
Ingredients:

- 1 cup of water - A pinch of salt
- 2 tablespoons of olive oil

- 1 tablespoon of chopped parsley
- 1 chopped red onion
- 2 chopped parsnips
- 12 oz. of turkey fillet, sliced

Instructions:

- In a medium-sized pan, heat the oil, then add the onion and cook for around 5 minutes. Add the turkey and continue to cook for another 5 minutes.
- Toss in the other ingredients, cover, and simmer for around 20 minutes.

213. Shrimp Nectarine Salad

(Preparation time: 10 minutes | Cooking time: 10 minutes | Difficulty: Easy | Servings: 4)
Per serving: Calories 110, Total fat 6g, Protein 10g, Carbs 4g

Ingredients:

- A pinch of salt
- 1/4 tsp. of ground black pepper
- 1 teaspoon of lemon juice
- 1 tablespoon of olive oil
- 1 teaspoon of olive oil
- 1 nectarine pitted and chopped
- 1 cup of spring mix salad greens
- 6 oz. of peeled shrimps

Instructions:

- In a small-sized saucepan, heat the oil over low flame.
- Mix salt, ground black pepper & shrimp.
- The shrimps should then be fried for around 5 minutes on each side in the heated oil. Place the cooked shrimp in a salad bowl.
- Spring mix salad greens, chopped nectarine, olive oil, & lemon juice. Toss the salad together and serve.

214. Quinoa and Salmon Salad Bowl

(Preparation time: 10 minutes | Cooking time: 30 minutes | Difficulty: Easy | Servings: 4)
Per serving: Calories 282, Total fat 11g, Protein 16g, Carbs 14g

Ingredients:

- A pinch of salt
- 1 tablespoon of lime juice
- 2 tablespoons of plus 1 tsp. of olive oil, divided
- 2 teaspoons of honey
- 2 tablespoons of minced fresh chives
- 2 chopped red onions
- 1 1/4 cups of fresh corn kernels
- 3 cups of cooked quinoa
- 3/4 pound of skinned salmon fillets

Instructions:

- Preheat the oven at 350°F. Line a baking pan using foil. Place the fish on a baking sheet lined with foil. Season with a dash of black pepper, salt and 1 tablespoon olive oil. To build a package, cover it with a second piece of foil, then seal it. Bake for around 25 minutes.
- Mix the 2 tablespoons of olive oil, lime juice, and honey. In a large-sized mixing dish, combine the quinoa, onions, and corn. Mix all of the ingredients. Before serving, flake the salmon and gently combine it with the quinoa before garnishing with chives.

215. Chunky Chicken Soup

(Preparation time: 10 minutes | Cooking time: 30 minutes | Difficulty: Easy | Servings: 4)
Per serving: Calories 287, Total fat 6g, Protein 30g, Carbs 19g

Ingredients:

- A pinch of salt
- 1 teaspoon of olive oil
- 1 chopped red onion
- 1 cup of carrots thinly sliced
- 3 cups of sliced kale/baby spinach
- 2 cups of no-salt-added diced tomatoes (around 14 oz.) - 1 cup of fat-free and reduced-sodium chicken broth
- 1 cup of diced and cooked chicken breast

Instructions:

- In a large-sized saucepan over medium-high flame, warm the oil. Cook, frequently turning, for about 5 minutes, or till the onion is golden brown. Bring the carrots and stock to a boil after adding them. Reduce the flame to low & cook for around 5 to 10 minutes, uncovered.
- After adding the tomatoes, cook for another 5 minutes, or till the carrots are soft. Cook, constantly tossing, till the chicken is cooked through. Stir in the kale till it has wilted.

216. Grilled COD and Blue Cheese

(Preparation time: 10 minutes | Cooking time: 10 minutes | Difficulty: Easy | Servings: 4)
Per serving: Calories 91, Total fat 7g, Protein 7g, Carbs 1g
Ingredients:

- A pinch of salt
- 1 tablespoon of olive oil
- 1 teaspoon of sesame oil
- 1/2 teaspoon of ground coriander
- 1 teaspoon of apple cider vinegar
- 1/2 teaspoon of sesame seeds
- 1 cup of chopped arugula
- 2 tablespoons of crumbled blue cheese
- 12 oz. of cod fillet

Instructions:

- Preheat the grill at 390°F.
- Meanwhile, toss the cod fillets with the apple cider vinegar, powdered coriander, salt, and olive oil.
- On the grill, cook the salmon fillets for 4 minutes on each side.
- In a salad dish, add chopped arugula, sesame seeds, blue cheese, & sesame oil.
- When the fish is done, finely slice it and combine it with the salad.
- Shake it up and serve.

217. Chili Chicken Soup

(Preparation time: 10 minutes | Cooking time: 10 minutes | Difficulty: Easy | Servings: 4)
Per serving: Calories 228, Total fat 5g, Protein 22g, Carbs 20g
Ingredients:

- A pinch of salt
- 1 teaspoon of ground cumin
- 1/4 teaspoon of pepper
- 1/2 teaspoon of dried oregano
- 1/2 cup of chopped bird's eye chilies
- 1 chopped red onion
- 2 cups of low-sodium chicken broth
- 2 cups of cooked cannellini beans
- 1 pound of lean ground chicken

Instructions:

- Cook chicken and onion in a large-sized saucepan over medium-high flame, breaking up chicken into crumbles for 6 to 8 minutes, or till chicken is no longer pink.
- One can of beans should be mashed gently in a small-sized bowl. Bring the chicken, mashed beans, seasonings, leftover can of beans, chilies, & broth to a boil. Reduce to a low flame & cook, covered, for around 12-15 minutes, or till the flavors have blended. Garnish with toppings as desired.

218. Fennel Bulb Salad

(Preparation time: 10 minutes | Cooking time: 0 minutes | Difficulty: Easy | Servings: 4)
Per serving: Calories 181, Total fat 14g, Protein 7g, Carbs 11g
Ingredients:

- A pinch of salt
- 1 tablespoon of olive oil
- 1 cup of chopped fresh parsley
- 2 chopped fennel bulbs
- 1/2 cup of chopped walnuts
- 2 tablespoons of crumbled low-fat feta cheese

Instructions:

- Combine all of the ingredients in a salad bowl.
- Stir all of the ingredients together thoroughly.

219. Brown Rice Salad with Chicken and Snap Pea

(Preparation time: 10 minutes | Cooking time: 25 minutes | Difficulty: Easy | Servings: 4)
Per serving: Calories 326, Total fat 20g, Protein 16g, Carbs 17g
Ingredients:

- A pinch of salt
- 1/2 teaspoon of black pepper
- 1/2 teaspoon of red pepper flakes
- 1 clove of minced garlic
- 2/3 cup of olive oil
- 1/2 cup of sliced green onion
- 1/2 cup of chopped fresh parsley
- 1/2 cup of sliced celery
- 3 tablespoons of Dijon mustard
- 3 tablespoons of tarragon vinegar
- 1 teaspoon of crumbled dried tarragon
- 1/2 pound of sugar snaps peas. remove the strings
- 1/2 cup of cooked brown rice
- 1/2 cup of toasted chopped walnuts
- 2 cups of cubed cooked chicken
- 1 tablespoon of sweetener

Instructions:

- Mix together mustard, vinegar, sweetener, garlic, black pepper, salt, dried tarragon, and red pepper flakes in a small-sized mixing bowl till smooth. Set aside the safflower oil, which should be poured into the dressing in a thin, steady stream and whisked vigorously till thoroughly absorbed.
- Toss the chicken, parsley, celery, & green onion with the cooled brown rice. Stir in the dressing till everything is well

mixed. Refrigerate the rice mixture for at least 4 hours or up to 24 hours.

- A small saucepan of water should be brought to a boil. Cook, uncovered, for 30 seconds or till the sugar snap peas are just tender. Drain in a sieve and immediately soak in ice water for several minutes to stop the cooking process.
- After the peas have cooled, drain them and cut them into 1-inch diagonal slices. Put it in the fridge till you're ready to serve it. Add the peas and roasted walnuts to the rice mixture just before serving.

220. Toasted Buckwheat Tabbouleh

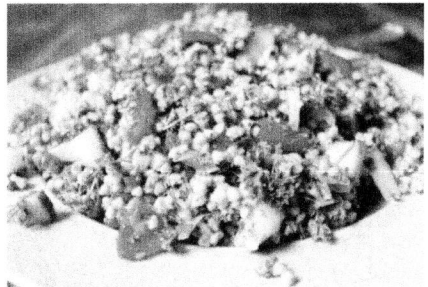

(Preparation time: 10 minutes | Cooking time: 15 minutes | Difficulty: Easy | Servings: 4)
Per serving: Calories 233, Total fat 5g, Protein 7g, Carbs 34g
Ingredients:

- A pinch of salt
- 1 juiced lemon
- 1 clove of minced garlic
- A pinch of dried mixed herbs
- 1 tablespoon of olive oil
- 2 peeled and chopped onions
- 3/4 cup of chopped fresh parsley
- 1 peeled and diced cucumber
- 6 tablespoons of chopped fresh mint
- 1 cup of kasha (toasted buckwheat groats)

Instructions:

- Buckwheat groats should be rinsed before cooking. Bring a pot of water to a boil, then add the buckwheat groats & simmer for 10 minutes, or till the buckwheat is tender. Drain the water and set it aside to cool.
- Heat the olive oil in a pan over medium flame, then sauté and stir the garlic and onions till the onion is transparent around 5 to 8 minutes. Allow cooling completely before serving.
- Toss cucumber, lemon juice, parsley, mint, salt & mixed herbs in a large-sized salad bowl till just combined; add cooked buckwheat and onion mixture.

221. Brown Rice and Mushroom Pilaf

(Preparation time: 10 minutes | Cooking time: 25 minutes | Difficulty: Easy | Servings: 4)
Per serving: Calories 163, Total fat 9g, Protein 4g, Carbs 19g
Ingredients:

- A pinch of salt
- 2 tablespoons of olive oil
- 2 tablespoons of chopped fresh parsley
- 1 chopped small onion
- 2 cups of low-sodium chicken broth
- 1/4 cup of chopped celery
- 1 1/2 cups of sliced mushrooms
- 2 cups of uncooked brown rice
- 1/2 cup of toasted and chopped walnuts

Instructions:

- Heat the oil in a medium-sized saucepan over medium flame. Cook for 3 minutes, or until onions & celery are crisp-tender, turning occasionally.
- Cook for 3 minutes, or till mushrooms are cooked, stirring occasionally. Add the broth and mix well. Bring the bring to the boil.

- Stir in the rice after covering it. Reduce the heat to medium-low and cook for another 5 minutes. Remove the pan from the flame and leave it aside for 5 minutes. Gently fold in the walnuts & parsley. Season using salt.

222. Shrimp Garlic Pasta

(Preparation time: 10 minutes | Cooking time: 25 minutes | Difficulty: Easy | Servings: 4)
Per serving: Calories 306, Total fat 32g, Protein 26g, Carbs 31g
Ingredients:

- A pinch of salt and black pepper to taste
- 1/2 teaspoon of red pepper flakes
- 4 cloves of finely chopped garlic
- 2 tablespoons of fresh lemon juice
- 2 tablespoons of olive oil extra-virgin
- 1/4 cup of parsley
- 1/4 cup of unsalted butter
- 1/2 cup of chicken broth
- 1 teaspoon of Old Bay seasoning
- 1 cup of uncooked buckwheat spaghetti
- 3/4 pound of medium shrimp, peeled and deveined
- 1/2 cup of half and half
- 2/3 cup of red wine

Instructions:

- Cook the buckwheat spaghetti as directed on the packet.
- Red pepper flakes, Old Bay seasoning, salt & pepper to taste are sprinkled over the shrimp.
- In a large-sized skillet, heat the oil. Cook for about 2 minutes with the shrimp and garlic, then turn & cook for another minute. Take the shrimp out of the pan and set them aside to cool.
- Deglaze the pan with red wine and fresh lemon juice. Combine the butter, chicken broth, & heavy cream. Cook for 5 minutes more, or till the liquid has reduced slightly.

- After draining the spaghetti, save one cup of the cooking liquid.
- Return the shrimp to the skillet & heat till cooked through. Mix parsley and cooked pasta. Cook, constantly stirring, until the pasta & parsley are done, adding more pasta water if necessary.

223. Baked Salmon Pasta with Lemon-Butter

(Preparation time: 10 minutes | Cooking time: 25 minutes | Difficulty: Easy | Servings: 4)
Per serving: Calories 316, Total fat 24g, Protein 30g, Carbs 29g
Ingredients:

- A pinch of salt and black pepper
- 3 tablespoons of fresh lemon juice
- 2 finely sliced garlic cloves
- 1 tablespoon of olive oil extra-virgin
- 4 tablespoons of margarine
- 1-pound of skinless and boneless salmon – one piece or multiple pieces

For the pasta:

- 1/4 cup of finely chopped parsley and dill
- 1/2 pound of buckwheat pasta

Instructions:

- Preheat the oven at 390°F.
- In a shallow baking dish, place the fish. Season using salt and pepper on both sides. Add the garlic & butter to the pan, along with a drizzle of olive oil and a squeeze of lemon juice.
- Bake for around 15 minutes or until the salmon is fully cooked.
- Allow it to cool before breaking it up into large chunks; tossing it will help it break up even more.

- In the same pan, combine the pasta & herbs. To coat the macaroni, gently toss it in the pan juices. If required, add more lemon. To taste, season with salt & pepper.

224. Pasta with Broccoli and Chicken

(Preparation time: 10 minutes | Cooking time: 20 minutes | Difficulty: Easy | Servings: 4)
Per serving: Calories 209, Total fat 21g, Protein 34g, Carbs 31g
Ingredients:

- A pinch of salt and black pepper
- 1 tablespoon of minced garlic
- 1/4 cup of olive oil
- 2 tablespoons of pesto
- 1 cup of chopped tomatoes
- 1/2 - a pound of fresh broccoli florets
- 1-pound of cooked and chopped boneless chicken breast halves
- 2 cups of buckwheat pasta
- 3/4 cup of low-fat grated Parmesan cheese

Instructions:

- In a large-sized saucepan of boiling water, cook buckwheat pasta till al dente. Drain. Blanch broccoli florets in a medium pot, then remove using a slotted spoon. In the same pan, sauté the minced garlic with pesto sauce for about 2 minutes in the olive oil. Add Place the chopped tomatoes and set them aside.
- In a large-sized mixing bowl, combine prepared pasta, cooked chicken, blanched broccoli, & garlic/tomato sauce. Add the grated Parmesan cheese, salt & freshly ground black pepper and stir to combine. Before serving, reheat the dish.

225. Herb-Crusted Pork Tenderloin

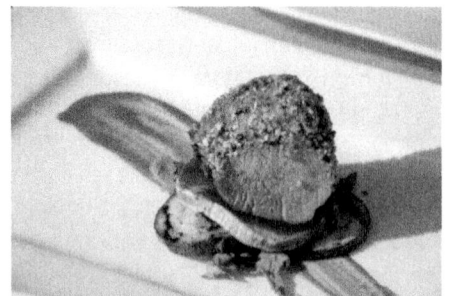

(Preparation time: 10 minutes | Cooking time: 25 minutes | Difficulty: Easy | Servings: 4)

Per serving: Calories 135, Total fat 7g, Protein 16g, Carbs 2g

Ingredients:

- A pinch of salt
- 1/4 teaspoon of ground black pepper
- 2 tablespoons of olive oil extra-virgin, divided
- 2 teaspoons of fresh parsley finely chopped - 2 teaspoons of fresh rosemary finely chopped
- 1 tablespoon of Dijon mustard
- 1 teaspoon of soy sauce
- 1 teaspoon of fresh thyme leaves
- 1-pound of pork tenderloin

Instructions:

- Preheat the oven at 390°F. Combine 1 tablespoon of olive oil, Dijon mustard, salt & soy sauce in a small cup. Coat the meat with a brush.
- Combine pepper, salt & fresh herbs in a small-sized cup. Season the pork using salt and pepper (or coat the pork in the mixture).
- In a skillet with 1 tablespoon of olive oil, brown the pork for about 2 minutes on each side over medium flame.
- Bake the pork for around 20 to 25 minutes.

CHAPTER 11:

Dinner Recipes

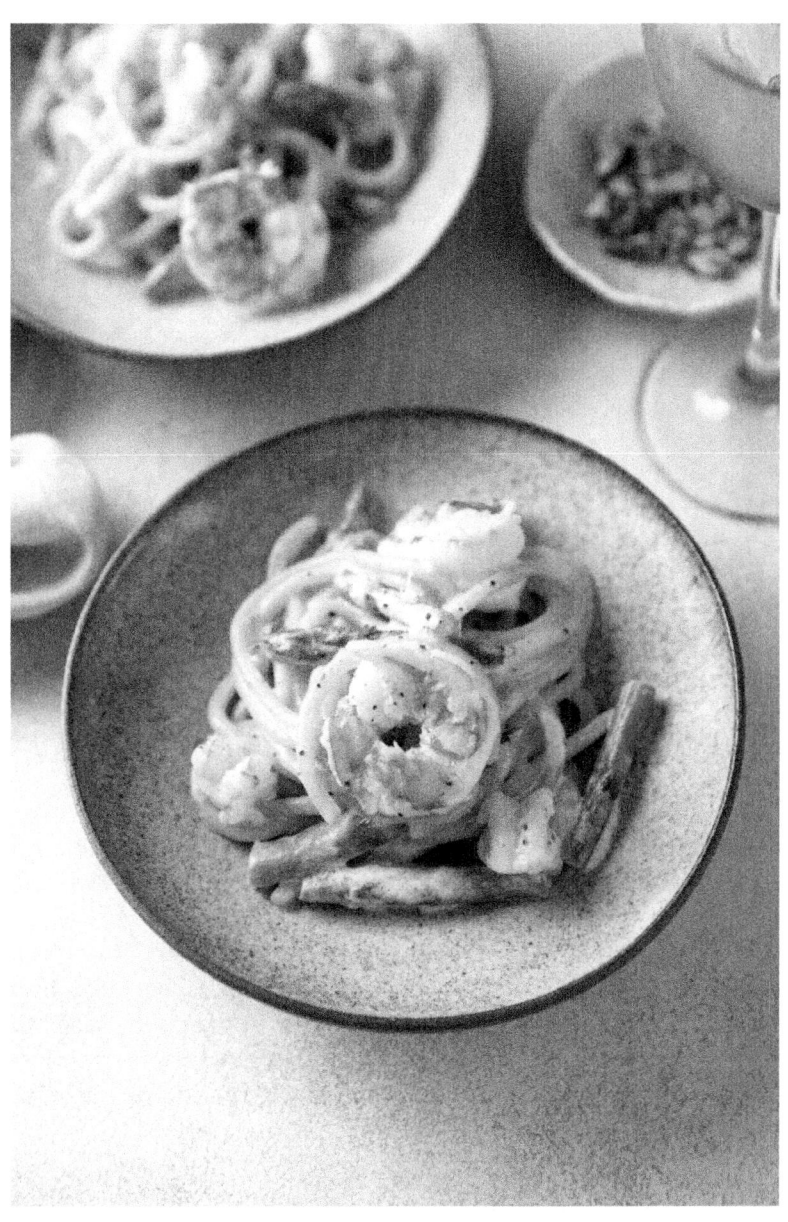

226. Roasted Sardines and Parsley

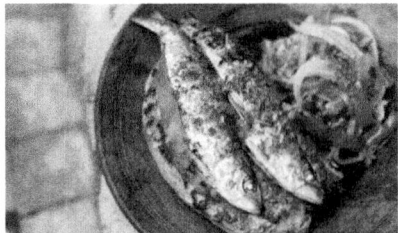

(Preparation time: 10 minutes | Cooking time: 20 minutes | Difficulty: Easy | Servings: 4)
Per serving: Calories 300, Total fat 17g, Protein 20g, Carbs 7g
Ingredients:
- Salt
- 1 teaspoon black pepper - 2 lemons zest
- 1 garlic clove, crushed
- 1 tablespoon of extra-virgin olive oil
- 1/4 cup of chopped parsley
- 2 tablespoons of red wine
- 400g of fresh sardines already cleaned

Instructions:
- Blend the parsley, pepper, garlic clove, and thinly grated lemon zest together to make the sauce. Add the red wine, lemon juice, and olive oil as well.
- Cook the sardines for one minute on each side in a nonstick pan (or grill).
- Spoon a little sauce on the platter, then arrange the sardines on top & season with the remaining sauce. Finish with a pinch of salt & strips of lemon zest.

227. Salmon with Caper Butter

(Preparation time: 10 minutes | Cooking time: 20 minutes | Difficulty: Easy | Servings: 4)
Per serving: Calories 270, Total fat 3g, Protein 10g, Carbs 21g
Ingredients:
- 1 tablespoon of salt and black pepper
- 2 tablespoons of extra virgin olive oil
- 2 tablespoons salted capers
- 3 tablespoons of butter
- 4 salmon steaks

Instructions:
- To make the caper butter for the salmon, first clean & dry the salmon steaks, then set them in a pan with two teaspoons of oil that has been heated.
- Cook for around 6-7 minutes on both sides over medium flame, seasoning using salt & pepper at the end of cooking. Meanwhile, in a saucepan over a low flame, melt the butter without cooking it. For a few minutes, season the desalted & well-dried capers.
- Transfer the salmon steaks to the serving plate once they've finished cooking. Serve your salmon steaks with caper butter right away after sprinkling the fish with the seasoned melted butter.

228. Tuscan Bean Stew

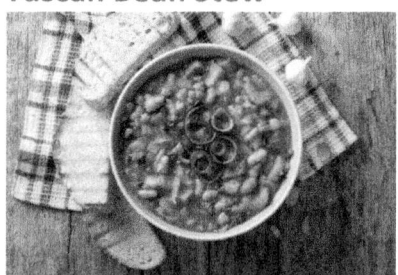

(Preparation time: 10 minutes | Cooking time: 40 minutes | Difficulty: Easy | Servings: 1)
Per serving: Calories 289, Total fat 2g, Protein 12g, Carbs 10g
Ingredients:
- 1 garlic clove, finely chopped
- 1 tablespoon of additional virgin olive oil
- 1 tablespoon of chopped parsley
- 1 teaspoon of herbs de Provence
- 1 teaspoon of tomato purée
- 1/4 cup of red onion, finely hacked
- 1/4 cup of carrot, stripped and finely chopped
- 1/4 cup of celery, cut and finely hacked
- 1/4 cup of kale, generally hacked

- 1 1/2 cups of vegetable stock
- ½ foot bean stew, finely slashed
- 1 x 400g tin of chopped Italian tomatoes
- 200g of tinned blended beans
- 1/4 cup of buckwheat

Instructions:

- In a medium-sized pan, gently sauté the onion, carrot, celery, garlic, chili, and herbs in the oil over low flame till the onion is tender but not browned.
- Bring to a boil the stock, tomatoes, & tomato purée. Cook the stew for 30 minutes after adding the beans.
- Cook for another 5-10 minutes, till the kale is tender, then add the parsley. Meanwhile, prepare the buckwheat as according to package directions, then serve and serve with the stew.

229. Pan-Fried Aubergine Olives and Capers

(Preparation time: 10 minutes | Cooking time: 20 minutes | Difficulty: Easy | Servings: 4)

Per serving: Calories 270, Total fat 3g, Protein 10g, Carbs 21g

Ingredients:

- Salt
- Black pepper
- 2 garlic cloves
- A sprig of parsley
- Extra virgin olive oil
- 2 onions
- 5 tomatoes
- 1 tablespoon of pitted olives
- 1 tablespoon of salted capers
- 1 tablespoon of vinegar
- 1 teaspoon of sweetener
- 4 small aubergines

Instructions:

- Begin by washing and drying the eggplant before cooking it in a pan with olives & capers.

- After removing the core area, which is particularly high in seeds, cut them into cubes. To get rid of some of the bitterness, soak them in salted water for half an hour.
- Rinse and dry the aubergine cubes after half an hour. Heat the oil in a saucepan, then add the icing-cut onions and whole garlic cloves.
- Remove the garlic cloves when they are slightly yellow & add the aubergine cubes, followed by the seeded and diced fresh tomatoes. Add salt & pepper to taste.
- Cook for about a quarter of an hour over medium flame, often stirring to prevent the eggplants and tomatoes from sticking to the bottom of the pan.
- Add the finely chopped parsley, olives rinsed and squeezed capers, vinegar, and sugar now.
- Allow it to absorb the flavor completely before tasting the aubergine to ensure that it has a sweet and sour flavor. If they're too sour, a pinch of sweetener can be added; if they're too sweet, a splash of vinegar can be added.
- Remove the eggplants from the flame after a few minutes and serve them in a skillet with olives & warm or lukewarm capers.

230. Beef with Herb-Roasted Potatoes and Red Wine

(Preparation time: 10 minutes | Cooking time: 55 minutes | Difficulty: Easy | Servings: 3)

Per serving: Calories 430, Total fat 32g, Protein 28g, Carbs 31g

Ingredients:

- 1 clove of garlic, finely chopped
- 1 tablespoon of extra virgin olive oil
- 1 tablespoon of parsley, finely chopped
- 1 teaspoon of tomato purée

- 1 teaspoon of corn flour dissolved in 1 tbsp. of water
- 1/4 cup of red onions, sliced into rings
- 1/4 cup of sliced kale
- 1/2 cup of potatoes, peeled, then cut into 2cm chunks
- 1/2 cup of beef stock
- 150g of beefsteak
- 1/4 cup of red wine

Instructions:

- Preheat the oven at 320°F.
- Drain the potatoes after 5 minutes of boiling.
- Put them in a roasting pan with a tablespoon of oil and roast for around 35 to 45 minutes.
- Make sure they're turned every ten minutes or so.
- Remove them from the oven and toss them with parsley.
- In a teaspoon of oil, sauté the onion for around 5 to 7 minutes over medium flame.
- Drain the kale after steaming it for around 2 to 3 minutes.
- In a teaspoon of oil, sauté the garlic for a minute, then add the kale and stir-fried for another 1 to 2 minutes.
- In 1/2 teaspoon of oil, smear on the meat, then fry in a heated pan over medium flame till done to your liking.
- Remove it and set them aside.
- Pour the wine into the hot pan & drop the flame to low to allow the wine to simmer till it is syrupy.
- Add the tomato purée & stock, bring to a boil and thicken with corn flour paste.
- Enjoy your beef with roast potatoes, onion rings, red wine sauce, & kale.

231. Salmon Salad with Mint Dressing

(Preparation time: 10 minutes | Cooking time: 30 minutes | Difficulty: Easy | Servings: 3)
Per serving: Calories 152, Total fat 11g, Protein 4g, Carbs 10g

Ingredients:

- 1 small handful of parsley, chopped roughly
- 1/4 cup of cucumber, cut into chunks
- 2 spring onions, trimmed, then sliced
- 1/4 cup of young spinach leaves
- 2 radishes, trimmed and thinly sliced
- 1/4 cup of mixed salad leaves
- 1 salmon fillet (around 130g)

For the dressing:

- Salt and freshly ground black pepper, to taste
- 2 mint leaves, finely chopped
- 1 tablespoon of natural yogurt
- 1 tablespoon of rice vinegar
- 1 tablespoon of low-fat mayonnaise

Instructions:

- Preheat the oven at 320°F. Place the salmon fillets onto a baking sheet and bake for around 16 to 18 minutes.
- Remove them from the oven and set them aside to cool (salmon is ok served hot or cold when added to the salad).
- After cooking, remove the skin from your salmon (if it has one).
- In a small-sized bowl, combine the mayonnaise, yogurt, mint leaves, rice wine vinegar, salt, & pepper; set aside for around 5 minutes to allow the flavors to meld.
- Place the salad leaves, spinach, & radishes on a plate, then top with the cucumber, spring onions, and parsley.

232. Baked Zesty Tilapia

(Preparation time: 10 minutes | Cooking time: 10 minutes | Difficulty: Easy | Servings: 4)
Per serving: Calories 276, Total fat 15g, Protein 35g, Carbs 3g
Ingredients:
- Kosher salt and black pepper to taste
- Zest of 1 lemon
- 2 tablespoons of freshly squeezed lemon juice to taste
- 3 cloves of garlic, minced
- 2 tablespoons of chopped fresh parsley leaves
- ¼ cup of unsalted butter, melted
- 4 tilapia fillets

Instructions:
- Preheat the oven at 425°F.
- Coat a baking dish using non-stick spray or lightly oil it.
- Set aside a small-sized bowl containing butter, garlic, lemon juice, and lemon zest.
- Season the fillets to taste using salt and pepper before placing them in the prepared baking dish & drizzling with the butter mixture.
- Place in the oven and bake for around 10 minutes, or till the fish flakes easily with a fork.
- Serve immediately with a parsley garnish.

233. Prawns with Asparagus

(Preparation time: 10 minutes | Cooking time: 15 minutes | Difficulty: Easy | Servings: 4)
Per serving: Calories 253, Total fat 13g, Protein 29g, Carbs 7g
Ingredients:
- Salt and black pepper, to taste
- 1 teaspoon of garlic, minced
- 1 teaspoon of fresh ginger, minced
- 2 tablespoons of lemon juice
- 3 tablespoons of olive oil
- 1 tablespoon of low-sodium soy sauce
- 1 lb. of asparagus, trimmed
- 1 lb. of prawns, peeled, and deveined

Instructions:
- Heat 2 tablespoons of oil in a wok over a medium-high flame and cook the prawns for around 5 minutes with salt and black pepper.
- Transfer the prawns to a bowl with a slotted spoon and set aside.
- Heat the remaining 1 tablespoon of oil in the same wok over medium-high flame & cook the asparagus, salt, ginger, garlic, and black pepper for around 7 minutes, turning often.
- Cook for 1 minute after adding the prawns & soy sauce.
- Remove the pan from the flame and stir in the lemon juice.
- Serve immediately.

234. Roast Beef with Grilled Vegetables

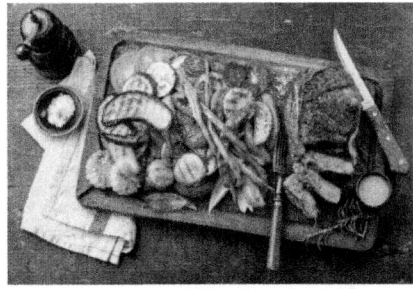

(Preparation time: 20 minutes | Cooking time: 1 hour 10 minutes | Difficulty: Easy | Servings: 5)
Per serving: Calories 347, Total fat 8g, Protein 32g, Carbs 31g
Ingredients:
- Garlic clove (squeezed)
- 1 tablespoon of olive oil
- 1 teaspoon of fresh rosemary
- 1 cup of carrots
- 2 cups of broccoli
- 2 cups of zucchini
- 500g roast beef

Instructions:

- Rub sweet pepper, garlic, salt, & rosemary into the roast beef.
- Cook the beef for around 20 minutes over a high flame or till brown spots emerge on all sides of the flesh.
- Wrap it in aluminum foil and set it aside for a few minutes.
- Cut the roast beef into thin slices before serving.
- Preheat the oven to 305°F. In a large-sized skillet, combine all of the vegetables.
- After a light coating of olive oil, season the vegetables using curry and paprika. Bake for around 30 minutes, or till the vegetables are soft and tender.

235. Spicy Ribs with Grilled Veggies

(Preparation time: 20 minutes | Cooking time: 4 hours 25 minutes | Difficulty: Easy | Servings: 5)
Per serving: Calories 151, Total fat 25g, Protein 41g, Carbs 38g
Ingredients:

- 2 garlic cloves
- 1 tablespoon of olive oil
- 2 tablespoons of honey
- 1 red pepper
- 1 green chili pepper
- 1/4 cup of spring onions
- 1 red onion
- 4 tablespoons of coconut-aminos
- 400g of spare ribs

For the roasted pumpkin:

- 1 tablespoon of olive oil
- 1 pumpkin
- 1 teaspoon of paprika powder

Instructions:

- The day before, marinate the ribs.
- Cut the ribs into four-rib sections apiece. In a mixing dish, combine the coconut amino, honey, & olive oil. Add the spring onions, garlic, and green

peppers once they have been chopped. Pour the marinade over the ribs and spread them out on plastic containers. Refrigerate them for at least one night.

- Place the onions, peppers, and peppers in the slow cooker cut them into pieces. Allow the ribs to cook for at least 4 hours, including the marinade.
- For the pumpkin, preheat the oven at 400°F.
- Cut the pumpkin into moons & lay them on a parchment-lined baking pan.
- Season using paprika, pepper, and salt on a baking sheet with a tablespoon of olive oil. Roast the pumpkin for around 20 minutes in the oven before serving with the spare ribs.

236. French-Style Chicken Thighs

(Preparation time: 20 minutes | Cooking time: 4 hours 10 minutes | Difficulty: Easy | Servings: 8)
Per serving: Calories 122, Total fat 35g, Protein 42g, Carbs 25g
Ingredients:

- 2 cloves of garlic
- 1 tablespoon of olive oil
- 2 tablespoons of fresh parsley
- 2 tablespoons of fresh rosemary
- 2 tablespoons of fresh thyme
- 2 red onions - 4 carrots
- 8 stems of celery
- 700g of chicken leg

Instructions:

- Rub the olive oil, pepper, & salt into the meat of the chicken.
- Add the onions, carrots, garlic, and celery to the slow cooker, roughly chopped. Finally, add the chicken and a few sprigs of rosemary, thyme, & parsley to the top. Allow for at least 4 hours of cooking time.
- Serve with a tasty salad and savor your dinner!

237. Chicken Curry with Pumpkin Spaghetti

(Preparation time: 20 minutes | Cooking time: 4 hours 20 minutes | Difficulty: Easy | Servings: 8)
Per serving: Calories 328, Total fat 39g, Protein 51g, Carbs 21g

Ingredients:

- 1 clove of garlic
- 2 teaspoons of olive oil
- 2 teaspoons of chili powder
- 2 tablespoons of fresh coriander
- 1/4 cup of spring onion
- 3 tablespoons of curry powder
- 1 red onion
- 1 red pepper
- 1 butternut squash
- 2 cups of pineapple
- 2 cups of mango
- 500g of chicken breast
- 2 cups of coconut milk

Instructions:

- Season the chicken with pepper, salt, & chili powder before cutting it into strips. The chicken should then be placed in the slow cooker.
- Add 2 teaspoons of olive oil, finely chop onion and garlic, lightly fry them for then add the curry powder.
- After a minute, deglaze with coconut milk. Allow 2 to 4 hours for the sauce to cook in the slow cooker with the pineapple, mango cubes, and chopped peppers.
- Cut the pumpkin into long pieces and use a spiralizer to produce spaghetti (it's not easy; a carrot works better).
- Cook the pumpkin spaghetti for a few minutes in the pan before spreading the chicken curry on top.
- Add thinly slice spring onions & chopped coriander for garnish.

238. Chicken Teriyaki with Cauliflower Rice

(Preparation time: 20 minutes | Cooking time: 4 hours 20 minutes | Difficulty: Easy | Servings: 8)
Per serving: Calories 280, Total fat 25g, Protein 28g, Carbs 25g

Ingredients:

- 1 lime
- 2 tablespoons of fresh ginger
- 2 cloves of garlic
- 1 tablespoon of olive oil
- 1 teaspoon of sesame oil
- 2 tablespoons of fresh coriander
- 1 onion - 2 red peppers - 1 leek
- 1 cauliflower (rice)
- 4 tablespoons of coconut amino
- 1 cup of Chinese cabbage
- 2 tablespoons of coconut blossom sugar
- 500g of chicken breast

Instructions:

- Chicken should be cut into cubes. In a small-sized bowl, combine coconut amino, coconut blossom sugar, olive oil, & sesame oil.
- Add the garlic and ginger to the marinade, finely chopped. Refrigerate the chicken in the marinade overnight.
- Add the Chinese cabbage, leek, garlic, & paprika to the slow cooker, roughly chopped. After that, add the marinated chicken & simmer for around 2 to 4 hours. Cut the cauliflower into small florets when the chicken is almost done. Then, to make rice, place the florets in a food processor & pulse quickly. Finely chop an onion and cook it in a pan with a teaspoon of oil. Then add the cauliflower rice & cook for a few minutes. Place the chicken & cauliflower rice on the dishes and top with a wedge of lime and some chopped coriander.

239. Turkey Escalope with Cauliflower Couscous

(Preparation time: 10 minutes | Cooking time: 50 minutes | Difficulty: Easy | Servings: 2)
Per serving: Calories 150, Total fat 10g, Protein 14g, Carbs 4g
Ingredients:

- Juice of a 1/4 lemon
- 2 teaspoons of turmeric
- 1 clove of garlic, finely chopped
- 1 teaspoon of chopped fresh ginger
- 2 tablespoons of extra virgin olive oil
- 2 tablespoons of parsley leaves
- 1 teaspoon of dried sage
- 1 tablespoon of capers
- 1 Thai chili, finely chopped
- 1 red onion, finely chopped
- 1/4 cup of dried tomatoes, finely chopped
- 1 cup of cauliflower, roughly chopped
- 150g of turkey escalope

Instructions:

- In a food processor, pulse the cauliflower till the individual pieces are about the size of a grain of rice.
- In a frying pan with a tablespoon of olive oil, cook the garlic, onions, chili, and ginger till they are slightly caramelized. Heat for about 1 minute after adding the turmeric and cauliflower. Remove from flame and stir in half of the parsley & all of the tomatoes.
- Combine the turkey escalope, oil, and sage. In a separate pan, heat the remaining oil and cook the scallops on both sides till done. Then add the lemon juice, capers, remaining parsley, and a tablespoon of water, and heat it briefly again. Serve with couscous made from cauliflower.

240. Honey Chili Squash

(Preparation time: 10 minutes | Cooking time: 50 minutes | Difficulty: Easy | Servings: 2)
Per serving: Calories 118, Total fat 7g, Protein 23g, Carbs 13g
Ingredients:

- Juice of 1 lime - 2 cloves of garlic
- 1 tablespoon of olive oil
- 2 bird's-eye chilies, finely chopped
- Juice of 1 orange - 2 teaspoons of honey
- 1-inch chunk of ginger root, finely chopped
- 2 red onions, roughly chopped
- 1/2 cup of vegetable stock broth
- 1 butternut squash, peeled and chopped

Instructions:

- In a pan, heat the oil and add the red onions, squash chunks, chilies, garlic, ginger, & honey to taste.
- Cook for around 5 minutes in the oven. Lime & orange juice should be squeezed in. Cook for around 15 minutes, till the stock broth, orange, and lime juice are soft.

241. Hot Chicory and Nut Salad

(Preparation time: 10 minutes | Cooking time: 40 minutes | Difficulty: Easy | Servings: 2)
Per serving: Calories 438, Total fat 8g, Protein 11g, Carbs 5g
Ingredients:
For the salad:

- 1 tablespoon of olive oil
- 2 tomatoes, chopped
- 1/2 cup of celery, chopped
- 1/2 cup of green beans
- 1/2 cup of red chicory, chopped if unavailable use yellow chicory
- 2 tablespoons of walnuts, chopped
- 2 tablespoons of plain peanuts, chopped - 2 tablespoons macadamia nuts, chopped

For the dressing:
- ½ teaspoon of turmeric
- 1 tablespoon of olive oil
- ½ teaspoon of mustard
- 2 tablespoons of red wine vinegar
- 2 tablespoons of fresh parsley, finely chopped

Instructions:
- Set aside the dressing ingredients after mixing them together. In a frying pan, heat a tablespoon of olive oil, then add the green beans, chicory, and celery.
- After the veggies have softened, add the chopped tomatoes and simmer for another 2 minutes.
- Toss in the prepared dressing and coat all of the vegetables thoroughly. Place the salad on plates and top with the nut mixture. Eat as soon as possible.

242. Stir-Fry Ginger Prawn

(Preparation time: 10 minutes | Cooking time: 30 minutes | Difficulty: Easy | Servings: 1)
Per serving: Calories 92, Total fat 10g, Protein 15g, Carbs 3g

Ingredients:
- 1 garlic clove, finely chopped
- 1 teaspoon of fresh ginger, finely chopped
- 2 tablespoons of extra virgin olive oil
- 1 bird's eye chili, finely chopped
- 2 tablespoons of soy sauce
- ½ small red onion, chopped
- 2 tablespoons of lovage or celery leaves
- 5-6 leaves of kale, chopped
- 2 stalks of celery, chopped
- 1 cup of green beans, chopped
- 1 cup of chicken stock or vegetable if you prefer
- 6 prawns or shrimp peeled and deveined - ½ packages of buckwheat noodles called Soba in Asian

Instructions:
- Cook the prawns in a little oil & soy sauce till they're done, then put aside for around 10-15 minutes).
- Boil the noodles as directed on the package (typically 6-8 minutes). Set them aside.In a small amount of oil, sauté the veggies, then add the red onion, garlic, ginger, & chili till soft and crisp but not mushy. Add the prawns and noodles and continue to cook on low for another 5-10 minutes.

243. Mussels in Red Wine Sauce

(Preparation time: 10 minutes | Cooking time: 50 minutes | Difficulty: Easy | Servings: 2)
Per serving: Calories 364, Total fat 3g, Protein 43g, Carbs 7g

Ingredients:
- Juice of 1 lemon
- 4 cloves of garlic, crushed
- 2 tablespoons of olive oil
- 1 tablespoon of fresh chives, chopped
- 1 tablespoon of fresh parsley, chopped
- 1 bird's-eye chili, finely chopped
- 2 cups of chopped tomatoes
- 800g of mussels
- 2 cups of red wine

Instructions:
- Remove the mussels' beards & set them aside after washing them. In a large-sized saucepan, heat the oil and add the red wine. Reduce the flame to low and mix in the parsley, chives, chili, & garlic.
- Combine the tomatoes, lemon juice, and mussels. Cook for around 2-3 minutes with the lid on the saucepan.
- Remove the saucepan from the flame and remove any mussels that have not yet opened. Serve and eat right away.

244. Chicken Thighs with Creamy Spinach Tomato Sauce

(Preparation time: 10 minutes | Cooking time: 25 minutes | Difficulty: Easy | Servings: 2)

Per serving: Calories 261, Total fat 37g, Protein 66g, Carbs 21g

Ingredients:

- ½ teaspoon of salt
- ¼ teaspoon of pepper
- 2 garlic cloves, minced
- 1 tablespoon of olive oil
- 4 leaves of fresh basil (or utilize ¼ teaspoon dried basil)
- 1 cup of tomato sauce
- 1/2 cup of spinach
- 1.5 lbs. of chicken thighs, boneless skinless - ½ cup of cream

Instructions:

- Heat the olive oil in a large-sized skillet over medium flame. Add salt & pepper boneless chicken. Place the top side down in the heated skillet.
- Cook over medium flame for around 5 minutes, or till the high side is delightfully browned. Turn the pan over to the other side and cook for another five minutes on medium flame.
- Remove the chicken out from the skillet and set it aside on a platter. To prepare a creamy tomato basil sauce, follow these steps: To the same, now-empty skillet, add tomato sauce, minced garlic, and a generous amount of cream. Bring to a boil, then combine. Reduce the flame to a gentle simmer. Toss in some fresh spinach and basil.
- Mix till the spinach wilts and shrinks in size. Taste the sauce and season using salt and pepper as needed. Return the cooked boneless skinless chicken thighs to the pan and turn the heat up to medium.

245. Horseradish Flaked Salmon with Kale

(Preparation time: 20 minutes | Cooking time: 30 minutes | Difficulty: Easy | Servings: 2)

Per serving: Calories 206, Total fat 7g, Protein 27g, Carbs 11g

Ingredients:

- A pinch of salt and pepper
- Juice of ¼ lemon
- ½ garlic clove, crushed
- 1 tablespoon of extra virgin olive oil
- 1 tablespoon of fresh chives, chopped
- 1 tablespoon of freshly chopped flat-leaf parsley
- 1 red onion, chopped
- 1/4 cup of green beans
- 1/4 cup of kale
- 200g of skinless, boneless salmon fillet
- 1 tablespoon of low fat crème fraiche
- 1 tablespoon of horseradish sauce

Instructions:

- Preheat the grill to high.
- Season a fillet of salmon using salt and pepper. Preheat the grill to medium-high and cook for around 10-15 minutes. Remove the flake and set it aside.
- Cook the kale & green beans for around 10 minutes in a steamer.
- Warm the oil in a skillet over a high flame. Fry for around 2-3 minutes with the garlic and red onion. Cook for a further 1-2 minutes after adding the kale and beans.
- Combine the chives, parsley, crème Fraiche, horseradish, lemon juice, & flakes salmon.
- Serve the greens and beans with the flakes of salmon that has been seasoned.

246. Prawn and Chili Pak Choi

(Preparation time: 15 minutes | Cooking time: 20 minutes | Difficulty: Easy | Servings: 1)

Per serving: Calories 403, Total fat 16g, Protein 17g, Carbs 25g

Ingredients:

- A pinch of salt and pepper
- 1 garlic clove, finely chopped
- 1 teaspoon of freshly grated ginger
- 1 tablespoon of extra virgin olive oil
- ½ bird's eye chili, finely chopped
- 1 tablespoon of freshly chopped flat-leaf parsley
- 1 tablespoon of soy sauce
- 1 red onion, finely chopped
- 1/4 cup of chicken stock
- 1 pak choi
- 1 teaspoon of five-spice
- 1/4 cup of brown rice
- 125g of shelled raw king prawns

Instructions:

- Cook the brown rice for around 25-30 minutes, or till softened, in a medium-sized saucepan of boiling water.
- Tear the pak choi leaves into small pieces. In a skillet over medium flame, warm the chicken stock and mix in the pak choi, simmering till the pak choi has somewhat wilted.
- Warm the olive oil in a separate skillet over a high flame. Fry for around 2-3 minutes with the ginger, chili, red onions, & garlic.
- Cook for around 6-8 minutes, or till prawns, five-spice, and soy sauce are cooked thoroughly. Drain the brown rice & return it to the skillet. Cook for around 2-3 minutes, stirring occasionally. Serve with pak choi and parsley as a garnish.

247. Sirtfood Cauliflower Couscous with Turkey Steak

(Preparation time: 15 minutes | Cooking time: 20 minutes | Difficulty: Easy | Servings: 2)

Per serving: Calories 362, Total fat 39g, Protein 17g, Carbs 9g

Ingredients:

- Juice of ½ lemon
- 2 teaspoons of ground turmeric
- 1 garlic clove, finely chopped
- 1 teaspoon of finely chopped fresh ginger
- 2 tablespoons of extra virgin olive oil
- 1 bird's eye chili, finely chopped
- 1 tablespoon of parsley
- 1 teaspoon of dried sage
- 1 tablespoon of capers
- 1 red onion, finely chopped
- 1/4 cup of sun-dried tomatoes, finely chopped
- 1/2 cup of cauliflower, roughly chopped
- 150g of turkey steak

Instructions:

- Using a food processor, disintegrate the cauliflower. Using 1-2 pulses, blend the cauliflower till it resembles breadcrumbs.
- Add 1 teaspoon of olive oil, garlic, chili, ginger, and red onion, fry in a skillet for around 2-3 minutes. Cook for another 1-2 minutes after adding the turmeric and cauliflower. Remove the pan from the flame and stir in the tomatoes and about half of the parsley.
- Dress the turkey steak in sage & oil. Cook the turkey steak in a pan over medium flame for around 5 minutes, stirring once. Add lemon juice, capers, and a splash of water after the steak is done. Stir in the couscous and serve.

248. Kale and Corn Succotash

(Preparation time: 10 minutes | Cooking time: 15 minutes | Difficulty: Easy | Servings: 2)

Per serving: Calories 137, Total fat 7g, Protein 10g, Carbs 4g

Ingredients:

- 1 teaspoon of sea salt
- 4 teaspoons of black pepper, ground
- 2 cloves of garlic, minced
- 1 tablespoon of extra virgin olive oil
- 2 tablespoons of parsley, chopped
- 1 red onion, finely diced
- 1 cup of grape tomatoes, sliced in half lengthwise
- 2 cups of kale, chopped
- 2 cups of corn kernels

Instructions:

- Pour the olive oil, red onion, & corn kernels into a large-sized skillet and cook till hot and soft, about four minutes.
- Cook till the kale has wilted, about 3 to 5 minutes, with the sea salt, garlic, and black pepper in the skillet.
- Toss in the parsley & fresh grape tomatoes after removing the large skillet from the flame. Warm the dish before serving.

249. Shrimp with Kale

(Preparation time: 10 minutes | Cooking time: 15 minutes | Difficulty: Easy | Servings: 4)

Per serving: Calories 270, Total fat 12g, Protein 28g, Carbs 15g

Ingredients:

- 4 garlic cloves, chopped finely
- 3 tablespoons of olive oil
- 1 bird's eye chili, sliced
- 1 red onion, chopped
- ¼ cup of low-sodium chicken broth
- 1-pound of fresh kale, tough ribs removed and chopped

- 1-pound of medium shrimp, peeled and deveined

Instructions:

- Heat 1 tablespoon of the oil in a large-sized nonstick wok over a medium-high flame and cook the shrimp for around 2 minutes per side.
- Transfer the shrimp to a plate using a spoon. Heat the remaining 2 tablespoons of oil in the same wok over medium flame and sauté the garlic & chili for 1 minute.
- Cook for 4–5 minutes, stirring regularly, after adding the greens and broth.
- Cook for around 5 minutes after adding the cooked shrimp.
- Serve immediately.

250. Chicken, Carrot and Kale Salad

(Preparation time: 10 minutes | Cooking time: 20 minutes | Difficulty: Easy | Servings: 4)

Per serving: Calories 330, Total fat 19g, Protein 25g, Carbs 16g

Ingredients:

For the Chicken:

- Salt and ground black pepper, to taste
- ¼ teaspoon of ground turmeric
- 1 tablespoon of olive oil
- 1 teaspoon of dried thyme
- ½ teaspoon of garlic powder
- ½ teaspoon of onion powder
- ¼ teaspoon of cayenne pepper
- 2 (7-ounce) of boneless, skinless chicken breasts, pounded into the ¾-inch thickness

For the Salad:

- 1½ cups of carrots, peeled and cut into matchsticks
- ¼ cup of pine nuts
- 5 cups of fresh kale, tough ribs removed and chopped

For the Dressing:

- 1 small garlic clove, minced

- 2 tablespoons of fresh lime juice
- 2 tablespoons of extra-virgin olive oil
- 1 teaspoon of raw honey
- ½ teaspoon of Dijon mustard

Instructions:

- Preheat the oven at 425ºF and prepare a baking pan using parchment paper.
- To make the chicken, combine the thyme, spices, salt, & black pepper.
- Drizzle the chicken breasts with oil, then massage generously with the spice mixture and finish with the oil.
- Arrange the chicken breasts in the baking dish that has been prepared.
- Bake for around 16–18 minutes.
- Remove chicken breasts from the pan and set them aside for 5 minutes on a chopping board.
- To make the salad, combine all of the ingredients in a salad bowl and toss well.
- To make the dressing, whisk together all of the ingredients in a separate dish till smooth.
- Each chicken breast should be cut into desired size slices.
- Serve the salad on each serving platter with chicken slices on top.
- Serve with a drizzle of dressing.

251. Tuna with Tomatoes

(Preparation time: 10 minutes | Cooking time: 20 minutes | Difficulty: Easy | Servings: 4)
Per serving: Calories 154, Total fat 4g, Protein 7g, Carbs 14g

Ingredients:

- 1 tablespoon of olive oil
- 1 red onion, chopped
- 1 cup of tomatoes, chopped
- 1 red pepper, chopped
- 1 teaspoon of sweet paprika
- 1 tablespoon of coriander, chopped

- 1-pound of tuna fillets, boneless, skinless and cubed

Instructions:

- Over medium flame, heat the oil in a skillet, then add the onions and pepper & cook for around 5 minutes.
- Cook for around 15 minutes with the fish and other ingredients, then divide amongst plates and serve.

252. Masala Scallops

(Preparation time: 10 minutes | Cooking time: 20 minutes | Difficulty: Easy | Servings: 4)
Per serving: Calories 281, Total fat 4g, Protein 17g, Carbs 11g

Ingredients:

- A pinch of salt and black pepper
- 2 tablespoons of olive oil
- 2 bird's eye chili, chopped
- ¼ teaspoon of cinnamon powder
- 1 teaspoon of cumin, ground
- 1 teaspoon of coriander, ground
- 1 teaspoon of garam masala
- 2 tablespoons of cilantro, chopped
- 1-pound of sea scallops

Instructions:

- Cook for around 10 minutes in a pan with the oil over medium flame, then add the chilies, cinnamon, and the remaining ingredients (except for the scallops).
- Toss in the other ingredients, simmer for another 10 minutes, then divide into bowls & serve.

253. Coriander Snapper Mix

(Preparation time: 10 minutes | Cooking time: 20 minutes | Difficulty: Easy | Servings: 4)
Per serving: Calories 251, Total fat 4g, Protein 7g, Carbs 14g

Ingredients:

- A pinch of salt and black pepper
- 2 garlic cloves, minced

- 2 tablespoons of olive oil
- ½ teaspoon of cumin, ground
- ½ teaspoon of rosemary, dried
- 1 tablespoon of coriander, chopped
- 1 tomato, cubed
- 1 zucchini, cubed
- 4 snapper fillets, boneless, skinless and cubed

Instructions:
- Over medium-high flame, heat the oil in a pan, then add the garlic, tomato, and zucchini & cook for around 5 minutes.
- Toss in the fish and the remaining ingredients, cook for another 15 minutes, then divide into bowls & serve.

254. Tempting Fish Soup

(Preparation time: 10 minutes | Cooking time: 30 minutes | Difficulty: Easy | Servings: 6)
Per serving: Calories 222, Total fat 3g, Protein 31g, Carbs 12g

Ingredients:
- 2 cloves of minced garlic
- 1/8 teaspoon of ground black pepper
- 1 teaspoon of dried basil
- 1/4 teaspoon of crushed fennel seed
- 2 bay leaves
- 1 chopped red onion
- 1/2 chopped green bell pepper
- 1/2 cup of orange juice
- 1 cup of tomato sauce
- 2 cups of diced tomatoes
- 2 cups of chicken broth
- 1/4 cup of mushrooms
- 1/4 cup of black olives sliced
- 1 pound of cubed cod fillets
- 1 pound of peeled and deveined medium shrimp
- 1/2 cup of dry white wine

Instructions:
- Toss the onion, tomatoes, green bell pepper, garlic, chicken broth, mushrooms, dried basil, tomato sauce, olives, orange juice, wine, bay leaves, fennel seeds, & pepper together in a pot. Cook the vegetables for 20 minutes, or till they are soft.
- Put the shrimp and cod. Cook for around 10 minutes, or till the shrimp are completely opaque. Bay leaves should be taken out and thrown away before serving.

255. Creamy Potato Bacon Soup

(Preparation time: 10 minutes | Cooking time: 25 minutes | Difficulty: Easy | Servings: 4)
Per serving: Calories 506, Total fat 40g, Protein 10g, Carbs 20g

Ingredients:
- Salt and pepper to taste
- Cayenne pinch
- 2 cloves of minced garlic
- 1/4 teaspoon of dried thyme
- 1 tablespoon of cornstarch
- 1/2 diced red onion
- 3 cups of chicken broth
- 2 diced ribs celery
- 2 cups of baking potatoes, peeled and diced
- 1 cup of heavy cream
- 8 slices of chopped bacon
- For garnishing sliced green onions and parmesan cheese

Instructions:
- Cook bacon in a large-sized saucepan over medium flame till crisp. Remove the bacon with a slotted spoon & set it aside.
- In the bacon fat with the garlic, onion, & celery, cook for around 3-4 minutes, or till the onion softens somewhat.
- Add the potatoes, thyme, and chicken broth. Bring to a boil, then reduce to a low flame and cook, covered, for 10 minutes, or till the potatoes are tender.

Cook for another 5 minutes after adding the cream.

- To form a slurry, combine one tablespoon of cornstarch with one tablespoon of water. 1/2 of the bacon should be added now, 1 minute after mixing into the boiling mixture. Season using pepper, salt, & cayenne pepper to taste.
- Serve in cups with grated parmesan cheese, green onions, and the rest of the bacon.

256. Cajun Crab Soup

(Preparation time: 10 minutes | Cooking time: 25 minutes | Difficulty: Easy | Servings: 8)
Per serving: Calories 420, Total fat 34g, Protein 15g, Carbs 14g
Ingredients:

- 1 teaspoon of salt
- 1/2 teaspoon of ground white pepper
- 1/4 teaspoon of ground cayenne pepper
- 1/4 teaspoon of dried thyme
- 2 cloves of minced garlic
- 1/4 cup of olive oil
- 1 chopped red onion
- 4 chopped green onions
- 1/4 cup of almond flour
- 1 package of frozen white corn (10 ounces)
- 2 cups of chicken broth
- 2 cups of heavy cream
- 2 cups of clam juice
- 1 pound of lump crabmeat, drained

Instructions:

- Heat the oil in a large-sized saucepan over medium flame. Cook the onion and garlic together till the onion is tender. After whisking in the flour, cook for 2 minutes. Bring the chicken broth & clam juice to a boil. Season with cayenne pepper, white pepper, thyme, salt, &

white pepper. Reduce to a low flame setting & cook for around 15 minutes.

- Combine the crab meat, cream, & green onions. Heat through, but do not boil, once the cream has been added.

257. Cabbage and Sausage Soup

(Preparation time: 10 minutes | Cooking time: 30 minutes | Difficulty: Easy | Servings: 6)
Per serving: Calories 307, Total fat 25g, Protein 8g, Carbs 12g
Ingredients:

- Salt & pepper to taste
- 3 tablespoons of olive oil
- 2 tablespoons of butter
- 1 tablespoon of fresh dill
- 2 tablespoons of fresh parsley
- 2/3 cup of chopped red onion
- 1 sliced carrot
- 1 sliced rib celery
- 2 cups of chicken broth low-sodium
- 2 cups of chopped cabbage
- 3/4 pound of diced potatoes (about 2 to 3 medium)
- 1/4 cup of buckwheat or almond flour
- 1/2 cup of heavy cream
- 1/2 cup of skim milk
- 1 pound of sliced smoked sausage

Instructions:

- Combine the onion, sausage, & butter in a small saucepan and cook till the onion is tender. Add the celery, cabbage, potato, carrot, & broth, and season with salt and pepper to taste.
- Bring them to a boil. Reduce flame to low, cover, and simmer for 10-15 minutes, or till potatoes are cooked.
- Butter should be melted in a small saucepan. After adding the flour, cook for 2 minutes on medium flame. In a separate bowl, whisk together the milk and cream until smooth. Whisk the sauce until it is thick and bubbling.

- Toss the soup with the cream mixture till the veggies are tender. Allow 5 minutes for the sauce to boil.
- Remove the pan from the flame and stir in the parsley and dill.

258. Creamy Chicken Noodles Soup

(Preparation time: 10 minutes | Cooking time: 30 minutes | Difficulty: Easy | Servings: 6)
Per serving: Calories 336, Total fat 19g, Protein 19g, Carbs 18g
Ingredients:

- 1 bay leaf
- Parsley for garnishing
- 1 tablespoon of olive oil
- 1 diced red onion
- 1 teaspoon of poultry seasoning
- 1 1/2 tablespoons of cornstarch
- 2 large sliced carrots
- 2 sliced ribs celery
- 4 cups of chicken broth
- 1 cup of heavy cream
- 1/2 cup of buckwheat spaghetti
- 2 cups of chopped cooked chicken

Instructions:

- Heat the oil in a medium-sized saucepan. Cook by adding the carrots, onion, & celery. Cook for around 3 to 4 minutes, or till the onion is softened.
- Season using salt, pepper, and bay leaf. Cook for around 10 minutes before serving.
- While the soup is boiling, cook the pasta according to package directions. Drain the water completely.
- Combine the cream & corn starch in a small-sized mixing dish. Cook for another 5 minutes after adding the chicken to the soup.
- Remove the bay leaf, add the pasta, and season using salt and pepper to taste.

259. Loaded Creamy Corn Soup

(Preparation time: 10 minutes | Cooking time: 30 minutes | Difficulty: Easy | Servings: 4)
Per serving: Calories 229, Total fat 16g, Protein 4g, Carbs 20g
Ingredients:

- Kosher salt & pepper, 1/2 teaspoon of each
- 2 minced cloves of garlic
- 1/2 chopped red onion
- 2 tablespoons of olive oil
- Chives for garnishing
- 1/2 teaspoon of fresh thyme leaves
- 1 tablespoon of buckwheat or almond flour
- 1 peeled and diced large potato
- 3 cups of chicken broth
- 2 finely diced ribs celery
- 1 cup of light cream
- 2 cups of corn kernels

Instructions:

- Combine the onion, olive oil, celery, & garlic in a saucepan. Cook, stirring periodically, for around 5 minutes, or till the onion softens.
- Combine the flour & thyme. Add another minute to the cooking time. Combine the corn and potatoes.
- Combine the broth, salt, cream, & pepper. Cook for around 15-20 minutes, uncovered, or till potatoes are tender.
- Sprinkle with chives before serving.

260. Chicken and Vegetable Stew

(Preparation time: 10 minutes | Cooking time: 35 minutes | Difficulty: Easy | Servings: 4)
Per serving: Calories 272, Total fat 9g, Protein 27g, Carbs 21g
Ingredients:

- 2 tablespoons of butter
- 1/2 teaspoon of dried basil
- 1/2 teaspoon of dried oregano
- 1 diced onion

- 2 teaspoons of chopped fresh parsley
- 1 tablespoon of buckwheat or almond flour
- 4 cups of chicken broth
- 2 cups of diced tomatoes with the juices
- 2 peeled potatoes and make 1/2" cubes
- 2 cups of frozen mixed vegetables
- 2 cups of cooked chicken

Instructions:

- Cook onion in oil for around 5 minutes on medium flame, till it begins to soften.
- After adding the potatoes, cook for a further 3-4 minutes. After adding the flour, cook for another minute.
- Combine the tomatoes, broth, & seasonings. Cook, occasionally stirring, for around 10 minutes, or till the potatoes are cooked.
- Combine the vegetables & chicken. Cook for an additional 5 minutes.
- To taste, season using salt and pepper.
- Serve with parsley on top.

261. Kale and Sausage Stew

(Preparation time: 10 minutes | Cooking time: 35 minutes | Difficulty: Easy | Servings: 4)
Per serving: Calories 369, Total fat 20g, Protein 21g, Carbs 29g
Ingredients:

- 1 tablespoon of olive oil extra-virgin
- 4 cloves of minced garlic
- 1 bay leaf
- 1 teaspoon of Italian seasoning
- Parmesan cheese for garnishing
- 1 large red chopped onion
- 2 cups of diced tomatoes with the juices
- 2 cups of chopped kale, packed
- 4 cups of chicken broth
- 3 medium of diced Yukon gold potatoes
- 2 cups of canned chickpeas or cannellini beans
- 1/2 pound of smoked sausage sliced

Instructions:

- Pour the olive oil into a pan. Combine the onion, potatoes, & sausage. Cook for around 4-5 minutes on medium flame, or till the onion is soft.
- Bring the rest of the ingredients to a boil. Reduce to a low flame and simmer for another 10-12 minutes, or till the potatoes are cooked. Remove the bay leaf out from the dish.
- Serve with bread and parmesan cheese if desired.

262. Shrimp Quinoa Salad

(Preparation time: 10 minutes | Cooking time: 15 minutes | Difficulty: Easy | Servings: 5)
Per serving: Calories 134, Total fat 9g, Protein 5g, Carbs 9g
Ingredients:

- Salt and ground black pepper, to taste
- 2 tablespoons of olive oil extra-virgin
- 1 lemon juice
- 1 teaspoon of oregano
- 1/4 chopped red onion
- 2 tablespoons of balsamic vinegar
- 3/4 chopped English cucumber
- 1/2 chopped green bell pepper
- 1 pint of grape tomatoes
- 1/2 chopped yellow bell pepper
- 1/4 cup of feta cheese crumbled
- 1/2 cup of chopped Kalamata olives
- 1/2 cup of cooked quinoa
- 1/2 cup of cooked shrimp

Instructions:

- Set aside for 15 minutes to marinate shrimp in a bowl with salt, fresh lemon juice, & black pepper.
- Combine tomatoes, cucumber, Kalamata olives, quinoa, yellow bell pepper, red onion, green bell pepper, and feta cheese in a large-sized mixing bowl.

- Whisk together the vinegar, olive oil, & oregano in a separate cup; add to the quinoa and vegetable mixture and stir well to combine.
- Serve the quinoa mixture with marinated shrimp on top.

263. Asian-Style Chicken Salad

(Preparation time: 10 minutes | Cooking time: 0 minutes | Difficulty: Easy | Servings: 4)
Per serving: Calories 336, Total fat 31g, Protein 14g, Carbs 21g
Ingredients:

- 1 sliced red bell pepper
- 1/4 cup of chopped cilantro
- 3 sliced green onions
- 1/2 sliced English cucumber
- 1 julienned large carrot
- 4 cups of shredded Napa cabbage
- 2 cups of green cabbage or coleslaw mix, finely grated
- 3 cups of cooked chicken, shredded

For the topping:

- 2 teaspoons of sesame seeds
- 1/4 cup of toasted chopped walnuts
- 1 cup of buckwheat noodles

Instructions:

- Combine all salad ingredients in a mixing bowl.
- Thoroughly combine the dressing and the vegetables.
- After dusting with toppings, serve immediately.

264. Red Potato Salad

(Preparation time: 10 minutes | Cooking time: 0 minutes | Difficulty: Easy | Servings: 4)
Per serving: Calories 160, Total fat 8g, Protein 2g, Carbs 15g
Ingredients:

- Salt and ground black pepper, to taste
- 2 crushed cloves of garlic
- 3 tablespoons of olive oil extra-virgin

- 2 tablespoons of white balsamic vinegar
- 1 cup of green onions sliced, with green
- 1/4 cup of shredded basil leaves
- 1/2 cup of celery sliced
- 2 teaspoons of Dijon mustard
- 1/2 pint of halved grape tomatoes
- 1 pound of cooked, cooled and unpeeled red potatoes

Instructions:

- In a large-sized mixing dish, combine the potatoes, tomatoes, basil, onions, & celery.
- In a small-sized cup, combine the garlic, salt, vinegar, oil, mustard, & pepper. Combine the potatoes and the dressing in a large mixing bowl. Keep refrigerated till ready to serve.

265. Chicken Cajun Pasta

(Preparation time: 10 minutes | Cooking time: 30 minutes | Difficulty: Easy | Servings: 6)
Per serving: Calories 366, Total fat 32g, Protein 36g, Carbs 24g
Ingredients:

- 1/2 teaspoon of salt divided
- 3 tablespoons of butter, divided
- 1 red pepper sliced
- 1/2 teaspoon of dried basil
- 3/4 teaspoon of smoked paprika
- 1/2 teaspoon of pepper, divided
- 1/4 teaspoon of garlic powder
- 1/2 diced yellow onion
- 1 sliced green pepper
- 1/3 cup of fresh parmesan cheese grated
- 4 teaspoons of Cajun seasoning, divided
- 1 1/2 cups of heavy cream
- 1 1/2 pounds of boneless skinless chicken breast cut into 1" pieces
- 1 cup of buckwheat pasta, cooked according to package instructions and drained

Instructions:

- In a large-sized skillet over medium-high flame, heat 2 tablespoons of oil.
- Combine 1/4 teaspoon of salt, 3 teaspoons of Cajun seasoning, and 1/4 teaspoon of pepper in a Ziploc bag. Add the chopped chicken to the bag, close it, and shake till the chicken is equally coated.
- Transfer the chicken to the heated pan and cook till golden brown and well done. Remove the chicken from the pan and set it aside on a platter.
- Allow the remaining tablespoon of oil in the pan to warm.
- Cook, occasionally stirring, till the onion and peppers begin to soften, around 4 minutes.
- Add heavy cream, 1 teaspoon of Cajun seasoning, smoked paprika, basil, garlic powder, and the remaining 1/4 teaspoon of salt and pepper. Bring to a boil, then reduce to a low flame and cook till the sauce has thickened, about 20 minutes.
- Add the parmesan cheese and stir till it melts. Return the cooked chicken and cooked pasta to the pan and mix well before dishing.

266. Herb-Crusted Pork Tenderloin

(Preparation time: 10 minutes | Cooking time: 30 minutes | Difficulty: Easy | Servings: 4)
Per serving: Calories 135, Total fat 7g, Protein 16g, Carbs 2g
Ingredients:

- A pinch of salt
- 1/4 teaspoon of ground black pepper
- 2 tablespoons of olive oil extra-virgin, divided
- 2 teaspoons of fresh parsley finely chopped

- 2 teaspoons of fresh rosemary finely chopped
- 1 teaspoon of fresh thyme leaves
- 1 teaspoon of soy sauce
- 1 tablespoon of Dijon mustard
- 1-pound of pork tenderloin

Instructions:

- Preheat the oven at 390°F. Combine 1 tablespoon of olive oil, Dijon mustard, & soy sauce in a small cup. Coat the meat with a brush.
- Combine pepper & fresh herbs in a small-sized cup. Season the pork using salt and pepper (or coat the pork in the mixture).
- In a skillet with 1 tablespoon of olive oil, brown the pork for about 2 minutes on each side over medium flame.
- Bake the pork for around 20 to 25 minutes.

267. Sirloin Steak Caesar Salad

(Preparation time: 10 minutes | Cooking time: 20 minutes | Difficulty: Easy | Servings: 4)
Per serving: Calories 180, Total fat 5g, Protein 28g, Carbs 2g
Ingredients:

- A pinch of salt
- 1/4 teaspoon of black pepper
- 1 tomato wedges
- 1 diced cucumber
- 1/2 cup of rocket leaves
- 2 cups of Romaine lettuce, roughly chopped
- 1 tablespoon of shredded low-fat parmesan cheese
- 2 tablespoons of light and low-sodium Caesar dressing
- 12 oz. of lean sirloin steak

Instructions:

- Season the sirloin steak using salt and black pepper on both sides and cook for around 6 minutes (or till the desired doneness). A grill pan can also be used on a cooktop over a medium flame.

- Plates should be stacked high with lettuce, tomato, rocket leaves, and cucumbers.
- Place the steak on top of the lettuce and slice it against the grain. Parmesan cheese and a mild dressing are strewn on top.

268. Pork Chops Topped with Sweet Apples

(Preparation time: 10 minutes | Cooking time: 25 minutes | Difficulty: Easy | Servings: 4)
Per serving: Calories 242, Total fat 9g, Protein 27g, Carbs 12g
Ingredients:

- 2 tablespoons of water
- A pinch of salt
- 2 minced or pressed cloves garlic
- Olive oil
- 1 tablespoon of cinnamon
- 2 teaspoons of fresh thyme
- 2 tablespoons of natural no-calorie sweetener
- 1 red onion, chopped in wedges
- 2 cored and sliced small apples
- 4 (4 oz.) of pork loin chops

Instructions:

- Pork should be seasoned using salt and black pepper. Cook the pork chops in a large-sized skillet sprayed with olive oil over medium-high flame. Cook for around 4 minutes on each side or till the internal temperature reaches 145°F. To keep the pork warm, remove it from the skillet & cover it using foil.
- Re-spray the skillet with cooking spray and add the apples, onions, & garlic. Cook, stirring periodically, for about 4-5 minutes.

- In the meantime, combine the thyme, sweetener, cinnamon, & water. Combine the apples and the dressing. After stirring to combine, cook for an additional 2 minutes.
- Serve the pork with an apple sauce dollop on top.

269. Stir-Fried Pork with Broccoli

(Preparation time: 10 minutes | Cooking time: 20 minutes | Difficulty: Easy | Servings: 4)
Per serving: Calories 120, Total fat 2g, Protein 15g, Carbs 7g
Ingredients:

- 3/4 cup of water - A pinch of salt
- 1 teaspoon of fresh ginger, minced optional - 4 cloves of minced garlic
- Olive oil - 1 cup of broccoli florets
- 1 cup of sliced mushrooms
- 1/4 cup of low-sodium oyster sauce
- 12 oz. of thinly sliced boneless pork chops

Instructions:

- 3/4 cup of water & 1/4 cup of oyster sauce should be combined in a small-sized bowl.
- Preheat a big skillet or a wok over a high flame. Using olive oil, coat the pan.
- Cook the pork for around 4 minutes on each side, or till golden brown. Place on a plate to cool. Add the broccoli, mushrooms, & garlic after another spray of oil. Cook for 2 minutes in total.
- Combine the ginger & oyster sauce. Cook for a further 3 minutes. Return the meat, along with any juices, to the pan. To properly cook the beef, stir it for 1 to 2 minutes. As needed, season using salt and black pepper.

270. Pork Loin Stuffed with Nuts

(Preparation time: 10 minutes | Cooking time: 25 minutes | Difficulty: Easy | Servings: 4)
Per serving: Calories 264, Total fat 18g, Protein 23g, Carbs 3g
Ingredients:

- A pinch of salt
- 1/2 teaspoon of ground black pepper
- 1 teaspoon of minced ginger
- 1 tablespoon of olive oil
- 1 teaspoon of ground paprika
- 1 tablespoon of low-fat yogurt
- 2 tablespoons of chopped nuts
- 2 tablespoons of chopped walnuts
- 1-pound of pork loin

Instructions:

- The pork loin is rubbed using minced ginger, ground paprika, salt & ground black pepper.
- Then, before rolling it up, mix the meat with almonds & walnuts.
- Secure the meat roll with toothpicks if necessary, and brush with yogurt & olive oil.
- Wrap the beef roll in foil & bake at 450°F for about 25 minutes.

271. Pork Loin Mandarin

(Preparation time: 10 minutes | Cooking time: 25 minutes | Difficulty: Easy | Servings: 4)
Per serving: Calories 340, Total fat 20g, Protein 32g, Carbs 6g
Ingredients:

- A pinch of salt
- 1 teaspoon of ground black pepper
- 1 teaspoon of minced garlic
- 1 tablespoon of olive oil
- 1 tablespoon of mustard
- 2 mandarins, peeled
- 1-pound of pork loin

Instructions:

- Mandarins are combined with chopped garlic, ground black pepper, mustard, salt and olive oil.
- The pork loin should then be properly coated in the mandarin mixture before being wrapped in foil.
- Wrap the leftover mandarin mixture around the meat.
- Preheat the oven at 450°F & bake for about 25 minutes.
- Remove the foil & slice the meat after that.

272. Shepherd Pie

(Preparation time: 10 minutes | Cooking time: 35 minutes | Difficulty: Easy | Servings: 4)
Per serving: Calories 139, Total fat 5g, Protein 14g, Carbs 10g
Ingredients:

- A pinch of salt
- 1 teaspoon of olive oil
- 1 teaspoon of chili powder
- 1 teaspoon of tomato paste
- 1 cup of mashed potatoes
- 1/2 cup of green peas
- 1/4 cup of low-fat yogurt
- 1 cup of lean ground beef

Instructions:

- Brown lean ground beef in a skillet.
- Add the olive oil, salt & chili powder.
- Cook for around 10 minutes with the beef.
- Stir in the tomato paste after that.
- Then, into the casserole mold, pour the mixture.
- On top, there are green peas & mashed potatoes.
- Flatten the potato as much as possible.
- Then, using foil and a dollop of yogurt, cover it.
- Preheat the oven to 400°F & bake the shepherd pie for around 25 minutes.

273. Ham Casserole

(Preparation time: 10 minutes | Cooking time: 30 minutes | Difficulty: Easy | Servings: 4)
Per serving: Calories 117, Total fat 2g, Protein 10g, Carbs 14g
Ingredients:

- A pinch of salt
- 1 teaspoon of Italian seasonings
- 1/4 cup of low-fat yogurt
- 1 cup of cooked kale
- 1/4 cup of low-sodium vegetable broth
- 1/2 cup of cooked red kidney beans
- 8 oz. of ham, chopped

Instructions:

- In a mixing bowl, combine the yogurt and ham. Italian spices, salt and pepper, are used to season the dish.
- Spoon the mixture into the casserole dish after that.
- On top, scatter the kale and red kidney beans. Cover with foil after pouring in the vegetarian broth. Preheat the oven to 450°F and bake for around 25 minutes.

274. Beef Sloppy Joe

(Preparation time: 10 minutes | Cooking time: 30 minutes | Difficulty: Easy | Servings: 4)
Per serving: Calories 134, Total fat 8g, Protein 7g, Carbs 8g
Ingredients:

- A pinch of salt
- 1 teaspoon of minced garlic
- 1 tablespoon of olive oil
- 1 tsp. of tomato paste
- 1/2 cup of tomato puree
- 1 cup of diced red onion
- 1/2 cup of diced sweet peppers
- 1 teaspoon of liquid honey
- 1 cup of lean ground beef

Instructions:

- Add olive oil & lean ground beef in a saucepan.

- Place the onion & sweet pepper and cook till everything is well incorporated.
- Cook for around 10 minutes in total.
- Stir in the honey, tomato puree, salt and tomato paste after that. Combine all of the ingredients thoroughly.
- Cook for around 20 minutes with the lid closed on a medium flame.

275. Fiesta Ground Beef

(Preparation time: 10 minutes | Cooking time: 25 minutes | Difficulty: Easy | Servings: 2)
Per serving: Calories 252, Total fat 9g, Protein 27g, Carbs 31g
Ingredients:

- A pinch of salt
- 1/2 teaspoon of turmeric
- 1 tablespoon of olive oil
- 1 teaspoon of cayenne pepper
- 1 teaspoon of dried rosemary
- 1/2 cup of tomato puree
- 1/2 cup of cooked white beans
- 1/2 cup of cooked corn kernels
- 1/2 cup of ground beef

Instructions:

- Brown the ground beef in a skillet.
- Add the olive oil, cayenne pepper, turmeric, salt and dried rosemary in a skillet.
- With the ingredients, cook for around 10 minutes. Then mix in the white beans, corn kernels, & tomato puree.
- Cook the dish over low flame for around 10 minutes with the lid closed.

276. Buckwheat Beef Patties

(Preparation time: 10 minutes | Cooking time: 25 minutes | Difficulty: Easy | Servings: 4)
Per serving: Calories 230, Total fat 7g, Protein 30g, Carbs 12g
Ingredients:

- Fresh ground black pepper and salt
- 1 clove of garlic

- 1/2 cup of chopped red onion
- 2 tablespoons of olive oil extra-virgin
- 1/4 cup of cilantro
- 1 package of ranch dressing mix
- 1 whole egg - 3/4 cup of whole-wheat or buckwheat breadcrumbs
- 1 cup of buckwheat cooked
- 1 pound of ground beef

Instructions:

- In a medium-sized mixing bowl, combine all of the ingredients and shape them into burger patties.
- In a nonstick pan with 2 tablespoons of olive oil, cook the patties for around 15 minutes on medium flame.

277. Pork Medallions with Blue Cheese Sauce

(Preparation time: 10 minutes | Cooking time: 25 minutes | Difficulty: Easy | Servings: 4)
Per serving: Calories 317, Total fat 23g, Protein 25g, Carbs 2g
Ingredients:

- Fresh ground black pepper and salt
- 2 tablespoons of olive oil extra-virgin
- 1 tablespoon of fresh parsley minced
- 2 teaspoons of steak seasoning
- 1 pork tenderloin (1 pound)
- 1/2 cup of half and half - 1/4 cup of low-fat blue cheese crumbled

Instructions:

- Season the pork with steak spice, salt and pepper after chopping it into equal slices. In a large-sized skillet, cook the medallions in the olive oil for about 15 minutes, rotating halfway through.
- In a skillet, bring the cream to a boil. Cook for around 2 to 3 minutes, or till the cream has thickened slightly. Add the cheese and stir till it's thoroughly melted. Toss with the pork and serve. Serve with a sprig of parsley on top.

278. Ginger-Soy Beef Skewers

(Preparation time: 10 minutes | Cooking time: 25 minutes | Difficulty: Easy | Servings: 4)
Per serving: Calories 232, Total fat 8g, Protein 27g, Carbs 10g
Ingredients:

- A pinch of salt
- 2 tablespoons of fresh lemon juice
- 1 clove of garlic minced
- 1/2 tablespoon of minced fresh ginger
- 1 tablespoon of olive oil extra-virgin
- 1 tablespoon of honey
- 1 red onion, sliced into large pieces
- 2 green onions thinly sliced
- 1/2 cup of soy leaves chopped
- 1 pound of sirloin steak cubed (or your favorite cut of beef)

Instructions:

- Combine olive oil, soy, honey, chopped green onions, salt, minced garlic, fresh lemon juice, & minced ginger in a zip lock bag.
- Meanwhile, marinate the steak cubes for 4 to 6 hours in the refrigerator.
- On each skewer, place one onion slice & one skewer of meat.
- Outside, preheat the grill to medium flame. Cook for around 15 to 20 minutes, turning the skewers halfway during the cooking time.

279. Spicy Peas Beef Strips

(Preparation time: 10 minutes | Cooking time: 30 minutes | Difficulty: Easy | Servings: 4)
Per serving: Calories 295, Total fat 13g, Protein 34g, Carbs 9g
Ingredients:

- A pinch of salt
- A pinch of ground black pepper
- 2 cloves of garlic minced
- 2 tablespoons of olive oil extra-virgin
- 1 red onion sliced
- 1 medium thinly sliced carrot

- 1 cup of frozen green peas, thawed
- 1 diagonally red hot pepper thinly sliced
- 1-pound of sirloin beef, thin strips

Instructions:

- Heat the 2 tablespoons of extra-virgin olive oil in a skillet or wok over medium flame. Cook for around 3 to 4 minutes with the garlic and onion.
- Cook for around 5 to 6 minutes in the pan, or till the meat strips are browned.
- After adding the green peas, carrot, & hot pepper, cook for another 3 minutes. Season using salt and pepper to taste, then cover and cook for around 15 minutes.

280. Garlic-Butter Steak Bites

(Preparation time: 10 minutes | Cooking time: 30 minutes | Difficulty: Easy | Servings: 4)
Per serving: Calories 213, Total fat 17g, Protein 37g, Carbs 2g
Ingredients:

- A pinch of salt
- 2 cloves of garlic minced
- 2 tablespoons of olive oil extra-virgin
- 2 tablespoons of butter
- 1 tablespoon of parsley
- 1/2 teaspoon of dried rosemary
- Steak spice, to taste
- 1 1/2 pounds of sirloin steak or strip loin

Instructions:

- The meat should be cut into small pieces. Combine the pepper and rosemary in a mixing bowl. Season using pepper and salt.
- Put 2 tablespoons of olive oil in the pan. Cook for approximately 10 to 15 minutes, flipping halfway through.
- In a skillet, combine the garlic & butter and cook for 1 minute, or till fragrant. Toss the parsley with the meat to coat it.

281. Sage Pork Chops with Cider Pan Gravy

(Preparation time: 10 minutes | Cooking time: 30 minutes | Difficulty: Easy | Servings: 4)
Per serving: Calories 249, Total fat 32g, Protein 29g, Carbs 10g
Ingredients:

- A pinch of salt - 1/4 teaspoon of pepper
- Minced fresh parsley
- 2 tablespoons of olive oil
- 2 tablespoons of unsalted butter
- 1/2 cup of apple cider or juice
- 3 tablespoons of dried sage leaves
- 1/4 cup of almond flour
- 1/2 cup of low-sodium chicken broth
- 1/4 cup of half and half
- 4 pork loin chops center-cut bone-in (6 oz. each)

Instructions:

- Season pork chops with salt, pepper, & sage. Toss in the flour gently to coat. Place in a nonstick pan with a drizzle of butter and oil on top.
- Cook for around 15 to 20 minutes over medium flame. In a skillet, bring the broth & cider to a boil. Stir in the cream and continue to cook, constantly stirring, till the cream has thickened. Reduce the flame to medium-low and toss in the cooked chops. Close the lid and cook for around 5 to 7 minutes. Before adding the parsley, allow for a 5-minute rest period.

282. Bake-Foil Packed Salmon and Asparagus

(Preparation time: 10 minutes | Cooking time: 20 minutes | Difficulty: Easy | Servings: 4)
Per serving: Calories 291, Total fat 34g, Protein 37g, Carbs 11g
Ingredients:

- 1 lemon juiced + 1 lemon sliced

- A pinch of salt
- 1 teaspoon of black pepper
- 1 tablespoon of garlic minced
- 1/4 cup of olive oil
- Fresh basil and lemon wedges for garnishing
- 1 teaspoon of garlic powder
- 1 teaspoon of paprika
- 2 teaspoons of fresh basil
- 1 pound of asparagus, trim the spears ends
- 4 fillets of salmon

Instructions:

- Cut four heavy-duty foil sheets 12 x 18 inches in half. Place two lemon slices on each piece of foil. Using garlic, paprika, salt and pepper, season the fish. Place a salmon fillet in the center of each lemon segment. On each foil sheet, cut the asparagus into four equal slices and arrange it next to the salmon.
- In a small cup, combine the fresh lemon juice, olive oil, garlic, & fresh basil. Evenly spread the butter mixture over the fish & asparagus.
- Wrap the salmon and asparagus in foil and seal the edges to produce a package.
- Arrange the foil packages on the baking sheet. Preheat the oven to 400°F and bake for around 12 to 15 minutes. Sprinkle the basil and lemon juice over the salmon just before serving.

283. Almond Pesto Salmon Fillets

(Preparation time: 10 minutes | Cooking time: 20 minutes | Difficulty: Easy | Servings: 2)
Per serving: Calories 333, Total fat 34g, Protein 23g, Carbs 4g
Ingredients:

- A pinch of salt and black pepper to taste
- 2 tablespoons of olive oil
- 1/4 cup of pesto marinade

- 1/4 cup of ground walnuts
- 8 oz. of salmon fillets skinless and boneless

Instructions:

- In a small mixing bowl, combine the walnuts, pepper, salt & pesto. Set the mixture aside.
- Using a brush, coat the fish in oil. Half of the pesto mixture should be spread on top of each fillet. Place the fillets in a heated nonstick pan.
- Cook for around 12 to 15 minutes. Serve immediately.

284. Salmon with Fennel Salad

(Preparation time: 10 minutes | Cooking time: 20 minutes | Difficulty: Easy | Servings: 4)
Per serving: Calories 264, Total fat 30g, Protein 38g, Carbs 9g
Ingredients:

- A pinch of salt
- 1 teaspoon of fresh lemon juice
- 1 clove of garlic grated
- 2 tablespoons of olive oil extra-virgin
- 1 teaspoon of finely chopped fresh thyme
- 2 teaspoons of finely chopped fresh flat-leaf parsley
- 2 tablespoons of chopped fresh dill
- 2 tablespoons of orange juice fresh (1 orange) - 2/3 cup of Greek yogurt
- 4 cups of thinly sliced fennel
- 4 skinless center-cut salmon fillets

Instructions:

- Combine the thyme, salt & parsley in a small mixing bowl. After spraying the salmon with oil, lightly sprinkle the herb mixture on top.
- Heat 2 tablespoons of oil in a large-sized skillet, place the salmon fillets. Cook for around 10–15 minutes.

- In a medium mixing bowl, combine the fennel, garlic, orange juice, dill, lemon juice, and yogurt while the salmon is cooking. Serve salmon fillets with a side of fennel salad.

285. Baked Orange-Pomegranate Salmon Packets

(Preparation time: 10 minutes | Cooking time: 20 minutes | Difficulty: Easy | Servings: 4)

Per serving: Calories 307, Total fat 19g, Protein 26g, Carbs 8g

Ingredients:

- A pinch of salt
- 2 tablespoons of olive oil extra-virgin
- 1 tablespoon of minced fresh dill
- 1 small red onion thinly sliced
- 1 medium navel orange thinly sliced
- 1 cup of pomegranate seeds
- 1 skinned salmon fillet (about 2-pounds)

Instructions:

- Place a 28x18-inch piece of heavy-duty foil in a baking tray. Arrange onion slices in a single layer on foil. Top with a slice of salmon. On top, arrange orange slices. Over the top, drizzle the oil & scatter the pomegranate seeds. On top of that, place the second piece of foil. To bind and seal the foil, crimp the edges together on both sides.
- Preheat the oven at 400°F and bake the foil bundles for around 12 to 15 minutes.

286. Baked Cod with Asparagus

(Preparation time: 10 minutes | Cooking time: 20 minutes | Difficulty: Easy | Servings: 4)

Per serving: Calories 141, Total fat 3g, Protein 23g, Carbs 6g

Ingredients:

- 2 tablespoons of fresh lemon juice
- 1 1/2 teaspoons of lemon zest grated

- A pinch of salt
- 2 tablespoons of olive oil - ¼ cup of soy
- 1-pint cherry tomatoes halved
- 1/4 cup of Romano cheese grated
- 1 pound of fresh thin asparagus, trimmed - 4 cod fillets

Instructions:

- Preheat the oven at 400°F.
- In a mixing dish, combine the lemon zest, salt, soy, lemon juice, & olive oil. After rubbing the fish and asparagus with the mixture, place them inside. Place the tomatoes cut side down in the pan. Shredded cheese should be sprinkled on top.
- Bake for around 15 minutes, or till the fish easily flakes with a fork.

287. Asian Cob Salad

(Preparation time: 10 minutes | Cooking time: 0 minutes | Difficulty: Easy | Servings: 4)

Per serving: Calories 195, Total fat 15g, Protein 3g, Carbs 16g

Ingredients:

- A pinch of salt
- 1 tablespoon of lemon zest, grated
- 1 tablespoon of olive oil
- 1 tablespoon of sesame seeds
- 3 tablespoons of balsamic vinegar
- 1/2 cup of chopped red onion
- 1 cup of grated carrot
- 2 cups of chopped lettuce
- 1 cup of peeled tangerines
- 1 sliced avocado

Instructions:

- To make the salad dressing, whisk together balsamic vinegar, sesame seeds, salt, lemon zest, and olive oil.
- Toss the remaining ingredients with the salad dressing in a mixing bowl.
- Give the salad a good shake before serving.

288. Pasta Salad with Summer Vegetables

(Preparation time: 10 minutes | Cooking time: 15 minutes | Difficulty: Easy | Servings: 4)
Per serving: Calories 250, Total fat 17g, Protein 17g, Carbs 15g
Ingredients:
- A pinch of salt and black pepper
- 4 tablespoons of extra-virgin olive oil
- 1 tablespoon of dried oregano
- 1/2 thinly sliced red onion
- 1 cucumber peeled and diced
- 2 cups of diced cherry tomatoes
- 1/4 cup of Kalamata olives
- ½ cup of crumbled feta cheese
- 1 package of buckwheat pasta
- 3 tablespoons of red wine

Instructions:
- In a big pot, bring 8 cups of water to a boil.
- Right away, add the buckwheat pasta. Cook for around 5-7 minutes (watch out for foam!), drain, and set aside to cool while you assemble the salad.
- Combine the tomatoes, cucumber, olives, onion, & feta cheese in a large-sized mixing dish. Toss in the oregano, salt, olive oil, and red wine to combine. After adding the cooled pasta, season with a pinch of salt and freshly ground black pepper to taste.

289. Creamy Broccoli Soup with Green Onions

(Preparation time: 10 minutes | Cooking time: 15 minutes | Difficulty: Easy | Servings: 4)
Per serving: Calories 115, Total fat 4g, Protein 7g, Carbs 16g
Ingredients:
- A pinch of salt
- A pinch of ground red pepper
- 1 tablespoon of olive oil

- 1/3 cup of finely chopped green onions
- 2 cups of chopped red onions
- 2 cups of chicken/vegetable broth
- 1 cup of fat-free (skim) milk
- 4 tablespoons of low-fat cream cheese
- 1 pound of broccoli florets fresh or frozen

Instructions:
- In a large-sized saucepan over medium-high flame, warm the oil. Cook, occasionally stirring, for 4 minutes, or till onions are transparent. Bring the broccoli and stock to the boil together. Reduce to a low flame, cover, and cook for 10 minutes, or till the broccoli is soft.
- In a food processor or blender, pulse the ingredients in batches till smooth. Return to the pot and continue to simmer over medium flame.
- Whisk the cream cheese in a separate dish till it is completely melted. Cook for another 2 minutes, or till cooked through, after adding the milk, salt and red pepper. Add the green onions on top.
- Serve and have fun.

290. Swiss Chard with Lentils

(Preparation time: 10 minutes | Cooking time: 15 minutes | Difficulty: Easy | Servings: 4)
Per serving: Calories 174, Total fat 5g, Protein 10g, Carbs 13g
Ingredients:
- A pinch of salt
- 2 tablespoons of olive oil
- 1/2 teaspoon of cayenne pepper
- 1 sliced red onion
- 1/2 teaspoon of dried sage
- 1 cup of chopped celery stalk
- 1 cup of green lentils
- 2 cups of low-sodium chicken broth
- 1 cup of Swiss chard, stemmed and chopped

Instructions:

- Chicken broth should be used to cook lentils. Cook for approximately 15 minutes. After that, add the cooked lentils to the salad plate and drizzle with 1 tablespoon of olive oil. Pour the remaining olive oil into the same skillet. Cook the red onion, diced, till golden brown. Toss the lentils with the onion that has been cooked.
- After that, add the celery stalk, Swiss chard, sage, salt and cayenne pepper.
- Toss the salad ingredients together.

291. Buckwheat Soup

(Preparation time: 10 minutes | Cooking time: 30 minutes | Difficulty: Easy | Servings: 4)
Per serving: Calories 119, Total fat 3g, Protein 18g, Carbs 13g
Ingredients:

- 6 cups of water - A pinch of salt
- 1 teaspoon of ground black pepper
- 1 tablespoon of olive oil
- 1 tablespoon of chopped fresh dill
- 1 diced yellow onion
- 1 chopped carrot 1/2 cup of buckwheat
- 1-pound of chopped chicken breast

Instructions:

- Cook the onion & carrot in olive oil for around 5 minutes in a saucepan. They should be stirred once in a while.
- Then, to taste, add the buckwheat, chicken breast, salt and black pepper.
- Close the lid and pour in the water.
- Cook the soup on low flame for about 25 minutes. After that, remove the pan from the flame and add the parsley. Allow for a 10-minute rest period.

292. Parsley Soup

(Preparation time: 10 minutes | Cooking time: 30 minutes | Difficulty: Easy | Servings: 4)
Per serving: Calories 46, Total fat 3g, Protein 2g, Carbs 5g

Ingredients:

- 6 cups of water
- A pinch of salt
- 2 teaspoons of olive oil
- 1 cup of chopped red onion
- 1 cup of chopped fresh parsley
- 1 cup of shredded carrot
- 1 cup of chopped celery
- 1/4 cup of grated low-fat parmesan

Instructions:

- Heat the oil in a skillet over medium-high flame, then add the onion, carrot, salt & celery, stir, and cook for about 10 minutes. Combine the water & the remaining ingredients.
- Cook the soup for another 10 minutes on medium flame.

293. Curry Stew

(Preparation time: 10 minutes | Cooking time: 30 minutes | Difficulty: Easy | Servings: 4)
Per serving: Calories 171, Total fat 12g, Protein 2g, Carbs 15g
Ingredients:

- 4 cups of water
- A pinch of salt
- 3 tablespoons of olive oil
- 1 chopped red onion
- 8 carrots, peeled and sliced
- 4 chopped celery stalks
- 2 teaspoons of curry paste

Instructions:

- In a saucepan, heat the oil & add the onion, celery, & carrots, frequently stirring for about 15 minutes.
- Add the curry paste, salt & water after that. Cook for a further 10 minutes, stirring frequently. Puree the stew till smooth once all of the components have softened, then cook for another minute and serve.

294. Berry Salad with Shrimps

(Preparation time: 10 minutes | Cooking time: 0 minutes | Difficulty: Easy | Servings: 4)

Per serving: Calories 283, Total fat 10g, Protein 29g, Carbs 20g

Ingredients:

- 1 tablespoon of lime juice
- A pinch of salt
- 2 tablespoons of olive oil
- 1 tablespoon of chopped parsley
- 1 cup of cooked corn kernels
- 1 shredded endive
- 1 cup of halved raspberries
- 1 cup of halved strawberries
- 1 pound of cooked shrimp

Instructions:

- Combine all of the ingredients from the list above in a salad dish & shake well.

295. Salmon Topped with Grated Beets

(Preparation time: 10 minutes | Cooking time: 15 minutes | Difficulty: Easy | Servings: 4)

Per serving: Calories 164, Total fat 10g, Protein 18g, Carbs 2g

Ingredients:

- A pinch of salt
- 1/2 teaspoon of minced garlic
- 1 teaspoon of olive oil
- 1 tablespoon of margarine
- 1 tablespoon of mustard
- 4 tablespoons of grated beetroot
- 1-pound of salmon fillet

Instructions:

- After smearing the fish with mustard, place it in the skillet.
- Cook the fish in oil for about 5 minutes per side.
- In the meantime, add the garlic, grated beetroot, salt & olive oil.
- The grilled salmon fillets are topped with grated beetroot.

296. Scallop Salad

(Preparation time: 10 minutes | Cooking time: 15 minutes | Difficulty: Easy | Servings: 4)

Per serving: Calories 255, Total fat 11g, Protein 15g, Carbs 18g

Ingredients:

- A pinch of salt
- 1/2 teaspoon of minced garlic
- 4 tablespoons of olive oil
- 1 tablespoon of dried cilantro
- 4 teaspoons of apple cider vinegar
- 1 cup of cooked green peas
- 1 cup of cooked quinoa
- 1 1/2 cups of sea scallops

Instructions:

- In a mixing bowl, combine the scallops, apple cider vinegar, & sesame oil.
- Heat a pan over medium flame, then add the scallops & cook for around 10 minutes, tossing regularly (4 minutes per side).
- Thoroughly combine the remaining ingredients. Cook the salad for around 5 minutes on low flame.

297. Fish Salsa

(Preparation time: 10 minutes | Cooking time: 0 minutes | Difficulty: Easy | Servings: 4)

Per serving: Calories 67, Total fat 3g, Protein 7g, Carbs 4g

Ingredients:

- A pinch of salt
- 3 tablespoons of lemon juice
- 2 tablespoons of olive oil
- 1/4 cup of chopped parsley
- 1/2 cup of chopped red onion
- 1 cup of chopped tomatoes
- 1/2 cup of chopped tomatillos
- 1 cup of chopped mango
- 1 cup of watermelon, seedless and chopped

- 1-pound of salmon, cooked and chopped

Instructions:
- Combine all of the ingredients in a mixing bowl.
- Set aside for at least 5 minutes to cool after thoroughly stirring the salsa.

298. Crab Celery Salad

(Preparation time: 10 minutes | Cooking time: 0 minutes | Difficulty: Easy | Servings: 4)
Per serving: Calories 79, Total fat 2g, Protein 10g, Carbs 3g
Ingredients:
- A pinch of salt
- 1/4 teaspoon of white pepper
- 1 teaspoon of olive oil
- 1/4 teaspoon of dried rosemary
- 1/4 cup of low-fat yogurt
- 1 cup of chopped celery stalk
- 1 cup of cooked and chopped crab meat

Instructions:
- Combine all of the ingredients in a salad bowl.
- Place the salad in the refrigerator for around 5-10 minutes before serving.

299. Carrot, Salmon, And Zucchini Patties

(Preparation time: 15 minutes | Cooking time: 15 minutes | Difficulty: Easy | Servings: 4)
Per serving: Calories 192, Total fat 10g, Protein 14g, Carbs 8g
Ingredients:
- A pinch of salt and pepper, to taste
- 2 tablespoons of olive oil
- 2 tablespoons of parsley chopped
- 1/2 cup of fresh chives chopped
- 2 whole eggs beaten - 1 carrot grated
- 1 grated zucchini medium
- 1/4 cup of buckwheat or almond flour
- 3/4 cup of whole-wheat breadcrumbs

- 16 oz. of canned flaked pink salmon drained and flaked

Instructions:
- Combine the salmon, eggs, zucchini, breadcrumbs, carrots, parsley, buckwheat or almond flour, and chives in a large-sized mixing bowl. Mix thoroughly after finishing with a dusting of salt and pepper.
- In a nonstick pan, warm two tablespoons of olive oil, then shape 1/2 cup of the ingredients into patties and set in the pan. Repeat with the remaining mixture.
- Cook, stirring periodically, for about 15 minutes, or till lightly browned. Halfway through cooking, flip the patties.

300. Tomato, Garlic, And Herb Prawns

(Preparation time: 15 minutes | Cooking time: 15 minutes | Difficulty: Easy | Servings: 4)
Per serving: Calories 210, Total fat 9g, Protein 26g, Carbs 5g
Ingredients:
- A pinch of salt and ground black pepper
- 1 tablespoon of garlic thinly sliced
- 2 tablespoons of olive oil
- 2 tablespoons of parsley fresh
- 1 cup of cherry tomatoes halved
- 1-pound of tiger prawns trimmed
- 1/4 cup of red wine vinegar

Instructions:
- Combine the olive oil, parsley, red wine, salt and garlic in a medium-sized mixing dish. Preheat a medium nonstick skillet over medium flame.
- Add the prawns & tomatoes to the same pan, after tossing to coat, season with salt and black pepper.
- Cook for around 10–12 minutes, or till prawns are cooked through. During the cooking process, turn them once.

301. Turkey Meatloaf

(Preparation time: 15 minutes | Cooking time: 25 minutes | Difficulty: Easy | Servings: 4)
Per serving: Calories 233, Total fat 15g, Protein 23g, Carbs 5g
Ingredients:
- A pinch of salt
- 1 teaspoon of olive oil
- 1 teaspoon of Italian seasonings
- 1 tablespoon of semolina
- 1 tablespoon of potato starch
- 1/4 cup of corn kernels
- 4 tablespoons of chopped walnuts
- 1-pound of ground turkey

Instructions:
- In a mixing dish, combine ground turkey, walnuts, Italian seasonings, semolina flour, potato starch, salt and corn kernels.
- Fill the meatloaf form with the turkey mixture after coating it with olive oil.
- Wrap it in foil and flatten it out.
- Preheat the oven to 425°F and bake the meatloaf for approximately 25 minutes.

302. Chicken Breast Stuffed with Parsley

(Preparation time: 15 minutes | Cooking time: 25 minutes | Difficulty: Easy | Servings: 4)
Per serving: Calories 166, Total fat 6g, Protein 24g, Carbs 2g
Ingredients:
- A pinch of salt
- 1 teaspoon of ground black pepper
- 1 teaspoon of minced garlic
- 1 tablespoon of olive oil
- 2 tablespoons of basil leaves
- 1 sliced tomato - 1-pound of chicken breast, skinless and boneless

Instructions:
- Make a lengthwise cut in the chicken breast.
- Following that, the chicken breasts are coated with minced garlic, salt and black pepper powder, then packed with basil leaves and tomato slices.
- To keep the cut secure, toothpicks are utilized. After that, rub the chicken breast with olive oil & wrap it in foil.
- Preheat the oven at 450°F and roast the chicken for around 25 minutes.

303. Chicken and Artichoke Stew

(Preparation time: 15 minutes | Cooking time: 25 minutes | Difficulty: Easy | Servings: 4)
Per serving: Calories 274, Total fat 10g, Protein 30g, Carbs 15g
Ingredients:
- A pinch of salt
- 2 tablespoons of olive oil
- 1/2 teaspoon of chili flakes
- 1 cup of chopped tomatoes
- 1 cup of chopped kale, chopped
- 4 chopped artichoke hearts
- 1-pound of chicken breast, chopped

Instructions:
- In a medium-high-heat pan, heat the oil, then add the chicken & chili flakes and cook for around 5 minutes per side.
- With the other ingredients, cook the stew for about 15 minutes on medium flame.

304. Creamy Turkey with Soy

(Preparation time: 10 minutes | Cooking time: 25 minutes | Difficulty: Easy | Servings: 4)
Per serving: Calories 160, Total fat 5g, Protein 21g, Carbs 7g
Ingredients:
- A pinch of salt
- 1 tablespoon of olive oil
- 1 teaspoon of curry powder
- 3 tablespoons of soy leaves
- 2 cups of chopped broccoli

- 1 cup of soy milk
- 12 oz. of turkey fillet, chopped

Instructions:
- Heat the oil in a pan over medium-high flame, then add the turkey, curry powder, salt, soy & broccoli. Stir the ingredients together for 10 minutes.
- Cook for another 15 minutes after adding the soy milk.

305. Chicken and Parsley Soup

(Preparation time: 10 minutes | Cooking time: 25 minutes | Difficulty: Easy | Servings: 4)
Per serving: Calories 136, Total fat 3g, Protein 21g, Carbs 7g
Ingredients:
- 5 cups of water
- A pinch of salt
- 1/2 teaspoon of chili powder
- 1 tsp. of smoked paprika
- 1 cup of chopped red onion
- 1 cup of shredded carrot
- 1/2 cup of chopped fresh parsley
- 1-pound of chicken breast, skinless and boneless, chopped

Instructions:
- Fill a pot halfway with water and add the chicken.
- Except for the parsley, cook the soup for around 30 minutes on medium flame with the remaining ingredients.
- During the last 5 minutes of cooking, add the parsley.

306. Tahini Chicken Skewers

(Preparation time: 10 minutes | Cooking time: 25 minutes | Difficulty: Easy | Servings: 4)
Per serving: Calories 147, Total fat 4g, Protein 14g, Carbs 15g
Ingredients:
- A pinch of salt
- 1 tablespoon of fresh lemon juice
- 1/2 teaspoon of ground black pepper

- 2 teaspoons of chili paste
- 2 tablespoons of toasted sesame seeds
- 2 tablespoons of tahini
- 8 cloves of garlic crushed and peeled
- 8 green onions diced
- 1/2 cup of stevia
- 5 chicken breasts, boneless and skinless (3/4-inch strips)
- 1/4 cup of red wine

Instructions:
- Combine the soy sauce, garlic, sugar, red wine, fresh lemon juice, tahini, chili paste, salt and pepper in a food processor. Blend till the mixture is completely smooth.
- In a zip-top bag, combine the chicken, toasted sesame seeds, & green onions with the marinade. Marinate into the refrigerator for approximately 3 hours or for overnight.
- In the meantime, soak the wooden skewers in a container with water for approximately 2 hours.
- After threading the chicken onto the skewers, place them on the grill.
- Cook for around 15 to 20 minutes on the grill, flipping halfway through.

307. Gorgonzola Stuffed Chicken

(Preparation time: 10 minutes | Cooking time: 25 minutes | Difficulty: Easy | Servings: 4)
Per serving: Calories 337, Total fat 18g, Protein 38g, Carbs 3g
Ingredients:
- A pinch of salt
- A pinch of ground black pepper to taste
- 1 clove of garlic minced
- 2 tablespoons of fresh parsley minced
- 2 tablespoons of shallot minced
- 1/4 cup of Gorgonzola cheese crumbled
- 4 turkey bacon thick slices
- 2 halves chicken breast boneless and skinless

Instructions:

- Preheat the oven to 390°F.
- Using a sharp knife, cut a slit about 2 inches long & 1 1/2 inches deep on the thick side of each chicken breast.
- Combine the fresh parsley, crumbled Gorgonzola cheese, minced shallot, salt and garlic in a small-sized mixing dish; season with salt and black pepper. Fill one-half of the filling into each chicken breast. Each breast should be wrapped in two pieces of turkey bacon and secured with toothpicks. On a baking pan, arrange the chicken breasts.
- Bake for around 20 to 25 minutes.

308. Portobello Chicken Baked Roll-Ups

(Preparation time: 10 minutes | Cooking time: 25 minutes | Difficulty: Easy | Servings: 4)
Per serving: Calories 342, Total fat 14g, Protein 40g, Carbs 12g
Ingredients:

- A pinch of salt
- 1 teaspoon of garlic minced
- 1 tablespoon of olive oil extra-virgin
- 1/2 teaspoon of dried oregano
- 1 large red bell pepper, make into strips
- 1 cup of low-fat milk
- 1 can of low sodium cream of mushroom soup (10 1/2 oz.)
- 8 asparagus spears trimmed
- 1 Portobello mushroom cap, make 1/2-inch slices
- 4 (6 oz.) of halves chicken breast, skinless and boneless

Instructions:

- Preheat the oven at 380°F.
- Heat the olive oil in a medium-sized saucepan. Cook, frequently stirring, for around 1 minute, or till the garlic turns golden brown. Add Combine the red pepper, mushroom, and asparagus. When the mushroom, red pepper, and asparagus have softened, season with salt and oregano. After putting the mixture into a pan, set it aside to cool.
- Pound each chicken breast to a thickness of 1/4 inch using two pieces of plastic wrap. Arrange the Portobello, red pepper, & asparagus on the chicken breasts in an equal layer. To hide it, roll it up and secure it with toothpicks. Place the cookies on a baking sheet and bake them for around 25 to 30 minutes.
- Combine cream of mushroom soup & milk in a medium-high-heat pot. While the chicken cooks, bring to a gentle boil, then cover and keep heated.
- Remove the toothpicks from the chicken & cut each piece in half at an angle before serving. Serve with a dollop of mushroom cream soup on top.

309. Turkey Herbed Meatballs

(Preparation time: 10 minutes | Cooking time: 25 minutes | Difficulty: Easy | Servings: 4)
Per serving: Calories 214, Total fat 9g, Protein 34g, Carbs 11g
Ingredients:

- A pinch of salt
- 1 teaspoon of garlic minced
- 2 tablespoons of olive oil extra-virgin
- 1 tablespoon of fresh parsley leaves chopped
- 1 tablespoon of fresh rosemary chopped - 1/4 cup of red onion chopped
- 1 whole egg
- 1/2 cup of buckwheat breadcrumb
- 1-pound of lean ground turkey breast
- 1/4 cup of Parmesan cheese grated

Instructions:

- Combine all of the ingredients in a mixing bowl. Toss everything together till it is evenly distributed.

- With around two tablespoons of the meat mixture, make little balls.
- Pour two tablespoons of olive oil onto a nonstick pan.
- In a pan over medium flame, brown the meatballs. Cook, stirring periodically, for about 15 minutes, or till golden brown.

310. Chicken Tikka

(Preparation time: 10 minutes | Cooking time: 25 minutes | Difficulty: Easy | Servings: 4)
Per serving: Calories 205, Total fat 6g, Protein 31g, Carbs 3g
Ingredients:

- A pinch of salt
- 2 teaspoons of fresh lemon juice
- 1 tablespoon of garlic crushed
- 1 tablespoon of ginger grated
- 1 teaspoon of cayenne pepper and paprika - 1 teaspoon of garam masala
- 2 tablespoons of olive oil extra-virgin
- 1/2 cup of Greek yogurt plain
- 1/4 cup of fresh parsley chopped
- 2-pounds of chicken tenders, sliced in half
- For garnish chopped fresh cilantro

Instructions:

- In a non-reactive mixing bowl, combine the chicken, chopped parsley, Greek yogurt, ginger, garlic, cayenne pepper, garam masala, turmeric, paprika, salt, olive oil, & fresh lemon juice. Everything should be completely combined. After covering, refrigerate for at least 2 hours.
- Cook the chicken in a nonstick skillet with 2 tablespoons of olive oil for around 20 to 25 minutes, flipping halfway through.
- Serve with a garnish of cilantro on a serving platter.

311. Chicken Salad with Kale

(Preparation time: 10 minutes | Cooking time: 25 minutes | Difficulty: Easy | Servings: 4)
Per serving: Calories 218, Total fat 4g, Protein 23g, Carbs 4g
Ingredients:

- A pinch of salt
- Olive oil cooking spray
- Assorted fresh greens (optional)
- 8 thin slices of red onion, separated into rings
- 1 large-sized grapefruit, peeled and sectioned
- 4 cups of shredded stemmed spinach
- 2 cups of washed and torn romaine lettuce - 3/4 pound of chicken tenders
- 1/4 cup of low-sodium homemade Italian salad dressing
- 2 tablespoons of crumbled blue cheese

Instructions:

- Chicken should be cut into 2 1/2-inch chunks. Cook over medium flame in a large nonstick skillet sprayed with cooking spray. Cook, stirring periodically, for about 5 minutes, or until the chicken is no longer pink in the center. Remove the pan from the heat.
- In 4 salad plates, combine the spinach, cheese, lettuce, grapefruit, salt, onion, and chicken. Combine the citrus blend concentrate and the Italian dressing in a mixing bowl and sprinkle over the salads.

312. Chicken with Kale and Artichokes

(Preparation time: 10 minutes | Cooking time: 25 minutes | Difficulty: Easy | Servings: 2)
Per serving: Calories 328, Total fat 11g, Protein 37g, Carbs 18g
Ingredients:

- A pinch of salt

- 1/8 tsp. of black pepper
- 1/2 tsp. of minced garlic
- 1/4 cup of chopped red onions
- 1 cup of chopped kale
- 1 cup of chopped and cooked chicken pieces
- 2 cups of artichoke hearts, drained and chopped
- 1/4 cup + 2 tablespoons of grated low-fat Parmesan cheese, divided
- 1/4 cup of fat-free mayonnaise

Instructions:
- Preheat the oven to 375°F.
- Using nonstick cooking spray, coat a 1-quart casserole.
- In a medium mixing bowl, combine spinach, artichoke hearts, 2 tablespoons of cheese, garlic, salt, mayonnaise, onions, and pepper. In the prepared dish, evenly distribute the spinach mixture over the chicken. Add the remaining 1/4 cup of cheese on top.
- Bake for around 25 minutes, or till the cheese is golden brown.

313. Turkey with Creamy Broccoli

(Preparation time: 10 minutes | Cooking time: 25 minutes | Difficulty: Easy | Servings: 2)
Per serving: Calories 165, Total fat 11g, Protein 10g, Carbs 8g
Ingredients:
- A pinch of salt
- 2 garlic cloves, minced
- 1 tablespoon of olive oil
- 2 red onions, chopped
- 1 tablespoon of chopped cilantro
- 1 tablespoon of chopped parsley
- 2 cups of broccoli florets
- 1 big turkey breast, skinless, boneless and cubed
- 1/2 cup of half and half

Instructions:
- In a medium-high-heat pan, heat the oil, then add the meat, onions, and garlic, tossing to coat. Cook for approximately 5 minutes.
- Stir in the broccoli & the additional ingredients, then cook for about 20 minutes on medium heat before dividing.
- Divide the dish between two plates.

314. Lamb Curry

(Preparation time: 10 minutes | Cooking time: 30 minutes | Difficulty: Easy | Servings: 2)
Per serving: Calories 306, Total fat 36g, Protein 32g, Carbs 12g
Ingredients:
- A pinch of salt
- 1/2 teaspoon of turmeric
- 4 finely chopped garlic cloves
- 2 tablespoons of olive oil
- 2 teaspoons of ground cumin
- 1/2 teaspoon of ground coriander
- 1 tablespoon of finely chopped parsley
- 1 finely chopped onion
- 1 large finely chopped tomato
- 2 carrots, chopped into 1/2-inch slices
- 2 cups of low-sodium hot chicken stock
- 10 oz. of cubed lean lamb

Instructions:
- In a large-sized saucepan, heat the oil over medium-high flame.
- Add the lamb when it's heated & brown it all over. This should take no more than 5 minutes. Cook for 3 minutes after adding the onion & finely chopped garlic. Add the carrots, cumin, heated chicken stock, turmeric, salt and ground coriander at this point.
- Bring everything to a boil.
- Reduce the flame to low and cook, covered, for about 15 minutes.

- Cook for another 2 minutes after adding the chopped tomato & parsley.
- To taste, season using salt and black pepper.

315. Strawberry and Arugula Salad

(Preparation time: 10 minutes | Cooking time: 0 minutes | Difficulty: Easy | Servings: 4)

Per serving: Calories 355, Total fat 32g, Protein 47g, Carbs 21g

Ingredients:
- 1/4 cup lemon juice
- 1/4 teaspoon of paprika
- 1/2 cup of olive oil
- 1 bag of fresh arugula - chopped, washed and dried
- 2 tablespoons of black sesame seeds
- 1 tablespoon of poppy seeds
- 1 ½ cup of strawberries, sliced

Instructions:
- Combine the sesame seeds, olive oil, poppy seeds, paprika, lemon juice, & onion in a mixing bowl. Refrigerate.
- Combine the arugula, strawberries, and walnuts in a large-sized mixing bowl. Dress the salad with the dressing. 15 minutes before serving, toss and chill.

316. Garlic Chicken Burgers

(Preparation time: 10 minutes | Cooking time: 10 minutes | Difficulty: Easy | Servings: 2)

Per serving: Calories 355, Total fat 32g, Protein 47g, Carbs 21g

Ingredients:
- 1 clove garlic, crushed
- 3 teaspoons of extra virgin olive oil
- ¼ red onion, finely chopped
- 1 cup of cherry tomatoes
- 1 cup of arugula
- 1 handful of parsley, finely chopped
- ½ orange, chopped
- 8 oz. of chicken mince

Instructions:
- In a mixing bowl, combine the chicken mince, onion, garlic, parsley, and salt & pepper. Make 2 patties and set them aside for 5 minutes to rest.
- Cook 3 minutes per section in a pan with olive oil when it is extremely hot.
- If you want to grill them, brush them with a little oil immediately before cooking.
- Place the arugula on two dishes, top with the cherry tomatoes and orange, then drizzle with the remaining olive oil and salt. Serve with the patties on top.

317. Buckwheat Gallo Pinto

(Preparation time: 10 minutes | Cooking time: 10 minutes | Difficulty: Easy | Servings: 1)

Per serving: Calories 250, Total fat 15g, Protein 9g, Carbs 17g

Ingredients:
- 1 teaspoon of ground turmeric
- 1 teaspoon of paprika
- 2 teaspoons of extra virgin olive oil
- 1 chopped bird's eye chili
- 1 tablespoon of chopped coriander
- 1/4 cup of diced red onion
- 1/4 cup of celery, diced
- 2 tablespoons of kale, chopped
- 2 medium-sized eggs
- 1/4 cup of boiled buckwheat
- 1/4 cup of canned black beans or kidney beans, drained

Instructions:
- Place a small pot on the stovetop over low to medium flame. Sauté the red onions, celery, kale, & chilies in 1 teaspoon of olive oil for 2-3 minutes, or till soft. Cook for another minute after adding the spices. Fry thoroughly with the buckwheat, beans, and a dash of water. Toss in the coriander. Prepare the eggs in the meantime.

- Heat the remaining teaspoon of olive oil in a pan over medium heat and fry the eggs to your satisfaction.
- Serve with buckwheat and beans.

318. Kale and Roasted Walnut Soup

(Preparation time: 10 minutes | Cooking time: 55 minutes | Difficulty: Easy | Servings: 1)
Per serving: Calories 260, Total fat 22g, Protein 12g, Carbs 18g
Ingredients:

- 1 clove of minced garlic
- 2 teaspoons of olive oil
- 1 teaspoon of dried thyme
- 1/4 cup of chopped red onion
- 1/4 cup of chopped celery
- 1/4 cup of kale
- 4 chopped walnut halves
- 2 cups of vegetable broth
- 1/2 cup of canned or homemade white beans such as cannellini or haricot

Instructions:

- Heat 1 teaspoon olive oil in a medium-sized skillet over medium flame and cook the red onions, celery, and garlic for around 2-3 minutes. Bring the thyme, beans, & broth to a boil after the onions are tender.
- Simmer for around 25 minutes on low flame, then add the greens & cook for another 10 minutes. Blend the mixture till smooth once all of the vegetables have been cooked thoroughly. If your soup is too thick, you may need to add more water. If it appears to be very runny before mixing, simply increase the heat and allow it to boil until it thickens.
- Preheat your oven to 320°F and roast your walnuts for 10-15 minutes, or till pleasantly roasted, while the soup is heating. Keep an eye on them since they can quickly go from roasted to charred.

Drizzle the remaining teaspoon of olive oil over the soup and top with the roasted walnuts.

319. Spicy Lentil and Veggie Stew

(Preparation time: 10 minutes | Cooking time: 30 minutes | Difficulty: Easy | Servings: 1)
Per serving: Calories 120, Total fat 7g, Protein 8g, Carbs 14g
Ingredients:

- 1 clove of garlic- 1 bird's eye chili
- 1 teaspoon of ground turmeric
- 1 teaspoon of extra virgin olive oil
- 1 teaspoon of curry powder
- 1 teaspoon of chopped parsley
- 1 red onion - 1/4 cup of celery
- 1/4 cup of carrot
- 2 cups of vegetable broth
- 1/4 red lentils

Instructions:

- Heat the olive oil in a small-sized saucepan over low to medium flame and cook the onion, celery, and carrot for 2-3 minutes, till tender. Cook for another minute after adding the chili, garlic, and seasonings. Bring the vegetable stock & lentils to a boil. Simmer for 30 minutes, occasionally stirring to ensure nothing sticks to the bottom.
- Stir in the parsley and a dash of extra virgin olive oil till the lentils have broken down & have a beautiful soupy consistency.

320. Bean Seaweed Salad with Miso Dressing

(Preparation time: 10 minutes | Cooking time: 0 minutes | Difficulty: Easy | Servings: 1)
Per serving: Calories 120, Total fat 11g, Protein 3g, Carbs 13g
Ingredients:

- 1 chopped red onion

- 1/4 cup of diced cucumber
- 2 tablespoons of chopped celery
- 1/4 cup of rocket
- 1/2 cup of canned or homemade mixed beans(drained)
- 5g of arame or wakame, prepared according to the instructions on the package

For the miso dressing:

- 1 teaspoon of extra virgin olive oil
- 1 teaspoon of chopped coriander
- 1 teaspoon of sesame seeds
- 1 teaspoon of rice vinegar
- 1 tablespoon of miso paste

Instructions:

- To begin, make the dressing by whisking together all of the ingredients and setting it aside. Except for the rocket, combine all salad ingredients in a dish.
- Serve on a bed of rockets with the miso dressing.

321. Chicory Tofu and Chili with Walnut Arugula Salad

(Preparation time: 10 minutes | Cooking time: 30 minutes | Difficulty: Easy | Servings: 1)
Per serving: Calories 330, Total fat 21g, Protein 26g, Carbs 11g
Ingredients:

- 1 clove of garlic, chopped
- 1 teaspoon of extra virgin olive oil
- 1 bird's eye chili, chopped
- 1 tablespoon of chopped parsley
- 1 teaspoon of thyme
- 1 red onion, diced
- 1/4 cup of celery, diced
- 1 × 400 g can of tomatoes
- 2 heads of chicory, quartered lengthways
- 150g of silken tofu, cut into small cubes

For the salad:

- 1 teaspoon of balsamic vinegar
- 1 teaspoon of extra virgin olive oil

- 1 teaspoon of capers
- 1/4 cup of rocket
- 6 walnut halves, chopped

Instructions:

- Preheat the oven at 400°F. Heat the olive oil in a medium-sized saucepan over medium flame, then sauté the red onions, celery, garlic, chilies, & thyme for around 2-3 minutes, or till soft.
- Bring to the boil with the tomatoes. Pour the liquid from the can into the pan after cleaning it with a little water.
- Allow 10–15 minutes to simmer. Carefully fold in the tofu & parsley, being careful not to damage it.
- In a baking dish, place the chicory. Preheat the oven at 400°F.
- Bake for around 8-10 minutes, till the chicory, is wilted and cooked, after pouring the hot sauce over it.
- Meanwhile, combine all of the salad ingredients in a bowl and serve with the chicory.

322. Stuffed Portobello Mushrooms with Braised Celery

(Preparation time: 10 minutes | Cooking time: 1 hour 20 minutes | Difficulty: Easy | Servings: 1)
Per serving: Calories 250, Total fat 15g, Protein 7g, Carbs 23g
Ingredients:

- 1 clove of garlic, chopped
- 1 teaspoon of extra virgin olive oil
- 1 teaspoon of parsley
- 1/2 red onion, chopped
- 1 tablespoon of sunflower seeds
- 2 tablespoons of chopped kale
- 2 tablespoons of rocket for serving
- 2 walnut halves
- 1 large Portobello mushroom
- 1/4 cup of canned or homemade white beans such as cannellini or haricot

For the celery:
- 1 clove of garlic
- 1 teaspoon of dried thyme
- 1 teaspoon of ground turmeric
- 3-4 celery stalks
- 1 cup of vegetable stock

Instructions:
- Preheat the oven at 360°F. Simply combine all of the ingredients in an ovenproof bowl for the celery. Bake for around 30 to 40 minutes, till soft, covered with a lid or foil.
- Prepare your mushroom while the celery is cooking so that it may be baked for the last 20 minutes of the celery's cooking time.
- To complete the filling.
- In a food processor, combine the beans, parsley, & walnuts.
- If you don't have a food processor, mash the beans using the back of a fork & coarsely chop the parsley and walnuts.
- Combine the sunflower seeds and fold them in. In a small-sized pan, heat the olive oil and gently sauté the red onion, kale, and garlic till tender.
- Remove the pan from the flame and add the bean mixture. Place the mushroom onto a baking sheet and fill it with it.
- Place in the oven for the last 20-25 minutes with the celery. The mushroom's top should be beautifully browned. Serve the mushrooms alongside arugula and braised celery.

323. Grilled Sweet Potato with Coriander Dressing

(Preparation time: 10 minutes | Cooking time: 15 minutes | Difficulty: Easy | Servings: 3)
Per serving: Calories 220, Total fat 38g, Protein 3g, Carbs 31g
Ingredients:
- 1 tablespoon of olive oil

- 2 sweet potatoes

For the Dressing:
- 2 ½ tablespoons of olive oil
- ½ red pepper
- 1 hand of fresh coriander
- 1 tablespoon of natural vinegar

Instructions:
- Wash the sweet potato & cut it lengthwise into 1 cm thick slices.
- Place the slices in a bowl & drizzle with olive oil. Mix in a pinch of salt and thoroughly combine.
- Grill the sweet potato till it is cooked through.
- Meanwhile, make the dressing by combining all of the ingredients in a food processor and blending till smooth.
- Toss the sweet potato with the dressing before serving.

324. Salad with Ham and Melon

(Preparation time: 10 minutes | Cooking time: 20 minutes | Difficulty: Easy | Servings: 4)
Per serving: Calories 127, Total fat 29g, Protein 19g, Carbs 21g
Ingredients:
- 4 tablespoons of lime juice
- 3 cloves of garlic (pressed)
- 3 tablespoons of olive oil
- 1 tablespoon of balsamic vinegar
- 2 sweet potatoes (peeled and diced)
- 5 slices of bacon

Instructions:
- Preheat the oven to 400°F and line a baking sheet using parchment paper.
- Place the bacon on a baking pan and roast in the oven till crispy (approx. 20 minutes).
- Remove the bacon from the baking pan, set it aside to cool, and then cut it.
- On the same baking sheet, combine the sweet potato cubes with the garlic,

sprinkle with a little mild olive oil, and bake for about 30 minutes.

- In a mixing dish, combine olive oil, vinegar, & lime juice to make a dressing.
- Remove the potato cubes from the oven and combine them with the bacon bits before drizzling the dressing over them.
- Finish with rocket and/or pine nuts if desired.

325. Pasta with Kale and Black Olives

(Preparation time: 10 minutes | Cooking time: 40 minutes | Difficulty: Easy | Servings: 3)
Per serving: Calories 327, Total fat 28g, Protein 4g, Carbs 21g
Ingredients:

- 2 tablespoons of oil
- ½ chili pepper
- Six leaves of washed curly kale
- 20 black olives
- 1/2 cup of buckwheat pasta
- 1/4 cup of whole-wheat pasta

Instructions:

- Cut the curly kale leaves into 4 cm broad strips and simmer for 5 minutes in salted boiling water. Add the spaghetti to the pan as well. While the pasta is cooking, heat the oil and olives in a nonstick pan.
- Drain the pasta & spaghetti, reserving some of the cooking water, and combine with the olives.
- Mix thoroughly, adding a little cooking water if necessary. Add the chili pepper and stir to combine.

326. Shitake and Tofu Soup

(Preparation time: 10 minutes | Cooking time: 20 minutes | Difficulty: Easy | Servings: 4)
Per serving: Calories 137, Total fat 7g, Protein 5g, Carbs 12g
Ingredients:

- 1 bird's eye chili, chopped
- 2 spring onions

- 1-liter vegetable stock
- 1 cup of shitake mushrooms, sliced
- 2 cups of natural tofu, cut into cubes
- 1/2 cup of miso paste
- 1 tablespoon of dried Wakame algae (instant)

Instructions:

- Bring the stock to the boil, then add the mushrooms and continue to cook for another 2 minutes. Meanwhile, dissolve the miso paste in a bowl with some heated stock, then return it to the saucepan with the tofu and turn off the flame.
- Soak the Wakame according to the package directions, then stir in the spring onions & Tai Chi before serving.

327. Bok Choy and Mushrooms Stir-Fry

(Preparation time: 10 minutes | Cooking time: 10 minutes | Difficulty: Easy | Servings: 4)
Per serving: Calories 77, Total fat 5g, Protein 4g, Carbs 5g
Ingredients:

- Ground black pepper, to taste
- 2 garlic cloves, chopped
- 1 teaspoon of fresh ginger, minced
- 4 teaspoons of olive oil
- 2 tablespoons of soy sauce
- 1/2 cup of fresh mushrooms, sliced
- 1-pound of baby bok choy
- 2 tablespoons of red wine

Instructions:

- Trim the bottoms of the bok choy leaves and detach the outer leaves from the stalks, keeping only the tiny interior leaves intact. Heat the oil in a big cast-iron wok over a medium-high flame and cook the ginger and garlic for 1 minute. Cook, often stirring, for 4–5 minutes after adding the mushrooms. Cook, tossing with tongs, for about 1 minute

after adding the bok choy leaves & stalks. Cook for 2–3 minutes, occasionally tossing, after adding the wine, soy sauce, & black pepper.
- Serve immediately.

328. Tofu with Kale and Chickpeas

(Preparation time: 10 minutes | Cooking time: 20 minutes | Difficulty: Easy | Servings: 4)
Per serving: Calories 370, Total fat 20g, Protein 17g, Carbs 25g
Ingredients:
- ¼ cup of water
- 2 tablespoons of olive oil
- 1 tablespoon of red pepper flakes
- 1 tablespoon of soy sauce
- 1 teaspoon of maple syrup
- 1 1/2 cups of tofu, drained, pressed, and cut into 1-inch cubes

For the Chickpeas & Kale:
- Salt and ground black pepper, to taste
- ¼ teaspoon of ground turmeric
- 2 tablespoons of olive oil
- 1 teaspoon of sesame seeds
- 6 cups of fresh baby kale
- 2 cups of chickpeas, rinsed and drained

Instructions:
- To make the tofu, heat the olive oil in a large cast-iron wok over medium flame and cook the tofu cubes for around 8–10 minutes, or till golden on all sides. Cook for another 2-3 minutes after adding the other ingredients.
- Meanwhile, prepare the chickpeas combination by heating the oil in a separate wok over medium flame and cooking the chickpeas, turmeric, salt, & black pepper for 2–3 minutes.
- Remove the chickpeas from the can and place them in a large mixing dish.
- Stir in the tofu and kale till everything is well combined.
- Serve with sesame seeds as a garnish.

329. Tofu Thai Curry

(Preparation time: 10 minutes | Cooking time: 40 minutes | Difficulty: Easy | Servings: 2)
Per serving: Calories 346, Total fat 26g, Protein 20g, Carbs 21g
Ingredients:
- Juice of 1 lime
- 2 cloves of garlic, crushed
- 1 tablespoon of virgin olive oil
- 5 cm of fresh ginger root, peeled and finely chopped - 1 teaspoon of cumin
- 2 tablespoons of tomato puree
- 2 red onions, chopped
- 2 bird's eye chilies - 1 tablespoon of fresh coriander, chopped
- 1 cup of vegetable stock (broth)
- 1 stalk of lemongrass, inner stalks only
- 1 cup of sugar snaps peas
- 2 cups of tofu, diced
- 1 cup of coconut milk

Instructions:
- In a frying pan, heat the oil, then add the onion & cook for around 4 minutes. Cook for 2 minutes after adding the chilies, cumin, ginger, & garlic.
- Cook for 2 minutes after adding the tomato puree, lemongrass, sugar snap peas, lime juice, and tofu. Simmer for 5 minutes with the stock (broth), coconut milk, & coriander (cilantro).
- Serve with brown rice or buckwheat on the side, as well as a handful of rocket (arugula) leaves.

330. Beans and Kale Soup

(Preparation time: 10 minutes | Cooking time: 30 minutes | Difficulty: Easy | Servings: 6)
Per serving: Calories 270, Total fat 5g, Protein 11g, Carbs 22g
Ingredients:
- Salt and ground black pepper, as required - 6 cups of water
- 4 garlic cloves, minced

- 2 tablespoons of olive oil
- 2 red onions, chopped
- 1-pound of kale, tough ribs removed and chopped - 2 cups of cannellini beans, rinsed and drained

Instructions:

- Heat the oil in a big pan over medium flame and cook the garlic and onions for around 4-5 minutes.
- Cook for 1-2 minutes after adding the kale. Bring the beans, water, salt, & black pepper to a boil.
- Cook for 15-20 minutes, partially covered.
- Serve immediately.

331. Greens and Lentils Stew

(Preparation time: 10 minutes | Cooking time: 55 minutes | Difficulty: Easy | Servings: 6)
Per serving: Calories 167, Total fat 5g, Protein 10g, Carbs 22g

Ingredients:

- 5½ cups water
- Salt and ground black pepper, as required
- 2 tablespoons of fresh lemon juice
- 3 garlic cloves, minced
- 1 teaspoon of ground turmeric
- 1 tablespoon of olive oil
- 1½ teaspoon of ground cumin
- ¼ teaspoon of red pepper flakes
- 1 medium red onion, chopped
- 2 carrots, peeled and chopped
- 2 celery stalks, chopped
- 2 cups of diced tomatoes
- 1 cup of red lentils, rinsed
- 2 cups of fresh mustard greens, chopped

Instructions:

- In a large-sized skillet over medium flame, heat the olive oil & sauté the celery, carrots, and onion for around 5-

6 minutes. Sauté for 1 minute after adding the garlic and seasonings.
- Cook for around 2-3 minutes after adding the tomatoes.
- Bring the lentils & water to a boil, stirring constantly.
- Reduce the flame to low and cook for about 35 minutes, covered.
- Cook for 5 minutes after adding the greens. Remove from the flame after adding the salt, black pepper, & lemon juice.
- Serve immediately.

332. Egg Fried Buckwheat

(Preparation time: 10 minutes | Cooking time: 45 minutes | Difficulty: Easy | Servings: 2)
Per serving: Calories 167, Total fat 2g, Protein 6g, Carbs 24g

Ingredients:

- 2 cloves of minced garlic
- 1 teaspoon of grated ginger
- 2 tablespoons of olive oil, divided
- 2 eggs, beaten
- 2 thinly sliced green onions
- 1 diced red onion
- 1/5 cup of frozen peas
- 2 diced carrots
- 2 teaspoons of sriracha sauce
- 2 tablespoons of tamari sauce
- 3 cups of cooked buckwheat groats

Instructions:

- In a large-sized skillet or wok placed over medium flame, heat half of the olive oil and add the egg, continually turning till it is fully cooked. Remove the egg & place it in a separate dish.
- Toss in the peas, carrots, then onion with the remaining olive oil in the wok. Cook for four minutes, or till the carrots & onions are softened. Cook for another minute, till the grated ginger & minced garlic, are aromatic.

- In a wok, combine the sriracha sauce, tamari sauce, & cooked buckwheat groats. Cook the buckwheat groats & stir the mixture for another two minutes, or till the buckwheat is completely warmed through and the flavors have merged.
- Toss in the cooked eggs & green onions in the wok to mix, and serve immediately.

333. Aromatic Turmeric Ginger Buckwheat

(Preparation time: 10 minutes | Cooking time: 55 minutes | Difficulty: Easy | Servings: 2)
Per serving: Calories 37, Total fat 3g, Protein 23g, Carbs 7g
Ingredients:

- 1.75 cups of water
- 1 teaspoon of sea salt
- 3 minced garlic cloves
- 1 tablespoon of grated ginger
- 1 tablespoon of lemon juice
- 1 teaspoon of turmeric
- 1 tablespoon of extra virgin olive oil
- 1/3 cup of chopped parsley
- 1/5 cup of dried cranberries
- 1/4 cup of toasted pine nuts
- 1 cup of buckwheat groats rinsed and drained

Instructions:

- Add the buckwheat groats, garlic, water, olive oil, ginger, turmeric, lemon juice, & sea salt to a medium-sized pot. Bring the water to a boil in the pot and then cover it with a lid. Allow it to simmer for around 20 minutes over a medium-low flame or till all of the liquid has been absorbed.
- The dried cranberries into the buckwheat sir around fifteen minutes into the cooking time allows them to

plump up the last few minutes of the cooking period.
- Before serving, sprinkle the pine nuts & parsley over the buckwheat.

334. Zucchini Salad with Lemon Salad

(Preparation time: 10 minutes | Cooking time: 25 minutes | Difficulty: Easy | Servings: 2 to 3)
Per serving: Calories 125, Total fat 30g, Protein 41g, Carbs 5g
Ingredients:

- 1 lemon
- 2 tablespoons of olive oil
- 1 red onion
- 1 cherry tomatoes - 1 zucchini
- 2 chicken breasts

Instructions:

- To make the chicken fillets as thin as possible, use a meat mallet or a heavy pan.
- Fill a bowl halfway with the fillets.
- Pour the olive oil over the chicken and squeeze the lemon over it. Cover and set aside for at least 1 hour to marinate.
- Cook the chicken in a pan over medium-high flame till it is cooked through and browned.
- Salt & pepper to taste.
- Put the zucchini in a bowl and make zucchini out of it.
- Toss in the zucchini and quartered tomatoes. Place the chicken fillets on the salad after slicing them diagonally.
- Season the salad using salt and pepper after drizzling it with olive oil.

335. Arugula with Fruits and Nuts

(Preparation time: 10 minutes | Cooking time: 10 minutes | Difficulty: Easy | Servings: 2 to 3)
Per serving: Calories 68, Total fat 1g, Protein 4g, Carbs 13g
Ingredients:

- 1/2 red onion

- 1/2 cup of arugula
- 2 peaches
- A handful of pecans
- A handful of blueberries
- For the Dressing:
- A pinch of salt and black pepper
- 2 tablespoons of olive oil
- 1 sprig of fresh basil
- 1/2 peach - 2 tablespoons of red wine

Instructions:

- Remove the core from the two peaches and cut them in half.
- Using a knife, cut the pulp into small pieces.
- Preheat a grill pan & cook the peaches on both sides for a few minutes.
- Thinly slice the red onion into half-rings.
- Chop the pecans coarsely.
- Warm a pan and toast the pecans in it till fragrant. Spread the arugula over the peaches, red onions, blueberries, and roasted pecans on a platter. In a blender or food processor, combine all of the dressing ingredients and pulse till smooth. Drizzle the dressing over the salad and toss to combine.

336. Spinach Salad with Salmon and Asparagus

(Preparation time: 10 minutes | Cooking time: 10 minutes | Difficulty: Easy | Servings: 2 to 3)
Per serving: Calories 108, Total fat 32g, Protein 46g, Carbs 23g
Ingredients:

- ½ lemon - 1 teaspoon of olive oil
- 2 eggs - 1/2 cup of cherry tomatoes
- 2 hands of spinach
- 1/2 cup of Asparagus tips
- 120g of smoked salmon

Instructions:

- Make the eggs any way you like them.
- Fry the asparagus tips al dente in a skillet with a little oil.

- Cherry tomatoes should be cut in half.
- Arrange the asparagus tips, cherry tomatoes, & smoked salmon on top of the spinach on a dish. Prepare the eggs by scaring, peeling, and halving them. Toss them in with the salad. Drizzle some olive oil over the lettuce and squeeze some lemon over it. Season the salad using salt and pepper to taste.

337. Tuna Salad

(Preparation time: 10 minutes | Cooking time: 0 minutes | Difficulty: Easy | Servings: 2)
Per serving: Calories 251, Total fat 13g, Protein 2g, Carbs 11g
Ingredients:

- 2 tablespoons of fresh parsley, chopped
- 2 hard-boiled eggs, peeled and quartered
- 2 tablespoons of garlic vinaigrette
- 1 red onion, chopped
- 2 tomatoes, chopped
- 1 celery stalk - 1/2 cup of cucumber
- 1/4 cup of rocket
- 6 Kalamata olives, pitted
- 1/2 cup of red chicory
- 1 tablespoon of capers
- 150g of tuna flakes in brine, drained

Instructions:

- In a mixing dish, combine all of the ingredients and serve.

338. Crowning Celebration Chicken Salad

(Preparation time: 5 minutes | Cooking time: 10 minutes | Difficulty: Easy | Servings: 1)
Per serving: Calories 314, Total fat 13g, Protein 2g, Carbs 25g
Ingredients:

- Juice of 1/4 of a lemon
- 1 teaspoon of ground turmeric
- 1 red onion diced
- 1 teaspoon of coriander, cleaved

- 1 finely shredded Medjool date
- 1/4 cup of rocket
- 1/2 teaspoon of mild curry powder
- 6 walnut parts, finely chopped
- 1/2 cup of yogurt - 1 bird's eye bean stew - 100g of cooked chicken bosom, cut into scaled-down pieces

Instructions:

- In a mixing dish, combine the yogurt, lemon juice, coriander, and flavors.
- Combine the remaining ingredients and serve over a bed of rockets.

339. Sirt Super Salad

(Preparation time: 10 minutes | Cooking time: 0 minutes | Difficulty: Easy | Servings: 1)
Per serving: Calories 314, Total fat 13g, Protein 2g, Carbs 25g
Ingredients:

- juice of 1/4 lemon
- 1 tablespoon of olive oil
- 1/4 cup of parsley chopped
- 1/8 cup of chopped red onion
- 1/2 cup of chopped celery
- 1/4 cup of arugula
- 1/8 cups of pecans, shredded
- 1 Medjool date, chopped and hollowed
- ½ cup of avocado, stripped, stoned, and chopped - 1 tablespoon of escapades
- 1/4 cup of endive leaves
- 100g of smoked salmon cuts

Instructions:

- Place the leaves of the mixed greens on a plate or in a large-sized bowl.
- Combine the remaining ingredients and pour over the lettuce leaves.

340. Poached Pear Salad with Dijon Vinegar Dressing

(Preparation time: 15 minutes | Cooking time: 0 minutes | Difficulty: Easy | Servings: 1)
Per serving: Calories 88, Total fat 11g, Protein 8g, Carbs 22g

Ingredients:
For The Dressing:

- A pinch of salt and black pepper to taste
- 3 tablespoons of olive oil
- 1 tablespoon of red wine vinegar
- 3 tablespoons of walnut oil
- 1 tablespoon of Dijon mustard

For The Salad:

- Few rocket leaves - 2 bay leaves
- Small bunch of thyme
- 2 ripe pears (peeled and cored) cut into quarters - 3 tablespoons of sweetener
- 1/2 cup of walnuts
- 1 cup of gorgonzola cheese, finely sliced
- 1 cup of red wine

Instructions:

- In a saucepan, bring the wine to a boil. Add bay leaves, sweetener, and thyme. Simmer on a low flame setting.
- Poach the pear for ten minutes in the boiling liquid. Remove the pan from the flame and set it aside to allow the pears to cool in the poaching liquid.
- Whisk together the mustard, salt, vinegar, & pepper in a mixing bowl till thoroughly combined; gently drizzle in the oil, whisking constantly.
- Drizzle the dressing over the salad components on a serving platter.

341. Steak Arugula and Strawberry Salad

(Preparation time: 10 minutes | Cooking time: 20 minutes | Difficulty: Easy | Servings: 4)
Per serving: Calories 306, Total fat 37g, Protein 23g, Carbs 17g
Ingredients:

- 1/2 tablespoon of extra virgin olive oil
- Montreal steak seasoning
- 2 Beef tenderloin steaks

For the Salad:

- 1/2 cup of blueberries
- 1/2 cup of raspberries

- 3 cups of arugula
- 1/2 cup of sliced strawberries
- 1/4 cup of crumbled feta cheese
- 1/8 cup of slivered walnuts

For the Balsamic Vinaigrette:
- A pinch of salt and pepper
- 1/8 cup of olive oil
- 1/8 cup of balsamic vinegar
- 1 1/2 teaspoons of sweetener
- 1/4 teaspoon of Dijon mustard

Instructions:
- **Steak:** Season the steak using Montreal steak seasoning and set aside for around 5-10 minutes.
- In a cast-iron skillet, heat the oil over medium-high flame. Once it's simmering, add the steak and cook for around 5-7 minutes; flip & cook for 3-4 minutes on the other side, or till it's cooked to your liking.
- Place the steak on a plate and set aside for 5 minutes to cool before slicing into strips.
- **Salad:** In a large-sized mixing bowl, combine all of the salad ingredients.
- Combine all vinaigrette ingredients in a small shaker and shake till well combined. Toss the salad in the dressing to evenly coat it.
- **To Assist:** Place the salad in two bowls and top with the meat.

342. Sirt Salmon and Lentil Salad

(Preparation time: 10 minutes | Cooking time: 0 minutes | Difficulty: Easy | Servings: 1)
Per serving: Calories 400, Total fat 25g, Protein 10g, Carbs 20g
Ingredients:
- Juice of 1/4 of a lemon
- 1 tablespoon of extra virgin olive oil
- 1 tablespoon of chopped parsley
- 1 sliced red onion
- 1/4 cup of sliced celery

- 1/2 cup of rocket
- 1 large Medjool date, remove pit and chopped
- 1/2 cup of avocado, peeled, pitted and sliced
- 1/2 cup of tinned green lentils or cooked Puy lentils
- 1 tablespoon of chopped lovage
- 1 tablespoon of capers
- 1/4 cup of chicory leaves
- 2 tablespoons of chopped walnuts

Instructions:
- Place the salad greens on a big plate.
- To serve, combine the remaining ingredients and distribute them over the leaves.

343. Fancy Chicken Salad

(Preparation time: 10 minutes | Cooking time: 10 minutes | Difficulty: Easy | Servings: 1)
Per serving: Calories 340, Total fat 5g, Protein 36g, Carbs 20g
Ingredients:
- Juice of 1/4 of a lemon
- 1 teaspoon of ground turmeric
- 1 bird's eye chili
- 1/2 diced red onion
- 1 teaspoon of chopped coriander
- 1/4 cup of rocket
- 1/2 teaspoon of mild curry powder
- 1 finely chopped Medjool date
- 1/2 cup of natural yogurt
- 100g of cooked chicken breast, chopped into bite-sized chunks
- 6 finely chopped Walnut halves

Instructions:
- Combine the lemon juice, yogurt, spices, and coriander in a mixing dish. Mix in the remaining ingredients till thoroughly combined.
- Serve on top of a bed of rockets.

344. Sesame Soy Chicken Salad

(Preparation time: 10 minutes | Cooking time: 0 minutes | Difficulty: Easy | Servings: 2)
Per serving: Calories 304, Total fat 6g, Protein 33g, Carbs 25g
Ingredients:

- ½ finely sliced red onion
- 1 tablespoon of sesame seeds
- Large handful of chopped parsley (20g)
- 1 peeled cucumber, slice in half lengthwise, remove seed and cut into slices
- 1/4 cup of bok choy, very finely shredded
- 1/2 cup of roughly chopped baby kale
- 150g of cooked chicken, shredded

For the dressing:

- Juice of 1 lime
- 1 tablespoon of extra virgin olive oil
- 1 teaspoon of sesame oil
- 2 teaspoons of soy sauce
- 1 teaspoon of clear honey

Instructions:

- After thoroughly cleaning and drying your frying pan, roast the sesame seeds in the pan for around 2 minutes, or till fragrant & lightly browned. Set aside to cool on a plate.
- **To Make Dressing:** In a small-sized bowl, combine the lime juice, soy sauce, olive oil, sesame oil, & honey.
- In a large-sized mixing dish, carefully combine the kale, cucumber, parsley, red onion, & bok choy. Pour the dressing over the salad and toss to combine.
- Divide the salad between two dishes and top with shredded chicken. Sprinkle sesame seeds on top just before serving.

345. Salmon Chicory Rocket Super Salad

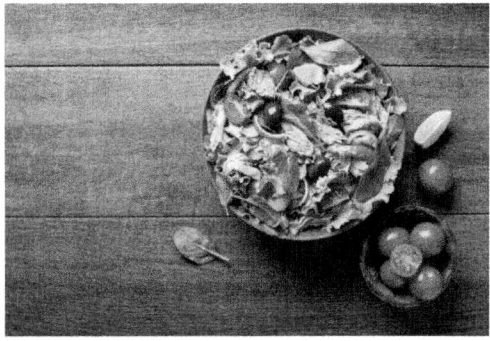

(Preparation time: 15 minutes | Cooking time: 0 minutes | Difficulty: Easy | Servings: 1)
Per serving: Calories 300, Total fat 21g, Protein 20g, Carbs 25g
Ingredients:

- Juice ¼ lemon
- 1 tablespoon of extra-virgin olive oil
- 1 tablespoon of chopped parsley
- 1/2 sliced red onion
- 2 tablespoons of chopped lovage or celery leaves
- 1/4 cup of rocket
- 1/4 of sliced celery
- 1 large Medjool date, pitted and chopped
- 1 tablespoon of capers
- 1/4 cup of chicory leaves
- 1/4 cup of chopped walnuts
- 1/2 cup of avocado, peeled, sliced
- 100g of smoked salmon slices or cooked chicken breast

Instructions:

- Place the salad greens on a big plate.
- To serve, combine the remaining ingredients and distribute them over the leaves.

346. Fresh Chopped Salad with Vinegar

(Preparation time: 15 minutes | Cooking time: 20 minutes | Difficulty: Easy | Servings: 8)
Per serving: Calories 113, Total fat 10g, Protein 1g, Carbs 5g
Ingredients:

- 1/2 teaspoon of salt
- Freshly ground pepper
- 4 tablespoons of extra-virgin olive oil
- 1/2 cup of chopped scallions
- 1/2 cup of fresh parsley, coarsely chopped
- 4 medium seeded and diced tomatoes
- 2 cups of diced seedless cucumber
- 1/2 cup of Kalamata olives, pitted and chopped coarsely
- 2 tablespoons of red wine

Instructions:

- In a medium mixing bowl, combine all of the ingredients and toss to blend coarsely.
- Within an hour, serve.

347. Creamy Asparagus Soup

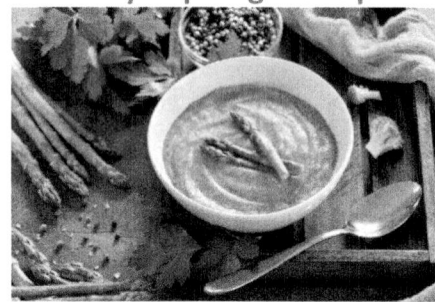

(Preparation time: 15 minutes | Cooking time: 30 minutes | Difficulty: Easy | Servings: 4)
Per serving: Calories 38, Total fat 2g, Protein 2g, Carbs 4g
Ingredients:

- A pinch of salt
- 1 chopped garlic clove
- 1 teaspoon of olive oil
- 1 teaspoon of dried oregano

- 2 cups of low-sodium chicken stock
- 1 cup of chopped broccoli
- 1 cup of chopped asparagus
- 2 tablespoons of low-fat sour cream

Instructions:

- Heat the olive oil in the pot for one minute. Continue to roast for 1 minute more after adding the garlic.
- Close the lid and add the remaining ingredients from the list above.
- On low flame, cook the soup for about 25 minutes. Then purée the soup with an immersion blender till it's completely smooth. Cook the soup for an additional 5 minutes.

348. Buckwheat Pasta Soup

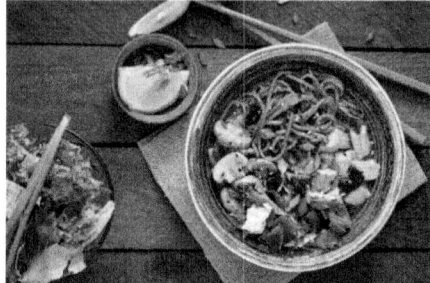

(Preparation time: 15 minutes | Cooking time: 20 minutes | Difficulty: Easy | Servings: 2)
Per serving: Calories 263, Total fat 3g, Protein 12g, Carbs 20g
Ingredients:

- A pinch of salt
- 1 teaspoon of ground black pepper
- 3 tablespoons of shredded carrot
- 1/2 cup of chopped celery stalk
- 1/2 cup of corn kernels
- 2 cups of low-sodium chicken stock
- 1/4 cup of buckwheat pasta

Instructions:

- Bring the chicken stock to the boil, then add the celery stalks and shredded carrots. On low flame, cook the liquid for around 5 minutes.

- Toss in the corn kernels, black pepper, salt and buckwheat pasta after that.
- Mix the soup thoroughly.
- On a medium temperature, cook for about 15 minutes.

349. Edamame and Tangerine Salad

(Preparation time: 10 minutes | Cooking time: 15 minutes | Difficulty: Easy | Servings: 4)
Per serving: Calories 113, Total fat 5g, Protein 4g, Carbs 16g
Ingredients:

- 2 cups of water
- A pinch of salt
- 1/2 teaspoon of ground black pepper
- 1 tablespoon of olive oil
- 1 teaspoon of chili flakes
- 1/2 cup of chopped Italian parsley
- 1 cup of cooked corn kernels
- 1 cup of peeled tangerines
- 1/2 cup of soaked edamame beans

Instructions:

- Fill the kettle halfway up with water. Boil the edamame beans for around 10 minutes. Before putting the edamame beans in the salad plate, drain and rinse them. Cook together the corn kernels, parsley, & tangerines.
- Then toss the salad with ground black pepper, salt, chili flakes, and olive oil.
- Toss the salad ingredients together.

350. South-Western White Bean Soup

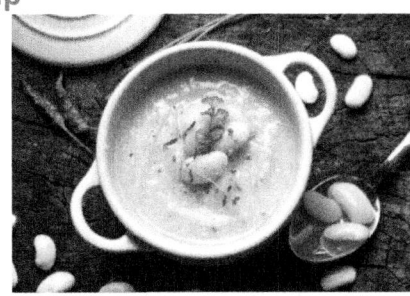

(Preparation time: 10 minutes | Cooking time: 15 minutes | Difficulty: Easy | Servings: 4)
Per serving: Calories 276, Total fat 4g, Protein 16g, Carbs 10g
Ingredients:

- A pinch of salt
- 3 minced garlic cloves
- 1 tablespoon of olive oil
- 2 tablespoons of chopped parsley
- 2 seeded and diced bird's eye chilies
- 1/2 cup of diced red onion
- 2 cups of low-salt diced tomatoes
- 1 cup of low-salt chicken broth
- 3 cups of cooked and drained white beans
- 1 1/2 diced assorted bell peppers
- 2 tablespoons of red wine

Instructions:

- Around 1 cup of cooked beans & the entire beans should be blended in a blender.
- In a soup pan, heat the oil over medium flame. Sauté the onions, chilies, bell peppers, and garlic for 4 to 5 minutes, or till the onions are transparent.
- Combine the bean mixture with broth. Stir for another 3 to 4 minutes, or till the beans are completely heated.
- Stir in the tomatoes and wine once the mixture is heated, then turn off the flame. Just before serving, add the parsley.

CHAPTER 12:

Snacks Recipes

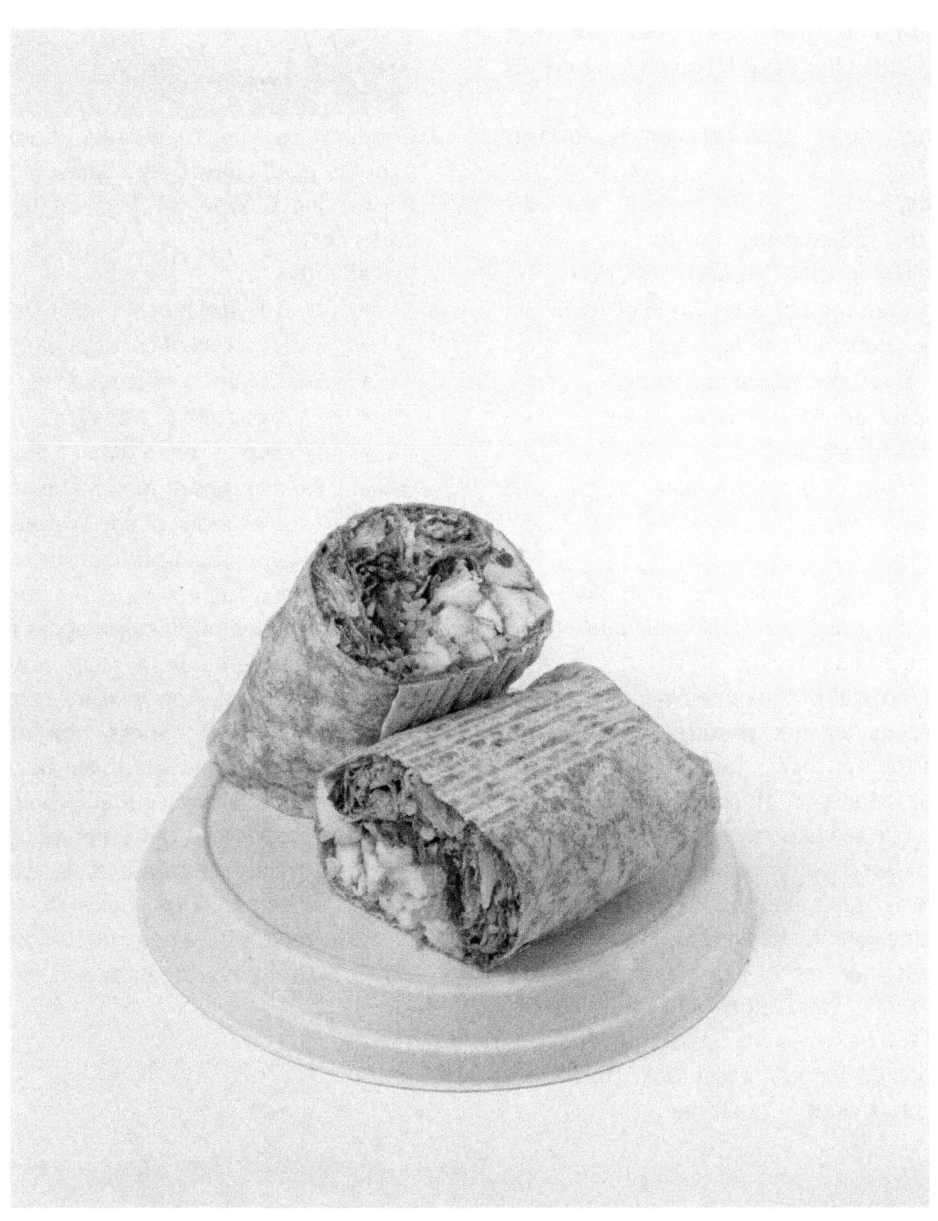

351. Sirtfood Bites

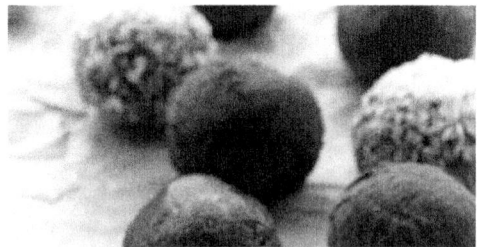

(Preparation time: 10 minutes | Cooking time: 0 minutes | Difficulty: Easy | Servings: 15 to 20 bites)

Per serving: Calories 100, Total fat 3g, Protein 6g, Carbs 11g

Ingredients:

- 1 to 2 tablespoons of water
- 1 tablespoon of ground turmeric
- 1 tablespoon of extra virgin olive oil
- 1 teaspoon of vanilla extract
- 1 tablespoon of cocoa powder
- 2 cups of Medjool dates, pitted
- 1 cup of walnuts
- 1/4 cup of dark chocolate (85 percent cocoa solids), broken into pieces

Instructions:

- In a food processor, combine the walnuts and chocolate and pulse till a fine powder forms.
- Blend in all of the remaining ingredients, except for the water, till the dough forms a ball. Depending on the consistency of the mixture (you don't want it to be too sticky), you may or may not need to add water.
- Form the mixture into bite-size balls using your hands and store in an airtight container for at least 1 hour before eating. If you choose, you can roll some of the balls in more cocoa powder or dry coconut for a different look. They'll last up to a week in the fridge.

352. Matcha Protein Bites

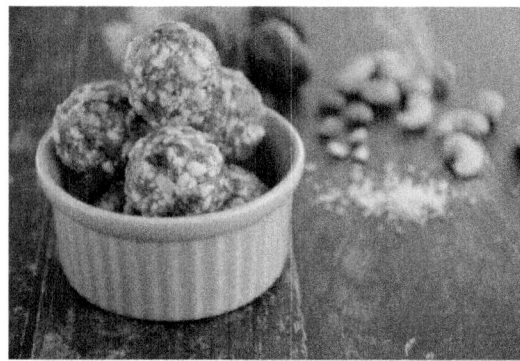

(Preparation time: 10 minutes | Cooking time: 0 minutes | Difficulty: Easy | Servings: 12 bites)

Per serving: Calories 34, Total fat 3g, Protein 1g, Carbs 2g

Ingredients:

- 1/4 teaspoon of sea salt
- 2 teaspoons of coconut oil
- 1 tablespoon of chia seeds
- 1 tablespoon of honey
- 1/5 cup of rolled oats
- 2 teaspoons of matcha powder
- 2 tablespoons of soy protein isolate
- 1/4 cup of almond butter

Instructions:

- Combine all of the matcha protein bite ingredients in a food processor and process till the mixture resembles wet sand and sticks together when squashed between your fingers.
- Make twelve equal amounts of the mixture. You can estimate by eye or use a digital kitchen scale for accurate portions. Form balls by rolling each amount between your palms.
- Refrigerate the bites and serve.

353. Chocolate-Covered Strawberry Trail Mix

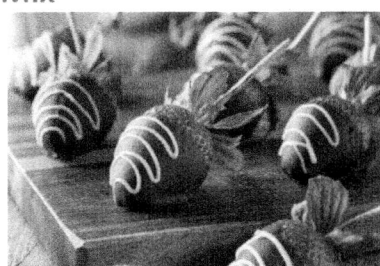

(Preparation time: 10 minutes | Cooking time: 0 minutes | Difficulty: Easy | Servings: 10)
Per serving: Calories 74, Total fat 7g, Protein 2g, Carbs 2g
Ingredients:
- 1 cup of strawberries
- 1/4 cup of roasted almonds
- 1/4 cup of roasted cashew
- 1 cup of walnuts
- 1/4 cup of dark chocolate chunks

Instructions:
- In a big glass jar, combine all of the trail mix ingredients, then divide each portion into its own transportable plastic bag. Keep for up to a month in the refrigerator.

354. Yogurt with Chopped Walnuts, Dark Chocolate and Mixed Berries

(Preparation time: 10 minutes | Cooking time: 0 minutes | Difficulty: Easy | Servings: 1)
Per serving: Calories 180, Total fat 7g, Protein 12g, Carbs 15g
Ingredients:
- 1 1/3 cups of mixed berries
- 2/3 cup of plain Greek yogurt
- 1/4 cup of chopped walnuts
- 1 1/2 tablespoons of grated dark chocolate (85% cocoa solids)

Instructions:
- Toss your favorite berries into a bowl, then top with yogurt. Walnuts and chocolate should be sprinkled on top.

355. Garlic Mashed Potatoes

(Preparation time: 10 minutes | Cooking time: 25 minutes | Difficulty: Easy | Servings: 1)
Per serving: Calories 177, Total fat 1g, Protein 6g, Carbs 20g
Ingredients:
- A pinch of salt
- 6 minced garlic cloves
- 4 russet potatoes
- 1 cup of vegetable broth
- 4 tablespoons of chopped parsley
- ½ cup of skim milk

Instructions:
- Potatoes should be cut into medium-sized bits.
- In the Instant Pot, combine the pieces, garlic, & broth.
- Cook for 5 minutes at high pressure with the lid closed.
- When the cooking is finished, let the pressure naturally release.
- Carefully open the cover and mash the potato with a handheld masher.

356. Salmon Fritters

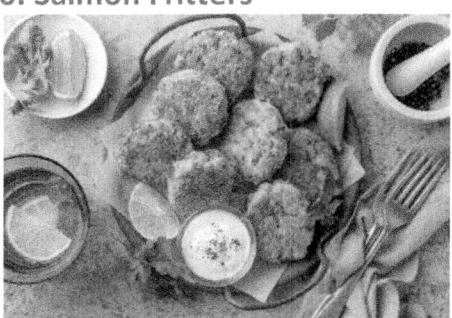

(Preparation time: 10 minutes | Cooking time: 20 minutes | Difficulty: Easy | Servings: 2)
Per serving: Calories 320, Total fat 7g, Protein 27g, Carbs 18g
Ingredients:
- Salt and pepper to taste
- 1 clove of garlic, crushed
- 2 teaspoons olive oil

- 1 tablespoon of buckwheat or almond flour
- ½ red onion, finely chopped
- 2 eggs
- 2 cups of arugula
- 6 oz. of salmon, canned

Instructions:

- Separate the egg whites from the yolks and whisk them together. Combine the salmon, flour, salt, pepper, onion, garlic, onion, & yolks in a separate bowl.
- Slowly incorporate the egg whites into the mixture. Preheat a pan to medium-high flame. When the oil is hot, add 1 teaspoon of salmon and create fritters with a spoon.
- Cook till golden brown on both sides (about 4 minutes per side) & serve with arugula salad seasoned with salt, pepper, and 1 tablespoon olive oil.

357. Turmeric and Chili Hummus

(Preparation time: 10 minutes | Cooking time: 0 minutes | Difficulty: Easy | Servings: 2)
Per serving: Calories 80, Total fat 5g, Protein 3g, Carbs 12g
Ingredients:

- 1/4 cup of water
- 1 lemon
- 1 teaspoon of ground turmeric
- 1 tablespoon of extra virgin olive oil juice
- 1 chopped bird's eye chili, chopped
- 2 tablespoons of tahini
- 1 × 400g can of chickpeas, drained

Instructions:

- In a food processor, combine all ingredients and process for 2-3 minutes, till smooth paste forms.
- Depending on how thick you prefer your hummus, you can add a little extra water. Serve alongside fresh vegetables.

358. Paleo-Force Bars

(Preparation time: 15 minutes | Cooking time: 0 minutes | Difficulty: Easy | Servings: 10)
Per serving: Calories 267, Total fat 33g, Protein 18g, Carbs 29g
Ingredients:

- 1/4 cup of coconut oil
- 10 pieces Medjoul dates (cored)
- 1/2 cup of grated coconut
- 1/2 cup of crushed linseed
- 1/3 cup of Cashew nuts

Instructions:

- In a food processor, combine all ingredients & pulse till a sticky, granular dough forms.
- Using parchment paper, line a small baking sheet.
- Spread the mixture on the baking sheet's bottom & firmly press it down.
- Place them in the freezer for a few hours to solidify and harden.
- Cut the mixture into bars once it has firm.
- Wrap the bars in cling film or baking paper if you wish to pack them as individual snacks.

359. Hearty Cashew and Almond Butter

(Preparation time: 10 minutes | Cooking time: 15 minutes | Difficulty: Easy | Servings: 1)
Per serving: Calories 205, Total fat 1g, Protein 6g, Carbs 31g
Ingredients:

- 1/2 teaspoon of cinnamon
- 2 tablespoons of coconut oil
- 1/3 cup of cashew nuts
- 1 cup of almonds, blanched

Instructions:

- Preheat the oven at 350°F.
- Almonds and cashews should be baked for approximately 12 minutes.

- Allow them to cool.
- Add the remaining ingredients to the food processor and pulse till smooth.
- Blend in the oil till it is completely smooth.
- Serve and have fun!

360. Chocolate Bites

(Preparation time: 10 minutes | Cooking time:0 minutes | Difficulty: Easy | Servings: 15)
Per serving: Calories 104, Total fat 5g, Protein 3g, Carbs 14g
Ingredients:

- 1 tablespoon of chia seeds
- 3 tablespoons of almond butter
- 1 cup of Medjool dates, pitted
- 2/3 cup of gluten-free rolled oats
- ¼ cup of unsweetened dark chocolate, chopped roughly
- ½ cup of cacao powder

Instructions:

- Place dates in a food processor and pulse till finely chopped.
- Pulse in the remaining ingredients, excluding the cacao powder, till just blended. From the mixture, make 1-inch balls. Place the cacao powder on a small-sized plate. Coat the balls in cacao powder and place them on a baking sheet lined using parchment paper.
- Before serving, freeze for 15 minutes or till totally set.

361. Asian Slaw

(Preparation time: 15 minutes | Cooking time: 0 minutes | Difficulty: Easy | Servings: 2)
Per serving: Calories 179, Total fat 12g, Protein 8g, Carbs 11g
Ingredients:

- 1 teaspoon of sea salt
- 1/2 teaspoon of ground black pepper
- 1 clove of garlic minced
- 2 teaspoons of grated ginger

- 2 tablespoons extra virgin olive oil
- 1 tablespoon of sesame seeds
- 1 red onion, finely sliced
- 5 teaspoons of sesame seed oil
- 2 teaspoons of honey
- 2 teaspoons of Sriracha
- 1 red bell pepper, finely sliced
- 2 tablespoons of peanut butter, natural
- 2 tablespoons of tamari sauce
- 1/4 cup of peanuts, chopped
- 1/4 cup of cilantro, chopped
- 1 cup of carrots shredded
- 2 cups of red cabbage, shredded
- 2 cups of broccoli florets, chopped
- 1/4 cup of rice wine vinegar

Instructions:

- Toss the vegetables, cilantro, & peanuts in a large-sized salad bowl.
- Whisk together the remaining ingredients in a separate bowl till emulsified. Toss the vegetables in the dressing till they are evenly coated.
- To blend the flavors, chill the slaw for at least 10 minutes. Refrigerate the Asian slaw up to a day ahead of time for added flavor.

362. Cinnamon Apple Chips

(Preparation time: 10 minutes | Cooking time: 2 hours | Difficulty: Easy | Servings: 4)
Per serving: Calories 80, Total fat 1g, Protein 4g, Carbs 7g
Ingredients:

- Cooking spray
- 2 teaspoons of cinnamon powder
- 2 apples, cored and thinly sliced

Instructions:

- Arrange apple slices on a baking sheet lined using parchment paper, drizzle with cooking oil, sprinkle with cinnamon, and bake for around 2 hours at 300°F. Serve as a snack by dividing the mixture into bowls.

363. Greek-Style Party Dip

(Preparation time: 10 minutes | Cooking time: 0 minutes | Difficulty: Easy | Servings: 4)
Per serving: Calories 100, Total fat 1g, Protein 3g, Carbs 8g
Ingredients:

- Black pepper to the taste
- 1 teaspoon of sweet paprika
- 2 teaspoons of parsley, chopped
- 2 teaspoons of chives, chopped
- 2 teaspoons of dill, dried
- 2 teaspoons of thyme, dried
- 1 cup of fat-free Greek yogurt
- 2 teaspoons of no-salt-added sun-dried tomatoes, chopped
- ½ cup of coconut cream

Instructions:

- Combine cream, yogurt, dill, thyme, paprika, tomatoes, parsley, chives, & pepper in a mixing bowl. Stir well, divide into smaller bowls, and serve as a dip.

364. Shrimp Muffins

(Preparation time: 10 minutes | Cooking time: 45 minutes | Difficulty: Easy | Servings: 6)
Per serving: Calories 140, Total fat 2g, Protein 14g, Carbs 4g
Ingredients:

- Cooking spray Black pepper to the taste
- 1 garlic clove, minced
- 1 teaspoon of parsley, dried
- 1 spaghetti squash, peeled and halved
- 1 ½ cups of almond flour
- 1 cup of low-fat mozzarella cheese, shredded
- 2 tablespoons of avocado mayonnaise
- 8 ounces of shrimp, peeled, cooked and chopped

Instructions:

- Place the squash on a prepared baking sheet and bake for around 30 minutes at 375°F. Scrape the flesh into a bowl

and toss in the pepper, parsley flakes, flour, shrimp, mayo, and mozzarella.
- Divide the mixture into muffin tins sprayed with cooking spray, bake for around 15 minutes, and serve cold as a snack.

365. Zucchini Bowls

(Preparation time: 10 minutes | Cooking time: 20 minutes | Difficulty: Easy | Servings: 12)
Per serving: Calories 120, Total fat 1g, Protein 6g, Carbs 12g
Ingredients:

- Cooking spray
- Black pepper to the taste
- 2 garlic cloves, minced
- 1 red onion, chopped - 1 egg
- ½ cup of dill, chopped
- 3 zucchinis, grated
- ½ cup of whole wheat flour

Instructions:

- Mix zucchinis with garlic, onion, flour, pepper, egg, & dill in a mixing bowl, stirring well. Form tiny bowls out of this mixture, lay on a lined baking sheet and coat using cooking spray.
- Bake for around 20 minutes at 400°F, flipping halfway through, then divide into bowls & serve as a snack.

366. Cheesy Mushroom Caps

(Preparation time: 10 minutes | Cooking time: 20 minutes | Difficulty: Easy | Servings: 20)
Per serving: Calories 120, Total fat 1g, Protein 7g, Carbs 11g
Ingredients:

- Black pepper to the taste
- 1 garlic clove, minced
- A drizzle of olive oil
- 2 red onions, chopped
- 2 tablespoons of non-fat yogurt
- 3 tablespoons of parsley, chopped
- 20 white mushroom caps

- ½ cup of low-fat parmesan, grated
- ¼ cup of low-fat mozzarella, grated

Instructions:

- Heat some oil in a pan over medium flame, then add the onion and garlic, stir, and cook for 10 minutes before transferring to a bowl.
- Stir in the black pepper, garlic, parmesan, parsley, mozzarella, and yogurt, then stuff the mushroom caps using the mixture, place them on a lined baking sheet, and bake for around 20 minutes at 400°F. Serve as a snack.

367. Cauliflower Mozzarella Bars

(Preparation time: 10 minutes | Cooking time: 40 minutes | Difficulty: Easy | Servings: 12)
Per serving: Calories 140, Total fat 1g, Protein 6g, Carbs 6g
Ingredients:

- Black pepper to the taste
- 1 teaspoon of Italian seasoning
- ¼ cup of egg whites
- 1 big cauliflower head, riced
- ½ cup of low-fat mozzarella cheese, shredded

Instructions:

- Spread the cauliflower rice on a prepared baking sheet and bake for around 20 minutes at 375°F. Transfer to a bowl, add the black pepper, cheese, seasoning, and egg whites, combine well and spread into a rectangle pan.
- Preheat the oven at 375°F, bake for around 20 minutes, then cut into 12 bars & serve as a snack.

368. Strawberry and Nut Granola

(Preparation time: 10 minutes | Cooking time: 50 minutes | Difficulty: Easy | Servings: 12)
Per serving: Calories 291, Total fat 1g, Protein 8g, Carbs 3g
Ingredients:

- 1½ teaspoons of ground ginger

- 1½ teaspoons of ground cinnamon
- 4 tablespoons of olive oil
- 2 tablespoons of honey
- 1/2 cup of walnuts, chopped
- 1/2 cup of almonds, chopped
- 1/2 cup of dried strawberries
- 1 cup of oats
- 1 cup of buckwheat flakes

Instructions:

- Mix together the oats, buckwheat flakes, almonds, ginger, & cinnamon in a mixing bowl. Warm the oil & honey in a saucepan. Stir till the honey is completely melted.
- In a large-sized mixing bowl, pour the heating oil into the dry ingredients and stir well. Spread the mixture out on a big baking tray (or two) & bake for around 50 minutes at 300°F, or till brown.
- Allow time for it to cool. Add the dried berries to the mix until ready to use, store in an airtight container. As a convenient snack, it can be served with yogurt, milk, or even dry.

369. Yogurt Crunch with Fruit and Nut

(Preparation time: 10 minutes | Cooking time: 0 minutes | Difficulty: Easy | Servings: 1)
Per serving: Calories 296, Total fat 4g, Protein 9g, Carbs 5g
Ingredients:

- 1/4 cup of strawberries, chopped
- 6 walnut halves, chopped
- 1/2 cup of plain Greek yogurt
- A sprinkling of cocoa powder

Instructions:

- Half of the sliced strawberries should be added to the yogurt.
- Using a glass, place a layer of yogurt with a dusting of strawberries & walnuts, followed by another layer of

the same till you reach the top of the glass.
- Serve with walnuts and a sprinkling of cocoa powder on top.

370. Apple Pastry

(Preparation time: 10 minutes | Cooking time: 25 minutes | Difficulty: Easy | Servings: 1)
Per serving: Calories 238, Total fat 8g, Protein 4g, Carbs 28g
Ingredients:
- A pinch of salt
- A pinch of each ground nutmeg and ground cinnamon
- 2 teaspoons of margarine
- 1 small apple
- 1 tablespoon of plain low-fat yogurt
- 2 teaspoons of reduced-calorie apricot spread
- 3 tablespoons of almond or buckwheat flour

Instructions:
- Combine all of the ingredients.
- Preheat the oven at 350°F.
- Core, pare, & thinly slice the apple; lay slices over the dough in a decorative pattern and season using nutmeg and cinnamon. Bake for around 20 to 30 minutes, or till the crust is brown.

371. Cinnamon-Apricot Bananas

(Preparation time: 10 minutes | Cooking time: 25 minutes | Difficulty: Easy | Servings: 1)
Per serving: Calories 130, Total fat 2g, Protein 2g, Carbs 25g
Ingredients:
- 1/4 teaspoon of ground cinnamon
- 1 medium banana, peeled and cut into squares
- 2 teaspoons of shredded coconut
- 1 tablespoon plus 1 teaspoon of reduced-calorie apricot spread

- 4 graham crackers, made into crumbs half lengthwise

Instructions:
- Toast the crumbs, coconut, and cinnamon being careful not to burn them; transfer on a sheet of wax paper or a paper plate, and leave aside.
- Heat the apricot spread in the same skillet till it melts, then remove it from the flame. Roll each banana half in the spread, then roll in the crumb mixture rapidly, pressing the crumbs into the banana; place coated halves on a platter, cover lightly, and chill till cooled.

372. Eggplant Pesto

(Preparation time: 10 minutes | Cooking time: 25 minutes | Difficulty: Easy | Servings: 2)
Per serving: Calories 144, Total fat 9g, Protein 5g, Carbs 12g
Ingredients:
- A pinch of salt and ground black pepper
- 1 small garlic clove, mashed
- 1 tablespoon of olive oil
- 1 medium eggplant
- 2 tablespoons of each chopped fresh basil and grated parmesan cheese

Instructions:
- Combine the remaining ingredients in a small-sized bowl;
- Cover each eggplant slice with an equal amount of the mixture. Transfer to the oven and bake for another 15 minutes, or until the slices are heated through.

373. Chilled Eggplant Relish

(Preparation time: 10 minutes | Cooking time: 25 minutes | Difficulty: Easy | Servings: 4)
Per serving: Calories 113, Total fat 7g, Protein 3g, Carbs 13g
Ingredients:
- 1 teaspoon of salt
- 2 garlic cloves
- 1 tablespoon of olive oil

- 1 cup of thinly sliced red onions
- 3 cups of eggplant
- 1 cup of each diced celery and chopped tomatoes - 1 teaspoon of sweetener
- 8 black olives
- 1 tablespoon of capers
- 2 teaspoons of red wine

Instructions:

- Heat the oil over medium flame, then add the garlic and onions and cook for 3 to 5 minutes, or till the onions are transparent. Cook, occasionally turning, till eggplant begins to soften, approximately 5 minutes; toss in celery and tomatoes, cover, and cook till celery is tender about 5 minutes.
- Cook for another 5 minutes, uncovered, after adding the wine and sweetener. Remove from the flame and toss in the olives and capers to incorporate; move to glass, plastic, or stainless-steel container, cover, & chill until completely cooled.

374. Crunchy Potato Bites

(Preparation time: 10 minutes | Cooking time: 25 minutes | Difficulty: Easy | Servings: 3)
Per serving: Calories 112, Total fat 1g, Protein 1g, Carbs 1g
Ingredients:

- 1 tablespoon of extra virgin olive oil
- 1 potato, sliced
- 1 small avocado, pitted and cubed
- 2 bacon slices, already cooked and crumbled

Instructions:

- Place potato slices on a baking sheet that has been lined.
- Toss them using extra virgin olive oil.
- Preheat the oven at 350°F and bake for around 20 minutes. Serve as a snack by arranging on a dish and topping each slice with avocado & crumbled bacon.

375. Dates Wrapped in Parma Ham Blanket

(Preparation time: 10 minutes | Cooking time: 25 minutes | Difficulty: Easy | Servings: 12)
Per serving: Calories 149, Total fat 1g, Protein 1g, Carbs 1g
Ingredients:

- 12 Medjool dates
- 2 slices of Parma ham, cut into strips

Instructions:

- Wrap a strip of Parma ham around each date. It can be served both hot and cold.

376. Spicy Pumpkin Seeds Bowl

(Preparation time: 10 minutes | Cooking time: 25 minutes | Difficulty: Easy | Servings: 6)
Per serving: Calories 50, Total fat 1g, Protein 1g, Carbs 0.8g
Ingredients:

- 2 teaspoons of lime juice
- ½ tablespoon of chili powder
- ½ teaspoon of cayenne pepper
- 2 cups of pumpkin seeds

Instructions:

- Toss pumpkin seeds with lime juice, cayenne pepper, and chili powder on a prepared baking sheet.
- Place it in the oven & bake for 20 minutes at 275°F.
- Serve as a snack by dividing the mixture into small bowls.

377. Apple and Pecan Bowls

(Preparation time: 10 minutes | Cooking time: 0 minutes | Difficulty: Easy | Servings: 4)
Per serving: Calories 60, Total fat 1g, Protein 1g, Carbs 0.5g
Ingredients:

- 2 teaspoons of lemon juice
- 4 big apples, cored, peeled and cubed
- ¼ cup of pecans, chopped

Instructions:
- Toss apples with lemon juice & pecans in a mixing bowl.
- Serve as a snack by dividing the mixture into small bowls.

378. Herbed Mixed Nuts

(Preparation time: 10 minutes | Cooking time: 25 minutes | Difficulty: Easy | Servings: 12)
Per serving: Calories 221, Total fat 2g, Protein 2g, Carbs 16g
Ingredients:
- ½ teaspoon of garlic salt
- 1 tablespoon of butter, melted
- 2 teaspoons of dried basil and/or oregano, crushed
- 1 tablespoon of Worcestershire sauce
- 3 cups of walnuts, soy nuts, and/or almonds - 2 tablespoons of grated Parmesan cheese

Instructions:
- Preheat the oven at 325°F.
- In a mixing bowl, combine the garlic salt, herb, Worcestershire sauce, & melted butter, then add the nuts and toss to coat.
- Line a 15x10x1-inch baking sheet with foil, then spread the nuts evenly in the pan. Place the parmesan on top and mix till it is evenly distributed.
- Allow it to bake for around 15 minutes, stirring twice. Allow time for it to cool. Cover tightly and keep refrigerated for up to one week.

379. Almonds with Rosemary and Cayenne

(Preparation time: 10 minutes | Cooking time: 15 minutes | Difficulty: Easy | Servings: 16)
Per serving: Calories 80, Total fat 2g, Protein 2g, Carbs 13g
Ingredients:
- ¼ to ½ teaspoon of salt

- ¼ teaspoon of ground red pepper
- 1½ teaspoons of margarine or butter
- 1½ teaspoons of sweetener
- 1 tablespoon of finely snipped fresh rosemary - 2 cups of unblanched almonds or pecan halves

Instructions:
- Preheat the oven at 350°F.
- Arrange the almonds or pecans in a single layer on the baking tray.
- Allow it to bake for around 10 minutes, or till fragrant and toasted.
- Meanwhile, in a medium-sized saucepan over medium flame, melt the margarine or butter till it sizzles. Remove it from the flame. Combine the red pepper, salt, sweetener, and rosemary.
- Toss the nuts in the butter mixture till they are well coated.
- Allow it to cool somewhat before serving.

380. Plum and Pistachio Snack

(Preparation time: 10 minutes | Cooking time: 0 minutes | Difficulty: Easy | Servings: 1)
Per serving: Calories 275, Total fat 1g, Protein 3g, Carbs 20g
Ingredients:
- 1 plum - ¼ cup of unsalted dry-roasted pistachios (measured in shell)

Instructions:
- Pistachios should be hulled & served with plums.

381. Chocolate Bark

(Preparation time: 15 minutes | Cooking time: 3 hours | Difficulty: Easy | Servings: 2)
Per serving: Calories 323, Total fat 38g, Protein 21g, Carbs 18g
Ingredients:
- 2 teaspoons of flaky sea salt
- 1 thin peel orange

- 1 cardamom pod, finely crushed and sieved
- 1 tablespoon of chia seeds
- 1 tablespoon of sesame seeds, toasted and cooled
- 1 teaspoon of grated orange peel
- ¼ cup of pumpkin seeds, toasted and chilled
- ¾ cup of pistachio nuts, roasted, chilled and chopped into large pieces
- ¼ cup of hazelnuts, toasted, chilled, peeled and chopped into large pieces
- 1 1/2 cups of tempered, dairy-free dark chocolate (85% cocoa content)
- Candy or candy thermometer

Instructions:

- Preheat the oven at 300°F. Using parchment paper, line a baking sheet.
- Place the orange on the prepared baking sheet, finely sliced crosswise. Bake for around 2 to 3 hours, or till the mixture is dry but still a little sticky. Allow it to cool after removing it from the oven.
- When the orange slices have cooled enough to handle, split them into shards and lay them aside.
- Mix the nuts, seeds, & grated orange peel in a large-sized mixing dish till well blended. Place the mixture on a baking sheet lined using kitchen parchment in a single layer. Set them aside.
- Melt the chocolate, then pour it over the nut mixture to completely cover it.
- Sprinkle sea salt and orange chunks on top of the chocolate when it's semi-cold but still sticky.
- Place the crust in a cool part of your kitchen or in the refrigerator till it is completely cool, then cut it into bite-size pieces.

382. Candy Wraps

(Preparation time: 15 minutes | Cooking time: 0 minutes | Difficulty: Easy | Servings: 4)
Per serving: Calories 90, Total fat 1g, Protein 3g, Carbs 21g
Ingredients:

- 1 (10 inches) whole wheat tortilla
- 1 teaspoon of pure maple syrup
- 1 teaspoon of orange marmalade

Instructions:

- Place the tortilla on a clean surface or dinner plate. On one half, spread orange marmalade, and on the other, maple syrup. Roll the tortilla firmly from end to end, starting with the syrup & ending with the marmalade.
- If necessary, secure it with toothpicks or wrap it in plastic wrap. Allow it to chill for a few hours before cutting into 1" pieces to serve.

383. Spicy Almonds

(Preparation time: 15 minutes | Cooking time: 25 minutes | Difficulty: Easy | Servings: 4)
Per serving: Calories 230, Total fat 20g, Protein 3g, Carbs 9g
Ingredients:

- 1-1/2 teaspoons of kosher salt
- 1/2 teaspoon of ground cinnamon
- 1/4 teaspoon of cayenne pepper
- 1 teaspoon of paprika
- 1/2 teaspoon of ground coriander
- 1/2 teaspoon of ground cumin
- 1 tablespoon of stevia
- 1 tablespoon of olive oil
- 2-1/2 cups of unblanched almonds

Instructions:

- In a small-sized mixing dish, combine the first seven ingredients. In a separate small bowl, combine the oil and almonds.
- Drizzle with the spice mixture and toss to coat.

- Place the mixture in a 15x10x1-inch foil-lined baking sheet greased using cooking spray. Bake at 325° for around 15 to 20 minutes, or till gently browned, stirring twice. Allow cooling completely. Keep the container sealed.

384. Rosemary Walnuts

(Preparation time: 10 minutes | Cooking time: 20 minutes | Difficulty: Easy | Servings: 8)
Per serving: Calories 188, Total fat 18g, Protein 4g, Carbs 6g
Ingredients:
- 1 teaspoon of salt
- 2 cloves of garlic, minced
- 1 tablespoon of extra-virgin olive oil
- 1 tablespoon of minced fresh rosemary
- 1 tablespoon of honey 2 cups of walnuts

Instructions:
- Preheat the oven at 350°F. Line your baking pan using parchment paper and set it aside.
- Combine honey, rosemary, salt, garlic, walnuts, & olive oil in a clean bowl. Transfer the walnuts to the prepared baking pan after mixing till they are completely coated.
- Bake the walnuts for around 10 minutes or till they are lightly browned.

385. Gluten-Free Snack Mix

(Preparation time: 10 minutes | Cooking time: 25 minutes | Difficulty: Easy | Servings: 8)
Per serving: Calories 110, Total fat 1g, Protein 1g, Carbs 16g
Ingredients:
- 1/2 teaspoon of ground cinnamon
- 1/3 cup of butter, cubed
- 1/3 cup of honey
- 8 cups of popped popcorn
- 2 cups of cereal
- 1/2 cup of dried cherries

Instructions:
- In a large-sized ungreased roasting pan, combine cherries, cereal, and popcorn. In a small-sized saucepan, melt the butter. Cook and whisk in the cinnamon and honey till thoroughly cooked. Drizzle the oil over the popcorn mixture & toss well to coat.
- Preheat oven to 325°F and bake for around 15 minutes, stirring every 5 minutes. Allow cooling completely. Keep it in an airtight container.

386. Corn Spread

(Preparation time: 10 minutes | Cooking time: 10 minutes | Difficulty: Easy | Servings: 6)
Per serving: Calories 192, Total fat 5g, Protein 8g, Carbs 11g
Ingredients:
- ½ teaspoon of chili powder
- 1 bird's eye chili, chopped
- 2 green onions, chopped
- 3 cups of canned corn, drained
- ½ cup of coconut cream

Instructions:
- Incorporate the corn, green onions, chilies, and chili powder in a small-sized saucepan, stir to combine, bring to a simmer, and cook for 10 minutes over medium flame, stirring occasionally. Remove from the flame, whisk in the coconut cream, divide into small bowls, and serve alongside buckwheat bread and vegetables.

387. Black Bean Salsa

(Preparation time: 10 minutes | Cooking time: 0 minutes | Difficulty: Easy | Servings: 6)
Per serving: Calories 181, Total fat 5g, Protein 7g, Carbs 14g
Ingredients:
- ½ teaspoon of cumin, ground
- 1 tablespoon of coconut amino

- 1 cup of salsa - 6 cups of romaine lettuce leave, torn
- 1 cup of canned black beans, no-salt-added, drained and rinsed
- ½ cup of avocado, peeled, pitted, and cubed

Instructions:

- Blend the beans, amino, cumin, salsa, lettuce, & avocado in a dish, toss to combine, divide into small bowls, and serve as a snack.

388. Chocolate Energy Balls

(Preparation time: 10 minutes | Cooking time: 0 minutes | Difficulty: Easy | Servings: 4)
Per serving: Calories 184, Total fat 12g, Protein 9g, Carbs 12g
Ingredients:

- 6 pitted Medjool dates
- 1/3 cup of cocoa powder
- 1 cup of raw hemp seeds

Instructions:

- Grind hemp seeds to a powder in a food processor; add dates and chocolate powder, and process till smooth. Roll the dough into a tight ball to make balls.

389. Vanilla Granola

(Preparation time: 10 minutes | Cooking time: 30 minutes | Difficulty: Easy | Servings: 4)
Per serving: Calories 131, Total fat 4g, Protein 4g, Carbs 20g
Ingredients:

- Non-stick cooking spray
- 1/4 teaspoon of ground cinnamon
- 4 teaspoons of vanilla extract
- 2 tablespoons of sweetener
- 1 cup of chopped walnuts
- 4 cups of rolled oats
- 1 cup of applesauce
- 1/2 cup of granular brown sugar replacement

Instructions:

- Preheat the oven at 300°F. A big baking sheet should be lightly coated using non-stick cooking spray.
- Combine the oats, walnuts, sweetener, & cinnamon in a large-sized mixing bowl.
- Combine applesauce & sweetener in a small-sized saucepan; bring to a boil over medium flame and remove from flame immediately. In a mixing dish, combine the applesauce and vanilla; spoon over the oats mixture & toss to coat. Fill the prepared baking dish halfway with the mixture.
- Cook for around 20 to 30 minutes, or until golden brown. To finish cooling the granola, place the baking sheet on a cooling rack.

390. Honey Nutters

(Preparation time: 10 minutes | Cooking time: 0 minutes | Difficulty: Easy | Servings: 4)
Per serving: Calories 166, Total fat 9g, Protein 4g, Carbs 21g
Ingredients:

- 1 cup of coconut
- 1/2 cup of non-fat dry milk powder
- 16 graham crackers
- 1 cup of crunchy peanut butter
- 2/3 cup of honey

Instructions:

- Smash the graham crackers between two pieces of wax paper with a rolling pin or a food processor.
- Combine honey, graham cracker crumbs, peanut butter, & powdered milk in a large mixing dish. Make a thorough mix.
- Form the mixture into little balls and place them on wax paper. Before serving, roll the balls in shredded coconut.

391. Pumpkin Almond Bites

(Preparation time: 10 minutes | Cooking time: 0 minutes | Difficulty: Easy | Servings: 4)

Per serving: Calories 158, Total fat 12g, Protein 5g, Carbs 10g

Ingredients:
- 1/2 teaspoon of ground cinnamon
- 1/4 teaspoon of ground cloves
- 1/4 teaspoon of ground nutmeg
- 1 packet of stevia
- 1/2 teaspoon of almond extract
- 1/4 cup of almond butter
- ½ cup of almond flour
- 1/4 cup of pumpkin puree
- 1/2 cup of rolled oats gluten-free

Instructions:
- Blend the oats, almond butter, almond flour, pumpkin puree, stevia sugar replacement, almond extract, cinnamon, cloves, & nutmeg in a food processor till smooth.
- After forming the dough into balls and spreading them on a dish or baking sheet, chill for at least 30 minutes.

392. Three Ingredient Cookies

(Preparation time: 10 minutes | Cooking time: 15 minutes | Difficulty: Easy | Servings: 4)

Per serving: Calories 56, Total fat 2g, Protein 1g, Carbs 11g

Ingredients:
- 2 ripe bananas
- 1/4 cup of dark chocolate chips
- 1/2 cup of oats

Instructions:
- Preheat the oven at 350°F.
- Mash the bananas using a fork in a mixing bowl till no lumps remain. Combine the oats & chocolate chips in a mixing bowl.
- Drop little amounts of batter onto the nonstick baking sheet with a tiny scoop.

- In a preheated oven, bake for around 15 minutes, or till golden brown. Allow each serving to cool for 2 to 5 minutes.

393. Spiced Peanut Butter Apples

(Preparation time: 10 minutes | Cooking time: 30 minutes | Difficulty: Easy | Servings: 4)

Per serving: Calories 206, Total fat 12g, Protein 6g, Carbs 20g

Ingredients:
- 1/8 teaspoon of ground cardamom
- 1/2 teaspoon of vanilla extract
- 1/8 teaspoon of ground cloves
- 6 tablespoons of peanut butter
- 4 Granny Smith apples

Instructions:
- Preheat the oven at 350°F.
- Remove the tops of the apples using a sharp knife. Remove the cores from the apples with an apple core while keeping the bottoms intact.
- Stuff 1 1/2 tablespoons of peanut butter + a dash of vanilla extract in the cored apples. In a baking pan, sprinkle cardamom & cloves over the apples.
- In a preheated oven, bake for about 30 minutes, or till apples are mellow and aromatic.

394. Chia Power Balls

(Preparation time: 15 minutes | Cooking time: 0 minutes | Difficulty: Easy | Servings: 4)

Per serving: Calories 236, Total fat 11g, Protein 7g, Carbs 21g

Ingredients:
- 1 cup of honey
- 1/2 cup of ground flax seed
- 1 cup of chia seeds
- 1 cup of peanut butter
- 1/2 cup of diced dried mango
- 1/2 cup of shredded coconut
- 1 cup of pumpkin seeds
- 2 cups of oats

- 1/2 cup of wheat germ
- 1 cup of diced dried pineapple
- 1/2 cup of dried blueberries

Instructions:

- Combine oats, chia seeds, peanut butter, pumpkin seeds, pineapple, coconut, honey, mango, flax, blueberries, & wheat germ in a large-sized mixing dish; roll into 1-inch balls refrigerate till firm, around 1 hour.

395. Black Bean Hummus without Tahini

(Preparation time: 10 minutes | Cooking time: 0 minutes | Difficulty: Easy | Servings: 4)

Per serving: Calories 62, Total fat 2g, Protein 31g, Carbs 9g

Ingredients:

- ¼ cup of lime juice
- 4 cloves of garlic
- 1 tablespoon of sesame oil
- 1/4 cup of fresh parsley
- 1 teaspoon of ground cumin
- 1/4 teaspoon of cayenne pepper
- 1/4 teaspoon of ground paprika
- 1 bird's eye chili, trimmed and seeded
- 1 cup of no-salt-added black beans, drained and rinsed

Instructions:

- Combine black beans, sesame oil, parsley, lime juice, chilies, paprika, garlic, cumin, & cayenne pepper in a food processor or blender; mix till smooth.

396. Mandarin Pumpkin

(Preparation time: 5 minutes | Cooking time: 0 minutes | Difficulty: Easy | Servings: 4)

Per serving: Calories 46, Total fat 1g, Protein 1g, Carbs 11g

Ingredients:

- 2 stalks of celery

- 10 peeled, pith removed mandarin or clementine oranges

Instructions:

- Cut the celery into small pieces & insert one inside each peeled mandarin orange.

397. Creamed Swiss Chard

(Preparation time: 5 minutes | Cooking time: 10 minutes | Difficulty: Easy | Servings: 4)

Per serving: Calories 128, Total fat 12g, Protein 2g, Carbs 4g

Ingredients:

- A pinch of salt
- 1/4 teaspoon of black pepper
- 2 cloves of minced garlic
- 1 teaspoon of olive oil
- 1/2 cup of half and half
- 1 bunch of Swiss chard

Instructions:

- Chard should be rinsed and dried before cooking. Make a separation between the leaves and the stalks. Stems should be cut into 1/2-inch lengths. "Slicing Leaves" should be cut up into large 1-inch chunks.
- Heat the olive oil in a big skillet over a high flame. Cook for around 30 seconds, or till garlic begins to smell fragrant.
- After adding the stems, cook for around 3-4 minutes, or till tender-crisp.
- Cook for 3 minutes, or till slightly thickened, after adding the half-and-half and pepper. Cook for an additional 2-3 minutes, or till the leaves are wilted. Season with black pepper to taste.

398. Garden Fresh Bruschetta

(Preparation time: 5 minutes | Cooking time: 10 minutes | Difficulty: Easy | Servings: 4)

Per serving: Calories 86, Total fat 3g, Protein 2g, Carbs 6g - **Ingredients:**

- 1/2 teaspoon of black pepper (or to taste)

- 1 clove of minced garlic
- 2 tablespoons of olive oil
- 1/4 cup of finely chopped fresh basil
- 1 tablespoon of red wine vinegar
- 2 to 3 Roma fresh tomatoes (diced small)

For serving:
- Olive oil and fresh garlic clove for toasting
- 1 whole-wheat baguette

Instructions:
- Tomatoes should be peeled and sliced into 1/4-inch pieces, then drained gently.
- In a mixing bowl, combine all ingredients and set them aside for at least 1 hour at room temperature.
- Slice the baguette, spray it with olive oil, then toast or broil it till lightly browned. Rub each toasted slice of bread with a raw garlic clove.
- Distribute the tomato mixture on top.

399. Grilled Marinated Pineapple

(Preparation time: 5 minutes | Cooking time: 5 minutes | Difficulty: Easy | Servings: 4)
Per serving: Calories 132, Total fat 5g, Protein 1g, Carbs 12g
Ingredients:
- 1/4 teaspoon of ground ginger
- 2 tablespoons of olive oil
- 2 tablespoons of brown sugar replacement
- 1 fresh pineapple

Instructions:
- Heat the grill to a medium-high setting.
- Remove the pineapple skin and slice it into 1/2" discs.
- Combine the olive oil, brown sugar substitute, and ginger in a small-sized bowl. Add to pineapple, toss to coat, and leave away to marinate for at least 30 minutes.

- Remove the pineapple from the marinade first, and season it using salt and black pepper.
- Grill pineapple for around 4 to 5 minutes on each side or till it caramelizes on the grill.

400. Whipped Feta with Roasted Tomatoes

(Preparation time: 5 minutes | Cooking time: 20 minutes | Difficulty: Easy | Servings: 4)
Per serving: Calories 95, Total fat 8g, Protein 3g, Carbs 2g
Ingredients:
For the dip:
- 2 tablespoons of Greek yogurt or sour cream
- 3 tablespoons of softened cream cheese
- 4 oz. block of feta cheese

For the tomatoes:
- A pinch of salt and black pepper
- 1 clove of minced garlic
- 1 teaspoon of olive oil
- 1/2 cup of cherry tomatoes or grape tomatoes

For serving:
- Fresh dill
- Whole-wheat pita bread

Instructions:
- After removing the feta from the brine, thoroughly rinse it in cold water. Pat dry with a paper towel.
- Put the feta block in a food processor and pulse till it is broken up.
- Mix the cream cheese and sour cream together. Pulse till creamy, about 3 minutes, scraping down the sides as needed. Before serving, chill for at least 30 minutes or up to 24 hours.
- Preheat the oven at 400°F.
- Combine all of the tomato ingredients in a small-sized bowl. Cook for about 20

minutes, or till the potatoes are soft and splitting. Allow for some cooling time.

- Place the whipped feta in a small bowl or platter. Serve with roasted tomatoes on top, along with their juices. Sprinkle with olive oil if preferred.
- Serve with chopped fresh dill on top of warm pita wedges.

401. Pineapple Salsa

(Preparation time: 10 minutes | Cooking time: 0 minutes | Difficulty: Easy | Servings: 4)
Per serving: Calories 50, Total fat 1g, Protein 1g, Carbs 8g
Ingredients:

- 1/2 lime juiced
- 1/2 tablespoon of olive oil
- 1/2 teaspoon of cumin
- 1 seeded and minced bird's eye chili
- 1 diced red pepper
- 3 tablespoons of chopped parsley
- 1/4 cup of minced red onion
- 2 cups of diced pineapple

Instructions:

- All of the ingredients should be whisked together well in a mixing dish.
- Before serving, let 30 minutes for the dish to come to room temperature.

402. Roasted Garlic Parmesan Asparagus

(Preparation time: 10 minutes | Cooking time: 10 minutes | Difficulty: Easy | Servings: 4)
Per serving: Calories 69, Total fat 5g, Protein 4g, Carbs 5g
Ingredients:

- A pinch of salt and black pepper
- 1 clove of minced garlic
- 1 tablespoon of olive oil
- 3 tablespoons of grated parmesan cheese
- 1 bunch of asparagus spears around 1 pound

Instructions:

- Preheat the oven at 425°F.
- Rinse and pat dry the asparagus after cleaning it. Remove the woody ends.
- Toss asparagus with olive oil, garlic, salt and pepper on a baking sheet.
- Bake for around 6 to 10 minutes in the oven, or till crisp and tender. After adding the parmesan cheese, broil for 1 minute.

403. Frozen Grape Bites

(Preparation time: 10 minutes | Cooking time: 0 minutes | Difficulty: Easy | Servings: 4)
Per serving: Calories 110, Total fat 11g, Protein 1g, Carbs 3g
Ingredients:

- Olive oil cooking spray
- 12 frozen green grapes
- 1 cup of heavy whipping cream

Instructions:

- Coat mini muffin cups in cooking spray.
- Add 1 tablespoon of cream to each muffin cup. In each muffin cup, place one grape & swirl it in the cream to coat it.
- Freeze the grape mixture for 1 hour or until it is completely solid.

404. Maple Pecan Granola

(Preparation time: 10 minutes | Cooking time: 25 minutes | Difficulty: Easy | Servings: 2)
Per serving: Calories 202, Total fat 11g, Protein 4g, Carbs 15g
Ingredients:

- 2 teaspoons of ground cinnamon
- 1/3 cup of olive oil
- 1/2 cup of chopped walnuts
- 1/2 cup of ground flax seed
- 1/2 cup of chopped pecans
- 2 cups of old-fashioned oats
- 2/3 cup of pure maple syrup
- 1 teaspoon of maple flavoring

Instructions:

- Preheat the oven at 400°F.
- Line a baking sheet using parchment paper.
- Combine oats, flaxseed, pecans, walnuts, and cinnamon in a large-sized mixing bowl.
- Combine the olive oil, maple syrup, and maple flavoring in a small-sized mixing bowl; pour over the oat mixture & toss to coat evenly.
- Spread the resulting mixture out equally on the prepared baking sheet.
- In a preheated oven, bake for about 25 minutes, or till lightly browned.
- Allow the granola to cool completely before slicing it. Keep the container tightly closed.

405. Summer Time Cucumber Sandwiches

(Preparation time: 10 minutes | Cooking time: 0 minutes | Difficulty: Easy | Servings: 4)
Per serving: Calories 136, Total fat 11g, Protein 2g, Carbs 6g
Ingredients:

- 1 large cucumber, peeled and sliced
- 1/2 cup of Greek yogurt
- 2 tablespoons of fresh dill
- 2 tablespoons of parsley
- 1 cup of softened cream cheese
- 1/2 cup of low-fat mayonnaise
- 6 slices of whole-wheat rye bread

Instructions:

- Cream together cream cheese, mayonnaise, salt, Greek yoghurt, and fresh dill in a mixing dish with a fork till smooth; chill for at least 1 hour to blend flavors.
- To soften the cream cheese mixture, take it out of the refrigerator 10 minutes before serving.
- Spread about 1 tablespoon of the cream cheese mixture evenly on each piece of whole-wheat rye bread, top with a cucumber slice, & sprinkle with parsley.

406. High Protein Snack Bars

(Preparation time: 10 minutes | Cooking time: 0 minutes | Difficulty: Easy | Servings: 4)
Per serving: Calories 95, Total fat 4g, Protein 5g, Carbs 10g
Ingredients:

- A pinch of cinnamon
- 2 scoops of protein chocolate-flavored powder -1/2 cup of golden raisins
- 1 cup of rolled oats quick-cooking
- 1/3 cup of chopped and unsalted peanuts
- 1/2 cup of smooth peanut butter
- 1/2 cup of unsweetened almond milk

Instructions:

- Combine the protein powder, cinnamon powder, oats, peanuts, & raisins in a large-sized mixing dish. Combine the almond milk & peanut butter.
- Half-fill a 6x6-inch baking pan with the batter. If covered, refrigerate for 3 hours to overnight. Serve by cutting the dough into bars.

407. Watermelon and Feta Skewers

(Preparation time: 10 minutes | Cooking time: 0 minutes | Difficulty: Easy | Servings: 4)
Per serving: Calories 195, Total fat 5g, Protein 6g, Carbs 15g
Ingredients:

- Toothpicks
- 3 sprigs of fresh mint, chopped
- 1/2 watermelon, make bite-sized cubes
- 1/2 package of feta cheese (4 oz.), make 1/2-inch cubes

Instructions:

- Attach 1 feta cheese square on a watermelon cube with a toothpick. Rep with the remaining feta cheese and watermelon. On top, mint leaves are strewn.

408. Crispy Dijon Smashed Potato

(Preparation time: 10 minutes | Cooking time: 30 minutes | Difficulty: Easy | Servings: 4)

Per serving: Calories 136, Total fat 5g, Protein 2g, Carbs 20g

Ingredients:
- Salt and ground black pepper to taste
- 3 cloves of garlic minced
- 1/2 teaspoon of dried thyme
- 1/2 teaspoon of dried rosemary
- 2 teaspoons of honey
- 24 ounces of red baby potatoes
- 1 tablespoon of whole-grain Dijon mustard 2 tablespoons of Dijon mustard

Instructions:
- Preheat the oven at 400°F. Coat a baking sheet using the baking spray.
- Bring the potatoes to a boil, then remove them from the water.
- Combine Dijon mustard, olive oil, whole grain mustard, honey, chopped garlic, rosemary, & thyme in a small-sized mixing cup, and season to taste using salt and pepper.
- Spray a baking tray using cooking spray and place the potatoes on it. Gently smash the potatoes with a potato masher to flatten them while keeping them whole. All of the potatoes should be brushed with the mustard mixture.
- Potatoes should be baked for around 18 to 20 minutes, or till golden and crisp.

409. Baked Chipotle Asparagus

(Preparation time: 10 minutes | Cooking time: 20 minutes | Difficulty: Easy | Servings: 3)

Per serving: Calories 115, Total fat 1g, Protein 2g, Carbs 4g

Ingredients:
- 1/2 teaspoon of salt

- Olive oil cooking spray
- 1 teaspoon of Chipotle powder seasoning
- 10 whole Asparagus spears

Instructions:
- Remove the bottoms of the asparagus spears and discard.
- Using nonstick cooking spray, coat the baking sheet. Arrange the asparagus spears flat on the baking sheet, not overlapping them.
- Season the asparagus evenly with the seasonings.
- Preheat the oven to 350°F and bake for around 10 minutes.
- The asparagus should be fully cooked at this point, but if you want them crispier, simmer for another 5 minutes.

410. Crispy Potato and Kale Nuggets

(Preparation time: 10 minutes | Cooking time: 20 minutes | Difficulty: Easy | Servings: 4)

Per serving: Calories 40, Total fat 1g, Protein 3g, Carbs 15g

Ingredients:
- 1/4 teaspoon of sea salt
- 1/8 teaspoon of ground black pepper
- 1 clove of garlic minced
- 1 teaspoon of olive oil extra-virgin
- Olive oil as required
- 2 cups of russet potatoes boiled
- 4 cups chopped and loosely packed kale
- 1/8 cup of almond milk

Instructions:
- Heat one teaspoon of olive oil in a large-sized skillet over medium-high flame. Cook the garlic till it turns a golden brown color. Sauté for around 2 to 3 minutes with the kale. Place in a large-sized mixing dish.
- Salt, milk, & pepper the boiling potatoes, then mash them using a fork or a potato masher. Mix the mashed

potatoes & cooked greens together in a large-sized mixing bowl. Preheat the oven at 390°F.

- Make 1-inch nuggets out of the potato & kale mixture. Squirt the olive oil into the baking sheet. Cook the nuggets for around 12 to 15 minutes, shaking after 6 minutes, till golden brown.

411. Roasted Celery Sticks

(Preparation time: 10 minutes | Cooking time: 20 minutes | Difficulty: Easy | Servings: 6)
Per serving: Calories 162, Total fat 4g, Protein 8g, Carbs 21g
Ingredients:

- Cooking oil spray
- 1/2 teaspoon of Kosher salt
- 1/2 teaspoon of onion powder
- 1/2 teaspoon of garlic powder
- 2 whole eggs
- 1 teaspoon of lemon pepper
- 1/2 cup of almond or buckwheat flour for dusting
- 1/4 cup of parmesan cheese grated
- 1 cup of whole-wheat breadcrumbs
- 4 celery stalks, trimmed and sliced into 3-inch pieces

Instructions:

- Preheat the oven at 400°F.
- Set aside the eggs, which have been beaten with salt and lemon pepper, in a small-sized cup.
- Combine the flour, breadcrumbs, parmesan cheese, onion powder, & garlic powder on a separate plate.
- Dip each stick in the egg, then roll in the breadcrumbs till well coated on all sides.
- Place the celery pieces on the baking sheet after coating them in oil.
- Bake for around 15 minutes, or till golden brown on both sides, rotating halfway through.

412. Tasty Cheesy Cauliflower Tots

(Preparation time: 10 minutes | Cooking time: 20 minutes | Difficulty: Easy | Servings: 4)
Per serving: Calories 181, Total fat 9g, Protein 13g, Carbs 6g
Ingredients:

- 1/4 teaspoon of garlic powder
- 1/4 teaspoon of dried parsley
- 1/4 teaspoon of onion powder
- 1 egg large-sized
- 1/2 cup of grated mozzarella cheese
- 1 large head of cauliflower
- 1.50 oz. 100% cheese crisps

Instructions:

- Fill a large pot halfway with water and place a steamer basket on top of it on the stovetop. Bring the water to a rolling boil.
- Cut the cauliflower into florets after removing the core and leaves. Place the florets in the steamer basket with care, then cover.
- Cook for 5 minutes or till the cauliflower is tender.
- Remove the steamer basket from the pan & set it aside to cool for 10 minutes. Suck out as much excess moisture as possible with a cheesecloth or a clean kitchen towel draped over the sink. If not enough water is extracted, the tots may become soggy.
- In a food processor, combine the grated mozzarella, cauliflower, cheese crisps, garlic powder, egg, parsley, & onion powder. Process for 1 minute on low, scraping down the sides as necessary. When molded, the mixture should be slightly moist but retain its shape.
- To make a tot, roll 2 teaspoons of the mixture into a ball in your hands. Continue in the same manner with the rest of the mixture. Prepare a baking

sheet by cutting a piece of parchment paper and lining it with it.

- Place the tots in the oven with a tot on each edge to keep the parchment from blowing away and the tots from cooking evenly.
- Preheat the oven at 320°F and bake the tots for around 12 minutes, flipping halfway through.

413. Spinach and Cheese Stuffed Mushrooms

(Preparation time: 10 minutes | Cooking time: 20 minutes | Difficulty: Easy | Servings: 4)
Per serving: Calories 223, Total fat 18g, Protein 6g, Carbs 9g
Ingredients:

- 3 cloves of garlic minced
- 1 onion chopped
- 4 tablespoons of butter
- 4 tablespoons of dry bread crumbs
- 4 tablespoons of grated Parmesan cheese
- 1 cup of mushrooms, stems removed
- 1 cup of chopped frozen spinach
- 1 cup of softened cream cheese
- 4 tablespoons of Italian-style salad dressing

Instructions:

- Apply Italian dressing on both sides of each mushroom cap.
- Preheat oven at 390°F and bake for around 5 minutes, or till mushrooms are tender. Remove the mushrooms from the oven while keeping the oven on.
- Melt butter in a skillet over a medium-high flame and cook onion and garlic for 6 minutes, or till onion softens. Combine the spinach, parmesan cheese, melted cream cheese, & 3 tablespoons bread crumbs.
- Before topping with the remaining bread crumbs, evenly spread the

spinach mixture among the mushroom caps. Return the mushrooms to the oven for a final 10 minutes of baking, or till golden brown on top.

414. Crispy Ring Onions

(Preparation time: 10 minutes | Cooking time: 20 minutes | Difficulty: Easy | Servings: 4)
Per serving: Calories 147, Total fat 3g, Protein 5g, Carbs 22g
Ingredients:

- 1/2 teaspoon of salt and black pepper
- 1/2 teaspoon of paprika
- 1/2 teaspoon of parsley
- 1 tablespoon of olive oil extra-virgin
- 2 red eggs
- 2 large onions
- 2 cups of whole-wheat bread crumbs
- 1/2 cup + 2 tablespoons of almond flour
- 2 cups of buttermilk, divided

Instructions:

- Peel and slice the onions into 1/2-inch thick rings. Freeze the sliced onions and one cup of butter in a freezer bag for at least 30 minutes.
- Preheat the oven at 400°F.
- Whisk together the eggs, buttermilk, & two tablespoons of flour in a large-sized mixing dish till smooth. Set the mixture aside.
- Combine bread crumbs, spices, and olive oil in a separate mixing bowl.
- Drain the onions thoroughly after removing them from the freezer bag. Toss the onion with 1/2 cup flour in a flour bag and toss well to coat.
- To coat the onions, put the panko mixture in a small-sized bowl and dip each onion one at a time into the egg mixture and then the panko mixture.
- Place the onion rings on a non-stick baking sheet. In a preheated oven, bake

for around 20 to 25 minutes, till crispy and golden.
- Serve the onion rings with ketchup and additional spice.

415. Mediterranean Stuffed Mini Sweet Peppers

(Preparation time: 10 minutes | Cooking time: 15 minutes | Difficulty: Easy | Servings: 4)
Per serving: Calories 176, Total fat 13g, Protein 7g, Carbs 3g
Ingredients:
- 1/4 cup of grated cheddar cheese
- 8 sweet peppers mini
- 1/2 cup of cream cheese softened
- 4 of cooked and crumbled slices of bacon

Instructions:
- After removing the tops, cut each sweet pepper in half lengthwise. Remove the seeds and membranes using a tiny knife.
- Combine the bacon, softened cream cheese, & grated cheddar cheese in a small mixing dish.
- Fill each sweet pepper with three teaspoons of the mixture and smooth it out. Place it on the baking pan.
- Preheat oven at 400°F and bake for around 8 to 10 minutes.

416. Cheesy Pepperoni Pizza Puffs

(Preparation time: 10 minutes | Cooking time: 15 minutes | Difficulty: Easy | Servings: 10 puffs)
Per serving: Calories 160, Total fat 9g, Protein 9g, Carbs 10g
Ingredients:
- 1 teaspoon of baking powder
- 1 egg lightly whisked
- 1/2 teaspoon of basil
- 3/4 teaspoon of oregano
- 1/2 teaspoon of garlic powder
- 1/2 red or green pepper, diced
- 3/4 cup of almond flour

- 4 strings of mozzarella
- 3/4 cup of pepperoni mini
- 1/2 cup of store-bought pizza sauce
- 1 cup of grated cheese (cheddar or mozzarella)
- 3/4 cup of fat-reduced milk

Instructions:
- Preheat the oven at 370°F. Cooking oil should be used to grease a muffin tray. In a mixing bowl, combine the spices, flour, & baking powder. Whisk together the milk & egg in a separate bowl until fully combined.
- Combine the shredded cheese, red pepper, & pepperoni in a mixing bowl and leave aside for 10 minutes.
- Fill each muffin cup halfway with the mixture. Cut each cheese string into three pieces and place one in the center of each muffin. Place the muffin pan in the oven.
- In the oven, bake for around 15-20 minutes.

417. Almond-Garlic Crackers

(Preparation time: 10 minutes | Cooking time: 15 minutes | Difficulty: Easy | Servings: 12)
Per serving: Calories 72, Total fat 6g, Protein 3g, Carbs 3g
Ingredients:
- 1/2 cup of water
- 1/2 teaspoon of salt
- 1 teaspoon of garlic powder
- 1/2 cup of the almond meal
- 1/3 cup of Parmesan cheese grated
- 1/2 cup of the ground flax seed

Instructions:
- Preheat the oven at 400°F.
- In a medium mixing bowl, combine ground flaxseed, almond meal, water, grated Parmesan cheese, garlic powder, & salt. Allow 3–5 minutes for the water to settle and the dough to firm up.

- Cover the dough with waxed paper or plastic wrap and place it on the prepared baking sheet. With a rolling pin or your fingertips, flatten the dough to 1/8-inch thickness. Leaving waxed paper out of the equation. Using a knife, make indentations in the dough to demonstrate where the crackers will be torn apart.
- Bake for around 15 minutes, or till gently brown.

418. Cheesy Asparagus Tots

(Preparation time: 10 minutes | Cooking time: 15 minutes | Difficulty: Easy | Servings: 10 tots)
Per serving: Calories 78, Total fat 3g, Protein 7g, Carbs 7g
Ingredients:

- Cooking spray
- 12 ounces of asparagus trimmed and diced
- 1/2 cup of whole-wheat bread crumbs
- 1/4 cup of Parmesan cheese grated

Instructions:

- On medium flame, bring salted water to a boil. In a pot, bring the asparagus to a boil for around 5 minutes. Drain in a colander for 5 minutes or till cold enough to handle.
- In a large-sized mixing bowl, combine the asparagus, parmesan cheese, and breadcrumbs. Knead everything together with your hands till it forms a dough-like consistency. To make a tot, take one tablespoon of the mixture & roll it into a ball. Arrange the ingredients on a serving plate. Continue in the same manner with the rest of the mixture. Toasted tots should be frozen for 30 minutes.
- Preheat the oven at 400°F.

- Nonstick cooking oil should be sprayed on the baking sheet and the outsides of the tots. Bake for around 10 to 15 minutes in total.

419. Zucchini Bites

(Preparation time: 10 minutes | Cooking time: 25 minutes | Difficulty: Easy | Servings: 24 to 36 bites)
Per serving: Calories 51, Total fat 3g, Protein 2g, Carbs 4g
Ingredients:

- 1 tablespoon of olive oil extra-virgin
- 3 whole eggs- 1 chopped red onion
- 1 large grated carrot
- 1 large grated zucchini
- 3 slices of bacon finely sliced
- 1/4 cup of cream
- 1/2 cup of almond flour
- 1 cup of cheese grated

Instructions:

- In a large-sized skillet, heat the oil and sauté the onion till it is transparent. After the bacon has changed color, cook for 2 to 3 minutes before adding the zucchini and carrots. Allow a few minutes for it to cool.
- Whisk together the milk, eggs, and cheese in a separate medium-sized mixing bowl; add the egg mixture to the zucchini mixture & stir in the flour.
- Fill each floured & greased muffin cup halfway with the zucchini bits' mixture.
- Bake at 350°F for around 15 to 20 minutes, or till done.

420. Pizza Muffins

(Preparation time: 10 minutes | Cooking time: 20 minutes | Difficulty: Easy | Servings: 10)
Per serving: Calories 117, Total fat 8g, Protein 8g, Carbs 4g
Ingredients:

- 1/2 teaspoon of salt

- 1/2 teaspoon of black pepper
- 1 tablespoon of butter melted
- 2 large whole eggs
- 2 tablespoons of coconut flour
- 2 medium grated zucchini
- 1 1/4 cups of mozzarella grated

For the topping:
- 1 teaspoon of the Italian seasoning
- 2/3 cup of mozzarella grated
- 1 oz. slices of pepperoni
- 1/4 cup of marinara sauce

Instructions:
- Preheat the oven at 390°F. Using cooking spray, coat a muffin pan.
- In a large-sized mixing bowl, combine all of the ingredients listed above. Cut a piece of parchment paper to fit a baking sheet.
- Combine grated zucchini, coconut flour, grated mozzarella, black pepper, & sea salt in a large-sized mixing bowl. Combine the melted butter and eggs in a mixing bowl.
- Fill the muffin cups evenly with the zucchini mixture, packing it down the sides & smoothing the tops.
- In the oven, bake for around 15 to 20 minutes, or till firm and brown on top.
- Toss the muffin with a teaspoon of marinara sauce & the remaining mozzarella cheese. To taste, season with Italian spice and pepperoni slices.

421. Cauliflower and Cheddar Muffins

(Preparation time: 10 minutes | Cooking time: 20 minutes | Difficulty: Easy | Servings: 12)
Per serving: Calories 110, Total fat 8g, Protein 8g, Carbs 2g
Ingredients:
- 1/4 teaspoon of salt
- 1/4 teaspoon of ground black pepper
- 1/2 teaspoon of garlic powder
- 1/2 teaspoon of baking powder
- 2 tablespoons of melted butter
- 1 tablespoon of dried onion flakes
- 2 tablespoons bird's eye chili
- 2 large whisked eggs
- 2 cups of riced raw cauliflower
- 1 cup of grated mozzarella
- 1 cup of grated cheddar cheese
- 1/4 cup of coconut flour
- 1/3 cup of grated parmesan cheese

Instructions:
- Preheat the oven at 380°F. Grease a muffin tray using cooking spray.
- In a medium-sized mixing bowl, combine the chilies, cauliflower, eggs with melted butter. Combine the grated cheeses thoroughly.
- Combine the onion flakes, pepper, salt, garlic powder, baking powder, & coconut flour in a mixing bowl till everything is thoroughly blended. Divide the batter evenly among the 12 muffin cups in a prepared muffin tray.
- Cook for around 15-20 minutes, or till thoroughly done.

422. Basil Chicken Bites

(Preparation time: 10 minutes | Cooking time: 20 minutes | Difficulty: Easy | Servings: 2)
Per serving: Calories 168, Total fat 8g, Protein 24g, Carbs 1g
Ingredients:
- 1/8 teaspoon of salt (optional)
- 1/4 teaspoon of black pepper
- 1/4 teaspoon of garlic powder
- 1 tablespoon of extra-virgin olive oil
- 2 tablespoons of dried parsley

Instructions:
- Cut the tenderloins into 2-inch-long bite-size chunks. In a plastic bag, combine the pieces, salt, parsley, pepper, and garlic powder. Give it a good shake to coat it. Heat the olive oil

in a large-sized skillet over medium flame. Add the chicken to the mix. Sauté for 10–12 minutes over medium heat, tossing frequently, or till chicken is cooked through.

423. Chicken & Asparagus Crustless Tart

(Preparation time: 10 minutes | Cooking time: 40 minutes | Difficulty: Easy | Servings: 2)
Per serving: Calories 289, Total fat 25g, Protein 37g, Carbs 3g
Ingredients:

- 1 tablespoon of olive oil, plus extra for greasing - 2 eggs
- 2 cups of asparagus
- 2 spring onions, finely sliced
- 150g of cooked chicken, roughly chopped
- 4 tablespoons of low-fat ricotta
- 2 tablespoons of low-fat Parmesan, freshly grated

Instructions:

- Before you begin, preheat the oven at 350°F. Grease a 24cm round tart tin & line it with 3cm of greaseproof paper.
- Heat the oil in a frying pan over low heat & soften the spring onions and garlic.
- Before slicing the asparagus into 1cm sections, remove the woody tips and leave the tips whole. Place the asparagus in a pan and cook on low flame for a few minutes. Remove from the heat, season with salt and pepper to taste, drain, and chill. Asparagus tips should be arranged to the side.
- Meanwhile, in a mixing bowl, whisk together the eggs, milk, ricotta, and 2/3 of the Parmesan, seasoning to taste.
- Combine the chicken and the asparagus. Gently combine the ingredients, then spoon them into the tin, ensuring they are well distributed. Place the ends of

the tart on top of the mixture & gently press them in.

- Bake for around 20 to 25 minutes, or till the center is just about set, sprinkling the remaining Parmesan on top. If it isn't browned, place it under the grill for a few seconds.
- Allow cooling to room temperature before serving, garnished with extra chopped spring onion.

424. Turkey-Stuffed Peppers

(Preparation time: 10 minutes | Cooking time: 55 minutes | Difficulty: Easy | Servings: 2)
Per serving: Calories 263, Total fat 27g, Protein 19g, Carbs 2g
Ingredients:

- 1/4 cup of water
- Pinch of sea salt
- Pinch of ground black pepper
- 1 clove of garlic, chopped
- 1/2 tablespoon of olive oil
- 4 tablespoons of diced red onion
- 1 tablespoon of diced bird's eye chili, or to taste
- 1/4 cup of tomato sauce
- 1 cup of frozen cauliflower rice
- 1 large bell peppers, any color - cut in half lengthwise, cored & seeded
- 1/4 can of diced tomatoes, undrained
- 2 teaspoons of low-fat sour cream
- 4 tablespoons of shredded low-fat Colby-Jack cheese
- 2 (1 inch) cubes of low-fat Colby-Jack cheese
- 4 slices of pickled jalapeno peppers (Optional)
- 1/4 pound of ground turkey
- 1 teaspoon of chili paste

Instructions:

- Preheat the oven at 375°F. Coat a baking dish using cooking spray.

- Heat the olive oil in a large-sized skillet over medium flame. In a mixing bowl, combine the ground turkey, chilies, onion, and garlic. Cook, occasionally turning, for 8 to 10 minutes, or till the turkey is browned and the vegetables are tender. Drain the grease from the skillet after it has been removed from the heat. Toss in the tomato sauce, frozen riced cauliflower, tomatoes, salt, water, chili paste, and pepper till everything is well blended. Reduce the flame to low and continue to cook for another 5 minutes.
- Half of the bell pepper halves should be placed in the baking dish. Stuff 1 cheese cube and turkey mixture in each pepper half. On the plate, spoon the leftover turkey mixture around the peppers.
- Cover with aluminum foil and bake in a preheated oven for about 30 minutes. Remove each pepper's wrapping and cover with shredded cheese. Cover and bake for a further 10 minutes, or till the peppers are soft and the cheese has melted.
- Place a small portion of the turkey mixture on a platter and top with half of the bell pepper to serve. Top each meal with 1 teaspoon sour cream and 2 chili slices.

425. Feta Spinach Rolls

(Preparation time: 10 minutes | Cooking time: 20 minutes | Difficulty: Easy | Servings: 2)
Per serving: Calories 106, Total fat 3g, Protein 7g, Carbs 14g
Ingredients:
- A pinch of salt
- A pinch of freshly ground pepper
- 1/2 cup of spinach
- 1/2 cup of feta cheese crumbled
- Whole wheat roll dough

- 1/2 teaspoon of marjoram

Instructions:
- In a large-sized mixing dish, combine the spinach, salt, feta, marjoram, & pepper. On a floured surface, roll out the dough into a coarse rectangle.
- Leave a 12-inch border around the edges of the spinach mixture while covering it with dough.
- Roll the dough tightly into a log, starting on the longer side, and squeeze to seal the edge.Using baking parchment, cut the log into four pieces. Using a serrated knife may be more convenient.
- Preheat the oven at 380°F.
- The rolls should then be baked for around 18 to 20 minutes or till lightly browned. Allow the rolls to cool slightly before serving.

426. Tasty Eggplant Rolls Roasted

(Preparation time: 10 minutes | Cooking time: 20 minutes | Difficulty: Easy | Servings: 2)
Per serving: Calories 77, Total fat 3g, Protein 3g, Carbs 12g
Ingredients:
- A pinch of black pepper
- 1 tablespoon of fresh lemon juice
- 1 minced clove of garlic
- 1 teaspoon of olive oil
- 1/4 teaspoon of dried oregano
- 4 tablespoons of minced green onion
- 1/2 medium-sized eggplant
- 1 sun-dried tomato (packed in oil), drained, rinsed, & minced
- 4 stemmed fresh spinach leaves
- 1 tablespoon of sour cream fat-free
- 2 tablespoons of cream cheese fat-free
- 1/4 cup of meatless pasta sauce

Instructions:
- Preheat the oven at 450°F. Set aside 2 nonstick baking plates that have been sprayed using nonstick cooking spray.

Cut off the ends of the eggplants & discard them. Cut the eggplants into 1/4-inch thick slices lengthwise. On the exterior slices, the skin should be removed. Arrange the slices in a single layer on the baking sheets that have been prepared.

- In a separate dish, combine the lemon juice and olive oil and lightly brush all sides of the eggplant pieces. Bake for around 20 minutes, flipping once or till golden brown. On a plate, cool the eggplant slices.
- In a small-sized mixing bowl, combine cream cheese, garlic, green onion, sour cream, oregano, sun-dried tomatoes, & pepper.
- Take 1 tablespoon of cream cheese mixture, spread evenly on each eggplant slice. With a 1/2-inch boundary between them, place one spinach leaf on top of the other. Begin rolling from the tiniest point possible. Place the rolls on a serving platter, seam sides down.
- Cover and chill for up to 2 days if making ahead. Allow time for the dish to cool to room temperature before serving. Toss with the warmed pasta sauce just before serving.

427. Spinach and Roasted Garlic Spirals

(Preparation time: 10 minutes | Cooking time: 10 minutes | Difficulty: Easy | Servings: 2)
Per serving: Calories 139, Total fat 2g, Protein 6g, Carbs 18g
Ingredients:
- 1/4 teaspoon of black pepper
- 1/2 whole head of garlic
- 1/2 teaspoon of dried oregano
- 1/8 teaspoon of ground red pepper
- 1 cup of finely shredded spinach leaves

- 1/2 can of rinsed & drained white beans
- 2 whole-wheat tortillas

Instructions:
- Preheat the oven at 400°F. Garlic tops should be removed and discarded. Wrap the garlic head in foil after moistening it with water. After baking, allow it to cool fully or till the garlic has softened.
- Remove the skins from the garlic cloves and place them in a blender or food processor. To make a smooth sauce, add the beans, black pepper, oregano, and ground red pepper as needed. Thoroughly combine the spinach and the remaining ingredients.
- Fill the tortillas evenly with the filling and roll them up jelly-roll style. Refrigerate for 1 to 2 hours, covered.
- Trim 1/2 inch off the ends of the rolls before serving & discard. Using a knife, cut the rolls into 1-inch pieces.

428. BLT Cukes

(Preparation time: 15 minutes | Cooking time: 0 minutes | Difficulty: Easy | Servings: 2)
Per serving: Calories 26, Total fat 2g, Protein 2g, Carbs 2g
Ingredients:
- 1/8 teaspoon of salt
- 1/4 teaspoon of black pepper
- 1/2 cucumber large
- 1/4 cup of lettuce finely chopped
- 4 tablespoons of tomato finely diced
- 1/4 cup of baby spinach finely chopped
- 1 tablespoon+1/2 teaspoon of fat-free mayonnaise - 1 crisp-cooked & crumbled slice of bacon

Instructions:
- In a medium-sized mixing bowl, combine the spinach, lettuce, bacon, pepper, tomato, mayonnaise, & salt.

- Cut the cucumber in half lengthwise after peeling and trimming the ends. Remove and discard the seeds with a spoon.
- Mound the bacon mixture in the middle of the cucumber halves. Cut into 2-inch slices & garnish with parsley.

429. Stuffed tomatillos

(Preparation time: 15 minutes | Cooking time: 0 minutes | Difficulty: Easy | Servings: 2)
Per serving: Calories 90, Total fat 5g, Protein 4g, Carbs 7g
Ingredients:

- Chopped parsley
- 1 green onion, sliced
- 1/2 teaspoon of ground red chilies
- 4 tomatillos or large cherry tomatoes (1 1/2 inches in diameter)
- 1/4 cup of shredded, low-fat Cheddar cheese
- ·1/4 cup of frozen whole kernel corn, thawed
- 1/4 cup of cheese, softened

Instructions:

- Tomatillos or cherry tomatoes should have their tops removed and the core scooped out. In a mixing dish, combine the cheese, corn, onions, cheese, & ground red chilies. Fill each tomatillo or cherry tomato with the cheese mixture. Refrigerate till ready to serve. Garnish with chopped parsley before serving.

430. Fresh Lime Salsa Picante

(Preparation time: 10 minutes | Cooking time: 0 minutes | Difficulty: Easy | Servings: 2)
Per serving: Calories 12, Total fat 0g, Protein 0g, Carbs 7g
Ingredients:

- 1/3 cup of freshly squeezed lime juice
- 2 bird's eye chilies, seeded & minced
- 1 tablespoon of chopped fresh parsley
- 1 tablespoon of chopped fresh cilantro

- 1 large red onion, peeled & diced
- 4 ripe medium plum tomatoes

Instructions:

- Toss the tomatoes on a plate after cutting them up.
- Combine the onion, cilantro, lime juice, chilies, and parsley in a large-sized mixing bowl. Refrigerate till ready to serve, stirring thoroughly.
- Serve with low-carb baked chips or tortilla chips as a garnish or compliment.

431. Tempting Tapenade

(Preparation time: 10 minutes | Cooking time: 0 minutes | Difficulty: Easy | Servings: 12)
Per serving: Calories 75, Total fat 7g, Protein 1g, Carbs 2g
Ingredients:

- 1 tablespoon of fresh lemon juice
- 1 clove of minced garlic
- 2 tablespoons of extra-virgin olive oil
- 3 leaves of fresh basil
- 2 rinsed anchovy fillets
- 1 cup of pitted mixed olives
- 2 tablespoons of capers

Instructions:

- Combine olives, lemon juice, anchovy fillets, basil, olive oil, capers, & garlic in a food processor and process till the mixture has the consistency of a coarse paste, about 1 to 2 minutes total, scraping down the sides of the bowl with a spatula as needed to ensure ingredients are fully incorporated.

432. Brie and Artichoke Snack

(Preparation time: 10 minutes | Cooking time: 0 minutes | Difficulty: Easy | Servings: 12)
Per serving: Calories 200, Total fat 16g, Protein 12g, Carbs 2g
Ingredients:

- 2 cloves of garlic minced

- 6 slices of sun-dried tomatoes in oil, minced
- 3 artichoke hearts packed in oil, chopped and drained
- 1 round Brie cheese (around 1 1/2 pound)

Instructions:

- Preheat the oven at 350°F.
- In a medium-sized cup, combine the garlic, artichoke hearts & sun-dried tomatoes.
- Remove and discard the top portion of the rind from the Brie cheese.
- Place the brie in a round baking dish. On top, layer the tomato mixture.
- Before the cheese softens, bake for around 15 minutes in a preheated oven.

433. Cheese Balls

(Preparation time: 10 minutes | Cooking time: 20 minutes | Difficulty: Easy | Servings: 12)
Per serving: Calories 206, Total fat 15g, Protein 13g, Carbs 5g
Ingredients:

- 3 tablespoons of water
- 1 teaspoon of sea salt
- 1 1/2 teaspoons of garlic powder
- 3 tablespoons of cornstarch
- 1 tablespoon of Italian seasoning
- 2 whisked eggs
- 1 1/2 teaspoons of Parmesan grated
- 1 cup of Italian whole-wheat breadcrumbs seasoned
- 2 cups of grated mozzarella

Instructions:

- In a large-sized mixing bowl, combine the mozzarella, Parmesan, cornstarch, and water. Make a well-rounded combination.
- Form the dough into 1-inch bite-size balls & place on a parchment-lined baking sheet. Place in the freezer for 1 hour. The eggs should be whisked together in a small-sized cup. Combine breadcrumbs, Italian seasoning, garlic powder, & salt on a separate plate.

- To coat the cheeseballs, dip them in the eggs. Return to the baking sheet after rolling in the breadcrumb mixture. Return the sheet to the freezer for a further 20 minutes. Remove the cheese balls from the freezer and coat them in the egg mixture before re-rolling them in breadcrumbs.
- Preheat the oven to 360°F and bake for around 20 minutes.

434. Roasted Beetroot Crostini

(Preparation time: 10 minutes | Cooking time: 20 minutes | Difficulty: Easy | Servings: 2)
Per serving: Calories 126, Total fat 1g, Protein 4g, Carbs 20g
Ingredients:

- A pinch of salt and black pepper
- A few fresh chives
- 3 sprigs of fresh thyme
- 2 raw beetroots
- 2 slices of whole wheat bread
- 2 tablespoons of red wine
- 1 tablespoon of creamed horseradish

Instructions:

- Preheat the oven at 350°F.
- Before cutting the beets into wedges & placing them in a roasting dish, scrub them thoroughly.
- Combine the wine, thyme, and 4 tablespoons of water in a mixing bowl and toss to coat.
- Cover with tin foil and roast for 45 minutes or till cooked through.
- When you're ready to serve, toast the bread and sprinkle it with horseradish.
- Roasted beets, chives, & a bit of salt and pepper are sprinkled on top.

435. Asparagus with Mushroom Mayonnaise

(Preparation time: 10 minutes | Cooking time: 15 minutes | Difficulty: Easy | Servings: 2)
Per serving: Calories 105, Total fat 7g, Protein 6g, Carbs 3g
Ingredients:

- 1/2 tablespoon of olive oil
- 8 asparagus spears
- 4 tablespoons of Cheddar cheese
- 1/4 cup of broad beans
- 1/2 handful of watercress or rocket

Mushroom mayonnaise:

- 1/2 tablespoon of balsamic vinegar
- 1 cup of button mushrooms
- 4 tablespoons of mayonnaise, prepared with free-range eggs

Instructions:

- The day prior, make the mushroom mayonnaise. Combine the mushrooms, vinegar, & 1/2 teaspoon of sea salt in a food processor. In a colander, place a piece of cheesecloth and put it over a dish. Fill the cheesecloth with the mixture and strain the liquid overnight.
- The next day, lift the cheesecloth with the mixture inside and squeeze off the remaining liquid after removing the particles and whisking the mayonnaise into the liquid, set aside.
- Preheat a griddle pan to medium-high flame. Cook for 3 minutes, or till the asparagus spears start to brown, then flip and cook for 2 minutes more.
- Divide the asparagus across four bowls and pod the broad beans.
- Drizzle the oil on top & grate the cheese on top of it. Serve with a side of salad leaves and a dollop of mushroom mayonnaise.

436. Beetroot Crisps with Coriander Hummus

(Preparation time: 10 minutes | Cooking time: 15 minutes | Difficulty: Easy | Servings: 2)
Per serving: Calories 173, Total fat 10g, Protein 6g, Carbs 14g
Ingredients:

- 1 lemon
- 1 clove of garlic
- 2 sprigs of fresh thyme
- Extra virgin olive oil
- 1 teaspoon of smoked paprika
- 1/4 cup of coriander leaves
- 1/2 cup of large beetroot
- 1 x 400g tin of chickpeas
- 2 tablespoons of tahini

Instructions:

- Preheat the oven at 400°F.
- After peeling and finely slicing the beets, place them in a dish. After plucking the thyme leaves, toss them with 1 tablespoon of olive oil.
- Spread out on parchment paper-lined baking pans and roast for around 15 minutes, or till crisp. Allow for cooling time. Peel and crush the garlic cloves in a blender, then add the chickpeas & their liquids. Blitz the remaining ingredients, plus 1 tablespoon olive oil, in a food processor till smooth.
- Season, then combine with the chips in a small-sized bowl and drizzle with olive oil. In the fridge, any leftover hummus will last for about 4 to 5 days.

437. Crab Filled Deviled Eggs

(Preparation time: 10 minutes | Cooking time: 0 minutes | Difficulty: Easy | Servings: 16)
Per serving: Calories 321, Total fat 2g, Protein 2g, Carbs 21g
Ingredients:

- 2 tablespoons of Lemon juice

- 1/4 teaspoon of salt
- 1/8 teaspoon of cayenne pepper
- 1 tablespoon of chopped green onion
- 8 large hard-boiled eggs
- 3 tablespoons of fat-free mayonnaise
- 4 teaspoons of minced fresh tarragon
- 1/4 teaspoon of hot pepper sauce
- 1 can (6 oz.) crabmeat, drained, flaked, and cartilage removed

Instructions:

- Cut the eggs in half lengthwise.
- Remove the yolks, then set the 4 yolks & egg whites aside.
- In a large-sized mixing dish, mash the saved yolks. Cayenne, hot pepper sauce, lemon juice, salt, onion, tarragon, and mayonnaise are all mixed together.
- Mix in the crab till everything is nicely combined. It's then piped or stuffed into egg whites and chilled till ready to serve.

438. Cinnamon Toasties

(Preparation time: 10 minutes | Cooking time: 15 minutes | Difficulty: Easy | Servings: 4)
Per serving: Calories 231, Total fat 1g, Protein 1g, Carbs 24g
Ingredients:

- 1-1/2 teaspoons of ground cinnamon
- 3 tablespoons of sweetener
- 8 slices of whole-wheat bread
- 1/4 cup reduced-fat cream cheese
- Refrigerated butter-flavored spray

Instructions:

- Flatten the bread with a rolling pin.
- Half of the slices should be spread with cream cheese on one side, and the remaining bread should be placed on top.
- Cut each slice into four squares. Spritz both sides with butter-flavored spray.
- In a small-sized bowl, combine the cinnamon and sweetener; add the bread squares & flip to coat both sides.

- Place on a baking sheet. Preheat oven at 350°F and bake for around 8-10 minutes, or till golden and puffy. Serve immediately.

439. Garlic Spinach Balls

(Preparation time: 15 minutes | Cooking time: 25 minutes | Difficulty: Easy | Servings: 8)
Per serving: Calories 234, Total fat 1g, Protein 3g, Carbs 33g
Ingredients:

- 1/4 teaspoon of salt
- 1/4 teaspoon of pepper
- 1 garlic clove, minced
- 1-1/2 teaspoons of dried thyme
- 1 cup of finely chopped onion
- 4 large eggs, lightly beaten
- 3/4 cup of butter, melted
- 1/2 cup of grated Parmesan cheese
- 2 cups of crushed seasoned stuffing
- 2 packages (10 oz. each) of frozen chopped spinach, thawed and squeezed dry

Instructions:

- In a large-sized mixing bowl, combine the first nine ingredients.
- Mix in the spinach till everything is well mixed. It should be rolled into 1-inch balls and placed in a greased 15x10x1-inch baking sheet.
- Allow it to bake for around 15-20 minutes at 350°F, or till golden brown.

440. Stuffed Dates

(Preparation time: 15 minutes | Cooking time: 0 minutes | Difficulty: Easy | Servings: 10)
Per serving: Calories 200, Total fat 7g, Protein 6g, Carbs 6g
Ingredients:

- 2 teaspoons of grated orange zest
- 1/2 cup of reduced-fat cream cheese
- 1/4 cup confectioners' sugar
- 30 pitted Medjool dates

Instructions:

- In a small-sized mixing bowl, add the orange zest, confectioner's sugar, and cream cheese.
- Carefully cut a slit in the middle of each date, then stuff with the cream cheese mixture.
- Cover and refrigerate in the refrigerator for at least 1 hour before serving.

CHAPTER 13:

Dessert Recipes

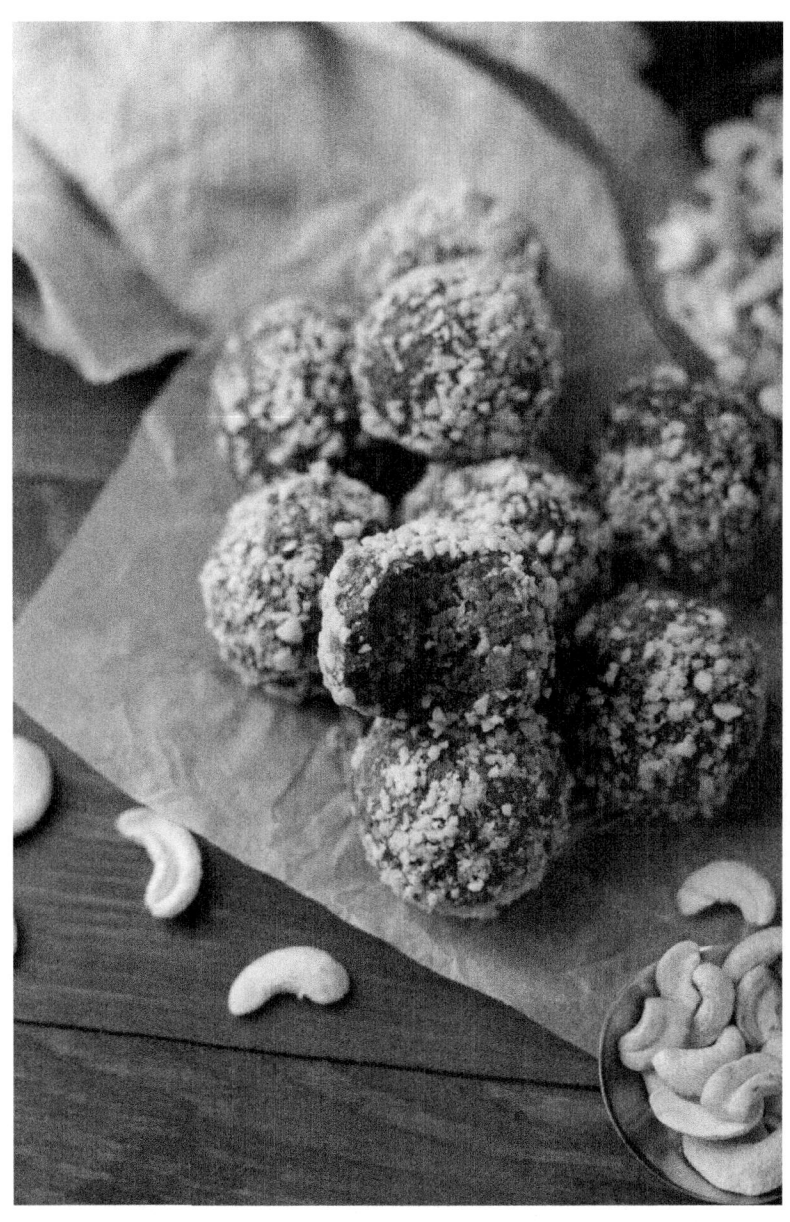

441. Vanilla Cake

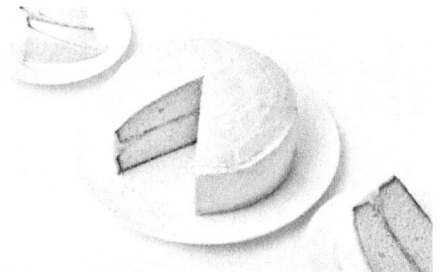

(Preparation time: 15 minutes | Cooking time: 25 minutes | Difficulty: Easy | Servings: 10)
Per serving: Calories 200, Total fat 8g, Protein 5g, Carbs 5g
Ingredients:
- 2 cups of water
- Cooking spray
- 1 tablespoon of lime juice
- 2 teaspoons of vanilla extract
- 1 cup of olive oil
- 3 teaspoons of baking powder
- 1 and 2/3 cup stevia
- 3 cups of almond flour
- 1 and ½ cup almond milk

Instructions:
- Whisk together the almond flour, baking powder, oil, and the remaining ingredients (excluding the cooking spray) in a mixing bowl.
- Pour the batter into a cake pan prepared using cooking spray, place in the oven, and bake for around 25 minutes at 370°F.
- Allow the cake to cool before cutting and serving!

442. Hearty Almond Crackers

(Preparation time: 15 minutes | Cooking time: 20 minutes | Difficulty: Easy | Servings: 40 crackers)
Per serving: Calories 130, Total fat 7g, Protein 11g, Carbs 5g
Ingredients:
- Salt and pepper to taste

- 1/8 teaspoon of black pepper
- ¼ teaspoon of baking soda
- 1 egg, beaten
- 3 tablespoons of sesame seeds
- 1 cup of almond flour

Instructions:
- Preheat the oven at 350°F.
- Line two baking pans using parchment paper and set them aside.
- In a large-sized mixing bowl, combine the dry ingredients & add the egg; stir well to combine and form a dough.
- Make two balls out of the dough.
- Between two pieces of parchment paper, roll out the dough.
- Cut the crackers into pieces and place them on the prepared baking sheet.
- Bake for around 15-20 minutes.
- Rep till you've used up all of the dough.
- Allow crackers to cool before serving.
- Enjoy!

443. Choc Bites

(Preparation time: 15 minutes | Cooking time: 0 minutes | Difficulty: Easy | Servings: 2)
Per serving: Calories 140, Total fat 3g, Protein 2g, Carbs 6g
Ingredients:
- 1-2 tablespoons of water
- 1 tablespoon of ground turmeric
- 1 tablespoon of extra-virgin olive oil
- 1 tablespoon of vanilla extract
- 1 cup of Medjool dates-pitted
- 1 tablespoon of cocoa powder
- 1/2 cup of walnuts

Instructions:
- In a food processor, combine the chocolate & walnuts and pulse till a fine powder forms. Process the remaining components (excluding the water) till a ball forms.

- You may or may not need to add water, depending on the consistency (we don't want it to be too sticky).
- Form bite-sized balls and place them in an airtight container in the refrigerator for about an hour before serving. If desired, roll the balls in desiccated coconut or cocoa powder. They'll last about a week in the fridge.

444. Raspberry and Blackcurrant Jelly

(Preparation time: 10 minutes | Cooking time: 10 minutes | Difficulty: Easy | Servings: 2)
Per serving: Calories 354, Total fat 5g, Protein 4g, Carbs 9g
Ingredients:
- 1 cup of water
- 2 leaves of gelatin
- 1/2 cup of washed raspberries
- 1/2 cup of washed blackcurrants (stalks removed)
- 2 tablespoons of sweetener (stevia)

Instructions:
- Divide the raspberries across two glasses or platters for serving. Place the gelatin leaves in a dish of cold water to soften them.
- In a small-sized saucepan, combine the blackcurrants, 1/2 cup of water, and the sweetener. Allow to come to a boil, then reduce to a low flame and continue to cook for five minutes before turning off the flame. Allow two minutes to stand.
- Squeeze the leaves to remove any extra water before adding them to the saucepan. Stir till the ingredients are completely dissolved, then add the remaining water and stir again. Store the liquid in the serving glasses or plates & place it in the refrigerator to set, ideally overnight or for at least 3 to 4 hours.

445. No-Bake Strawberry Flapjacks

(Preparation time: 15 minutes | Cooking time: 0 minutes | Difficulty: Easy | Servings: 1)
Per serving: Calories 123, Total fat 2g, Protein 2g, Carbs 11g
Ingredients:
- 1 tablespoon of coconut oil
- 1/2 cup of dates
- 1/4 cup of strawberries
- 1/4 cup of peanuts, unsalted
- 1/4 cup of walnuts
- 1/2 cup of porridge oats
- 2 tablespoons of 100% cocoa powder or cacao nibs

Instructions:
- In a blender, combine the ingredients and process them till they reach a soft consistency.
- Using a baking sheet or a small flat tin, spread the mixture out.
- Smooth out the mixture by pressing it down. It's ready to serve after being cut into 8 pieces.
- If desired, a sprinkle of cocoa powder can be added as a garnish.

446. Choco Nut Truffles

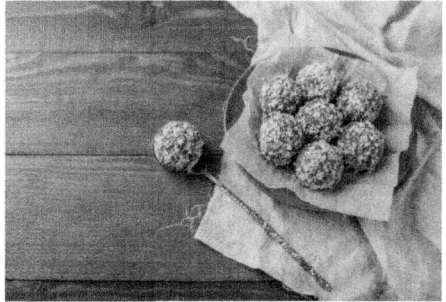

(Preparation time: 15 minutes | Cooking time: 0 minutes | Difficulty: Easy | Servings: 1)
Per serving: Calories 220, Total fat 2g, Protein 10g, Carbs 1g
Ingredients:
- 1 tablespoon of olive oil
- 4 Medjool dates

- 1/2 cup of desiccated shredded coconut
- 1/4 cup of walnuts, chopped
- 2 tablespoons of 100% cocoa powder or cacao nibs
- 1/4 cup of hazelnuts, chopped

Instructions:

- Blend the ingredients in a blender till smooth and creamy.
- Divide the mixture into bite-size pieces using a teaspoon, then roll it into balls.
- Before serving, place them in little paper cases, cover them, & chill for 1 hour.

447. Figs Pie

(Preparation time: 15 minutes | Cooking time: 1 hour | Difficulty: Easy | Servings: 8)
Per serving: Calories 200, Total fat 4g, Protein 8g, Carbs 7g
Ingredients:

- 4 eggs, whisked
- ½ teaspoon of vanilla extract
- 6 figs, cut into quarters
- ½ cup of stevia
- 1 cup of almond flour

Instructions:

- In the bottom of a spring form pan lined using parchment paper, spread the figs.
- Combine the remaining ingredients in a dish, whisk together, & pour over the figs.
- Bake for around 1 hour at 375°F, then flip the pie upside down and serve.

448. Green Tea and Vanilla Cream

(Preparation time: 15 minutes | Cooking time: 0 minutes | Difficulty: Easy | Servings: 4)
Per serving: Calories 120, Total fat 3g, Protein 4g, Carbs 7g
Ingredients:

- 1 teaspoon of vanilla extract
- 2 tablespoons of green tea powder
- 1 teaspoon of gelatin powder

- 3 tablespoons of stevia
- 2 cups of heavy cream
- 2 cups of almond milk, hot

Instructions:

- Combine the almond milk, green tea powder, and the remaining ingredients in a mixing bowl, whisk well, and set aside to chill.
- Divide the mixture into cups and chill for around 2 hours before serving.

449. Black Tea Cake

(Preparation time: 15 minutes | Cooking time: 35 minutes | Difficulty: Easy | Servings: 8)
Per serving: Calories 200, Total fat 6g, Protein 5g, Carbs 6g
Ingredients:

- 1 teaspoon of baking soda
- 3 teaspoons of baking powder
- 6 tablespoons of black tea powder
- 2 teaspoons of vanilla extract
- 4 eggs - 1 cup of avocado oil
- 2 cups of stevia 3 ½ cups of almond flour
- 2 cups of almond milk, warmed up

Instructions:

- Whisk together the almond milk, oil, stevia, & the remaining ingredients in a mixing bowl. Pour the mixture into a cake pan lined using parchment paper and bake for around 35 minutes at 350°F.
- Allow the cake to cool before slicing and serving.

450. Blackberry and Apple Cobbler

(Preparation time: 15 minutes | Cooking time: 30 minutes | Difficulty: Easy | Servings: 6)
Per serving: Calories 221, Total fat 6g, Protein 9g, Carbs 6g
Ingredients:

- ½ cup of water
- Cooking spray
- ¼ teaspoon of baking powder

- 1 tablespoon of lime juice
- 3 ½ tablespoons of olive oil
- ¾ cup of stevia
- 6 cups of blackberries
- ¼ cup of apples, cored and cubed
- ½ cup of almond flour

Instructions:

- Mix the berries with half of the stevia & lemon juice in a mixing bowl, then dust with flour, whisk, and pour into a buttered baking dish.
- In a separate basin, combine the flour, remaining sweetener, baking powder, water, and oil, and blend everything together using your hands.
- Spread the mixture over the berries & bake for around 30 minutes at 375°F. Warm the dish before serving.

451. Cold Lemon Squares

(Preparation time: 15 minutes | Cooking time: 30 minutes | Difficulty: Easy | Servings: 4)
Per serving: Calories 136, Total fat 3g, Protein 1g, Carbs 7g
Ingredients:

- A pinch of lemon zest, grated
- ¼ cup of lemon juice
- 1 tablespoon of honey
- 2 bananas, peeled and chopped
- 1 cup of olive oil

Instructions:

- Mix the bananas with the rest of the ingredients in a food processor, pulse till smooth, and spread on the bottom of a pan oiled with a drizzle of oil.
- Refrigerate for around 30 minutes before cutting into squares and serving.

452. Chocolate Fondue

(Preparation time: 15 minutes | Cooking time: 0 minutes | Difficulty: Easy | Servings: 1)
Per serving: Calories 220, Total fat 2g, Protein 10g, Carbs 2g

Ingredients:

- 2 apples, peeled, cored, and sliced
- 1 1/4 cups of strawberries
- 1 cup of cherries
- 1/2 cup of dark chocolate min 85% cocoa
- 1/4 cup of double cream, heavy cream

Instructions:

- Place the chocolate & cream in a fondue pot or saucepan and heat till smooth and creamy.
- Serve immediately in the fondue pot or in a serving bowl.
- Arrange the fruit in a serving dish to be dipped in the chocolate.

453. Tropical Chocolate Delight

(Preparation time: 15 minutes | Cooking time: 0 minutes | Difficulty: Easy | Servings: 1)
Per serving: Calories 185, Total fat 2g, Protein 10g, Carbs 2g
Ingredients:

- 1 mango, peeled & de-stoned
- 1/2 cup of fresh pineapple, chopped
- 1/4 cup of kale
- 1/4 cup rocket
- 1 tablespoon of 100% cocoa powder or cacao nibs
- 1/2 cup of coconut milk

Instructions:

- In a blender, combine all of the ingredients and blend till smooth. If it seems overly thick, thin it out with a little water.

454. Chocolate Coffee Cake

(Preparation time: 15 minutes | Cooking time: 40 minutes | Difficulty: Easy | Servings: 6 to 8)
Per serving: Calories 370, Total fat 20g, Protein 4g, Carbs 24g
Ingredients:

- 1/8 teaspoon of salt
- 1 teaspoon of baking soda

- ½ teaspoon of baking powder
- 3 teaspoons of cinnamon
- ½ teaspoon of ground nutmeg
- 1 cup of coconut oil, cold and solid
- 3 cups of almond or buckwheat flour
- ½ cup of Medjool dates, chopped
- ½ cup of mixed nuts or walnuts, chopped
- 4 teaspoons of unsweetened cocoa powder
- 2 cups of sweetener
- 2 cups of buttermilk

Instructions:

- Preheat oven at 350°F.
- Combine the flour and sweetener in a large-sized mixing dish.
- Cut in the solid coconut oil with a pastry knife until the mixture is crumbly. 1 cup of the crumbled mixture should be saved for topping.
- Add cocoa powder, baking soda, baking powder, cinnamon, nutmeg, & salt to the remaining ingredients and whisk till thoroughly blended.
- Toss in the dates and nuts.
- Make a well in the center of the cake mix and gradually pour in the buttermilk. Stir till the mixture is slightly moistened.
- Fill a greased 13-in. x 9-in. x 2-in. baking pan halfway with batter. Sprinkle with the crumb mixture that was set aside.
- Bake for around 35-40 minutes, or until a toothpick inserted in the center comes out clean.

455. Date Nut Loaf

(Preparation time: 15 minutes | Cooking time: 40 minutes | Difficulty: Easy | Servings: 4 to 6)
Per serving: Calories 70, Total fat 1g, Protein 1g, Carbs 15g
Ingredients:

- ½ teaspoon of salt

- 2 teaspoons of baking powder
- ¼ teaspoon of baking soda
- 1 tablespoon of coconut oil, melted
- ¾ cup of Medjool dates
- ¾ cup of milk
- 1 egg, slightly beaten
- ½ cup of sweetener
- 1 ¼ cups of almond flour
- 1 tablespoon of orange peel, grated
- 1 cup of walnuts, chopped
- 1 ¼ cups of buckwheat flour

Instructions:

- Place the dates on a cutting board and dust them with 1 tablespoon of flour. Finely chop the dates with a knife dipped in flour. To keep the cut-up fruit from sticking together, flour the knife frequently.
- In a large-sized mixing dish, sift the remaining flour, baking powder, baking soda, salt, & sweetener.
- Combine the milk, egg, orange peel, & oil in a separate dish.
- Add the buckwheat flour to the flour mixture, stir well, then fold in the dates, as well as any remaining flour on the cutting block and the walnuts, gently.
- Mix in the liquid components till they are completely blended.
- Place the dough in a greased and oiled baking pan.
- Preheat oven at 350°F and bake for around 35 to 40 minutes.

456. Apple Date Pudding

(Preparation time: 15 minutes | Cooking time: 40 minutes | Difficulty: Easy | Servings: 6 to 8)
Per serving: Calories 287, Total fat 9g, Protein 2g, Carbs 22g
Ingredients:

- 1/8 teaspoon of salt
- 1 teaspoon of baking powder
- ¼ teaspoon of Nutmeg

- 2 tablespoons of coconut oil, melted
- 1 egg, beaten
- 4-5 apples, diced
- ½ cup of Medjool dates, chopped
- 2 tablespoons of buckwheat flour
- ¾ cup of stevia, or less, to taste
- ½ cup of walnuts, toasted and chopped

Instructions:

- Combine apples, stevia, dates, & walnuts into a baking pan.
- Combine flour, baking powder, salt, & nutmeg in a large-sized mixing bowl, then fold into apple mixture.
- Pour the melted coconut oil over the batter & whisk one more.
- Incorporate the beaten egg.
- Preheat oven at 350°F and bake for around 35 to 40 minutes.

457. Strawberry and Rhubarb Crisp

(Preparation time: 15 minutes | Cooking time: 45 minutes | Difficulty: Easy | Servings: 6 to 8)
Per serving: Calories 242, Total fat 3g, Protein 3g, Carbs 28g

Ingredients:

- ½ lemon, juiced
- 1 cup of coconut oil, melted
- 3 cups of strawberries, sliced
- 3 cups of rhubarb, diced
- 1 cup of stevia
- ¼ cup of walnuts, chopped
- ½ cup of buckwheat flour + 3 tablespoons
- 1 cup of stevia
- ¾ cup of rolled oats
- ¼ cup of buckwheat groats

Instructions:

- Preheat the oven at 375°F.
- Combine stevia, 3 tablespoons of flour, strawberries, rhubarb, and lemon juice in a large-sized mixing dish. Fill a 9x13 inch baking dish halfway with the mixture.

- Mix 1/2 cup of flour, stevia, coconut oil, oats, buckwheat groats, and walnuts in a separate bowl till crumbly. For this, you might wish to use a pastry blender. On top of the rhubarb and strawberry mixture, crumble.
- Bake for around 45 minutes, or till crisp and lightly browned in a preheated oven.

458. Chocolate and Matcha Dipped Strawberries

(Preparation time: 15 minutes | Cooking time: 15 minutes | Difficulty: Easy | Servings: 4 to 6)
Per serving: Calories 88, Total fat 5g, Protein 1g, Carbs 10g

Ingredients:

- ¼ cup of coconut oil
- 1 teaspoon of Matcha green tea powder
- 20 – 25 large whole strawberries, stems on
- 4 tablespoons of cocoa butter
- 4 square of dark chocolate, at least 85%

Instructions:

- In a double boiler, melt the cocoa butter, dark chocolate, coconut oil, & Matcha till nearly smooth.
- Remove from the flame and stir till the chocolate has completely melted.
- Pour into a large glass bowl and whisk regularly for 2 to 5 minutes, or till chocolate thickens and loses its luster.
- Hold the strawberries by the stems and dip them into the chocolate matcha mixture to coat them one at a time. Allow any surplus liquid to drain back into the dish.
- Chill dipped berries on a parchment-lined baking sheet for around 20–25 minutes or until the shell is firm.
- If the matcha mixture starts to solidify before you've dipped all of the berries, you may need to reheat it.

459. Crunchy Chocolate Chip Coconut Macadamia Nut Cookies

(Preparation time: 15 minutes | Cooking time: 45 minutes | Difficulty: Easy | Servings: 4)
Per serving: Calories 257, Total fat 20g, Protein 32g, Carbs 18g
Ingredients:

- 1/2 teaspoon of salt
- 1/2 teaspoon of baking soda
- 1 tablespoon of butter, softened
- 1 egg - 1 cup of yogurt
- 1/2 cup of sweet coconut flakes
- 1 cup of firmly packed sweetener
- 1/2 cup of raisins
- 1/2 cup of sweetener
- 1/2 cup of dark chocolate chips
- 1/2 cup of coarsely chopped roasted walnuts macadamia nuts

Instructions:

- Preheat the oven at 325ºF.
- Whisk together the flour, oats, baking soda, & salt in a small-sized bowl, then set aside.
- Combine the butter, sweetener, and egg mixture in your mixer bowl.
- Stir in the chocolate chips, raisins, nuts, and coconut from the flour/oats mixture till just incorporated.
- On a parchment-lined cookie sheet, arrange sized chunks.
- Bake for around 3 to 5 minutes, or until the biscuits are just golden brown.
- Remove the cookie sheets from the oven and set them aside to cool for at least 10 minutes.

460. Lemon Ricotta Cookies with Lemon Glaze

(Preparation time: 15 minutes | Cooking time: 20 minutes | Difficulty: Easy | Servings: 2)
Per serving: Calories 123, Total fat 9g, Protein 12g, Carbs 18g

Ingredients:

- 3 tablespoons of lemon juice
- 1 lemon
- 1 teaspoon of salt
- 1 teaspoon of baking powder
- 1 tablespoon of unsalted butter softened
- 2 1/2 cups of almond flour
- 2 cups of stevia
- 2 cups of whole milk ricotta cheese

For the Glaze:

- 3 tablespoons of lemon juice - 1 lemon
- 1 1/2 cups of powdered sweetener

Instructions:

- Preheat oven at 375°F.
- Combine the salt, flour, & baking powder in a medium-sized mixing bowl. Set-aside.
- Using an electric mixer, cream the butter and sugar together in a large-sized mixing bowl till light & fluffy, about three minutes. 1 at a time, beat in the eggs till fully combined.
- Place the ricotta cheese, lemon juice, and lemon zest in a mixing bowl. To combine, beat the ingredients together. Add the dry skin and mix well.
- Line two baking pans using parchment paper. Place the dough on the baking sheets (about 2 teaspoons per cookie). Bake for 15 minutes or till the edges are slightly golden. Remove the cookies from the oven & set them aside. Cook for another 20 minutes on the remaining baking sheet.
- In a small-sized bowl, whisk together the powdered sweetener, lemon juice, and lemon peel till smooth. Spoon about 1/2 teaspoon onto each cookie and lightly spread with the back of the spoon. Allow two hours for the glaze to solidify. Fill a beautiful container halfway with biscuits.

461. Loaded Chocolate Fudge

(Preparation time: 15 minutes | Cooking time: 0 minutes | Difficulty: Easy | Servings: 3)
Per serving: Calories 258, Total fat 4g, Protein 8g, Carbs 5g
Ingredients:

- 1 teaspoon of vanilla
- 2 tablespoons of coconut oil, melted
- 1 cup of Medjool dates, chopped
- ¼ cup of unsweetened cocoa powder
- 1/2 cup of peanut butter
- ½ cup of walnuts

Instructions:

- Soak the dates for 20–30 minutes in warm water.
- Using coconut oil, lightly coat an 8" square baking pan.
- In a food processor, combine the dates, peanut butter, chocolate powder, and vanilla and pulse till smooth.
- Toss in the walnuts.
- Place the fudge in a prepared baking sheet and freeze for 1 hour, or till solid and firm.
- Cut into 16 or more bite-sized squares & store in the refrigerator in a semi-airtight container.

462. Plum Oat Bars

(Preparation time: 15 minutes | Cooking time: 0 minutes | Difficulty: Easy | Servings: 4)
Per serving: Calories 274, Total fat 12g, Protein 15g, Carbs 11g
Ingredients:

- 1/4 teaspoon of salt
- 1/5 teaspoon of cinnamon
- 1 teaspoon of baking powder
- 1/5 cups of rolled oats
- 2 tablespoons of soybean oil
- 1/5 cup of almond meal
- 2 cups of prunes

Instructions:

- Begin by preheating the oven to 350°F and prepping the prunes. Pour hot water over the prunes in a large-sized mixing bowl till they are completely soaked. Allow five minutes for the prunes to soften in the water.
- Reserving the water, remove the prunes from the water & place them in a blender or food processor. Blend in a small bit of the prunes' water that you had previously set aside till the prunes form a thick paste.
- In a medium kitchen bowl, combine two tablespoons of the prune puree, the oil, sea salt, baking powder, cinnamon, almond flour, & rolled oats. Mix everything together till it resembles a crumble, like wet sand. If the prune puree is too dry, add more.
- To make a crust, line a square baking dish with parchment paper and press three-quarters of the oat mixture into the bottom. Spoon the remaining prune puree on top of the crust, and then crumble the remaining oat mixture on top of the prune puree.
- Cook the bars in the oven for about 15 minutes, or till they are set and slightly browned. Remove the plum oat bars out from the hot oven & cool thoroughly in the pan. Slice the bars into nine bars after they have reached room temperature.

463. Blueberry Nut Bran Muffins

(Preparation time: 15 minutes | Cooking time: 20 minutes | Difficulty: Easy | Servings: 4)
Per serving: Calories 154, Total fat 8g, Protein 15g, Carbs 13g
Ingredients:

- 1/4 teaspoon of salt
- 1/4 teaspoon of baking soda
- 1/4 teaspoon of baking powder

- 1 teaspoon of cinnamon
- 1 tablespoon of apple cider vinegar
- 2 eggs
- 1 cup of blueberries
- 1/4 cup of chopped walnuts
- 1/5 cup of date sweetener
- 1/4 cup of soybean oil
- 1 cup of wheat bran
- 1 1/5 cups of whole wheat flour
- 1/4 cup of apple sauce unsweetened
- 1/4 cup of soy milk unsweetened

Instructions:

- Preheat your oven to 400°F in either a conventional or toaster oven. Line a 12-cup muffin tin with paper liners & coat using nonstick cooking spray.
- In a large mixing bowl, whisk together the eggs, applesauce, date sweetener, soybean oil, soy milk, & apple cider vinegar till thoroughly incorporated. Set them aside.
- In a separate clean bowl, combine the whole wheat flour, wheat bran, cinnamon, sea salt, baking soda, & baking soda. Fold the dry ingredients into the other prepared ingredients once they've been blended. Just till the blueberries and walnuts are incorporated, gently fold them in.
- Allow the blueberry nut bran muffin batter to bake in the prepared muffin liners for fifteen to eighteen minutes or till a toothpick inserted in the center comes out clean. Allow the muffins to cool for five minutes after taking them out of the oven before removing them from the pan.

464. Chocolate Maple Walnuts

(Preparation time: 15 minutes | Cooking time: 20 minutes | Difficulty: Easy | Servings: 4)
Per serving: Calories 154, Total fat 8g, Protein 15g, Carbs 13g

Ingredients:

- 1 tablespoonful of water
- 1 teaspoonful of vanilla extract
- 1 ½ tablespoons of coconut oil, melted
- 2 cups of raw, whole walnuts
- ½ cup pure maple syrup, divided
- 5 squares of dark chocolate, at least 85% - Sifted icing sweetener

Instructions:

- Using parchment paper, line a large-sized baking sheet.
- Combine the walnuts and 1/4 cup of maple syrup in a medium to a large skillet and simmer, constantly turning, till the walnuts are completely covered in syrup and brown in color, about 3 – 5 minutes. Pour the walnuts onto the parchment paper & use a fork to divide them into individual pieces. Allow at least 15 minutes for the mixture to cool fully. Meanwhile, melt the chocolate and coconut oil in a double boiler. Stir in the remaining maple syrup till everything is well mixed. When the walnuts have cooled, pour the melted chocolate syrup over them in a glass bowl. Mix carefully with a silicone spatula till the walnuts are well covered.
- Return the nuts to the parchment paper-lined baking sheet and divide them with a fork once more. Place the nuts in the fridge for around 10 minutes or the freezer for 3–5 minutes, till the chocolate has hardened fully. Refrigerate in an airtight container.

465. Warm Berries and Cream

(Preparation time: 15 minutes | Cooking time: 0 minutes | Difficulty: Easy | Servings: 1)
Per serving: Calories 193, Total fat 5g, Protein 2g, Carbs 15g
Ingredients:

- 1 tablespoon of honey

- 4 tablespoons of fresh whipped cream
- 1/2 cup of blueberries
- 1/2 cup of strawberries
- 1/4 cup of blackberries
- 1/4 cup of red currants

Instructions:

- In a mixing dish, combine all of the ingredients. Scoop a small amount of the mixture out and roll it into a ball.
- Set the ball aside after rolling it in cocoa powder. Rep with the rest of the mixture. It can be eaten right away or kept in the refrigerator.

466. Guilt-Free Banana Ice-cream

(Preparation time: 15 minutes | Cooking time: 0 minutes | Difficulty: Easy | Servings: 3)
Per serving: Calories 208, Total fat 3g, Protein 2g, Carbs 15g
Ingredients:

- 2 tablespoons of skim milk
- A couple of dark chocolate chips
- 3 quite ripe bananas - peeled and chopped

Instructions:

- Blend all of the ingredients in a food processor till smooth.
- Eat: Freeze for later enjoyment.

467. Apricot Oatmeal Cookies

(Preparation time: 10 minutes | Cooking time: 15 minutes | Difficulty: Easy | Servings: 3)
Per serving: Calories 132, Total fat 3g, Protein 2g, Carbs 14g
Ingredients:

- 1/2 teaspoon of cinnamon
- 1/4 teaspoon of salt
- 1/2 teaspoon of baking soda
- 1/2 teaspoon of vanilla extract
- 1/2 cup (1 stick) of butter, softened
- 1 egg
- 3/4 cup of yolks
- 2/3 cup of light brown sugar packed

- 3/4 cup of almond flour
- 1/2 cups of chopped oats
- 1/4 cup of sliced apricots
- 1/3 cup of slivered almonds

Instructions:

- Preheat the oven at 350°F.
- Combine the butter, sweetener, and egg in a large-sized mixing bowl till smooth.
- Combine the flour, baking soda, cinnamon, & salt in a separate bowl.
- Toss in the dry ingredients with the butter and sugar in a mixing dish.
- Combine the oats, raisins, apricots, and almonds in a mixing bowl.
- Scoop the biscuits onto a parchment-lined cookie sheet, spacing them about two inches apart (for easier removal and cleanup).
- Bake them for around 10 to 12 minutes.

468. Peach and Blueberry Pie

(Preparation time: 10 minutes | Cooking time: 25 minutes | Difficulty: Easy | Servings: 2)
Per serving: Calories 167, Total fat 4g, Protein 12g, Carbs 11g
Ingredients:

- 1 box of whole-wheat puff pastry dough

For the Filling:

- Juice of 1/2 lemon - 1 egg yolk, beaten
- 3 cups of strawberries
- 5 peaches, peeled and chopped (I used roasted peaches)
- 1/4 cup of whole-wheat bread
- 3/4 cup of sweetener

Instructions:

- Preheat the oven at 400°F.
- On a 9-inch pie plate, roll out the dough.
- Toss peaches, sugar, bread, and lemon juice together in a large mixing dish. Fill the pie plate to the rim, mounding the filling in the center.

- Simply take a portion of the bread and cut it into little pieces, then put the dough in a pie shirt and flatten the borders. Brush the egg wash on the crust before sprinkling the sweetener on top. Place on a baking sheet lined using parchment paper. Bake for around 20 minutes, or until the crust has browned around the edges.
- Reduce the oven temperature to 350°F and bake for another 40 minutes.
- Remove from the oven and set aside for at least 30 minutes.
- Serve with a scoop of vanilla ice cream.

469. Walnut and Date Cake

(Preparation time: 10 minutes | Cooking time: 0 minutes | Difficulty: Easy | Servings: 12)
Per serving: Calories 204, Total fat 3g, Protein 2g, Carbs 16g
Ingredients:

- 1 teaspoon of baking soda
- 1 medium banana, mashed
- 1/2 cup of Medjool dates, chopped
- 3 eggs - 1 cup of skim milk
- 1 cup of almond flour
- 1/4 cup of walnuts, chopped

Instructions:

- In a mixing dish, sift together the baking soda & flour.
- Combine all of the ingredients, including the banana, eggs, milk, and dates.
- Smooth the batter into a loaf pan lined using parchment paper.
- Sprinkle the walnuts over the top.
- Preheat the oven to 360°F and bake the loaf for around 45 minutes.

470. Chocolate Cream Fruity Cake

(Preparation time: 15 minutes | Cooking time: 0 minutes | Difficulty: Easy | Servings: 4)
Per serving: Calories 106, Total fat 5g, Protein 14g, Carbs 1g

Ingredients:

- Pinch of sea salt
- 2 tablespoons of coconut oil
- 2 tablespoons of cacao powder
- 1/2 cup of raw honey
- 1 cup of coconut flakes
- 1 avocado
- 1 teaspoon of ground vanilla bean
- ¼ cup of coconut milk

Fruits:

- 1 chopped banana
- 1 cup of pitted cherries

Instructions:

- Prepare the crust & press it into the pan's bottom.
- Combine all of the ingredients for the chocolate cream, fold in the fruits, and pour into the crust.
- Whip up the top layer, then spread it out and top with cacao powder.
- Refrigerate.

471. Carrot Cake

(Preparation time: 15 minutes | Cooking time: 0 minutes | Difficulty: Easy | Servings: 4)
Per serving: Calories 241, Total fat 13g, Protein 2g, Carbs 21g
Ingredients:

- Water, as needed
- Juice from 1 lemon
- 1 teaspoon cinnamon
- ½ teaspoon nutmeg
- 4 tablespoons of coconut oil
- 1/2 tablespoons of raw honey
- 1 teaspoon ground vanilla bean
- 4 carrots, chopped
- 2 cups of Medjool dates
- 1½ cups oats
- ½ cup dried coconut
- 1½ cups of cashews

Instructions:

- In a blender, combine all of the crust ingredients.

- Mix thoroughly and, if desired, add a few drops of water at a time to help the mixture hold together.
- In a small pan, press. Remove it from the oven and place it on a platter to freeze. In a blender, combine the frosting ingredients and, if necessary, add water. Refrigerate the crust after icing it.

472. Chocolate Pie

(Preparation time: 15 minutes | Cooking time: 0 minutes | Difficulty: Easy | Servings: 4)
Per serving: Calories 280, Total fat 18g, Protein 7g, Carbs 25g
Ingredients:
For the Crust:
- 1½ teaspoon of ground vanilla bean
- 2 teaspoons of chia seeds
- 1 banana - 1 cup of pitted dates, soaked overnight and drained
- 1 cup of chopped dried apricots
- 2 cups of almonds, soaked overnight and drained

For the Filling:
- 3 tablespoons of organic coconut oil
- 4 tablespoons of raw honey
- 6 tablespoons of raw cacao powder
- 2 ripe avocados
- 1/4 cup of almond milk (if needed, check for consistency first)

Instructions:
- In a food processor or blender, combine the almonds and banana.
- Blend till thick ball forms.
- In a blender, combine the vanilla, dates, & apricot pieces.
- Mix thoroughly and, if desired, add a few drops of water at a time to help the mixture hold together. Spread out in a 10-inch square dish. In a blender, combine the filling ingredients and, if necessary, add almond milk. Refrigerate the crust after adding the filling.

473. Peanut Butter Truffles

(Preparation time: 15 minutes | Cooking time: 0 minutes | Difficulty: Easy | Servings: 4)
Per serving: Calories 94, Total fat 8g, Protein 4g, Carbs 3g
Ingredients:
- A pinch of salt
- 1 cup of coconut oil
- 1 cup of raw honey
- 1 teaspoon of ground vanilla bean
- 5 cups of sunflower seed butter
- ¾ cup of almond flour
- 1 cup of flaxseed meal
- Hemp hearts (optional)
- 1 tablespoon of cacao butter
- ¼ cup of super-foods chocolate

Instructions:
- Mix till all of the ingredients are combined.
- Refrigerate for half an hour after rolling the dough into 1-inch balls and placing them on parchment paper (yield around 14 truffles).
- One by one, dip each truffle into the melted superfoods chocolate.
- Using parchment paper, return them to the pan or coat them with cocoa powder or coconut flakes.

474. Bounty Bars

(Preparation time: 15 minutes | Cooking time: 0 minutes | Difficulty: Easy | Servings: 4)
Per serving: Calories 70, Total fat 4g, Protein 1g, Carbs 7g
Ingredients:
"Peanut" butter filling:
- A Pinch of sea salt
- 1 teaspoon ground vanilla bean
- 3 coconut oil - melted
- 2 cups of desiccated coconut
- 1 cup of coconut cream - full fat
- 4 tablespoons of raw honey

Superfoods chocolate part:

- 2 tablespoons of raw honey
- ½ cup of cacao powder
- 1/3 cup of coconut oil (melted)

Instructions:

- Combine the coconut oil, coconut cream, honey, vanilla, & salt in a mixing bowl.
- Pour the liquid over the desiccated coconut and stir well.
- Freeze the coconut mixture in the form of balls or little bars similar to bounty. Alternatively, pour the entire mixture into a tray, freeze it, then cut it into little bars.
- Make a superfoods chocolate mixture, warm it up, and dip frozen coconut in it before placing it on a tray to freeze again.

475. Double Almond Raw Chocolate Tart

(Preparation time: 15 minutes | Cooking time: 0 minutes | Difficulty: Easy | Servings: 4)
Per serving: Calories 101, Total fat 9g, Protein 2g, Carbs 3g
Ingredients:

- ¼ cup of coconut oil, melted
- 1 raw honey or royal jelly
- ½ cup unsweetened shredded coconut
- 1½ cups of raw almonds
- 1 cup of dark chocolate, chopped
- 1 cup of coconut milk

Instructions:

- Crust:
- Combine ground almonds, melted coconut oil, and raw honey.
- Spread the mixture into the tart or pie pan with a spatula.
- Filling:
- In a mixing dish, place the chopped chocolate, heat the coconut milk, and

pour over the chocolate, whisking to combine.
- Fill the tart shell with filling.
- Refrigerate.
- Almond slivers chips are toasted and sprinkled over the dessert.

476. Chocolate Cashew Truffles

(Preparation time: 15 minutes | Cooking time: 0 minutes | Difficulty: Easy | Servings: 4)
Per serving: Calories 87, Total fat 6g, Protein 2g, Carbs 6g
Ingredients:

- ½ cup of coconut oil
- ¼ cup of raw honey
- 1 teaspoon of ground vanilla bean
- 1 cup of ground cashews
- 2 cups of cacao powder
- 2 cups of flax meal
- 2 cups of hemp hearts

Instructions:

- Make truffles by combining all of the components.
- On top, streusel with coconut flakes.

477. Chocolate Muffins

(Preparation time: 15 minutes | Cooking time: 15 minutes | Difficulty: Easy | Servings: 8)
Per serving: Calories 200, Total fat 35g, Protein 11g, Carbs 6g
Ingredients:

- ½ teaspoon of tartar baking powder
- 1 teaspoon of vanilla extract
- 3 bananas (ripe)
- 2 eggs
- 1/2 cup of chocolate chips
- 1 cup of almond paste

Instructions:

- Preheat the oven at 400°F and line a baking sheet using parchment paper or silicone muffin pans.
- In a food processor, combine all ingredients (except for the optional

chocolate chips) and pulse till a smooth, sticky dough forms.

- Optional: add chocolate bits and whisk
- Place the dough in muffin tins and bake for around 12-15 minutes, or till golden brown and done.

478. Cocoa Bars

(Preparation time: 15 minutes | Cooking time: 0 minutes | Difficulty: Easy | Servings: 12)
Per serving: Calories 198, Total fat 5g, Protein 89g, Carbs 10g
Ingredients:
- ½ cup of chia seeds
- 1 cup of unsweetened dark cocoa chips
- 1 cup of low-fat peanut butter
- 2 cups of rolled oats - ½ cup of raisins
- ¼ cup of coconut sugar
- ½ cup of coconut milk

Instructions:
- Process 1 and 1/2 cup of oats well in a blender; transfer to a dish; add the remainder of the oats, cocoa chips, chia seeds, raisins, sweetener, & milk; stir well; spread onto a square pan; press well; chill for 2 hours; slice into 12 bars & serve.

479. Chocolate Wraps with Fruit

(Preparation time: 15 minutes | Cooking time: 10 minutes | Difficulty: Easy | Servings: 2)
Per serving: Calories 355, Total fat 34g, Protein 20g, Carbs 25g
Ingredients:
- 1 tablespoon of olive oil (mild)
- 1 tablespoon of coconut oil
- 2 tablespoons of cocoa powder
- 4 eggs - 1 banana - 2 kiwi (green)
- 2 mandarins
- 2 tablespoons of maple syrup
- 2 tablespoons of arrowroot powder
- 4 tablespoons of chestnut flour
- 1/2 cup of almond milk

Instructions:
- To make an even dough, combine all ingredients (except the fruit and coconut oil).
- In a small-sized pan, melt some coconut oil and pour a fourth of the batter into it. Cook it on both sides like a pancake.
- Wrap the fruit in a wrap & serve it at room temperature.

480. Walnut Pie Crust Raw Brownies

(Preparation time: 15 minutes | Cooking time: 10 minutes | Difficulty: Easy | Servings: 2)
Per serving: Calories 299, Total fat 31g, Protein 14g, Carbs 31g
Ingredients:
- 1 ½ tsp. ground vanilla bean
- 1 cup of Medjool pitted dates
- 1 ½ cups walnuts
- 1/3 cup of unsweetened cocoa powder

Topping for Raw Brownies:
- 1/3 cup of walnut butter

Instructions:
- In a food processor or blender, combine walnuts. Mix till everything is finely ground. In a blender, combine the vanilla, dates, & cocoa powder. Mix thoroughly and, if desired, add a few drops of water at a time to help the mixture hold together.
- If a pie crust is required, spread it thinly in a 9-inch disc and top with filling.
- Transfer the mixture to a small plate and top with walnut butter if you want to make Raw Brownies. Freeze till set and serve.

481. Ganache Squares

(Preparation time: 15 minutes | Cooking time: 25 minutes | Difficulty: Easy | Servings: 10)
Per serving: Calories 141, Total fat 17g, Protein 8g, Carbs 21g
Ingredients:
- 1 pinch of salt

- ½ teaspoon of vanilla extract
- 1 ½ tablespoons of coconut oil
- 2 hands of pecans
- 1/2 cup of honey
- 1 cup of coconut milk
- 1 1/2 cups of pure chocolate (> 70% cocoa)

Instructions:

- In a saucepan, cook the coconut milk for around 5 minutes over medium flame.
- Cook for around 15 minutes after adding the vanilla extract, coconut oil, & honey. Stir in a pinch of salt thoroughly.
- Pour the boiling coconut milk over the broken chocolate in a bowl. Stir constantly till the chocolate has completely melted in the coconut milk.
- Meanwhile, coarsely cut the pecans. Roast the nuts in a pan without any oil.
- In a separate bowl, stir the pecans into the ganache.
- Allow the ganache to cool to room temperature before using. (You might be able to speed things up by submerging the bowl in cold water.)
- Preheat oven to 350°F. Line a baking pan with parchment paper. Fill it with the cooled ganache.
- Refrigerate the ganache for at least 2 hours to allow it to thicken.
- You may take the ganache out of the mold & cut it into the appropriate shape once it has solidified.

482. Date Candy

(Preparation time: 15 minutes | Cooking time: 5 minutes | Difficulty: Easy | Servings: 10)
Per serving: Calories 292, Total fat 20g, Protein 4g, Carbs 29g
Ingredients:

- 2 ½ tablespoons of grated coconut
- 1 handful of almonds

- 10 Medjoul dates
- 1/2 cup of pure chocolate (> 70% cocoa)

Instructions:

- In a water bath, melt the chocolate.
- Chop the almonds coarsely.
- Meanwhile, remove the core from the dates by cutting them lengthwise.
- Close the dates and fill the resultant cavity with the roughly chopped almonds.
- Place the dates onto a sheet of parchment paper & cover them with melted chocolate.
- Over the chocolate dates, sprinkle the grated coconut.
- Refrigerate the dates to let the chocolate to solidify.

483. Bars with Nuts and Dates

(Preparation time: 15 minutes | Cooking time: 0 minutes | Difficulty: Easy | Servings: 15)
Per serving: Calories 126, Total fat 29g, Protein 17g, Carbs 22g
Ingredients:

- 1 teaspoon of cinnamon
- 2 cups of Medjool dates
- ¼ cup of grated coconut
- ¼ cup of almonds - ¼ cup of walnuts

Instructions:

- Cut the dates into little pieces & soak them in warm water for around 15 minutes. Meanwhile, chop the almonds & walnuts coarsely.
- Dates should be drained.
- In a food processor, combine the dates, nuts, coconut, and cinnamon till they form an even mass. (but not for too long; crispy chunks or nuts add a lot of flavors)
- On two baking trays, roll out the dough into a 1 cm thick rectangle.
- Cut the rectangle into bars, then wrap each one in parchment paper.

484. Hazelnut Bars

(Preparation time: 15 minutes | Cooking time: 0 minutes | Difficulty: Easy | Servings: 15)
Per serving: Calories 130, Total fat 36g, Protein 26g, Carbs 32g
Ingredients:

- ½ teaspoon of vanilla extract
- 1 teaspoon of honey
- 2 tablespoons of cocoa powder
- 1/2 cup of dates
- 1/2 cup of hazelnuts

Instructions:

- In a food processor, crush the hazelnuts till you get hazelnut flour (you can also utilize ready-made hazelnut flour).
- Set aside the hazelnut flour in a mixing dish.
- Place the dates in a food processor and pulse till they form a ball.
- Pulse in the hazelnut flour, vanilla extract, cocoa, and honey till everything is well combined.
- Take the mixture out of the food processor & roll it into lovely balls.
- Keep the balls refrigerated.

485. Walnut Energy Bars

(Preparation time: 10 minutes | Cooking time: 25 minutes | Difficulty: Easy | Servings: 4)
Per serving: Calories 192, Total fat 4g, Protein 6g, Carbs 22g
Ingredients:

- 1 pinch of salt
- ½ teaspoon of vanilla extract
- 1 tablespoon of peanut butter
- 2 tablespoons of shredded coconut
- 1/2 cup of rolled oats
- 8 walnuts, chopped
- 3 tablespoons of agave syrup
- ½ cup of almond milk, unsweetened

Instructions:

- Combine all of the ingredients in a baking pan coated with parchment paper and bake at 325°F for around 20-25 minutes, or till golden and crisp.

486. No-Bake Choco Cashew Cheesecake

(Preparation time: 10 minutes | Cooking time: 25 minutes | Difficulty: Easy | Servings: 4)
Per serving: Calories 168, Total fat 11g, Protein 7g, Carbs 11g
Ingredients:

- ¼ teaspoon of ground cinnamon
- 1 teaspoon of vanilla extract
- ¼ cup of chopped dates
- ¼ cup of cocoa powder
- ¼ cup of agave syrup
- 2 cups of cashews - 1¼ cups of walnuts
- ¼ cup of coconut cream
- ¼ cup of almond meal

Instructions:

- Using parchment paper, line the bottoms of four 4-inch spring form pans.
- In a high-powered food processor, combine the cashews, coconut cream, cocoa powder, agave syrup, & vanilla. Repeat the process till the mixture is completely smooth, scraping the pieces with a rubber spatula as needed. Place the mixture in a medium-sized mixing dish and put it aside. Using a paper towel, wipe down the food processor or blender. This is the crème of the crop.
- Combine walnuts, dates, & cinnamon in a food processor and mix till smooth. This is the foundation.
- Fill a baking tin halfway with the base mixture. By pressing firmly, you may get an even layer. Pour in the cream & chill for at least 12 hours before serving.

487. Strawberry Sorbet

(Preparation time: 10 minutes | Cooking time: 0 minutes | Difficulty: Easy | Servings: 2)
Per serving: Calories 145, Total fat 3g, Protein 3g, Carbs 15g
Ingredients:

- Juice of 2 lemons
- 1/3 cup of coconut sugar
- 3 cups of fresh strawberries

Instructions:

- In a blender, puree the frozen strawberries. Mix in the lemon juice & coconut sugar thoroughly.
- Freeze for at least 4 hours before serving, then rapidly combine again.

488. Pistachio Fudge

(Preparation time: 10 minutes | Cooking time: 0 minutes | Difficulty: Easy | Servings: 6)
Per serving: Calories 280, Total fat 12g, Protein 4g, Carbs 15g
Ingredients:

- 2 tablespoons of water
- 1 cup of Medjool dates pitted
- 4 tablespoons of shredded coconut
- 1/4 cup of pistachio nuts shelled
- 2 tablespoons of oats

Instructions:

- In a food processor, combine the dates, almonds, coconut, oats, & water and process till well combined.
- Cut the mixture into 6 pieces by rolling it into a 1-inch thick roll. Refrigerate for around 2 hours before serving.

489. Chocolate Mousse

(Preparation time: 10 minutes | Cooking time: 0 minutes | Difficulty: Easy | Servings: 1)
Per serving: Calories 87, Total fat 1g, Protein 2g, Carbs 11g
Ingredients:

- 1 teaspoon of cocoa powder
- 1 teaspoon of agave syrup - ½ avocado

Instructions:

- Combine all ingredients in a blender, freeze till set & serve right away.

490. Chocolate Agave Walnuts

(Preparation time: 10 minutes | Cooking time: 20 minutes | Difficulty: Easy | Servings: 15)
Per serving: Calories 139, Total fat 10g, Protein 24g, Carbs 18g
Ingredients:

- 1 tablespoon of water
- 1 teaspoon of vanilla extract
- 1 ½ tablespoons of coconut oil, melted
- ½ cup of pure agave syrup,
- 2 cups of walnuts
- ½ cup of dark chocolate, at least 85%

Instructions:

- Using parchment paper, line a baking tray. In a skillet, combine the walnuts & 1/4 cup of agave syrup and simmer, constantly stirring, for 3 to 5 minutes, or till walnuts are completely covered in syrup and golden in color.
- Spread the walnuts onto the parchment paper & use a fork to divide them into individual pieces. Allow at least 15 minutes for thorough cooling.
- Meanwhile, melt the chocolate with the coconut oil, then stir in the remaining agave syrup till smooth. When the walnuts are cool enough to handle, place them in a glass bowl and drizzle with melted chocolate syrup.
- Mix carefully with a silicone spatula till the walnuts are well covered.
- Return the nuts to the parchment paper-lined baking sheet & divide them with a fork once more.
- Place the nuts in the fridge for around 10 minutes or the freezer for 3 to 5 minutes, till the chocolate has hardened. Refrigerate the leftovers in an airtight bag.

491. Strawberry Frozen Yogurt

(Preparation time: 15 minutes | Cooking time: 0 minutes | Difficulty: Easy | Servings: 4)
Per serving: Calories 100, Total fat 1g, Protein 4g, Carbs 19g
Ingredients:

- 1 tablespoon of honey (optional)
- Juice of 1 orange - 1 lb. of plain yogurt
- 1/2 cup of strawberries

Instructions:

- In a food processor, pulse the strawberries & orange juice till smooth.
- To remove the seeds, strain the mixture into a dish through a sieve. Combine the honey and yogurt.
- Fill an ice cream maker halfway with the mixture and process according to the manufacturer's instructions. Alternatively, pour the mixture into a freezer-safe container and freeze for one hour.
- Whisk it with a fork to break up any ice crystals, then freeze for another 2 hours.

492. Spiced Poached Apples

(Preparation time: 10 minutes | Cooking time: 10 minutes | Difficulty: Easy | Servings: 4)
Per serving: Calories 180, Total fat 1g, Protein 5g, Carbs 20g
Ingredients:

- 2 cinnamon sticks
- 2 tablespoons of honey
- ¼ cup of Greek yogurt
- 4 apples - 4-star anise
- 1 cup of green tea

Instructions:

- In a saucepan, combine the honey & green tea and bring to a boil. Combine the apples, star anise, & cinnamon. Reduce the flame to low and cook for around 15 minutes. With a dollop of Greek yogurt, serve the apples.

493. Matcha Green Tea Mochi

(Preparation time: 10 minutes | Cooking time: 20 minutes | Difficulty: Easy | Servings: 12 pieces)
Per serving: Calories 100, Total fat 8g, Protein 2g, Carbs 13g
Ingredients:

- 1 teaspoon of baking powder
- 2 tablespoons of butter melted
- 2 tablespoons of matcha powder
- 1 cup of superfine white rice flour
- 1 cup of coconut milk
- 1/2 cup of coconut sugar

Instructions:

- Preheat the oven at 325°F. Spray your baking pan using non-stick cooking spray. Combine all of the dry ingredients, including the sweetener.
- Add the coconut milk & melted butter and whisk to combine. Stir everything together thoroughly.
- Place the mixture in a muffin baking pan and bake for around 20 minutes.

494. Mango Mousse with Chocolate Chips

(Preparation time: 10 minutes | Cooking time: 0 minutes | Difficulty: Easy | Servings: 1)
Per serving: Calories 87, Total fat 1g, Protein 2g, Carbs 12g
Ingredients:

- ¼ teaspoon of vanilla extract
- 1 cup of mango - ½ cup of Greek yogurt
- 2 squares of dark chocolate, chopped

Instructions:

- Combine the mango, yogurt, & vanilla in a blender. Serve immediately with dark chocolate chips.

495. Fruit Skewers with Strawberry Dip

(Preparation time: 15 minutes | Cooking time: 0 minutes | Difficulty: Easy | Servings: 6)
Per serving: Calories 131, Total fat 1g, Protein 2g, Carbs 20g
Ingredients:
- 1 cup of strawberries
- 1/2 cup of red grapes
- 1 cup of pineapple, peeled and diced

Instructions:
- In a food processor, puree 1/2 cup of strawberries till smooth. Fill a serving bowl halfway with the dip. Using skewers, skewer the grapes, pineapple chunks, & leftover strawberries. Serve with the strawberry dip on the side.

496. Frozen Blackberry Cake

(Preparation time: 25 minutes | Cooking time: 0 minutes | Difficulty: Easy | Servings: 4)
Per serving: Calories 372, Total fat 18g, Protein 33g, Carbs 15g
Ingredients:
- 1⁄4 cup of coconut oil
- 3⁄4 cup of shredded coconut
- 15 Medjool dates - 2 egg whites
- 1/3 cup of pumpkin seeds
- 1 lb. of frozen blackberries
- Coconut whipped cream
- ¾ cup of agave syrup
- 1⁄4 cup of coconut cream

Instructions:
- Grease the cake tin using coconut oil and blend all of the base ingredients till a sticky ball forms. In a cake tin, press the foundation mixture. Freeze. Whip up some coconut whipped cream. Freeze.
- Blend the berries with the honey, coconut cream, & egg whites till smooth.
- Spread the center filling - coconut whipped cream - evenly. Freeze. Fill the tin halfway with the berry mixture, smooth it out, and top with blueberries & almonds before returning it to the freezer.

497. Dark Chocolate Mousse

(Preparation time: 15 minutes | Cooking time: 0 minutes | Difficulty: Easy | Servings: 4)
Per serving: Calories 175, Total fat 24g, Protein 5g, Carbs 18g
Ingredients:
- Mint leaves
- 1 teaspoon of pure vanilla extract
- ½ cup of unsweetened cocoa powder
- 2 cups of silken tofu, drained
- ½ cup of pure agave syrup
- ¼ cup of soy milk

Instructions:
- In a food processor, combine the tofu, agave syrup, & vanilla. Blend in the soy milk & cocoa till smooth. Chill for at least 2 hours after pouring the mousse into small glasses. Just before serving, garnish with fresh mint leaves.

498. Chocolate Pudding with Fruit

(Preparation time: 15 minutes | Cooking time: 0 minutes | Difficulty: Easy | Servings: 2)
Per serving: Calories 106, Total fat 5g, Protein 14g, Carbs 20g
Ingredients:
For the Chocolate cream:
- Pinch of sea salt - 2 teaspoons of honey
- 2 tablespoons of coconut oil
- 1 teaspoon of ground vanilla bean
- 1 avocado 3 teaspoons of cacao powder
- ¼ cup of coconut milk

Fruits:
- 1 tablespoon of coconut flakes
- 1 chopped banana
- 1 cup of pitted cherries

Instructions:

- Combine all of the ingredients for the chocolate cream and divide them into two cups. Sprinkle shredded coconut on top of the fruit chunks after placing them on top of chocolate cream.
- Refrigerate for at least two hours before serving.

499. Chocolate Cupcakes with Matcha Icing

(Preparation time: 15 minutes | Cooking time: 30 minutes | Difficulty: Easy | Servings: 12)
Per serving: Calories 220, Total fat 8g, Protein 4g, Carbs 23g

Ingredients:

- 3/8 cup boiling water
- 1/2 teaspoon of salt
- ½ teaspoon of vanilla extract - 1 egg
- 1/2 teaspoon of espresso coffee
- ¼ cup of vegetable oil
- 1/2 cup of almond flour
- 1/4 cup of cocoa - ½ cup of skim milk
- 1/2 cup of coconut sugar

For the icing:

- 1/2 teaspoon of vanilla bean paste
- 4 tablespoons of butter at room temperature
- 2 tablespoons of soft cream cheese
- 4 tablespoons of coconut sugar
- 1 tablespoon of matcha green tea powder

Instructions:

- Preheat the oven at 350°F. Use silicone or paper muffin cups to line a cupcake tin. In a large-sized mixing bowl, combine the flour, cocoa, sweetener, salt, & espresso powder.
- Beat the dry ingredients with an electric mixer till completely combined, adding the vanilla, vanilla extract, oil, and egg. Gradually pour in the hot water till everything is well combined.

- Continue mixing to incorporate air bubbles into the batter. The recipe will provide more liquid than a traditional cake batter. Pour the batter into the cupcake tins in an equal layer. It's important to remember that each seat can't be more than 3/4 occupied. Bake for around 15 to 18 minutes, or till the mixture bounces back when pressed. Before icing, remove the cake from the oven & allow it to cool completely. To prepare the frosting, mix together the sweetener and butter till smooth and creamy. Stir in the matcha powder and vanilla extract. The cupcakes should be iced.

500. Chocolate Cream

(Preparation time: 15 minutes | Cooking time: 0 minutes | Difficulty: Easy | Servings: 4)
Per serving: Calories 200, Total fat 4g, Protein 12g, Carbs 20g

Ingredients:

- Pinch of salt
- 1 teaspoon of ground vanilla bean
- 2 teaspoons of coconut oil
- 2 teaspoons of honey - 1 avocado
- ¼ cup of goji berries
- 2 teaspoons of cacao powder
- ¼ cup of almond milk

Instructions:

- In a food processor, combine all of the ingredients till smooth and thick.
- Distribute among four cups, garnish with goji berries, & chill overnight.

501. Chocolate Brownies

(Preparation time: 15 minutes | Cooking time: 35 minutes | Difficulty: Easy | Servings: 12)
Per serving: Calories 188, Total fat 12g, Protein 3g, Carbs 18g

Ingredients:

- ½ teaspoon of baking soda
- 3 tablespoons of melted coconut oil

- 2 teaspoons of vanilla essence
- 3 eggs
- 5 cups of Medjool dates pitted
- 1/2 cup of walnuts, chopped
- 1 cup of dark chocolate (min 85% cocoa)

Instructions:

- In a food processor, combine the dates, chocolate, eggs, coconut oil, baking soda, & vanilla extract and pulse till smooth.
- Combine the walnuts and the rest of the ingredients. Bake the mixture for around 25 to 30 minutes at 350°F in a prepared baking pan.
- Allow time for it to cool. Serve by slicing into pieces.

502. Pecan Banana Muffins

(Preparation time: 15 minutes | Cooking time: 45 minutes | Difficulty: Easy | Servings: 8)
Per serving: Calories 223, Total fat 9g, Protein 7g, Carbs 21g

Ingredients:

- 1 teaspoon of cinnamon
- 1 tablespoon of vanilla
- 3 tablespoons of butter softened
- 1 tablespoon of honey
- 1 tablespoon of instant yeast
- 4 ripe bananas
- 2 eggs
- ⅛ cup of orange juice, unsweetened
- 2 cups of almond flour
- 2 pecans, sliced

Instructions:

- Preheat the oven at 350°F. Dust a muffin tray using flour & lightly oil the sides and bottom. Remove any extra flour with a tap.
- Peel and mash the bananas in a mixing dish. Mix in the flour.
- Stir together the orange juice, butter, yeast, eggs, vanilla, & cinnamon.

- On a chopping board, coarsely chop the pecans and toss them in with the rest of the ingredients.
- Fill each muffin tray 3/4 full with batter and bake for around 40 minutes, or till golden.

503. Banana and Blueberry Muffins

(Preparation time: 15 minutes | Cooking time: 35 minutes | Difficulty: Easy | Servings: 12)
Per serving: Calories 250, Total fat 9g, Protein 4g, Carbs 29g

Ingredients:

- A pinch of cinnamon
- 1/2 teaspoon of salt
- 1 teaspoon of baking powder
- 1 teaspoon of baking soda
- 1 egg, lightly beaten
- 4 ripe bananas, mashed
- 2 cups of blueberries
- 1 cup of coconut, shredded
- 1/2 cup of peanut butter,
- 1/2 cup of almond flour
- 1/2 cup of applesauce
- 3/4 cup of coconut sugar

Instructions:

- In a mixing bowl, mash the banana. Mix in the sweetener and the egg thoroughly. Combine the peanut butter & blueberries.
- Mix lightly the dry components into the wet mixture.
- Bake for around 20 to 25 minutes at 350°F in 12 greased muffin cups.

504. Avocado Mousse

(Preparation time: 15 minutes | Cooking time: 0 minutes | Difficulty: Easy | Servings: 2)
Per serving: Calories 264, Total fat 20g, Protein 5g, Carbs 15g

Ingredients:

- 1 teaspoon of vanilla extract
- 2 teaspoons of stevia

- 1 tablespoon of cocoa powder
- 1 avocado, peeled and pitted
- 1/2 cup of low-fat milk

Instructions:

- In a food processor, pulse the avocado till it is finely chopped.
- Combine the milk, vanilla extract, stevia, and cocoa powder.
- Blend the ingredients till completely smooth.
- Prepared mousse should be half-filled in the glasses.

505. Milky Fudge

(Preparation time: 15 minutes | Cooking time: 10 minutes | Difficulty: Easy | Servings: 2)
Per serving: Calories 85, Total fat 8g, Protein 2g, Carbs 3g

Ingredients:

- 1 teaspoon of vanilla extract
- 1/2 cup of margarine
- 1 cup of low-fat milk
- 1/2 cup of cocoa powder

Instructions:

- Heat the milk in a medium-sized pot, then add the margarine, stir well, and cook for around 7 minutes.
- Take the pan from the flame and stir in the cocoa powder.
- After filling a lined square pan halfway with the mixture and smoothing it, chill for around 1 to 2 hours.

506. Pecan Brownies

(Preparation time: 15 minutes | Cooking time: 25 minutes | Difficulty: Easy | Servings: 2)
Per serving: Calories 174, Total fat 16g, Protein 5g, Carbs 5g

Ingredients:

- Cooking spray
- 1/2 teaspoon of baking powder
- 2 tablespoons of softened margarine
- 2 eggs, beaten

- 2 tablespoons of cocoa powder
- 5 chopped pecans
- 1 cup of almond meal

Instructions:

- Combine all ingredients in a food processor, except for the cooking spray, in a food processor.
- Then spray the square pan using cooking spray, pour in the brownie batter, smooth it out, and bake for around 25 minutes at 350°F.
- Cut the brownies into bars once they've cooled.

507. Coconut Mousse

(Preparation time: 10 minutes | Cooking time: 10 minutes | Difficulty: Easy | Servings: 2)
Per serving: Calories 53, Total fat 1g, Protein 2g, Carbs 10g

Ingredients:

- 3 tablespoons of corn starch
- 2 tablespoons of coconut flakes
- 3 cups of low-fat milk
- 3 tablespoons of stevia

Instructions:

- Bring the milk to the boil, then slowly whisk in the corn starch, stevia, and coconut flakes.
- Cook the mousse for around 2 minutes on a low flame.
- Allow for thorough cooling of the dessert.

508. Peach Crumble

(Preparation time: 15 minutes | Cooking time: 25 minutes | Difficulty: Easy | Servings: 2)
Per serving: Calories 197, Total fat 15g, Protein 2g, Carbs 15g

Ingredients:

- 1/2 teaspoon of ground cinnamon
- 1 teaspoon of ground nutmeg
- 1 teaspoon of olive oil
- 2 tablespoons of margarine softened

- 1 cup of chopped peach
- 4 tablespoons of grated oatmeal

Instructions:

- Combine margarine & oatmeal in a mixing bowl. Crumble the dough using your fingertips after it's been made smooth. After that, rub the peaches with olive oil and set them in a small roasting pan. Ground nutmeg& cinnamon are sprinkled over the peaches. Then sprinkle smashed dough on top of the fruits.
- Preheat the oven at 360°F and bake the dish for around 25 minutes, or till the crust is golden brown.

509. Raspberry and Raw Apple Tart

(Preparation time: 15 minutes | Cooking time: 0 minutes | Difficulty: Easy | Servings: 2)
Per serving: Calories 317, Total fat 32g, Protein 20g, Carbs 22g
Ingredients:

- 1/2 teaspoon of ground cinnamon
- 1/2 cup of apples, cut lengthways
- 6 soft dried dates
- A handful of raspberries
- 1/4 cup of pecan nuts
- 1/4 cup of raw almonds
- 1/4 cup of cashew nuts

Instructions:

- In a blender, pulse the pecan nuts, almonds, & cashew nuts till finely crushed.
- In a blender, combine the dates & cinnamon till fully combined and uniformly distributed.
- Add 4 tablespoons of water to the blender to completely incorporate the ingredients.
- Fill loose-bottomed tartlet cases halfway with the ingredients and firmly press them down.

- Serve with apple slices & a sprinkling of raspberries on top. Freeze and enjoy.

510. Chocolate and Raspberry Mousse

(Preparation time: 10 minutes | Cooking time: 15 minutes | Difficulty: Easy | Servings: 2)
Per serving: Calories 169, Total fat 15g, Protein 3g, Carbs 18g
Ingredients:

- 2 tablespoons of vanilla bean paste
- 4 tablespoons of stevia
- 1/2 cup of raspberries
- 1/4 cup of chocolate, at least 70% cocoa solids, roughly chopped
- 1/4 cup of soft silken tofu
- 3 tablespoons of coconut cream

Instructions:

- Half-fill a medium-sized saucepan with boiling water over a medium flame.
- Place a medium heatproof bowl on top of that, making sure the base is in contact with the water.
- Place the roughly chopped chocolate in a mixing dish and set it aside to melt, stirring occasionally.
- After draining excess water with a clean tea towel, mix the tofu, stevia, & vanilla bean paste in a food processor.
- Melt the chocolate and combine it with the coconut cream. Pulse till you have a velvety smooth texture. In a large-sized mixing dish, combine all of the ingredients.
- Fold the raspberries into a large-sized mixing bowl, reserving a couple for garnish. Chill for 30 minutes after dividing the mixture into individual bowls. Take it out of the refrigerator as a garnish, top with raspberries & a sprig of mint.

511. Strawberry Pie

(Preparation time: 10 minutes | Cooking time: 25 minutes | Difficulty: Easy | Servings: 2)
Per serving: Calories 228, Total fat 6g, Protein 7g, Carbs 15g
Ingredients:
- 1/4 teaspoon of baking powder
- 1/2 teaspoon of vanilla extract
- 1 1/2 tablespoons of margarine, softened - 1 egg, beaten
- 1 tablespoon of coconut flakes
- 1/4 cup of low-fat milk
- 1/2 cup of chopped strawberries
- 1 cup of whole wheat or almond flour

Instructions:
- Combine the flour, strawberries, & the remaining ingredients in a mixing bowl.
- Half-fill the baking pan with strawberry batter, flatten it evenly and bake at 365°F for about 25 minutes.

512. Walnut and Chocolate Loaf

(Preparation time: 10 minutes | Cooking time: 25 minutes | Difficulty: Easy | Servings: 2)
Per serving: Calories 66, Total fat 5g, Protein 3g, Carbs 1g
Ingredients:
- 1/8 cup of hot water
- A pinch of sea salt
- 1 teaspoon of baking powder
- 1 tablespoon of apple cider vinegar
- 4 tablespoons of stevia - 4 egg whites
- 4 tablespoons of grounded golden flaxseed (use coffee bean grinder or multi grinder to make powder)
- 1/4 cup of coconut flour
- 1/4 cup of melted dark chocolate
- 1/4 cup of walnuts chopped (reserved half for topping and half for loaf)

Instructions:
- Preheat the oven at 360°F. Using a baking spray, coat a loaf pan and line it using parchment paper. In a large-sized mixing dish, beat together all of the loaf ingredients, except for the walnuts, using an electric mixer till completely combined. In a separate bowl, fold half of the walnuts into the batter.
- Smooth the batter out evenly in the loaf pan that has been prepared.
- On top of the bread that has been left aside, sprinkle the walnuts.
- Cook for around 20 to 25 minutes in the oven. After that, use a wooden skewer to check whether the baked bread is done. You're done if it comes out clean.

513. Cherry Cobbler Layered with Hazelnut Topping

(Preparation time: 10 minutes | Cooking time: 20 minutes | Difficulty: Easy | Servings: 2)
Per serving: Calories 106, Total fat 7g, Protein 3g, Carbs 9g
Ingredients:
- 1/8 teaspoon of baking powder
- 1 1/2 tablespoons of butter melted
- 5 tablespoons of stevia, divided
- 1 tablespoon of egg white
- 1/4 cup of hazelnut flour or ground hazelnuts
- 1/4 cup of almond flour blanched
- 3 cups of pitted Sour cherries

Instructions:
- Preheat the oven at 350°F.
- In a mixing dish, combine half of the stevia & the sour cherries. Place the mixture on a foil-lined baking tray (or non-stick). Combine the almond flour, stevia, hazelnut flour, & baking powder.
- In a separate bowl, beat the egg whites till they are crumbly. Incorporate the melted butter completely. Crumble the flour mixture over the berries in an even layer. Bake for around 15 to 20 minutes, or till golden brown.

514. Zucchini and Chocolate Chip Muffins

(Preparation time: 10 minutes | Cooking time: 20 minutes | Difficulty: Easy | Servings: 2)
Per serving: Calories 181, Total fat 15g, Protein 5g, Carbs 8g
Ingredients:
- A pinch of sea salt
- 1/2 teaspoon of baking powder
- 1/8 teaspoon of vanilla extract
- 3 tablespoons of olive oil
- 3 eggs
- 1/4 cup of sugar-free dark chocolate chips
- 1/4 cup of stevia
- 4 oz. of grated zucchini
- 1/4 cup of coconut flour

Instructions:
- Preheat the oven at 350°F.
- In a large-sized mixing bowl, combine the stevia, coconut flour, baking powder, & sea salt. Mix the eggs, shredded zucchini, and vanilla extract. Toss together all of the ingredients till they're evenly distributed. Pour in the melted coconut oil and stir till it's completely smooth.
- Stir in the chocolate chips after combining the ingredients. Allow 5 minutes for the batter to thicken.
- Pour the batter in an equal layer into the parchment liners, almost to the top. If desired, more chocolate chips can be sprinkled on top.
- Preheat the oven at 350°F & bake for around 15 to 20 minutes.

515. Chewy Avocado Brownies

(Preparation time: 10 minutes | Cooking time: 20 minutes | Difficulty: Easy | Servings: 2)
Per serving: Calories 158, Total fat 15g, Protein 3g, Carbs 4g

Ingredients:
- 1/2 teaspoon of vanilla essence
- 4 tablespoons of butter
- 1/2 beaten egg
- 1/4 cup of stevia
- 1/4 avocado medium-sized
- 1/4 cup of blanched almond flour
- 2 tablespoons of cocoa powder unsweetened
- 1/2 cup of dark chocolate chips sugar-free

Instructions:
- Preheat the oven at 380°F. Use foil or parchment paper to line a glass baking dish and lightly butter it.
- Melt the butter & chocolate in a double boiler over low flame. (Bring a saucepan of water to a boil, then place the butter and chocolate in a heatproof bowl on top of the pot.) Cook, occasionally stirring, till the chocolate is melted.) Allow for some chilling time before serving. (You can do this in the microwave if you want.) Make sure it doesn't catch fire.)
- Combine the avocado, eggs, and vanilla in a high-powered blender or food processor. Puree till the mixture is completely smooth. One more time, puree the melted butter/chocolate mixture.
- In a small-sized mixing dish, combine the cocoa powder, almond flour, & sweetener. In a blender or food processor, combine the dry ingredients with a spatula. Pulse a few times more, scraping down the edges as required, till everything is well blended. (Be careful not to overmix the ingredients.)
- Spread the batter evenly in the prepared baking pan. Smooth the end with a spatula.

- Bake for around 15 minutes or till the brownies are barely set in the oven. Despite the fact that the top is no longer damp, it should still be soft. Allow for complete chilling before cutting.

516. Orange and Chocolate Mousse

(Preparation time: 10 minutes | Cooking time: 10 minutes | Difficulty: Easy | Servings: 2)
Per serving: Calories 270, Total fat 19g, Protein 5g, Carbs 18g
Ingredients:

- 1 egg, separated
- 2 tablespoons of butter melted
- 1 tablespoon of orange juice
- 3 teaspoons of stevia
- 1/2 cup of skimmed milk
- 4 tablespoons of unsweetened dark chocolate

Instructions:

- In a medium-sized saucepan, combine the chocolate & milk and boil over medium flame till the chocolate has melted. Combine the melted butter, egg yolks, and chocolate.
- Whisk the egg whites & stevia sweetener together in a separate bowl till stiff and glossy.
- Combine the two ingredients, along with the orange juice. Serve the completed concoction in four glasses after chilling it.

517. Walnut and Blueberry Muffins

(Preparation time: 10 minutes | Cooking time: 20 minutes | Difficulty: Easy | Servings: 2)
Per serving: Calories 256, Total fat 18g, Protein 6g, Carbs 19g
Ingredients:

- 1/2 egg
- 4 tablespoons of butter
- 1/8 teaspoon of baking soda
- 3 tablespoons of stevia

- 1/4 cup of blueberries
- 3 tablespoons of finely chopped walnuts
- 1/4 cup of whole-wheat flour
- 60ml of semi-skimmed milk
- 1/4 cup of almond flour
- 1/2 cup of full-fat cream cheese

Instructions:

- Preheat the oven at 380°F.
- In a skillet over a low flame, combine the stevia & butter.
- Allow for cooling on one side.
- While the mixture cools, soften the cream cheese in a bowl using a wooden spoon for a few minutes.
- In a mixing dish, whisk the eggs gently.
- Combine the eggs, milk, & cream cheese. After that, add the blueberries, walnuts, almond flour, whole-wheat flour, & baking soda. Fill muffin tins halfway with batter and place on a baking sheet. Bake for about 15 minutes in a preheated oven. Allow the muffins to cool for a few minutes after removing the baking tray from the oven.

518. Apple and Cranberry Muffins

(Preparation time: 10 minutes | Cooking time: 20 minutes | Difficulty: Easy | Servings: 2)
Per serving: Calories 192, Total fat 7g, Protein 1g, Carbs 25g
Ingredients:

- 1/2 teaspoon of ground cinnamon
- 1/2 large beaten eggs
- 1/4 cup of soft butter
- 1/2 cup of whole-wheat flour
- 1/4 cup of semi-skimmed milk
- 2 tablespoons of stevia
- 1 eating apple peeled, cored & sliced into small pieces
- 2 tablespoons of dried cranberries

Instructions:

- Preheat the oven at 400°F.
- On a baking sheet, place muffin tins.

- Sift together the flour, sweetener, & cinnamon in a large-sized mixing dish.
- In the middle of the dry ingredients, make a hole. In a mixing dish, whisk together the eggs, milk, & butter till smooth. Mix in the apple chunks thoroughly. Fill the muffin tins two-thirds of the way with batter. Bake for around 20 minutes, or till the muffins are golden brown, in the partially filled muffin tins.

519. Fig Pastry

(Preparation time: 10 minutes | Cooking time: 20 minutes | Difficulty: Easy | Servings: 4)
Per serving: Calories 303, Total fat 31g, Protein 14g, Carbs 27g
Ingredients:

- 1 tablespoon of butter melted
- 1/4 cup of roughly chopped fresh mint leaves - 1 cup of fresh figs
- 2 tablespoons of good fig jam
- 1/4 cup of roughly chopped walnuts
- 1 sheet of whole-wheat puff pastry, store-bought - 1/2 cup of goat cheese

Instructions:

- Preheat the oven at 375°F.
- Place the thawed puff pastry on a baking sheet lined using parchment paper and cut it into four rectangle parts. Spread goat cheese on each slice. Then add the jam, figs, & chopped walnuts. Brush the figs & puff pastry sides with melted butter. Slightly raise the pastry edges.
- Bake the pastry for around 18-20 minutes, or till golden and fluffy.
- Garnish with chopped mint leaves & more walnuts if desired.

520. Almond Stuffed Dates Covered in Chocolate

(Preparation time: 15 minutes | Cooking time: 10 minutes | Difficulty: Easy | Servings: 24 dates) **Per serving:** Calories 152, Total fat 5g, Protein 2g, Carbs 21g
Ingredients:

- 1 teaspoon of ground cinnamon
- 1 teaspoon of canola oil
- 24 Medjool dates
- 1 tablespoon of almonds and pistachios crushed
- 1 1/2 cups of dark chocolate chips
- 24 roasted almonds unsalted

Instructions:

- By cutting a slit in each date, you may remove the pit. In an almond, in the pit press's position. Place them on a tray or in a bowl, completely enclosing the dates and almonds.
- Combine the olive oil, chocolate chips, and ground cinnamon in a heat-safe container that can fit tightly on top of a saucepan with grain simmering water. Stir often till the chocolate has completely melted. Turn off the stove.
- Drop the dates into the melted chocolate one at a time and gently roll them to coat them. Remove with a spoon & set on a baking sheet lined using parchment paper. After the chocolate-covered dates have been placed on the tray, carefully sprinkle the crushed pistachios & almonds over them.
- Refrigerate the chocolate for at least 1 hour, or till it hardens. Before serving, let 10 minutes for the meal to come to room temperature.

521. Pumpkin Yogurt Parfait

(Preparation time: 15 minutes | Cooking time: 0 minutes | Difficulty: Easy | Servings: 6)
Per serving: Calories 102, Total fat 2g, Protein 1g, Carbs 15g
Ingredients:

- 2 teaspoons of ground cinnamon
- A pinch of nutmeg
- 1 teaspoon of vanilla extract
- Dark chocolate chips for garnishing
- Chopped walnuts for garnishing
- 2 1/2 tablespoons of stevia
- 1 1/4 cups of Greek yogurt low-fat
- 2 tablespoons of molasses, more for garnishing
- 2 cups of pumpkin puree
- 3 to 4 tablespoons of mascarpone cheese

Instructions:

- Combine the Greek yogurt, pumpkin puree, and the additional ingredients in a large-sized mixing dish (except the nuts & chocolate chips). With an electric hand mixer, blend everything together till it's smooth. Taste it and adjust the flavor to your preferences. Change the spices if you like more cinnamon or nutmeg.) Mix one more to ensure that everything is well-combined.
- Pour the pumpkin-yogurt mixture into tiny mason jars. Cover and chill for 30 minutes or overnight.
- When ready to serve, sprinkle each one with chocolate chips, molasses, & chopped walnuts.

522. Macadamia and Double Chocolate Biscotti

(Preparation time: 15 minutes | Cooking time: 20 minutes | Difficulty: Easy | Servings: 24 biscotti)
Per serving: Calories 267, Total fat 15g, Protein 3g, Carbs 20g

Ingredients:

- 1 tube of refrigerated chocolate chip cookie dough (around 18 ounces)
- 1/2 cup of thoroughly chopped macadamia nuts
- 1/2 cup of the vanilla/ chocolate chips

Instructions:

- Preheat the oven at 350°F.
- Combine the dough, nuts, & chips in a large-sized mixing dish. Knead everything together using your hands till everything is well incorporated. Set aside the dough, which has been divided into two equal parts.
- Prepare 13-inch greased baking sheets with a 2-inch thickness for each piece of dough. Bake for around 12 to 15 minutes, or till light brown.
- Cut biscotti diagonally into 1-inch slices; after cutting, divide each piece by 1/4 inch. Cook for another 4 to 5 minutes. Before serving, let the biscotti cool fully.

523. Oatmeal and Peanut Butter Bars

(Preparation time: 15 minutes | Cooking time: 20 minutes | Difficulty: Easy | Servings: 9 bars)
Per serving: Calories 293, Total fat 3g, Protein 9g, Carbs 27g
Ingredients:

- 1/2 teaspoon of salt
- 1 teaspoon of vanilla
- 1 teaspoon of baking soda
- 1/2 cup of skim milk
- 1/2 cup of stevia packed
- 1 cup of almond flour
- 1 cup of rolled oats
- 3/4 cup of peanut butter creamy
- 1/3 cup of dark chocolate chips

Instructions:

- Preheat the oven at 325°F.
- Cream the peanut butter, rolled oats, & sweetener together in a mixer till

smooth. Mix in the vanilla extract and milk till thoroughly combined.

- Combine flour, salt, and baking soda in a small-sized mixing dish, then stir in the prepared mixture. Add the chocolate chips and mix well.
- Bake the mixture for around 18 to 20 minutes on an 8x8 inch, prepared baking sheet. Before slicing the bar, allow it to cool slightly.

524. Oatmeal and Chia Seeds Cookies

(Preparation time: 15 minutes | Cooking time: 20 minutes | Difficulty: Easy | Servings: 12)
Per serving: Calories 262, Total fat 8g, Protein 3g, Carbs 21g
Ingredients:

- 1/2 teaspoon of salt
- 1/2 teaspoon of baking powder
- 1 teaspoon of ground cinnamon
- 1 teaspoon of baking soda
- 3 tablespoons of coconut oil
- 2 tablespoons of chia seeds
- 1 cup of stevia unpacked
- 1/2 cup of dark chocolate chips
- 1/4 cup of coconut grated and unsweetened - 2 cups of rolled oats
- 2/3 cup of whole wheat or almond flour
- 2/3 cup of the applesauce
- 1 cup of dried cranberries

Instructions:

- Preheat the oven at 350°F.
- In a large-sized mixing dish, combine sweetener, chia seeds, baking soda, oats, flour, cinnamon, baking powder, and salt. Combine the oat mixture, coconut oil, and applesauce in a mixing bowl till well combined. Gently mix the chocolate chips, grated coconut, & cranberries into the prepared dough.

Place the dough on a parchment paper-lined cookie sheet. In a preheated oven, bake for around 10 to 15 minutes, or till the edges are gently browned.

525. Chocolaty Nut Bars

(Preparation time: 15 minutes | Cooking time: 10 minutes | Difficulty: Easy | Servings: 2)
Per serving: Calories 148, Total fat 12g, Protein 4g, Carbs 11g
Ingredients:

- Pinch of sea salt
- 1/4 teaspoon of vanilla extract
- Butter for melting
- 5 tablespoons of cocoa powder
- 8 tablespoons of stevia
- 1/4 cup of butter unsalted
- 4 tablespoons of chopped almonds
- 1/4 cup of almond butter

Instructions:

- In a medium-sized saucepan, melt the butter over low flame.
- Combine the cocoa powder, unsalted butter, almond butter, sea salt, vanilla extract, stevia, & vanilla extract.
- Stir constantly till the mixture thickens.
- Stir the chocolate mixture vigorously for another 30 seconds, being careful not to overheat it; swirling it takes only a few seconds!
- Toss in the chopped almonds after removing the skillet from the flame.
- Using baking parchment, line the square baking tin.
- Spread the mixture evenly over the baking parchment while it is still warm.
- Refrigerate for about an hour after allowing the mixture to firm up.
- It's time to set the table with the chocolate nut bars!

CHAPTER 14:

Non-Alcoholic and Alcoholic Cocktails

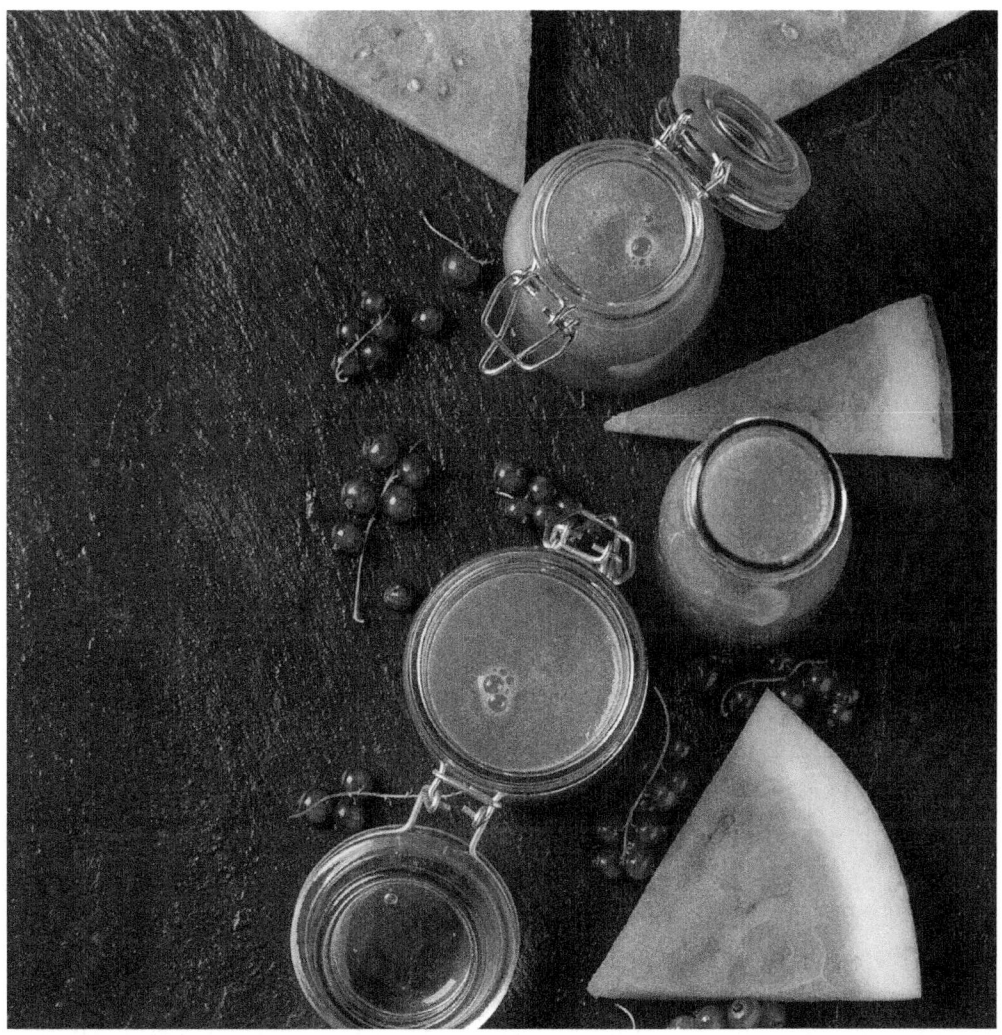

The Sirt green juice is indeed an important part of the Phase 1 diet, and it continues to be a staple throughout Phase 2. To increase your energy in the best way possible during Phase 1, adhere to the original Sirt green juice, which is the first recipe; however, as your sirtfood diet expands in Phase 2 and further on, you will be able to indulge in additional delicious green juices and cocktails.

526. Sirtfood Green Juice

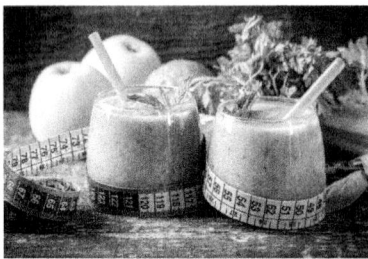

(Preparation time: 5 minutes | Cooking time: 0 minutes | Difficulty: Easy | Servings: 1)
Per serving: Calories 37, Total fat 1g, Protein 4g, Carbs 25g
Ingredients:

- Juice of ½ lemon
- ½ medium green apple
- 1 very small handful of parsley
- 1 large handful of rocket
- 2 large handfuls of kale
- 2 or 3 large stalks of green celery, including the leaves
- 1 very small handful of lovage leaves (optional) - ½ level teaspoon of matcha

Instructions:

- Juice the greens after thoroughly mixing them (to get about 50ml of juice).
- Juice the apple and celery, then peel and juice the lemon by hand.
- In a glass, pour a little of the juice, add the matcha powder, and vigorously stir. Pour it back into the juice after it has dissolved and whisk it in. If the blend is too powerful for you, add some water and serve.

527. Simple Celery Juice

(Preparation time: 10 minutes | Cooking time: 0 minutes | Difficulty: Easy | Servings: 2)
Per serving: Calories 42, Total fat 7g, Protein 27g, Carbs 35g
Ingredients:

- ½ cup filtered water
- Pinch of salt - 1 lemon, peeled

- 2 tablespoons of fresh ginger, peeled
- 8 celery stalks with leaves

Instructions:

- In a blender, add all of the ingredients and pulse till smooth.
- Strain the juice through a fine-mesh strainer and pour it into two glasses.
- Serve right away.

528. Kale Apple and Celery Juice

(Preparation time: 10 minutes | Cooking time: 0 minutes | Difficulty: Easy | Servings: 2)
Per serving: Calories 198, Total fat 2g, Protein 3g, Carbs 6g
Ingredients:

- 1/2 organic lemon with peel
- 1-inch piece of ginger with peel
- 1 medium cucumber 1/2 apple with skin
- 10 celery stalks with leaves
- A handful of kale stems removes

Instructions:

- All ingredients should be well washed and chopped to suit the juicer's feed funnel.
- Then slowly pour into the feed chute, allowing it to press out. If you make more juice ahead of time, it will keep in the refrigerator for one or two days.

529. White Wine Fruit Cocktail

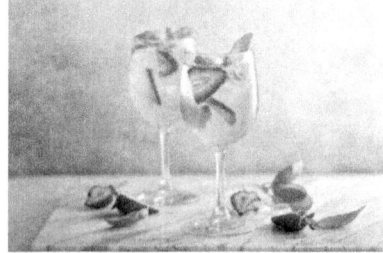

(Preparation time: 10 minutes | Cooking time: 15 minutes | Difficulty: Easy | Servings: 4)
Per serving: Calories 209, Total fat 1g, Protein 2g, Carbs 35g
Ingredients:

- 1 tablespoon of chopped fresh mint

- 1 pint of fresh strawberries, hulled & halved
- ⅓ cup of stevia
- 1 cup of seedless green grapes, halved
- ½ cantaloupe, cut into bite-size pieces
- 1 ¼ cups of dry white wine

Instructions:

- In a saucepan, combine the wine & sweetener. Bring the pot to a boil over medium flame, stirring to dissolve the sweetener. Remove the saucepan from the flame and stir in the mint.
- In a large-sized mixing dish, combine the cantaloupe, grapes, & strawberries. Pour the wine mixture over the fruit, tossing everything together till the wine mixture is well covered; cover and refrigerate. Refrigerate for up to eight hours before serving.

530. The Mojito Cocktail

(Preparation time: 10 minutes | Cooking time: 0 minutes | Difficulty: Easy | Servings: 1)
Per serving: Calories 250, Total fat 0.5g, Protein 1g, Carbs 30g
Ingredients:

- 1 ½ cups of ice
- 1 lime, halved
- 4 sprigs of fresh mint
- 1 sprig fresh mint
- 2 tablespoons of stevia
- 1 fluid ounce of club soda
- 2 fluid ounces of light rum
- 2 fluid ounces of club soda

Instructions:

- In a pint glass, muddle sweetener & mint with soda water. Squeeze both lime halves into the glass, leaving one hull behind. Fill with ice and stir in the rum. Add a splash of club soda to finish.
- Serve with a sprig of mint as a garnish.

531. Lemony Kale and Apple Juice

(Preparation time: 10 minutes | Cooking time: 0 minutes | Difficulty: Easy | Servings: 2)
Per serving: Calories 196, Total fat 1g, Protein 5g, Carbs 27g
Ingredients:

- Pinch of salt
- ½ cup of filtered water
- 1 lemon, peeled
- 1 tablespoon of fresh ginger, peeled
- 4 tablespoons of fresh parsley leaves
- 2 large green apples, cored and sliced
- 4 cups of fresh kale leaves

Instructions:

- In a blender, add all ingredients and pulse till smooth.
- Strain the juice through a fine-mesh strainer and pour it into two glasses.
- Serve right away.

532. Watermelon Juice

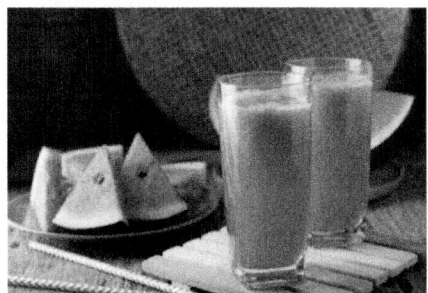

(Preparation time: 10 minutes | Cooking time: 0 minutes | Difficulty: Easy | Servings: 2)
Per serving: Calories 68, Total fat 1g, Protein 1g, Carbs 7g
Ingredients:

- 4 mint leaves
- Ice cubes
- ½ cucumber
- 1/4 cup of young kale leaves
- 1 cup of watermelon chunks

Instructions:

- Remove the kale stalks and roughly cut the leaves.

- If desired, peel the cucumber before halves and discard the seeds.
- In a blender or juicer, combine all of the ingredients and process till you reach the desired consistency. Serve right away.

533. Strawberry-Gin Cocktail

(Preparation time: 10 minutes | Cooking time: 0 minutes | Difficulty: Easy | Servings: 1)
Per serving: Calories 186, Total fat 0g, Protein 0.1g, Carbs 11g
Ingredients:

- Ice cubes
- 2 fresh basil leaves
- 1 fluid ounce of fresh lemon juice
- 1 strawberry - 2 teaspoons of stevia
- 3 fluid ounces of chilled club soda
- 2 fluid ounces of gin

Instructions:

- In a cocktail shaker, combine the strawberry stevia, basil leaves, then mash well using a cocktail muddler. Half of the ice should go into the cocktail shaker, & the rest should go into a tall glass. Fill the shaker halfway with gin & lemon juice, cover, then shake till the outside has frosted. To serve, strain into a chilled glass over ice, top with club soda and mix to combine.

534. The Greenest Cocktail

(Preparation time: 10 minutes | Cooking time: 0 minutes | Difficulty: Easy | Servings: 1)
Per serving: Calories 210, Total fat 0g, Protein 2g, Carbs 30g
Ingredients:

- 1 cup of baby spinach leaves (pull off stems if you would like)
- ½ ripe pear, cored
- 1 kiwi, peeled, halved
- ½ cup of pre-pressed apple juice
- ¼ avocado pitted and scooped out

Instructions:

- Simply juice all of the ingredients till they are completely smooth.
- Serve right away.

535. Kiwi Cocktail

(Preparation time: 10 minutes | Cooking time: 0 minutes | Difficulty: Easy | Servings: 2)
Per serving: Calories 210, Total fat 0g, Protein 2g, Carbs 10g
Ingredients:

- Ice cubes to chill and serve
- 2 limes
- All the seeds from 1 pomegranate
- 6 large Kiwis, peeled

Instructions:

- Remove the juice from the limes and set it aside.
- Pomegranate seeds should be juiced.
- After blending the kiwis with the lime juice, incorporate the pomegranate juice. To serve, add ice.

536. Strawberry Lemonade Cocktail

(Preparation time: 10 minutes | Cooking time: 0 minutes | Difficulty: Easy | Servings: 1)
Per serving: Calories 158, Total fat 0.1g, Protein 0.5g, Carbs 16g
Ingredients:

- ice
- 1 ½ fluid ounces of citron vodka
- 1 lemon slice
- 1 fluid ounce of strawberry puree
- 4 fluid ounces of lemonade

Instructions:

- Ice should be added to a shaker. In a shaker, combine the lemonade, citron vodka, and strawberry puree; shake quickly to blend. Pour the contents of the shaker into the pint glass & top with a lemon slice.

537. Blueberry-Ginger Fizz

(Preparation time: 10 minutes | Cooking time: 10 minutes | Difficulty: Easy | Servings: 1)
Per serving: Calories 307, Total fat 2g, Protein 3g, Carbs 40g
Ingredients:

- 1 cup of water - ¼ cup of crushed ice
- 1 slice of orange (Optional)
- 1 tablespoon of grated fresh ginger
- 2 tablespoons of orange juice
- 1-pint of blueberries
- ¼ cup of stevia - ¼ cup of club soda

Instructions:

- In a saucepan on a medium-high flame, bring blueberries, water, sweetener, and ginger to a boil. Reduce to a low flame & cook for around 5 minutes, mashing the blueberries with a potato masher as needed. Remove from flame and set aside for 10 minutes to cool. To remove the blueberry skins, run the mixture through the food mill or fine mesh sieve. Reserved 1/4 cup of syrup & keep the rest in the fridge for up to one week.
- In a glass, put crushed ice. Add the orange juice and the blueberry-ginger syrup you set aside. Stir in the club soda to mix everything. Serve with an orange slice as a garnish.

538. Strawberry-Mango Limonata

(Preparation time: 10 minutes | Cooking time: 0 minutes | Difficulty: Easy | Servings: 1)
Per serving: Calories 262, Total fat 1g, Protein 3g, Carbs 38g
Ingredients:

- ¼ cup of ice as needed
- 1 sliced strawberry
- 1 cup of strawberry puree
- 1 fluid ounce of lemonade concentrate
- 1 fluid ounce of lemon-lime soda
- 1 cup of mango puree

Instructions:

- In a cocktail shaker, combine strawberry puree, lemonade concentrate, mango puree, and strawberry slices. Shake vigorously for a few seconds. Over a few cubes of ice, put into a Weizen or Pilsner glass. Add a dash of lemon-lime soda to finish.

539. Matcha Green Tea Cocktail

(Preparation time: 10 minutes | Cooking time: 0 minutes | Difficulty: Easy | Servings: 1)
Per serving: Calories 112, Total fat 1g, Protein 0.3g, Carbs 3g
Ingredients:

- 1/2 cup of cold water
- 1 cup of ice
- Splash of vanilla or chai spice or some fresh mint
- 2 teaspoons of matcha powder
- 1/4 cup of chilled vanilla almond milk unsweetened

Instructions:

- Put ice into a shaker or bottle, then sift two tablespoons of matcha powder inside the shaker.
- Pour half a cup of cold water into the mixture, give it a good shake, and put into an ice-filled bottle. (The tea does not boil or dissolve; instead, it is mixed in.) If you leave it for a long time after shaking, the tea will settle on the edge, so mic it or even shake again fast to get it blended in!)
- When creating this latte, you can put 2-3 ounces of cold, vanilla almond milk in the glass &, depending on our mood, add a splash of coffee or chai spice—or some of the fresh mint!

540. Watermelon Fizz

(Preparation time: 10 minutes | Cooking time: 0 minutes | Difficulty: Easy | Servings: 1)
Per serving: Calories 82, Total fat 2g, Protein 1g, Carbs 20g
Ingredients:
- 1 teaspoon of stevia
- 1 cup of coconut water
- ½ cup of ice cubes, or as desired
- ½ cup of watermelon puree

Instructions:
- In a blender, combine watermelon, coconut water, & stevia till smooth.
- Load a cocktail shaker halfway with ice, then pour in the watermelon mixture. Cover shaker & shake till well chilled; strain into a small glass.

541. Tiki Cooler

(Preparation time: 10 minutes | Cooking time: 0 minutes | Difficulty: Easy | Servings: 4)
Per serving: Calories 150, Total fat 10g, Protein 2g, Carbs 17g
Ingredients:
- 4 pinches of ground nutmeg
- 3 limes, juiced
- Ice cubes
- 4 sprigs of fresh mint
- 1/2 cup of pineapple juice
- 4 lime wheels
- 1 cup of club soda, or as needed
- 6 fluid ounces coconut milk
- 2 tablespoons of almond-flavored syrup

Instructions:
- In a pitcher, combine a few ice cubes, pineapple juice, lime juice, coconut milk, & almond-flavored syrup, and stir till combined. Pour the mixture into four glasses after straining it.
- To make the mocktail foam up, pour club soda into each glass.

- Nutmeg should be sprinkled over each mocktail. Serve with a lime wheel and a mint sprig.

542. Cucumber Tea Spritzer

(Preparation time: 10 minutes | Cooking time: 0 minutes | Difficulty: Easy | Servings: 5)
Per serving: Calories 83, Total fat 0.1g, Protein 0.3g, Carbs 21g
Ingredients:
- 2 cups of water
- Ice cubes
- 1 lemon
- 1 cucumber, cut into 1/4-inch slices
- 2 green tea bags, or more to taste
- 5 cups of sparkling water, or as needed
- ½ cup of sweetener

Instructions:
- In a kettle, bring water to the boil. Fill a pitcher halfway with water. Sweetener should be stirred till it melts into a syrup. Allow 5 minutes for the tea bags to steep.
- Fill five glasses with ice cubes. Put some cucumber slices into the mix. Fill glasses with sparkling water to 3/4 capacity. Pour sweet tea into glasses in an equal layer. Add a squeeze of lemon juice to each drink & whisk well.

543. Raspberry Citrus Mocktail

(Preparation time: 10 minutes | Cooking time: 0 minutes | Difficulty: Easy | Servings: 1)
Per serving: Calories 62, Total fat 0.2g, Protein 0.6g, Carbs 18g
Ingredients:
- 1 cup ice cubes
- 6 tablespoons water, divided
- 1 lime halved - 1 teaspoon of honey
- 5 each fresh raspberries
- ¾ teaspoon of stevia
- ½ (12 fluid ounce) can of grapefruit-flavored seltzer

Instructions:

- In a small-sized bowl, crush raspberries using a fork or spoon. Add 2 tablespoons of water to the mix. Stir in the honey & sweetener till they are completely dissolved. Set aside after straining into another small-sized bowl.
- Ice should be added to a glass. Add the remaining water & seltzer to the mixture. Lime juice should be squeezed in. Pour the raspberry mixture in slowly; it will reach the bottom & create a lovely ombre appearance. Mix your drink prior to taking a sip to get the most raspberry taste.

544. Grape, Celery and Parsley Reviver

(Preparation time: 10 minutes | Cooking time: 0 minutes | Difficulty: Easy | Servings: 2)
Per serving: Calories 182, Total fat 2g, Protein 1g, Carbs 39g
Ingredients:

- Ice cubes
- 1 tablespoon of fresh parsley
- 1/2 cup of red grapes
- 3 sticks of celery
- 1 avocado, de-stoned and peeled
- ½ teaspoon of matcha powder

Instructions:

- Blend the ingredients in a blender till smooth and creamy, adding enough water to cover them. To have it even more refreshing, add crushed ice.

545. Mango, Rocket and Arugula Punch

(Preparation time: 10 minutes | Cooking time: 0 minutes | Difficulty: Easy | Servings: 2)
Per serving: Calories 220, Total fat 18g, Protein 3g, Carbs 25g
Ingredients:

- Juice of 1 lime

- 1/4 cup of fresh rocket arugula
- 1/2 cup of fresh mango, peeled, de-stoned and chopped
- 1 avocado, de-stoned and peeled
- ½ teaspoon of matcha powder

Instructions:

- In a blender, combine all of the ingredients with just enough water to cover them & blend till smooth. Enjoy with a couple of ice cubes.

546. Irish Coffee Cocktail

(Preparation time: 10 minutes | Cooking time: 0 minutes | Difficulty: Easy | Servings: 1)
Per serving: Calories 274, Total fat 11g, Protein 1g, Carbs 17g
Ingredients:

- 6 fluid ounces of hot coffee
- ¼ cup of whipped cream
- 1 tablespoon of stevia (Optional)
- 1 ½ fluid ounces of whiskey

Instructions:

- Sweetener should be placed on a plate or in a shallow bowl. Using a moistened paper towel, lightly moisten the rim of an Irish coffee glass. To coat the rim, dip it in sweetener. Pour the Irish whiskey into the glass that has been prepared. Fill within about 1/2 inch of the top with coffee. Stir in the sweetener. Whipped cream is served on top.

547. Turmeric and Ginger Mocktail

(Preparation time: 10 minutes | Cooking time: 0 minutes | Difficulty: Easy | Servings: 1)
Per serving: Calories 163, Total fat 1g, Protein 3g, Carbs 35g
Ingredients:

- Ice cubes - 1/2 lemon, peeled
- 1/2 teaspoon of ground turmeric
- 1 (1 inch) piece of fresh ginger
- 1 orange, peeled & divided
- 2 Fuji apples, cored & sliced

Instructions:

- Process the ginger, lemon, orange, ice cubes and apples in a juicer, then whisk in the turmeric till equally incorporated.

548. Alcohol-Free Mojitos

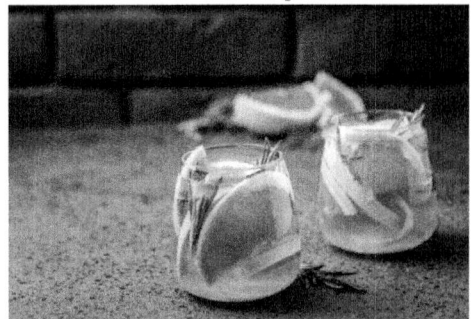

(Preparation time: 10 minutes | Cooking time: 10 minutes | Difficulty: Easy | Servings: 14)
Per serving: Calories 120, Total fat 1g, Protein 1g, Carbs 30g
Ingredients:

- 1 cup of water
- lime slices for garnish
- 2 cups of water
- 2 cups of mint leaves, chopped
- 1 cup of lime juice
- 1 ½ cups of stevia
- 2 cups of lime sherbet, softened
- 8 cups of club soda

Instructions:

- In a microwave-safe bowl, combine 2 cups of water & the sweetener; cook on High for 5 minutes. Allow 5 minutes after adding the mint to the water. Remove the mint leaves out from the syrup and set it aside.
- In a large pitcher, whisk together the lime juice, lime sherbet, and 1 cup of water till well blended. Combine the mint-infused syrup and the rest of the ingredients. Stir in the club soda. Serve with ice cubes. Serve with lime slices as a garnish.

549. Virgin Pina Colada

(Preparation time: 10 minutes | Cooking time: 0 minutes | Difficulty: Easy | Servings: 2)
Per serving: Calories 267, Total fat 23g, Protein 4g, Carbs 35g - **Ingredients:**

- 1 cup of ice - ½ cup of skim milk
- 2 tablespoons of stevia
- 1 ¼ cups of pineapple juice
- ½ cup of heavy cream

Instructions:

- Blend ice, cream, pineapple juice, milk, and sweetener in an electric blender. Blend till completely smooth.

550. Iced Tea

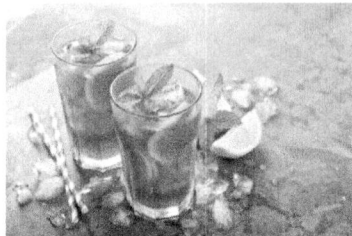

(Preparation time: 10 minutes | Cooking time: 0 minutes | Difficulty: Easy | Servings: 6)
Per serving: Calories 50, Total fat 0g, Protein 1g, Carbs 12g - **Ingredients:**

- Ice cubes - 6 tea bags
- 2 lemons, 1 juiced, 1 sliced
- 2 tablespoons of golden caster sugar
- A small bunch of mint leaves picked
- 1 orange, sliced - 1 tablespoon of runny honey, plus extra to serve

Instructions:

- In a large jug, combine the tea bags, sweetener, honey, and 1.5 liters of water. Allow 10 minutes for infusion before removing and discarding the tea bags. Refrigerate till ready to serve.
- Combine the lemon juice, orange slices, lemon slices, and mint leaves. Fill the pitcher with ice and swirl one more.
- Fill tall glasses halfway with ice & pour in the iced tea; top with honey to taste.

CHAPTER 15:

A Smart 21-Day Meal Plan to Jumpstart Your Weight Loss!

The First Phase

Phase One refers to the first seven days of the diet plan. A dieter must concentrate on calorie control and the use of green juices during this phase. These seven days are critical for kick-starting your weight reduction and normally result in a seven-pound decrease if the instructions are followed correctly. If you accomplish this goal, you are on the correct course.

The caloric intake for the first 3 days of Phase One is fixed at roughly 1,000 calories. The dieter must also consume green juice three times a day while doing so.

The caloric intake is raised to 1,500 calories per day over the next four days after the first three days. Green juices are limited to two per day over these four days, and each meal includes Sirtuin-rich meals.

The Second Phase

After the first week of the Sirtfood Diet, or Phase One, Phase Two begins. The second phase focuses on sticking to the diet, which becomes easier as your body adjusts to the new routine. The first week, according to the plan, allows the body to adjust to the change and begin working toward the weight reduction target, while the second week allows the body to continue dropping weight slowly & steadily. As a result, this period will last almost two weeks.

So, how does this phase vary from the first? There are no calorie restrictions during this

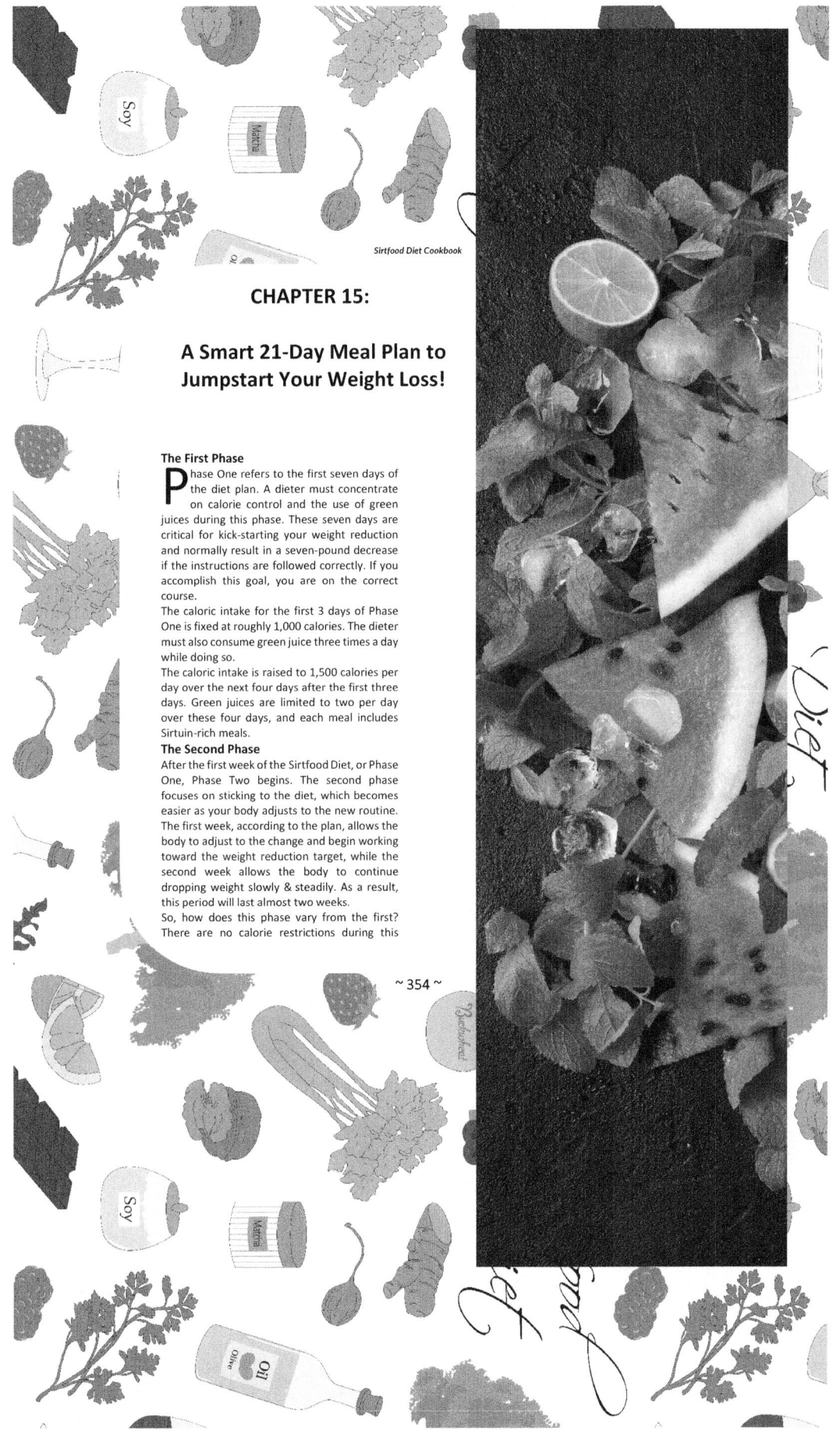

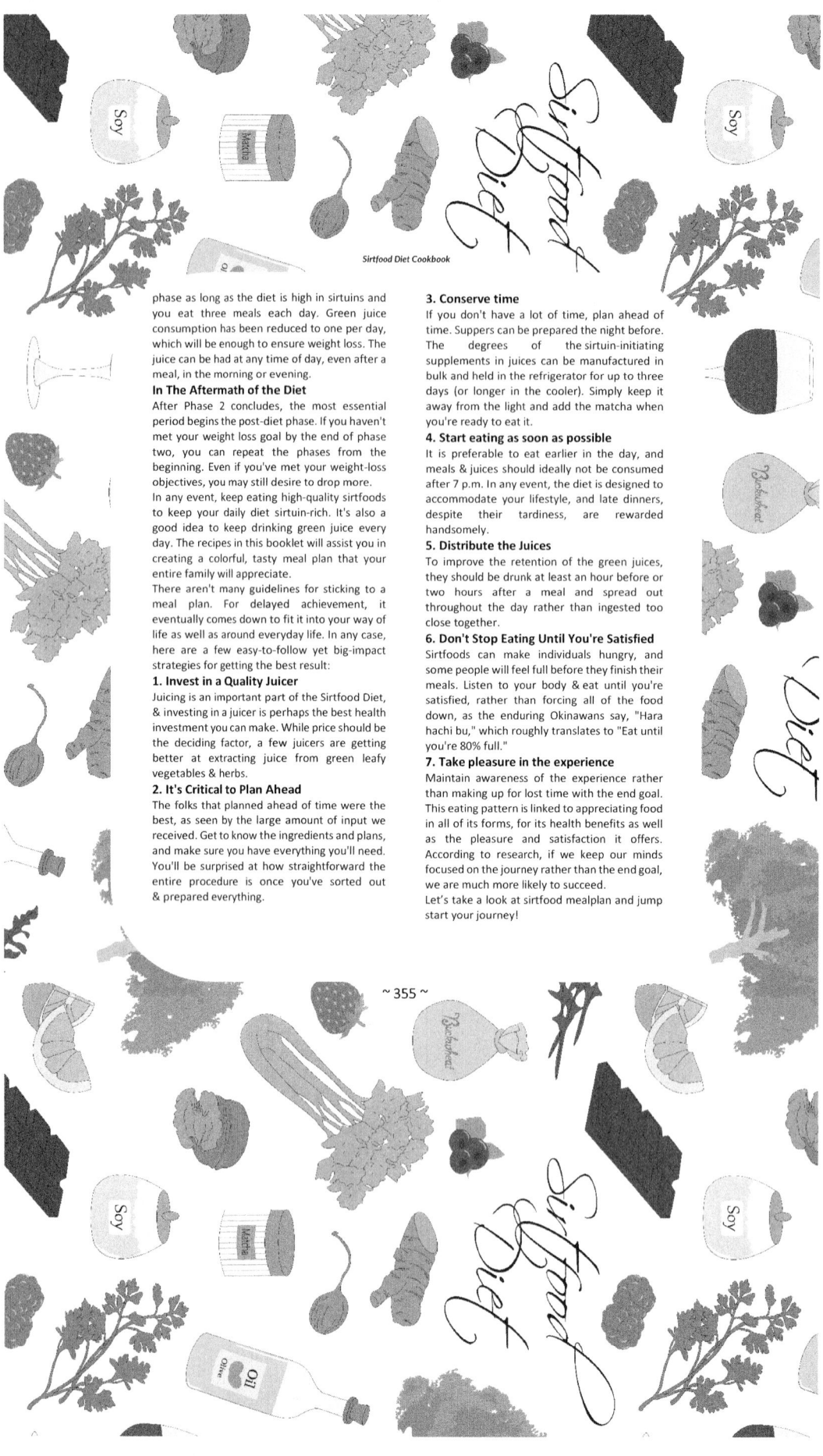

phase as long as the diet is high in sirtuins and you eat three meals each day. Green juice consumption has been reduced to one per day, which will be enough to ensure weight loss. The juice can be had at any time of day, even after a meal, in the morning or evening.

In The Aftermath of the Diet

After Phase 2 concludes, the most essential period begins the post-diet phase. If you haven't met your weight loss goal by the end of phase two, you can repeat the phases from the beginning. Even if you've met your weight-loss objectives, you may still desire to drop more.

In any event, keep eating high-quality sirtfoods to keep your daily diet sirtuin-rich. It's also a good idea to keep drinking green juice every day. The recipes in this booklet will assist you in creating a colorful, tasty meal plan that your entire family will appreciate.

There aren't many guidelines for sticking to a meal plan. For delayed achievement, it eventually comes down to fit it into your way of life as well as around everyday life. In any case, here are a few easy-to-follow yet big-impact strategies for getting the best result:

1. Invest in a Quality Juicer

Juicing is an important part of the Sirtfood Diet, & investing in a juicer is perhaps the best health investment you can make. While price should be the deciding factor, a few juicers are getting better at extracting juice from green leafy vegetables & herbs.

2. It's Critical to Plan Ahead

The folks that planned ahead of time were the best, as seen by the large amount of input we received. Get to know the ingredients and plans, and make sure you have everything you'll need. You'll be surprised at how straightforward the entire procedure is once you've sorted out & prepared everything.

3. Conserve time

If you don't have a lot of time, plan ahead of time. Suppers can be prepared the night before. The degrees of the sirtuin-initiating supplements in juices can be manufactured in bulk and held in the refrigerator for up to three days (or longer in the cooler). Simply keep it away from the light and add the matcha when you're ready to eat it.

4. Start eating as soon as possible

It is preferable to eat earlier in the day, and meals & juices should ideally not be consumed after 7 p.m. In any event, the diet is designed to accommodate your lifestyle, and late dinners, despite their tardiness, are rewarded handsomely.

5. Distribute the Juices

To improve the retention of the green juices, they should be drunk at least an hour before or two hours after a meal and spread out throughout the day rather than ingested too close together.

6. Don't Stop Eating Until You're Satisfied

Sirtfoods can make individuals hungry, and some people will feel full before they finish their meals. Listen to your body & eat until you're satisfied, rather than forcing all of the food down, as the enduring Okinawans say, "Hara hachi bu," which roughly translates to "Eat until you're 80% full."

7. Take pleasure in the experience

Maintain awareness of the experience rather than making up for lost time with the end goal. This eating pattern is linked to appreciating food in all of its forms, for its health benefits as well as the pleasure and satisfaction it offers. According to research, if we keep our minds focused on the journey rather than the end goal, we are much more likely to succeed.

Let's take a look at sirtfood mealplan and jump start your journey!

Week 1

Day	Breakfast	Lunch	Snack	Dinner	Dessert
1	Green juice	Green juice	Green juice	Asian King Prawn Stir-Fry with Buckwheat Noodles	A piece of dark chocolate
2	Green juice	Green juice	Green juice	Stir-Fried Tofu and Veggies in Ginger Sauce	A piece of dark chocolate
3	Green juice	Green juice	Green juice	Lemon Herb Sardines with Avocado, Rocket and Caper Salad	A piece of dark chocolate
4	Green juice	Caribbean Yellow and Green Split Pea Buckwheat	Green juice	Baked Cod with Asparagus	Walnut and Date Cake
5	Green juice	Shredded Chicken Bowls	Green juice	Spicy Asian Buckwheat Noodle Soup	Hearty Almond Crackers
6	Green juice	Chicken and Kale with Spicy Salsa	Green juice	Roasted Sardines and Parsley	Chocolate Muffins
7	Green juice	Smoked Trout with Curd Cheese and Caper Crackers	Green juice	Red Onion and Kale Dhal with Buckwheat	Bars with Nuts and Dates

Week 2

Day	Breakfast	Lunch	Snack	Dinner	Dessert
1	Matcha Pancakes	Salmon with Capers	Green juice	Creamy Turkey with Soy	Choco Nut Truffles
2	Nut and Date Millet Porridge	Fragrant Asian Hot Pot	Green juice	Chicken, Carrot and Kale Salad	Apple Date Pudding
3	Chia and Almonds Blueberry Bowl	Turmeric Turkey Breast with Cauli Rice	Green juice	Bake-Foil Packed Salmon and Asparagus	Sirtfood Bites
4	Scrambled Eggs with Parsley and Red Onion	Goat Cheese Salad with Walnut and Cranberries	Green juice	Chicken Teriyaki with Cauliflower Rice	Loaded Chocolate Fudge
5	Pancakes with Caramelized Strawberries	Chicken, Arugula, Avocado and Buckwheat Crackers	Green juice	Pan-Fried Aubergine Olives and Capers	Bounty Bars
6	Kale with Scrambled Egg	Quinoa, Chickpea and Turmeric Curry	Green juice	Chicory Tofu and Chili with Walnut Arugula Salad	No-Bake Strawberry Flapjacks
7	Blueberry Banana Buckwheat Pancakes	Baked Cod with Chicory, Kale and White Beans	Green juice	Sage Pork Chops with Cider Pan Gravy	Chocolate Maple Walnuts

~ 357 ~

Week 3

Day	Breakfast	Lunch	Snack	Dinner	Dessert
1	Date and Walnut Strawberry Porridge	Chicken Skewers with Buckwheat and Satay Sauce	Green juice	Turkey Escalope with Cauliflower Couscous	Chocolate and Matcha Dipped Strawberries
2	Buckwheat Granola	Cream of Kale and Broccoli Soup	Green juice	Steak Arugula and Strawberry Salad	Tropical Chocolate Delight
3	Apple Cinnamon Wraps	Buckwheat with Green Onions and Mushrooms	Green juice	Creamy Chicken Noodles Soup	Green Tea and Vanilla Cream
4	Scrambled Eggs with Kale, Red onion and Tomatoes	Grilled Turkey Schnitzel with Walnut, Herb and Cheddar Crust	Green juice	Beef with Herb-Roasted Potatoes and Red Wine	Crunchy Chocolate Chip Coconut Macadamia Nut Cookies
5	Buckwheat Pancakes	Beef and Kale Salad	Green juice	Spicy Lentil and Veggie Stew	Chocolate Pie
6	Smoked Salmon Omelet	Spicy Asian Buckwheat Noodle Soup	Green juice	Tuna Salad	Blackberry and Apple Cobbler
7	Matcha Overnight Oats	Sirt Chicken Salad	Green juice	Pork Chops Topped with Sweet Apples	Chocolate Cashew Truffles

~ 359 ~

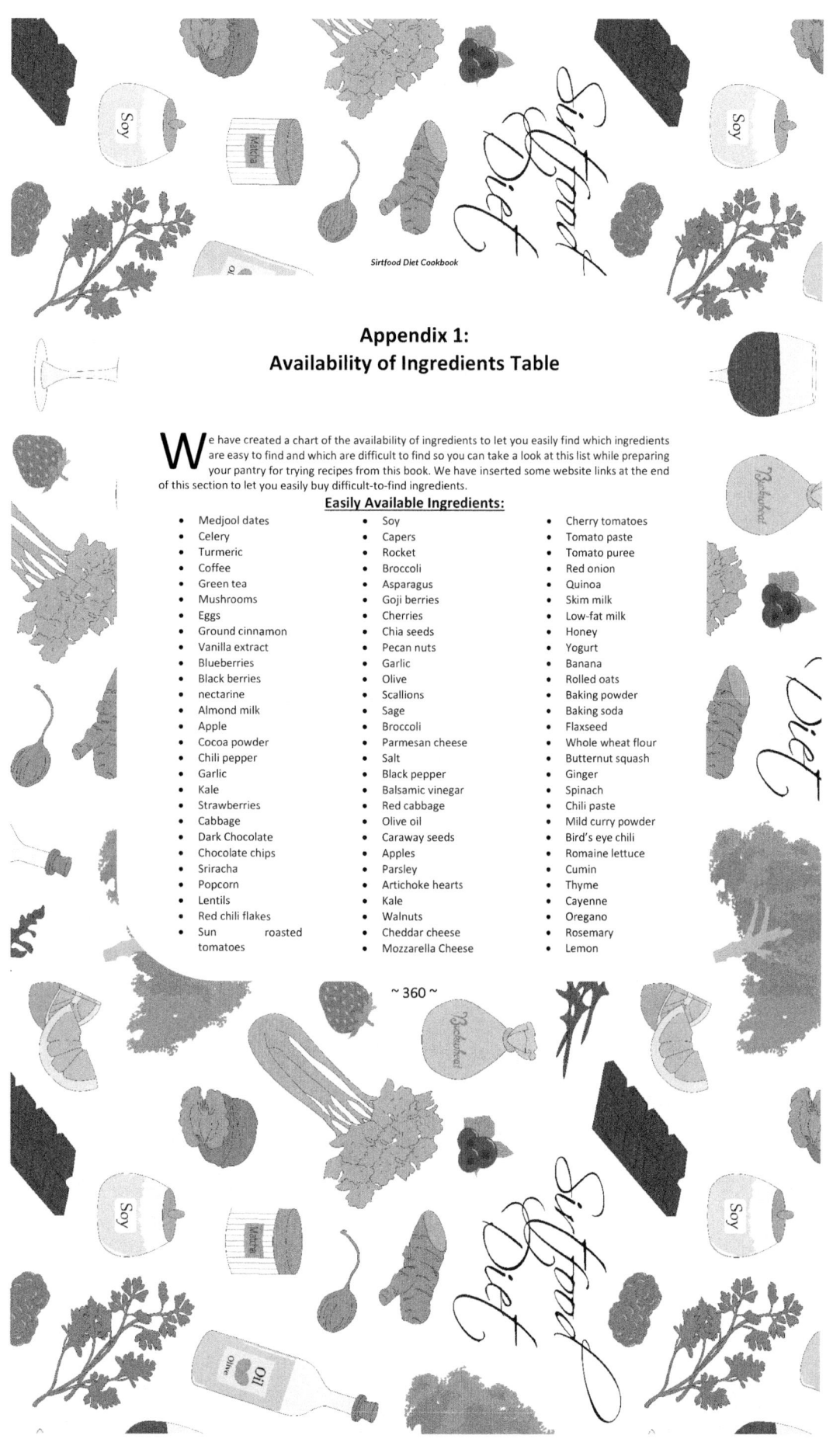

Appendix 1:
Availability of Ingredients Table

We have created a chart of the availability of ingredients to let you easily find which ingredients are easy to find and which are difficult to find so you can take a look at this list while preparing your pantry for trying recipes from this book. We have inserted some website links at the end of this section to let you easily buy difficult-to-find ingredients.

Easily Available Ingredients:

- Medjool dates
- Celery
- Turmeric
- Coffee
- Green tea
- Mushrooms
- Eggs
- Ground cinnamon
- Vanilla extract
- Blueberries
- Black berries
- nectarine
- Almond milk
- Apple
- Cocoa powder
- Chili pepper
- Garlic
- Kale
- Strawberries
- Cabbage
- Dark Chocolate
- Chocolate chips
- Sriracha
- Popcorn
- Lentils
- Red chili flakes
- Sun roasted tomatoes

- Soy
- Capers
- Rocket
- Broccoli
- Asparagus
- Goji berries
- Cherries
- Chia seeds
- Pecan nuts
- Garlic
- Olive
- Scallions
- Sage
- Broccoli
- Parmesan cheese
- Salt
- Black pepper
- Balsamic vinegar
- Red cabbage
- Olive oil
- Caraway seeds
- Apples
- Parsley
- Artichoke hearts
- Kale
- Walnuts
- Cheddar cheese
- Mozzarella Cheese

- Cherry tomatoes
- Tomato paste
- Tomato puree
- Red onion
- Quinoa
- Skim milk
- Low-fat milk
- Honey
- Yogurt
- Banana
- Rolled oats
- Baking powder
- Baking soda
- Flaxseed
- Whole wheat flour
- Butternut squash
- Ginger
- Spinach
- Chili paste
- Mild curry powder
- Bird's eye chili
- Romaine lettuce
- Cumin
- Thyme
- Cayenne
- Oregano
- Rosemary
- Lemon

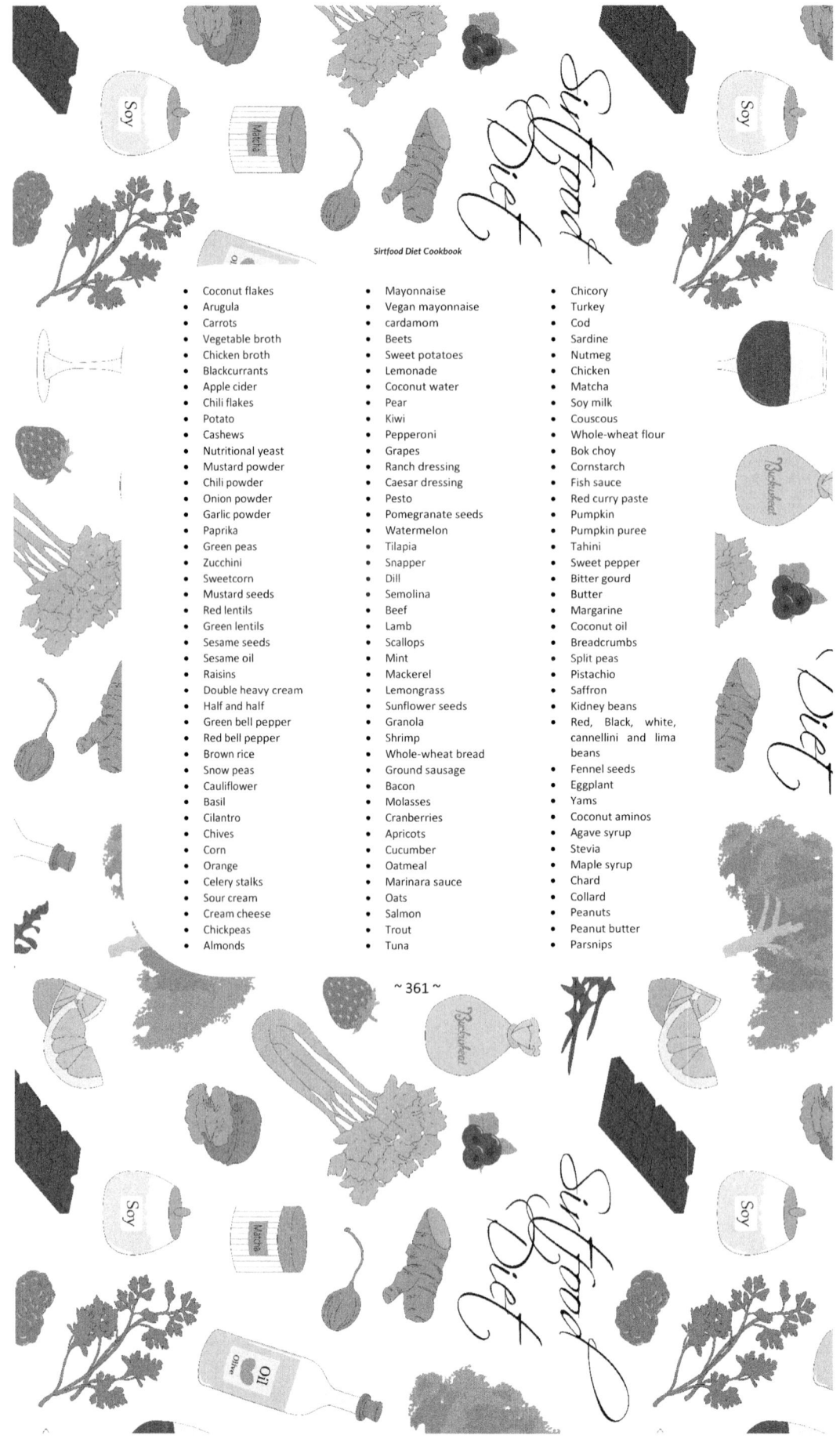

- Coconut flakes
- Arugula
- Carrots
- Vegetable broth
- Chicken broth
- Blackcurrants
- Apple cider
- Chili flakes
- Potato
- Cashews
- Nutritional yeast
- Mustard powder
- Chili powder
- Onion powder
- Garlic powder
- Paprika
- Green peas
- Zucchini
- Sweetcorn
- Mustard seeds
- Red lentils
- Green lentils
- Sesame seeds
- Sesame oil
- Raisins
- Double heavy cream
- Half and half
- Green bell pepper
- Red bell pepper
- Brown rice
- Snow peas
- Cauliflower
- Basil
- Cilantro
- Chives
- Corn
- Orange
- Celery stalks
- Sour cream
- Cream cheese
- Chickpeas
- Almonds

- Mayonnaise
- Vegan mayonnaise
- cardamom
- Beets
- Sweet potatoes
- Lemonade
- Coconut water
- Pear
- Kiwi
- Pepperoni
- Grapes
- Ranch dressing
- Caesar dressing
- Pesto
- Pomegranate seeds
- Watermelon
- Tilapia
- Snapper
- Dill
- Semolina
- Beef
- Lamb
- Scallops
- Mint
- Mackerel
- Lemongrass
- Sunflower seeds
- Granola
- Shrimp
- Whole-wheat bread
- Ground sausage
- Bacon
- Molasses
- Cranberries
- Apricots
- Cucumber
- Oatmeal
- Marinara sauce
- Oats
- Salmon
- Trout
- Tuna

- Chicory
- Turkey
- Cod
- Sardine
- Nutmeg
- Chicken
- Matcha
- Soy milk
- Couscous
- Whole-wheat flour
- Bok choy
- Cornstarch
- Fish sauce
- Red curry paste
- Pumpkin
- Pumpkin puree
- Tahini
- Sweet pepper
- Bitter gourd
- Butter
- Margarine
- Coconut oil
- Breadcrumbs
- Split peas
- Pistachio
- Saffron
- Kidney beans
- Red, Black, white, cannellini and lima beans
- Fennel seeds
- Eggplant
- Yams
- Coconut aminos
- Agave syrup
- Stevia
- Maple syrup
- Chard
- Collard
- Peanuts
- Peanut butter
- Parsnips

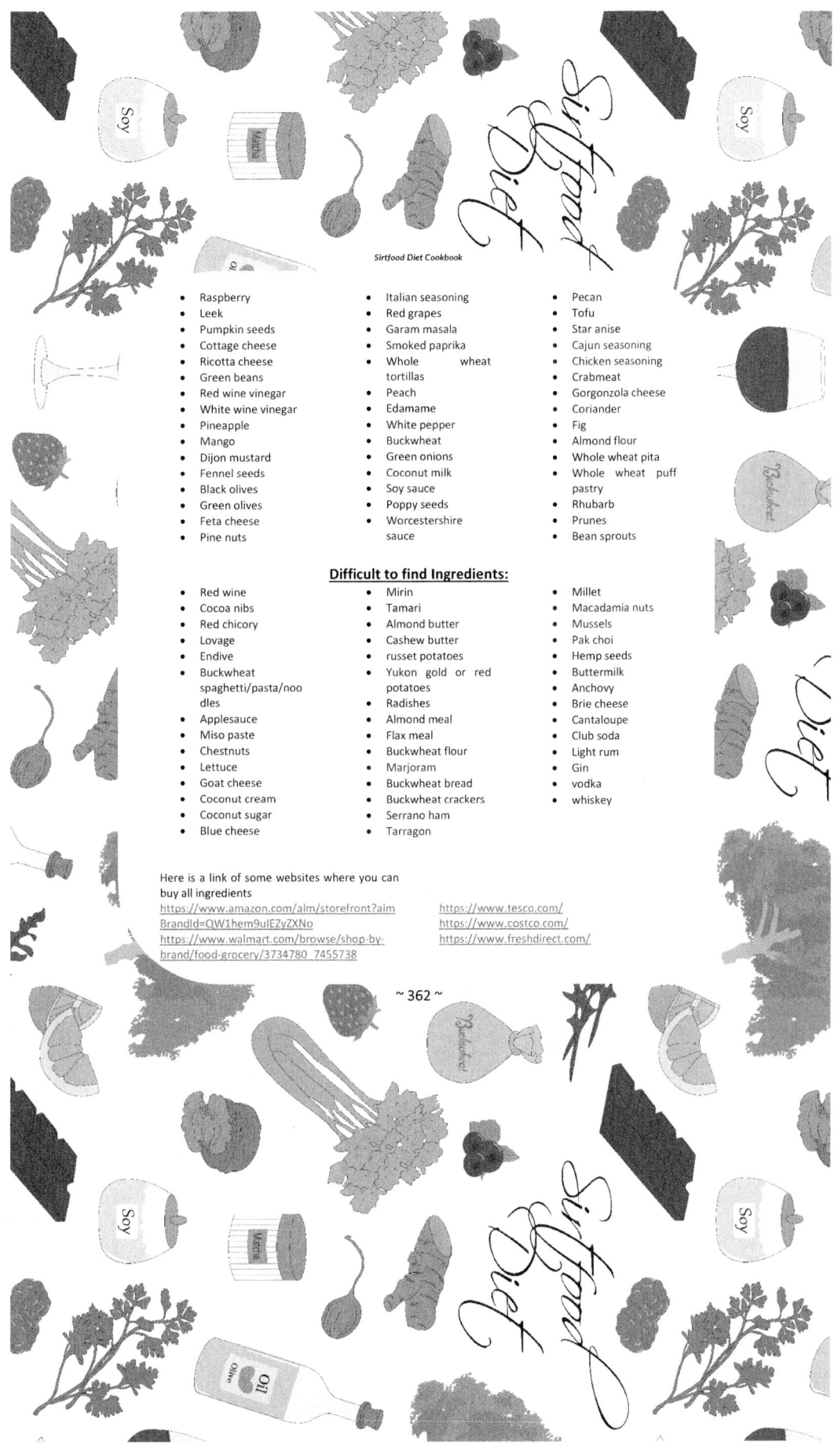

- Raspberry
- Leek
- Pumpkin seeds
- Cottage cheese
- Ricotta cheese
- Green beans
- Red wine vinegar
- White wine vinegar
- Pineapple
- Mango
- Dijon mustard
- Fennel seeds
- Black olives
- Green olives
- Feta cheese
- Pine nuts

- Italian seasoning
- Red grapes
- Garam masala
- Smoked paprika
- Whole wheat tortillas
- Peach
- Edamame
- White pepper
- Buckwheat
- Green onions
- Coconut milk
- Soy sauce
- Poppy seeds
- Worcestershire sauce

- Pecan
- Tofu
- Star anise
- Cajun seasoning
- Chicken seasoning
- Crabmeat
- Gorgonzola cheese
- Coriander
- Fig
- Almond flour
- Whole wheat pita
- Whole wheat puff pastry
- Rhubarb
- Prunes
- Bean sprouts

Difficult to find Ingredients:

- Red wine
- Cocoa nibs
- Red chicory
- Lovage
- Endive
- Buckwheat spaghetti/pasta/noodles
- Applesauce
- Miso paste
- Chestnuts
- Lettuce
- Goat cheese
- Coconut cream
- Coconut sugar
- Blue cheese

- Mirin
- Tamari
- Almond butter
- Cashew butter
- russet potatoes
- Yukon gold or red potatoes
- Radishes
- Almond meal
- Flax meal
- Buckwheat flour
- Marjoram
- Buckwheat bread
- Buckwheat crackers
- Serrano ham
- Tarragon

- Millet
- Macadamia nuts
- Mussels
- Pak choi
- Hemp seeds
- Buttermilk
- Anchovy
- Brie cheese
- Cantaloupe
- Club soda
- Light rum
- Gin
- vodka
- whiskey

Here is a link of some websites where you can buy all ingredients

https://www.amazon.com/alm/storefront?almBrandId=QW1hem9uIEZyZXNo
https://www.walmart.com/browse/shop-by-brand/food-grocery/3734780_7455738
https://www.tesco.com/
https://www.costco.com/
https://www.freshdirect.com/

~ 363 ~

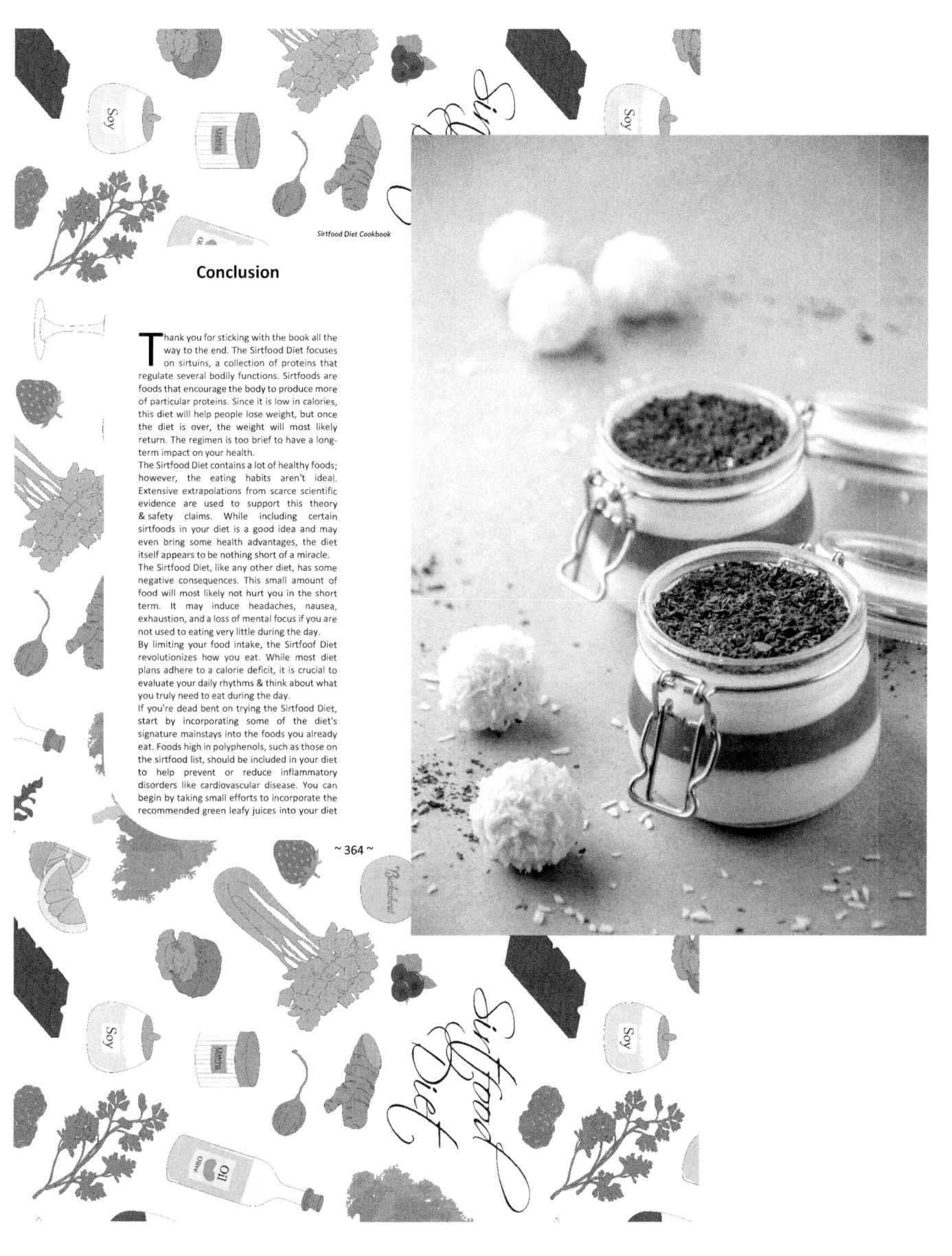

Conclusion

Thank you for sticking with the book all the way to the end. The Sirtfood Diet focuses on sirtuins, a collection of proteins that regulate several bodily functions. Sirtfoods are foods that encourage the body to produce more of particular proteins. Since it is low in calories, this diet will help people lose weight, but once the diet is over, the weight will most likely return. The regimen is too brief to have a long-term impact on your health.

The Sirtfood Diet contains a lot of healthy foods; however, the eating habits aren't ideal. Extensive extrapolations from scarce scientific evidence are used to support this theory & safety claims. While including certain sirtfoods in your diet is a good idea and may even bring some health advantages, the diet itself appears to be nothing short of a miracle.

The Sirtfood Diet, like any other diet, has some negative consequences. This small amount of food will most likely not hurt you in the short term. It may induce headaches, nausea, exhaustion, and a loss of mental focus if you are not used to eating very little during the day.

By limiting your food intake, the Sirtfoof Diet revolutionizes how you eat. While most diet plans adhere to a calorie deficit, it is crucial to evaluate your daily rhythms & think about what you truly need to eat during the day.

If you're dead bent on trying the Sirtfood Diet, start by incorporating some of the diet's signature mainstays into the foods you already eat. Foods high in polyphenols, such as those on the sirtfood list, should be included in your diet to help prevent or reduce inflammatory disorders like cardiovascular disease. You can begin by taking small efforts to incorporate the recommended green leafy juices into your diet

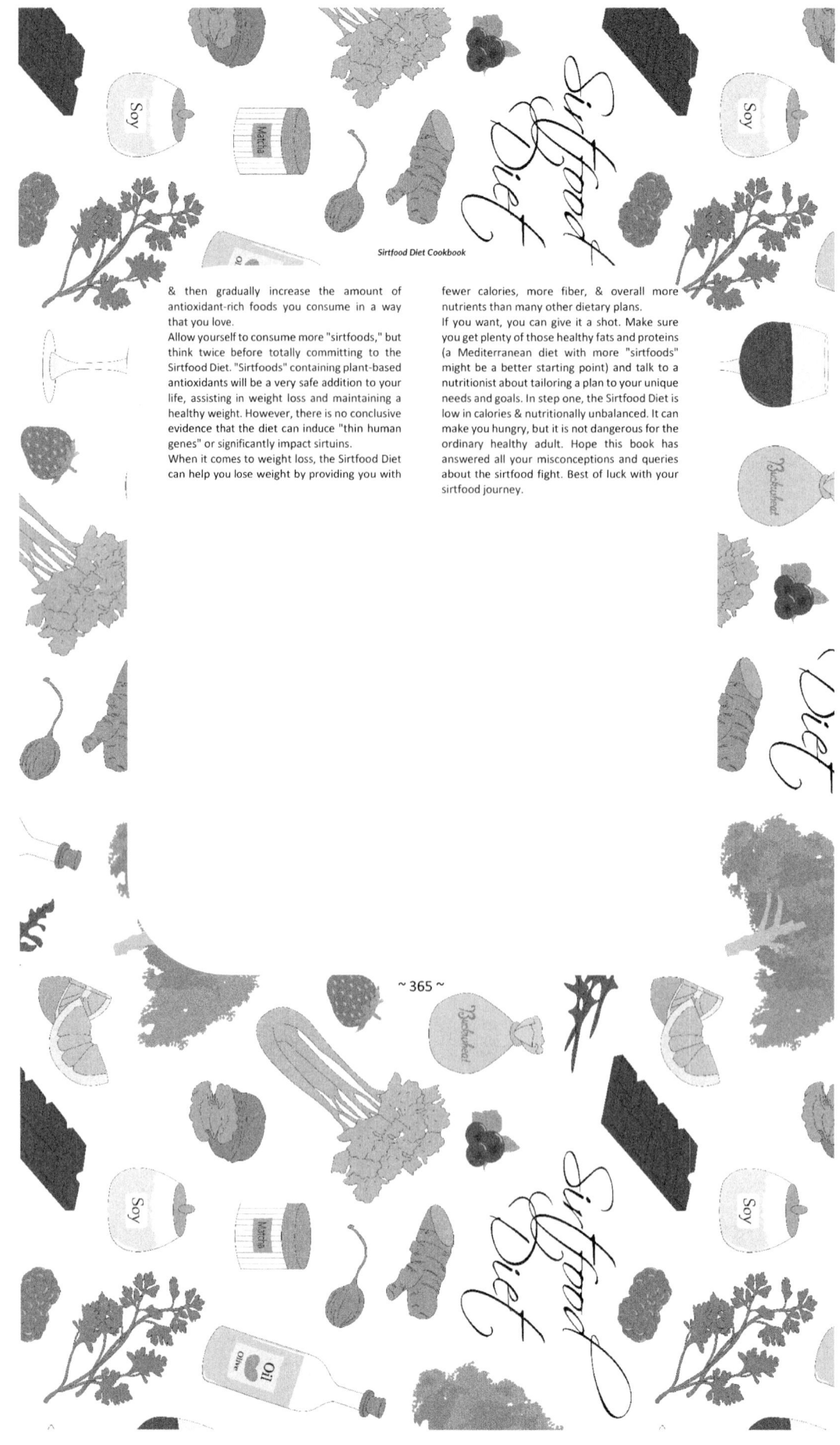

& then gradually increase the amount of antioxidant-rich foods you consume in a way that you love.

Allow yourself to consume more "sirtfoods," but think twice before totally committing to the Sirtfood Diet. "Sirtfoods" containing plant-based antioxidants will be a very safe addition to your life, assisting in weight loss and maintaining a healthy weight. However, there is no conclusive evidence that the diet can induce "thin human genes" or significantly impact sirtuins.

When it comes to weight loss, the Sirtfood Diet can help you lose weight by providing you with fewer calories, more fiber, & overall more nutrients than many other dietary plans.

If you want, you can give it a shot. Make sure you get plenty of those healthy fats and proteins (a Mediterranean diet with more "sirtfoods" might be a better starting point) and talk to a nutritionist about tailoring a plan to your unique needs and goals. In step one, the Sirtfood Diet is low in calories & nutritionally unbalanced. It can make you hungry, but it is not dangerous for the ordinary healthy adult. Hope this book has answered all your misconceptions and queries about the sirtfood fight. Best of luck with your sirtfood journey.

Printed in Great Britain
by Amazon